Atlas of Single-Incision Laparoscopic Operations in General Surgery

Shuodong Wu • Ying Fan • Yu Tian
Editors

Atlas of Single-Incision Laparoscopic Operations in General Surgery

Springer

Editors
Shuodong Wu
Ying Fan
Yu Tian
Minimal Invasive Surgery and Bile Duct Surgery
Shengjing Hospital
China Medical University
Shenyang
China

ISBN 978-94-007-6954-0 ISBN 978-94-007-6955-7 (eBook)
DOI 10.1007/978-94-007-6955-7
Springer Dordrecht Heidelberg New York London

Library of Congress Control Number: 2013944056

Printed on acid-free paper

Springer is part of Springer Science+Business Media (www.springer.com)

Preface

With the development and improvement of laparoscopic equipment, conventional laparoscopic operation techniques have become standardized and are the mainstream of surgical operations all over the world. Taking 1987 as the year of the introduction of minimally invasive surgery, in the course of 25 years it has experienced twists and turns. We are the generation of surgeons witnessing the rapid development of science and technology and I feel great joy and pride and am honored to participate in this great medical reform, and in persistently pursuing and exploring the possibilities. But I always remind myself not to be complacent or vain, or stop improving. It is a doctor's duty to serve patients by relieving pain and facilitating fast recovery. The concept of natural orifice transluminal endoscopic surgery (NOTES) or "no scar surgery" is a reflection of this point. We are going forward with continuous improvement and development. Since 2008, single-incision laparoscopic technique has been well-known all over the world. "Atlas of single-incision laparoscopic operations in general surgery" is the summary and accumulation of the experience of more than 1,000 cases and 40 categories of operations carried out by the chief editors and their team. This book provides HD video pictures in the arrangement of operation steps and description in words to facilitate observation and understanding. Tips and tricks, together with complications and management, are also discussed to help readers to carry out these operations in the clinic.

Like any other science or technology, any type of minimally invasive technique will never be the best, only better than before. So I hope my limited experience in single-incision laparoscopic surgery will help this technique to flourish. Guidance and criticism are cordially welcomed.

In the process of compiling this book, chief editors Ying Fan and Yu Tian spent valuable time on information collection, selection, and arrangement, and processing the text. Associate professor Hong Yu and lecturer Yu Xiaopeng and others sacrificed a great deal of spare time in editing the pictures. I express my sincere gratitude and regards to all of them for helping to publish this book.

Shenyang City, Liaoning Province, China

Shuodong Wu

Contents

Contributors

Yong-Sheng Chen Minimal Invasive Surgery and Bile Duct Surgery, Shengjing Hospital, China Medical University, Shenyang, China

Jin-Yan Han Minimal Invasive Surgery and Bile Duct Surgery, Shengjing Hospital, China Medical University, Shenyang, China

Jing Kong Minimal Invasive Surgery and Bile Duct Surgery, Shengjing Hospital, China Medical University, Shenyang, China

Yong-Nan Li Minimal Invasive Surgery and Bile Duct Surgery, Shengjing Hospital, China Medical University, Shenyang, China

Chao Lv Minimal Invasive Surgery and Bile Duct Surgery, Shengjing Hospital, China Medical University, Shenyang, China

Dian-Bo Yao Minimal Invasive Surgery and Bile Duct Surgery, Shengjing Hospital, China Medical University, Shenyang, China

Hong Yu Minimal Invasive Surgery and Bile Duct Surgery, Shengjing Hospital, China Medical University, Shenyang, China

Xiao-Peng Yu Minimal Invasive Surgery and Bile Duct Surgery, Shengjing Hospital, China Medical University, Shenyang, China

Sketch of Single-Incision Laparoscopic Surgery (SILS)

1

Abstract

Single-incision laparoscopic surgery (SILS) is developed based on that of conventional laparoendoscopic surgery with a better cosmetic outcome and more minimal invasiveness. Compared with natural orifice transluminal endoscopic surgery(NOTES), SILS is more applicable and practical at present for surgeons. In the recent 3 years, we have finished more than 1,000 cases of SILS operations (more than 40 types) of general surgery. General anesthesia and herringbone position is often used during SILS. Though the so-called "Chopsticks effect"exists during the surgery, we believe most of the operations performed by us during our daily clinic practice can be successfully completed by SILS technique. More experience accumulation and learning curve training are needed to further develop this technique. We expect this technique would be a powerful weapon of our surgeons in the near future.

Keywords

Single-incision laparoscopic surgery (SILS) • Natural orifice transluminal endoscopic surgery (NOTES) • Chopsticks effect

The techniques of single-incision laparoscopic surgery (SILS) is developed based on that of conventional laparoendoscopic surgery. At first, surgeons attempted to find a method for visceral surgery with no incision on body's surface, which is called natural orifice transluminal endoscopic surgery (NOTES). As we know, soft endoscopies, such as gastroscope, enteroscope and choledochoscope, were used only for diagnosis and treatment of diseases in mucosa or submucosa of digestive lumen. Since the appearance of NOTES, the operations aimed at the sickness of appendix, gallbladder and spleen have been performed gradually, based on these further improved soft endoscopies. For several years of clinical practice, doctors have achieved a gratifying progress and harvest. However, the technique still reached its developmental bottleneck. Research and development of instrument cannot meet the need of clinical necessity. Other available methods are time-consuming, strenuous and inefficient. Compared to NOTES, SILS is easier, safer, more applicable and convenient for surgeons to master. Why it is difficult for NOTES to develop now? The main reason is that physicians, but not surgeons always use endoscopies. However, laparoscope has been a tool for surgeons for a long time. So, it is not an insurmountable problem to perform operations through three close packed ports. What's more, the way to use chopsticks is similar to that of SILS. As Chinese people, we are born with a unique advantage. In the recent 3 years, we have finished more than 1,000 cases of SILS operations (more than 40 types) of general surgery. Its learning curve goes with a swing. Now, we display a table to compare the advantages and disadvantages between SILS, conventional laparoscopic surgery and open surgery (Table 1.1).

What's the characteristics of body position for patients, position between surgeon and assistant, and operation technique? The anesthesia of patients is the same to that in traditional laparoscopic surgery and herringbone position is often used. SILS is operated mainly by the surgeon himself, and his assistant co-operates closely. To avoid much disturbance, it seems reasonable for surgeon and assistant to stand slightly apart. However, for multi-port laparoscopic surgery, it requires the second assistant to perform some pulling and

S. Wu et al. (eds.), *Atlas of Single-Incision Laparoscopic Operations in General Surgery*,
DOI 10.1007/978-94-007-6955-7_1, © Springer Science+Business Media Dordrecht 2013

Table 1.1

	Single port	Multiple port	Open
Cholecystectomy	★★★	★★	★
Appendectomy	★★★	★★	★
Common bile duct exploration (without operation history)	★★	★★	★
Cholecystojejunostomy	★★★	★★	★
Cholangiojejunostomy	★	★★★	★★
Splenectomy (non-giant spleen)	★★★	★★	★
Splenectomy (portal hypertension)	★★	★★	★★
Sigmoid colon, rectum	★★	★★	★
Esophageal surgery	★★★	★★	★
Partial gastrectomy	★★★	★★	★
Subtotal gastrectomy (BII)	★★★	★★	★
Radical gastrectomy	★★	★★★	★★
Proximal or total gastrectomy	★	★★	★★
Liver cyst fenestration	★★★	★★	★
Partial hepatectomy	★★	★★	★
Semi-hepatectomy	★	★★	★★
Pancreaticoduodenectomy		★	★★★
Distal pancreatectomy (benign)	★★	★★	★★
Distal pancreatectomy (malignant)	★	★	★★★
Hernioplasty	★★	★★	★
Breast	★★	★★	★
Thyroidectomy	★	★★	★★

grasping movements, therefore the assistant holding the laparoscope has to stand at the same side with the surgeon. We need to fix the patient on the operating bed to avoid the patient body slipping while reaching an excellent exposure. The typical characteristic of SILS operation is that the two operation ports are close to the observation port (the distance between them can be less than 10 mm), and they often form a triangle (an inverted triangle in upper abdominal operation and an equilateral one in lower abdominal operation). These three ports interfere with each other, influencing exposure of the operation fields and effective tissue separation, which is called "Chopsticks effect". Except for complicated operations such as pancreaticoduodenectomy, lesions in right posterior liver, frozen Calot's triangle in cholecystitis and so on, many operations can be performed successfully by the use of SILS technique. As for operations like cholecystectomy, appendectomy and hernioplasty, operative time and amounts of intra-operative bleeding are similar by using SILS or traditional laparoscopic surgery technique. Surgery of spleen, liver and stomach may cost more time by the former one. It requires surgeons to accumulate more experience on these surgeries. All in all, the SILS results in a better cosmetic outcome and more minimally invasive. More popularity has taken on a booming appearance in a few years. We expect this technique would be a powerful weapon of our surgeons in the near future.

Esophageal Surgery

2

Abstract

Laparoscopic Heller myotomy has proved to be superior to endoscopic techniques in improving symptoms and duration of effect for achalasia (Campos et al., Ann Surg 249:45–57, 2009). The addition of an anterior fundoplication decreases symptoms of acid reflux without exacerbating or promoting dysphagia (Rebecchi et al., Ann Surg 248:1023–1030, 2008; Tapper et al., Am Surg 74:626–634, 2008). It has also been proved that laparoscopic hiatus hernioplasty and Nissen fundoplication is superior to open surgery in medical cost and postoperative complications with similar anti-reflux effect (Siddiqui et al., Pediatr Surg Int 27:359–366, 2011; Ostlie et al., J Laparoendosc Adv Surg Tech A 17:493–496, 2007).

Recent publications confirm the rapid increase in the use of SILS for a wide range of laparoscopic procedures (Fan et al., Surg Innov 18:185–188, 2011; Fan et al., J Laparoendosc Adv Surg Tech A 21:243–247, 2011; Joseph et al., Am Surg 78:119–124, 2012). However, application of SILS technique in Heller myotomy and Dor fundoplication or hiatus hernioplasty and Nissen fundoplication is still in its infancy due to its technical difficulties (Huang et al., Obes Surg 19:1711–1715, 2009; Sakaguchi et al., Surg Endosc 22:2532–2534, 2008; Gianni et al., Obes Surg 22:190–191, 2012). So far, we have performed single incision laparoscopic fundoplication in more than ten cases with good results (Fan et al., J Laparoendosc Adv Surg Tech A 23:356–360, 2013).

Keywords

Hiatal hernia • Hiatus hernioplasty • Nissen fundoplication • Achalasia • Heller myotomy • Dor fundoplication

S. Wu et al. (eds.), *Atlas of Single-Incision Laparoscopic Operations in General Surgery*,
DOI 10.1007/978-94-007-6955-7_2, © Springer Science+Business Media Dordrecht 2013

2.1 Laparoscopic Hiatus Hernioplasty and Nissen Fundoplication

2.1.1 Indications and Case Selection

1. Patients with type II/III/IV esophageal hiatal hernia.
2. Patients with type I esophageal hiatal hernia complicating with esophageal reflux, but medication is ineffective.
3. Patients complicating with severe peptic esophagitis, hemorrhage, recurrent aspiration pneumonia, etc.

2.1.2 Contraindications

1. Absolute contraindications
   (a) severe cardiorespiratory dysfunction.
   (b) inability to tolerate general anesthesia or pneumoperitoneum.
   (c) refractory coagulopathy.
2. Relative contraindications
   (a) extensive previous surgery, or previous peritonitis leading to severe adhesion.
   (b) morbid obesity.
   (c) pregnancy (during first and third trimesters).

2.1.3 Major Instruments or Energy Sources

1. Laparoscopy System.
2. Holding forceps, non-traumatic intestinal clamps, needle holder etc.
3. Harmonic scalpel.

2.1.4 Team Setup, Anesthesia and Position

The procedures were performed under general anesthesia with the patients in the supine position with legs parted, left shoulder raised 15–20°. The viewing monitor was placed above the patient's left shoulder, with the surgeon standing between the patient's legs and the camera operator on the patient's right side (Fig. 2.1).

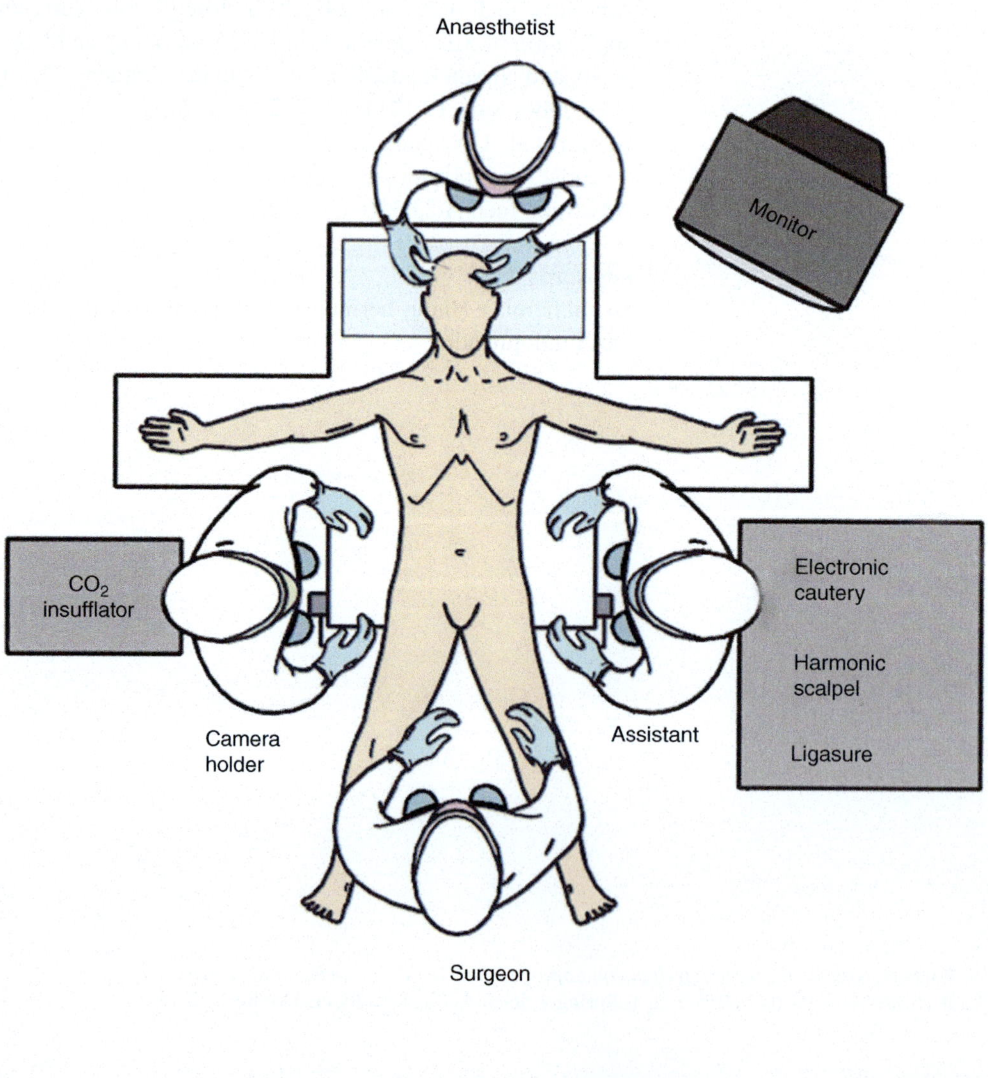

Fig. 2.1

2.1.5 Key Steps

1. Establishment of Pneumoperitoneum and Placement of Trocars.
2. Abdominal Exploration.
3. Division of lower esophagus and bilateral crura.
4. Division of the cardia and fundus of the stomach.
5. Hernioplasty.
6. Fundoplication.
7. Placement of the suction drainage.

2.1.6 Surgical Techniques

1. Establishment of Pneumoperitoneum and Placement of Trocars.
2. Abdominal Exploration.

   The fundus of the stomach was retracted to expose the hiatus and the degree of hiatus hernia was judged (Fig. 2.2).

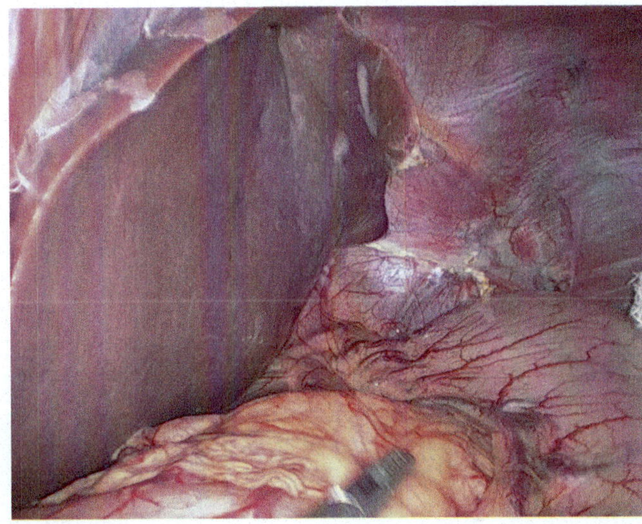

Fig. 2.2

3. Division of lower esophagus and bilateral crura.
   The right crura were retracted laterally with a roticulated grasper, and peritoneum was incised with Harmonic scalpel. The hernia sac was dissected and totally mobilized in a standard fashion from right to left. Then, the gastrosplenic ligament was divided. The esophagus was retracted upwards, thus exposing the posterior crus of the diaphragm (Fig. 2.3a–o).

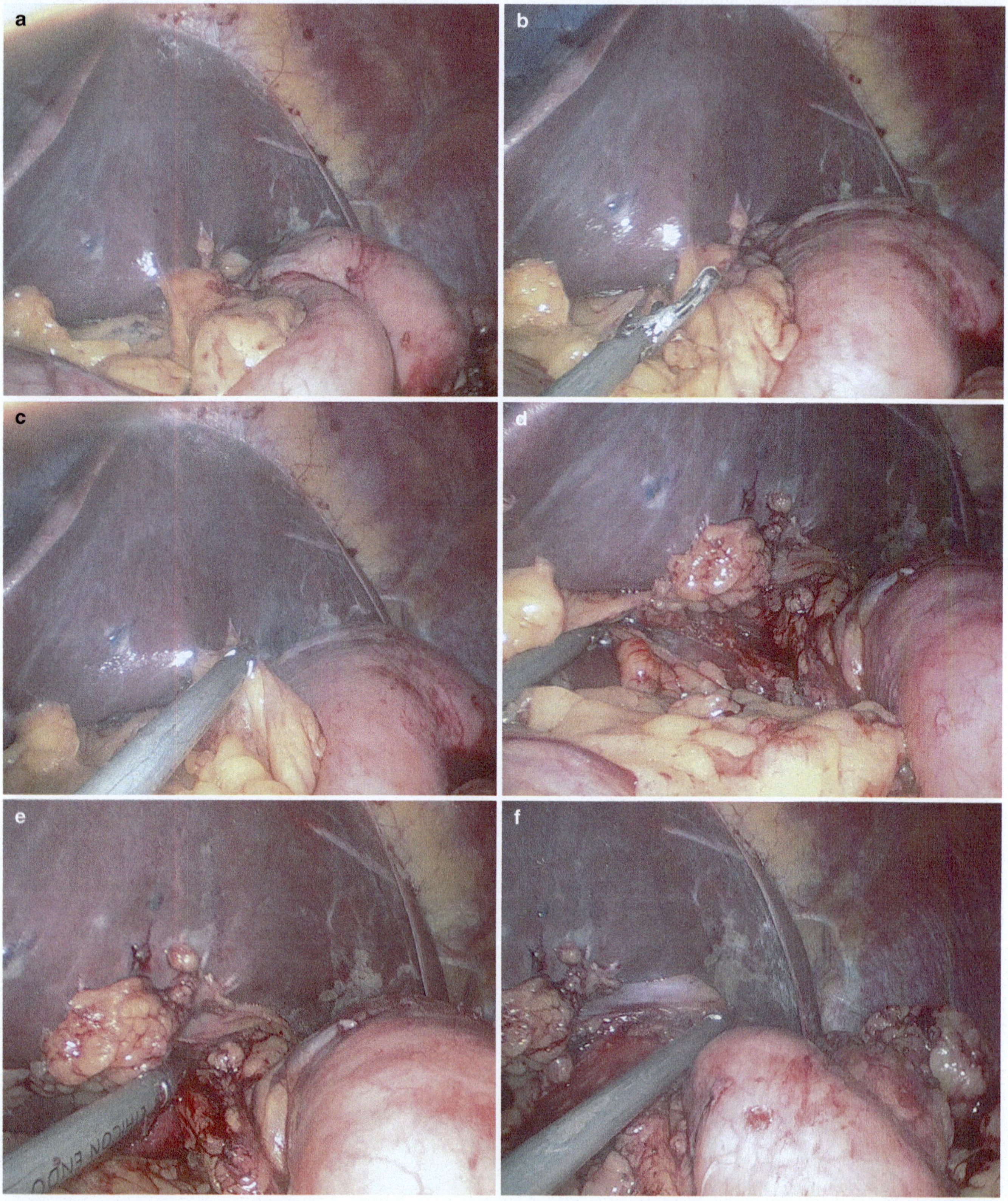

Fig. 2.3

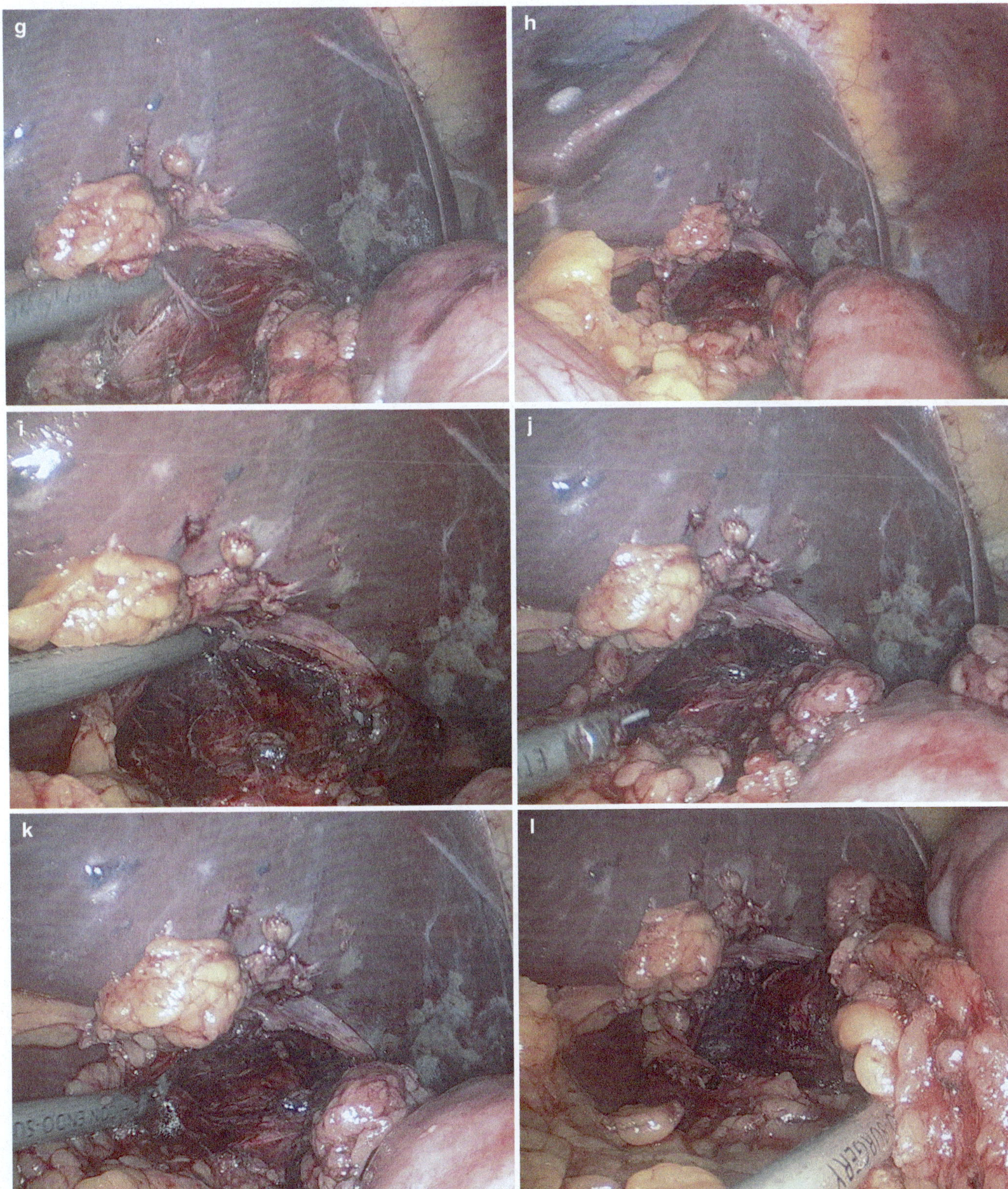

Fig. 2.3 (continued)

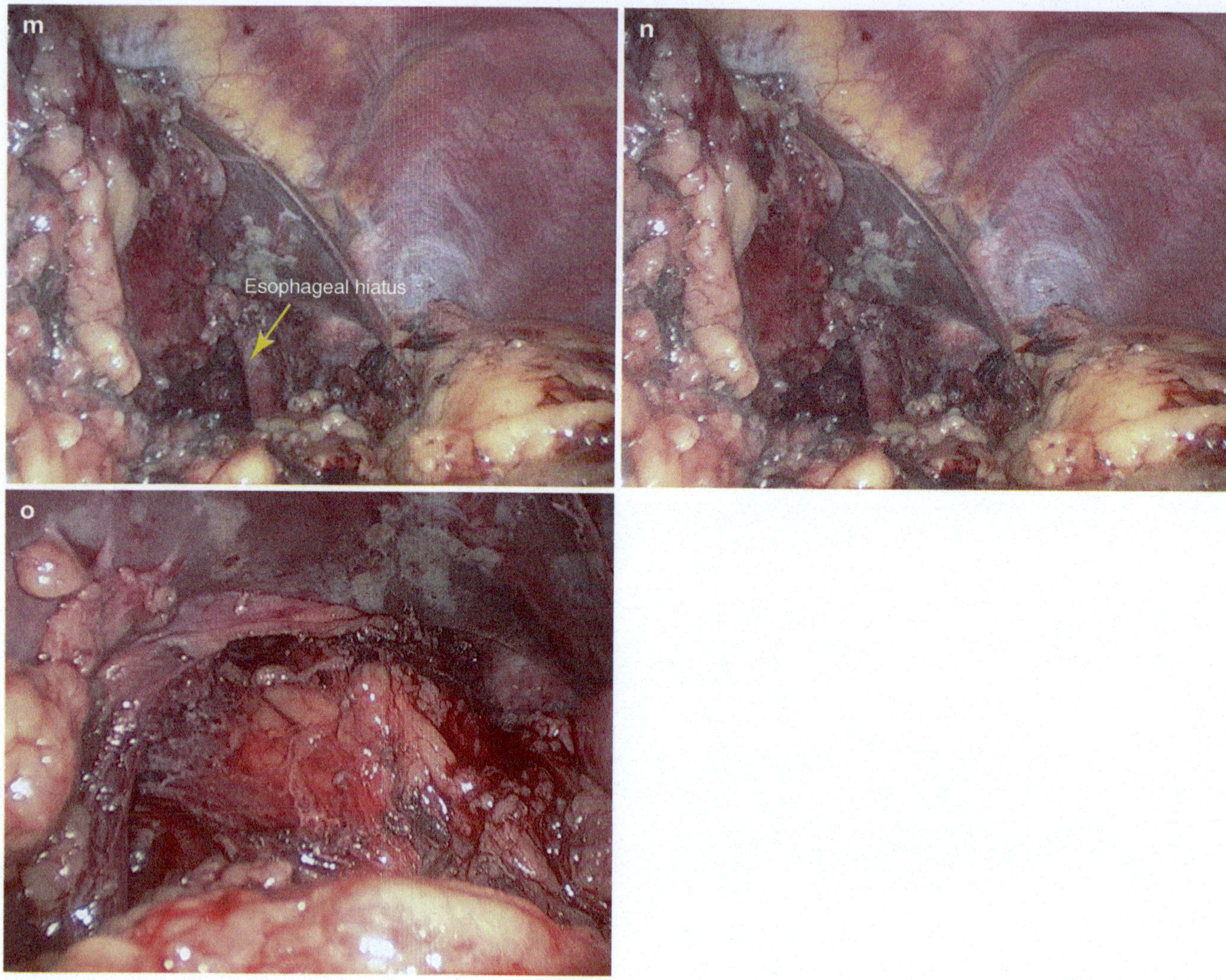

Fig. 2.3 (continued)

4. Division of the cardia and fundus of the stomach.
   Then, the gastrocolic and gastrosplenic ligament was divided to free the fundus of the stomach (Fig. 2.4a–j).

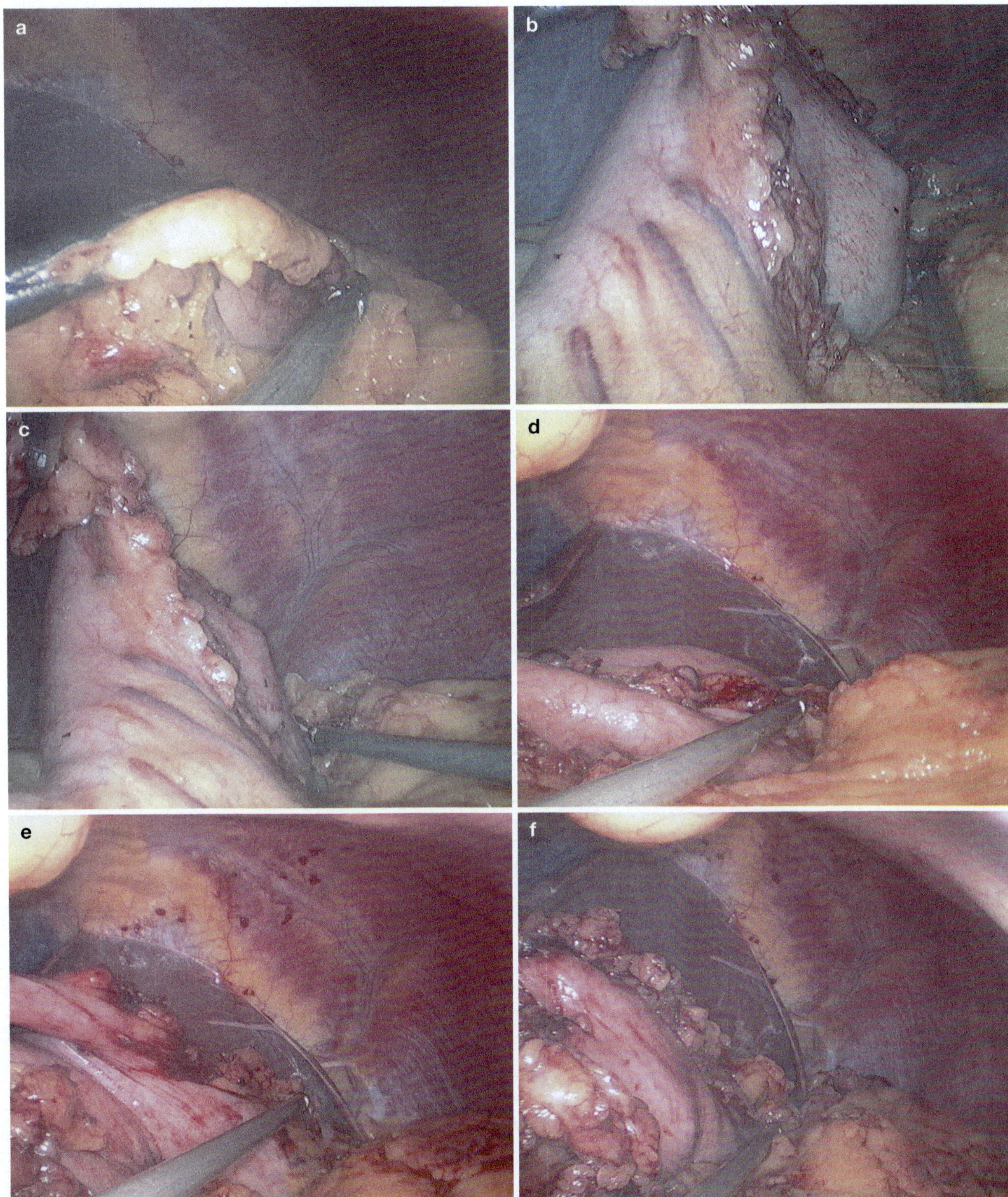

Fig. 2.4

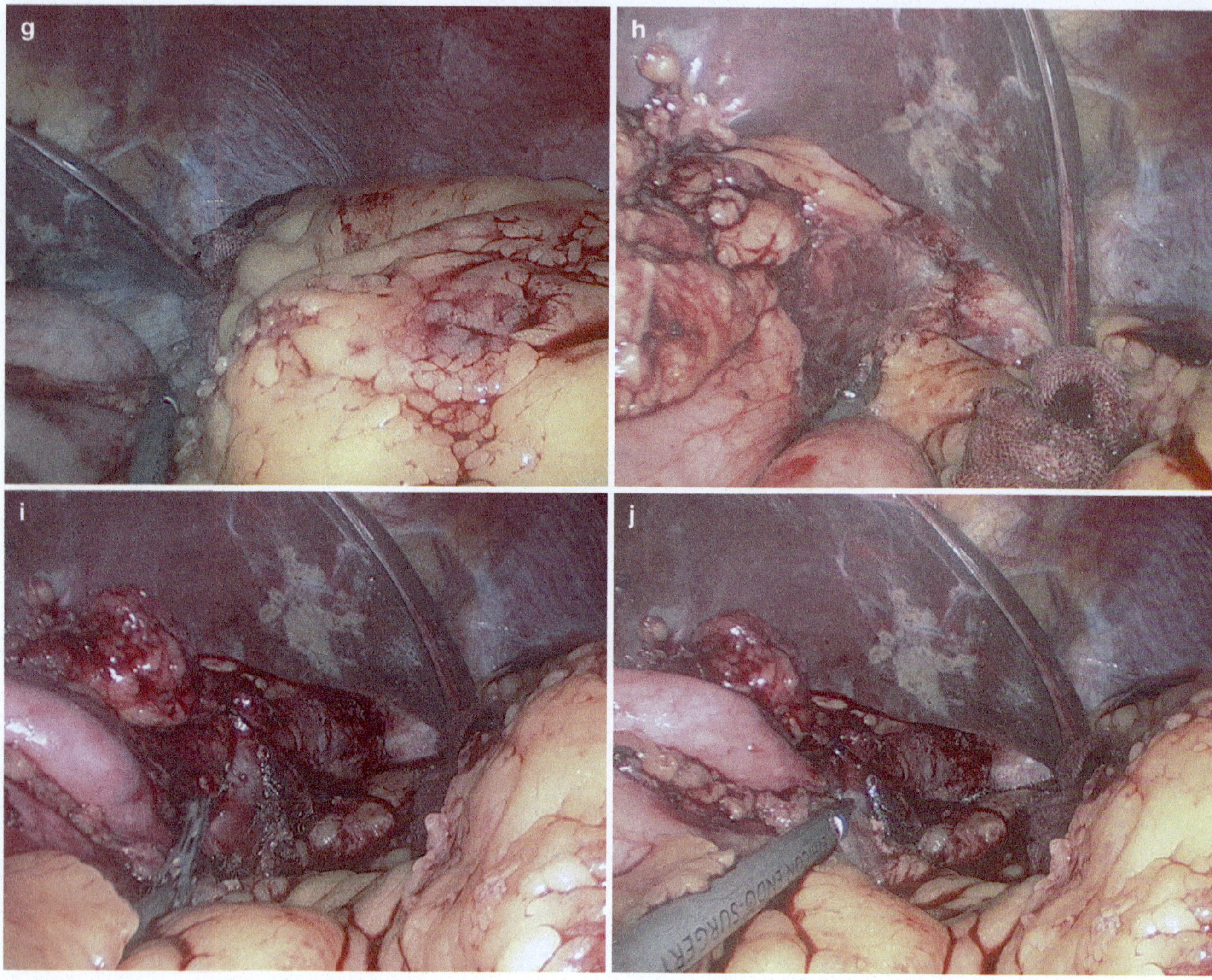

Fig. 2.4 (continued)

5. Hernioplasty.

   After completion of dissection and removal of the whole hernia sac, a gauze strip was introduced into the abdomen and placed behind the esophagus to encircle the esophagus thus exposing the posterior crus of the diaphragm. Prolene (polypropylene) suture w/wo needle was used to close the hiatus to 0.5–1.0 cm (Fig. 2.5a–l).

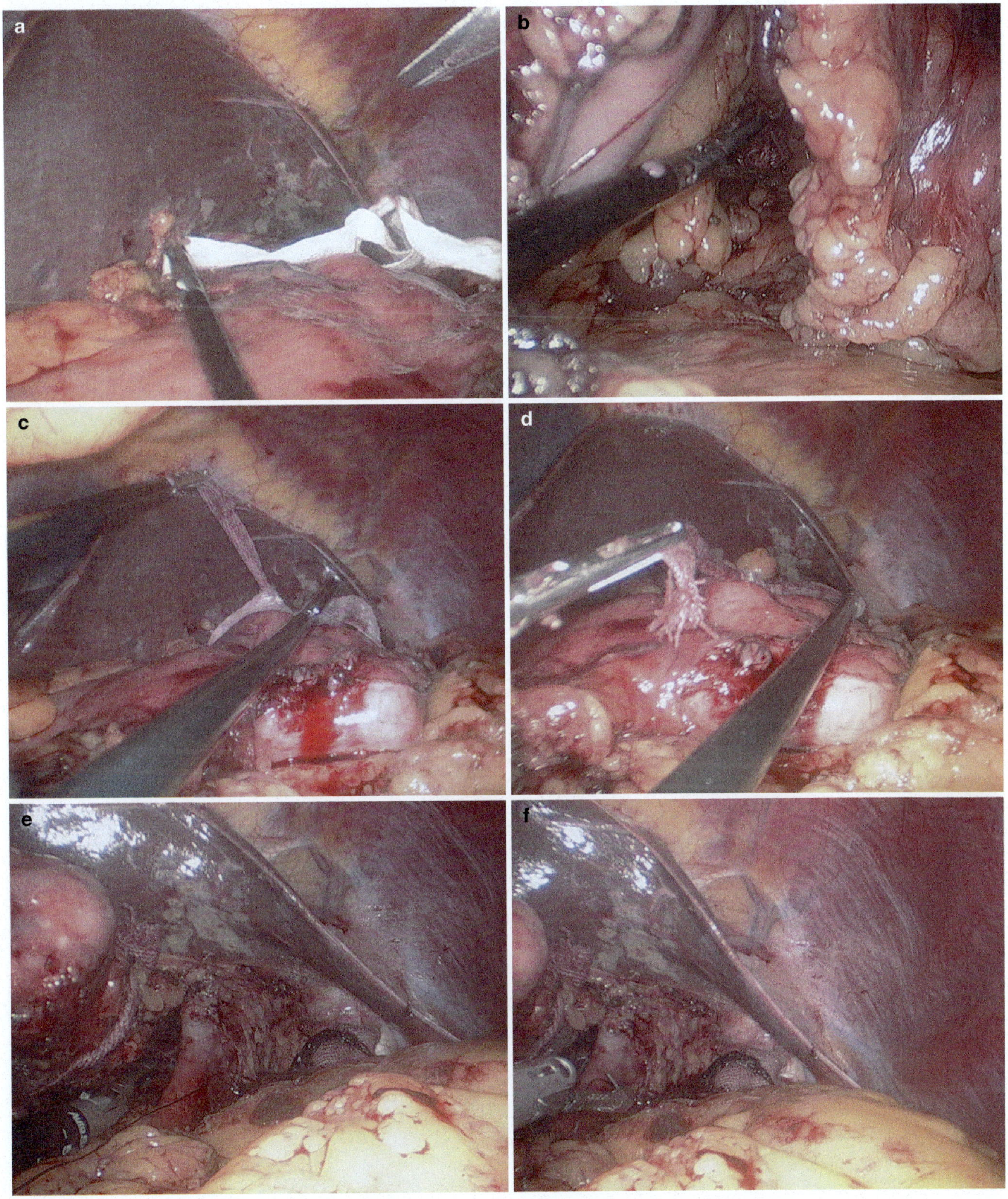

Fig. 2.5

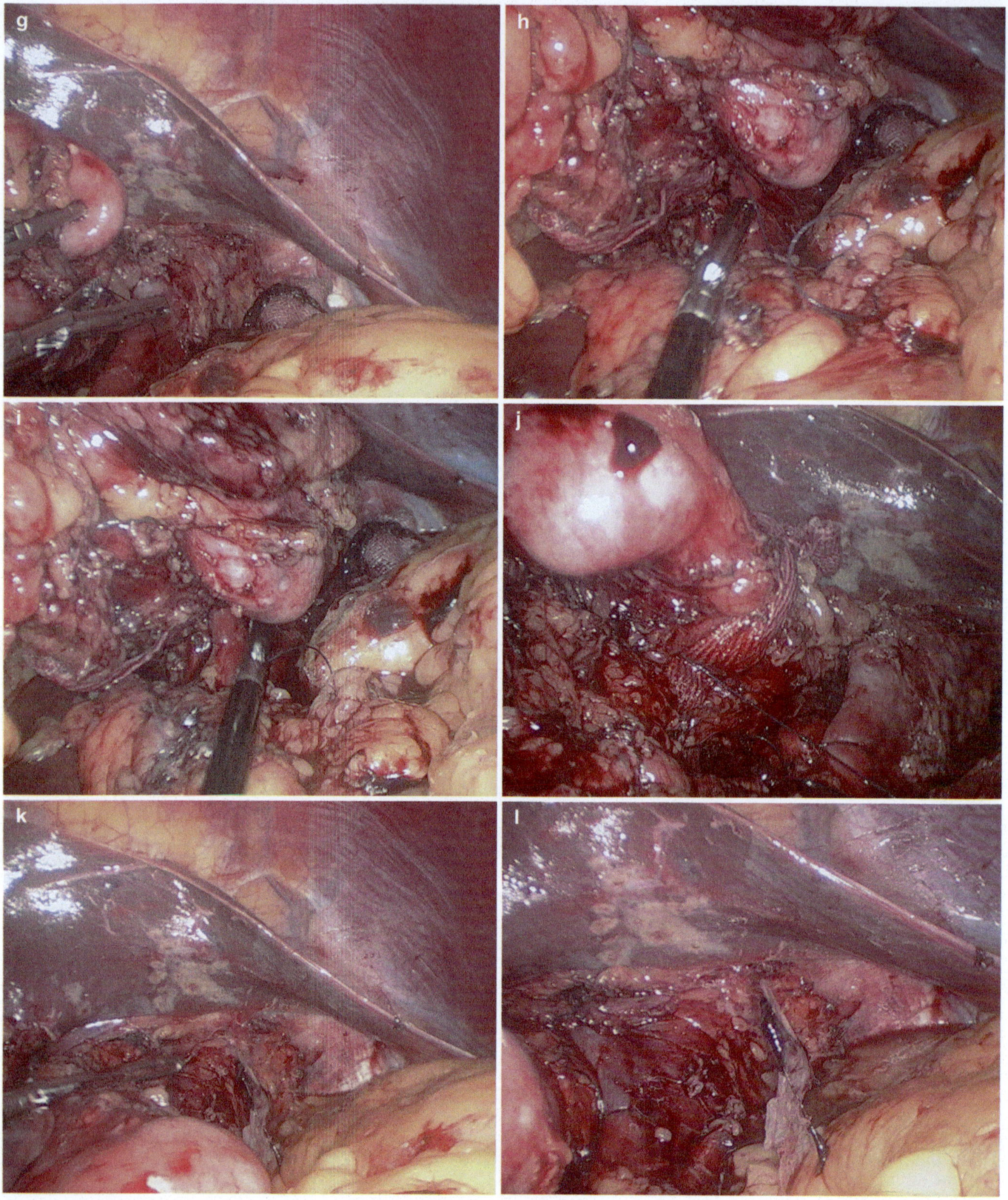

Fig. 2.5 (continued)

6. Fundoplication.

   The fundus was then brought behind the esophagus creating a 360° wrap. Nissen fundoplication was created the same as conventional laparoscopic multiple-incision procedure. The sutures were tied using the intracorporeal technique. The length of the wrap was approximately 3–4 cm (Fig. 2.6a–j).

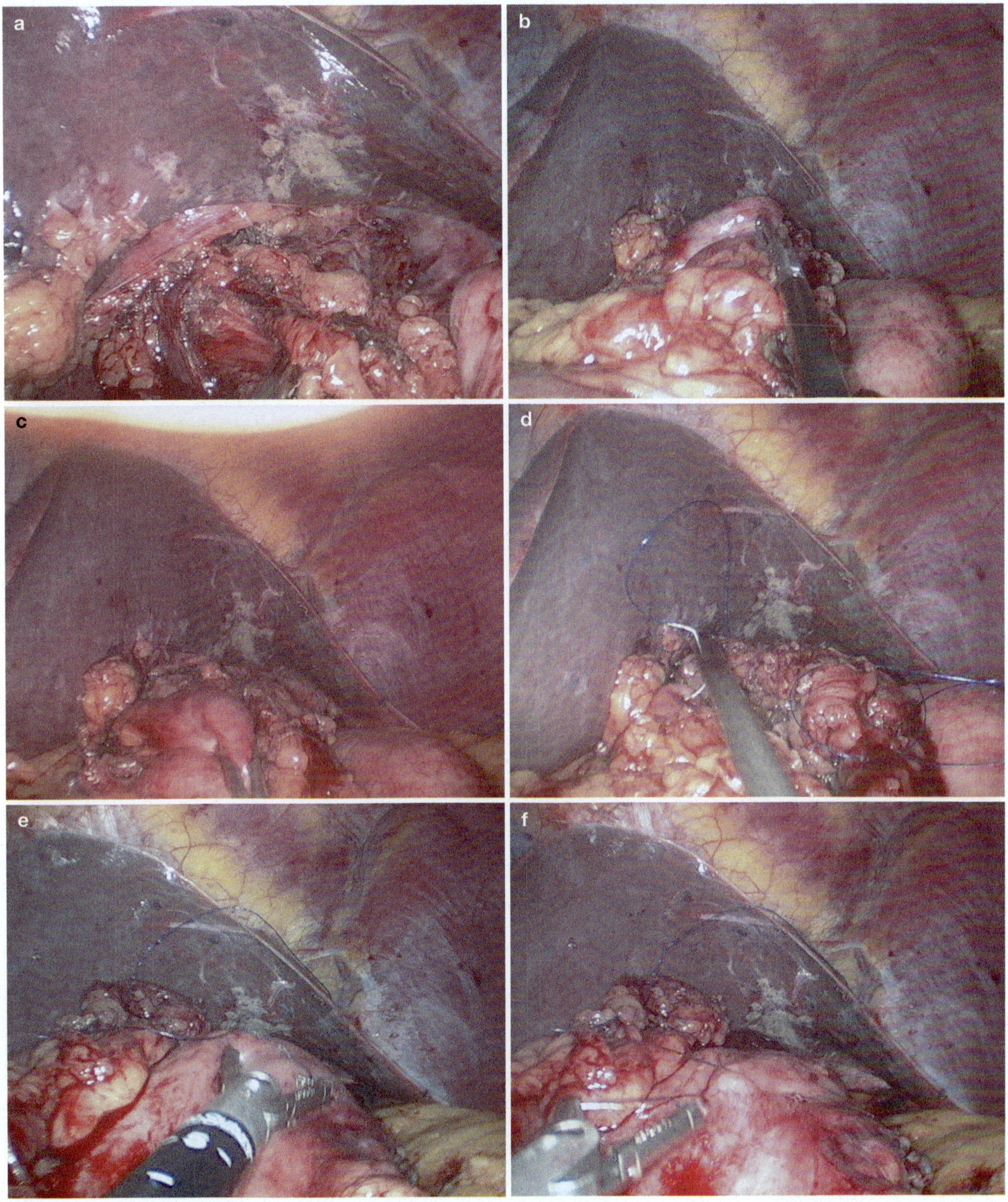

Fig. 2.6

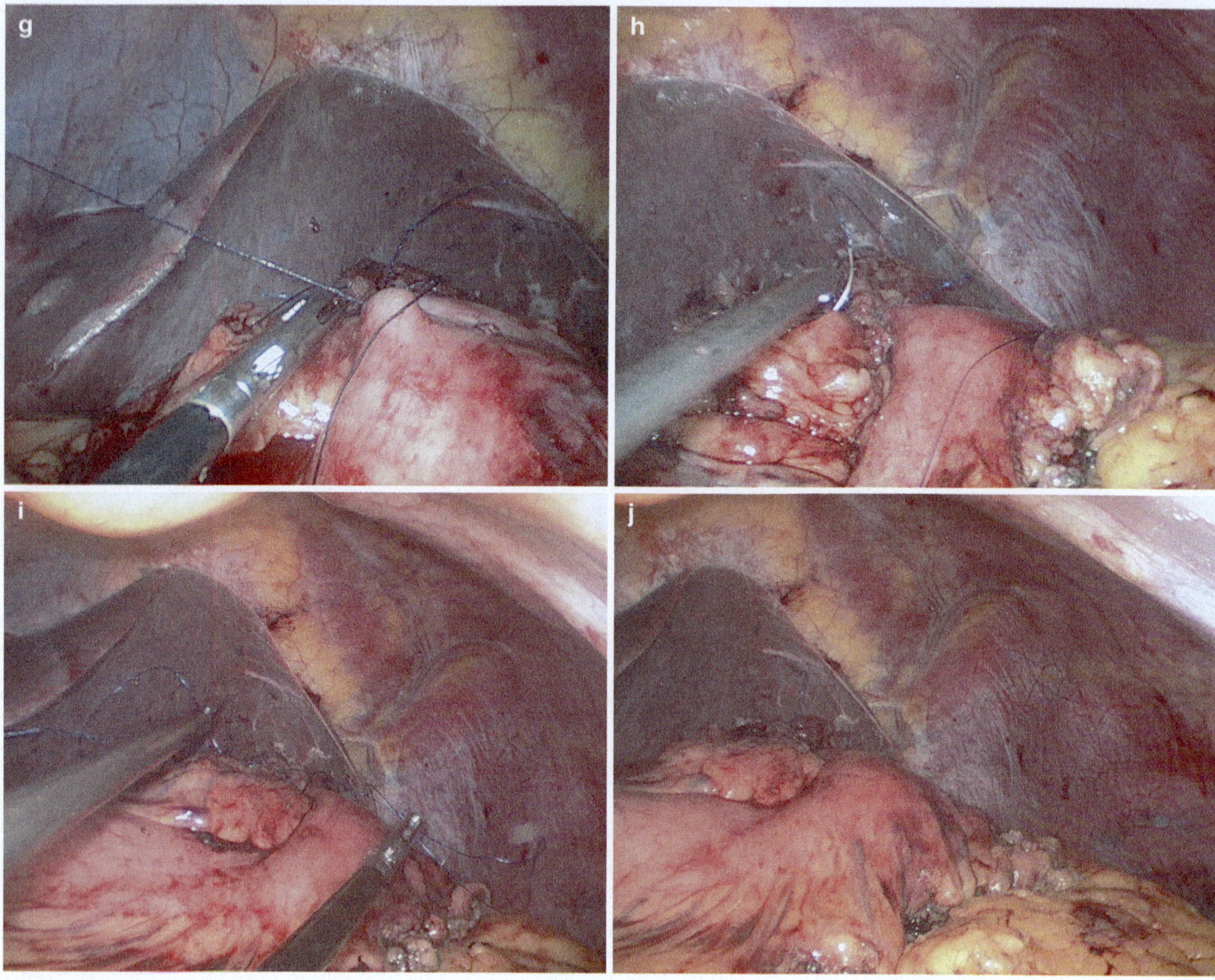

Fig. 2.6 (continued)

7. Placement of the suction drainage.
After adequate flushing of the operative field, a closed suction drain was placed into the surgical field through the umbilical incision (Fig. 2.7a–d).

2.1.7 Tips and Tricks

1. To achieve adequate retraction of the liver, without resorting to the standard trocar placement, some methods have been invented to overcome this obstacle, such as a Jackson–Pratt drainage penetrated with a 2-0 Prolene and fixed with Kelly clamps at the skin, a Penrose drain tied with two silk sutures of 10 cm in length and fixed at the skin or utilizing a 15-cm Veress needle, etc. As described, additional puncture of the abdominal wall or incision is needed during the techniques mentioned above. In our procedure, adequate retraction of the liver was achieved by binding the lateral left lobe of the liver to the diaphragm with Cyanoacrylate glue.
2. The dissection should start with the division of Leimer ligament. The right crura was retracted laterally with a grasper, and peritoneum was incised with harmonic scalpel.
3. The hernia sac should be dissected and totally mobilized by using harmonic ace in a standard fashion from right to left. Esophagus was further mobilized in the thorax, and the gastrosplenic ligament was divided.

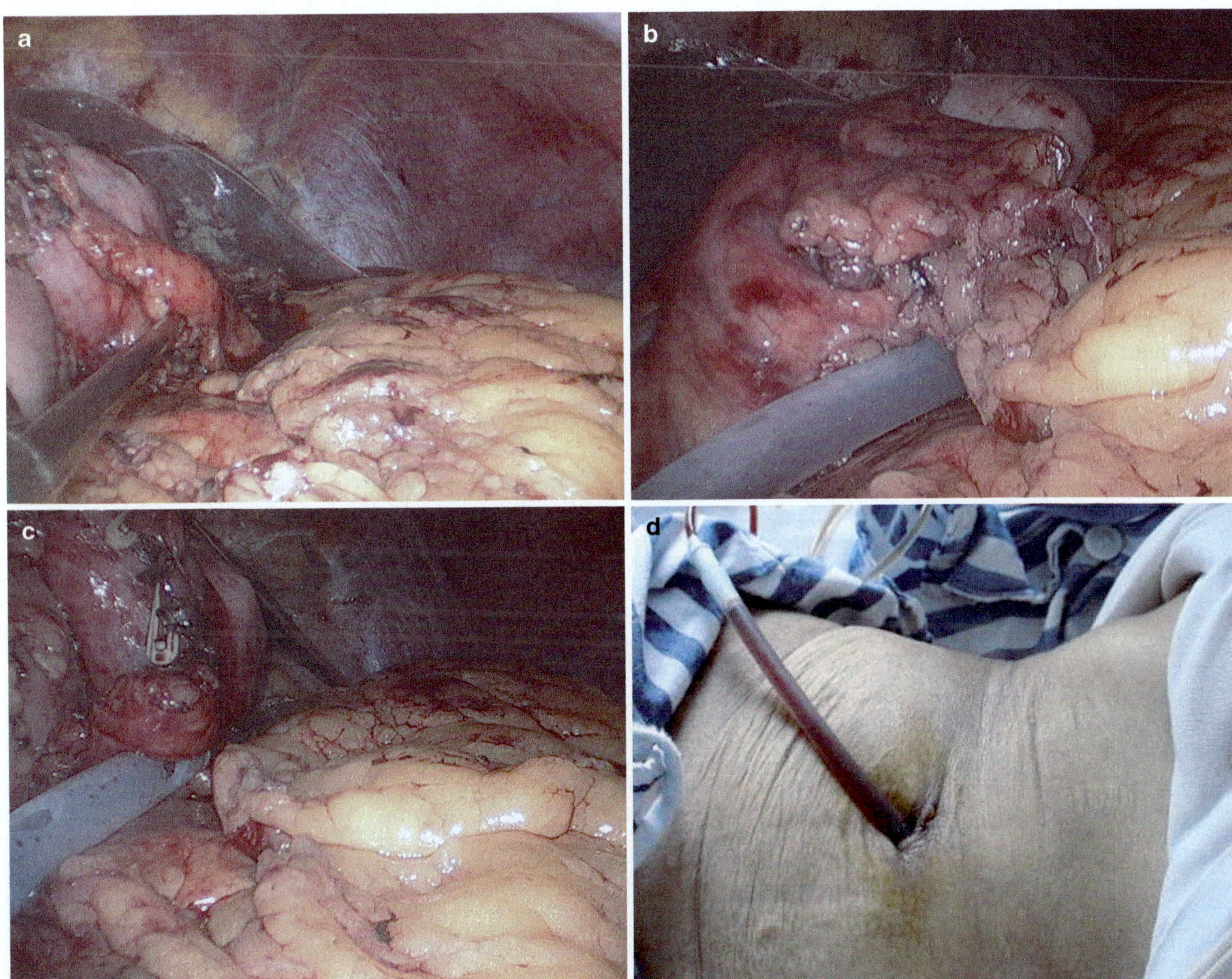

Fig. 2.7

2.2 Laparoscopic Heller Myotomy and Dor Fundoplication

2.2.1 Indications and Case Selection

1. Patients with moderate or severe achalasia of cardia.
2. Patients with achalasia of cardia, but it's ineffective when treated by bouginage of esophagus.
3. Partial fundoplication is indicated for isolated hypertensive lower esophageal sphincter, while Nissen fundoplication should be performed in patients with hypertensive lower esophageal sphincter with GERD/type III hiatal hernia.

2.2.2 Contraindications

1. Absolute contraindications
   (a) severe cardiorespiratory dysfunction.
   (b) inability to tolerate general anesthesia or pneumoperitoneum.
   (c) refractory coagulopathy.
   (d) complicated with esophageal malignancies, or documented diffuse esophageal spasm.
2. Relative contraindications
   (a) extensive previous surgery, or previous peritonitis leading to severe adhesion.
   (b) morbid obesity.
   (c) pregnancy (during first and third trimesters).

2.2.3 Major Instruments or Energy Sources

1. Laparoscopy System.
2. Holding forceps, non-traumatic intestinal clamps, needle holder etc.
3. Harmonic scalpel.

2.2.4 Team Setup, Anesthesia and Position

The same as Sect. 2.1.4.

2.2.5 Key Steps

1. Establishment of Pneumoperitoneum and Placement of Trocars.
2. Abdominal Exploration.
3. Division of lower esophagus and bilateral cruras.
4. Division of the cardia and fundus of the stomach.
5. Hernioplasty.
6. Fundoplication.
7. Placement of the suction drainage.

2.2.6 Surgical Techniques

1. Establishment of Pneumoperitoneum and Placement of Trocars.
2. Abdominal Exploration.
   The gastroesophageal junction was retracted to expose the cardia and fundus of the stomach. Careful checking for adhesions and ruling out other factors of stenosis were performed (Fig. 2.8a, b).

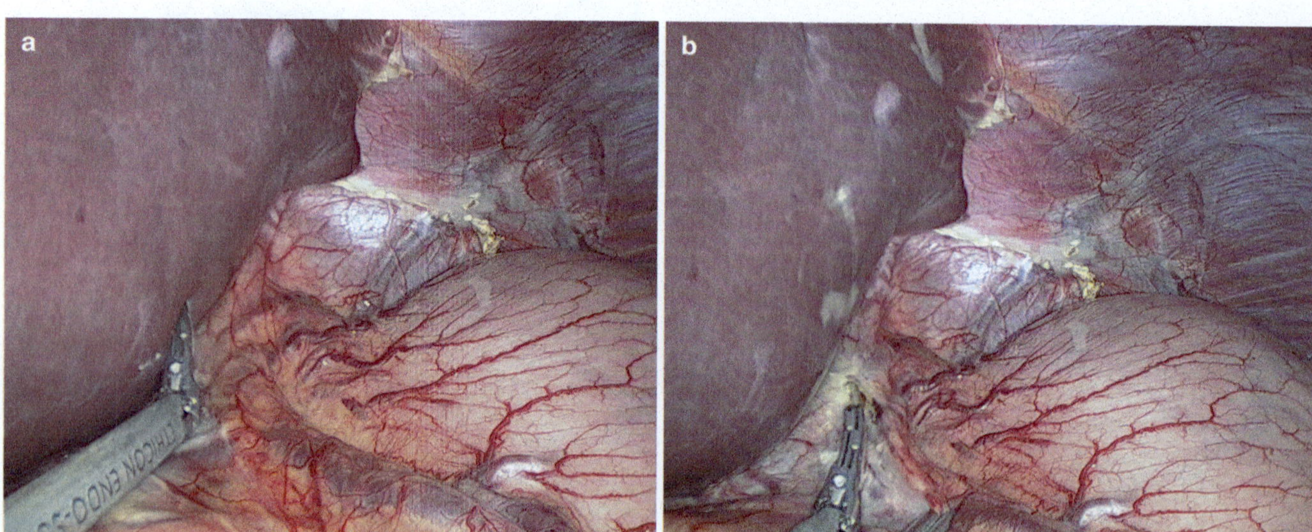

Fig. 2.8

3. Division of bilateral cruras, lower esophagus and cardia of stomach.

   The right crura was retracted laterally with a roticulated grasper, and peritoneum was incised with Harmonic scalpel to expose the right margin of the abdominal segment of the esophagus (Fig. 2.9a–f).

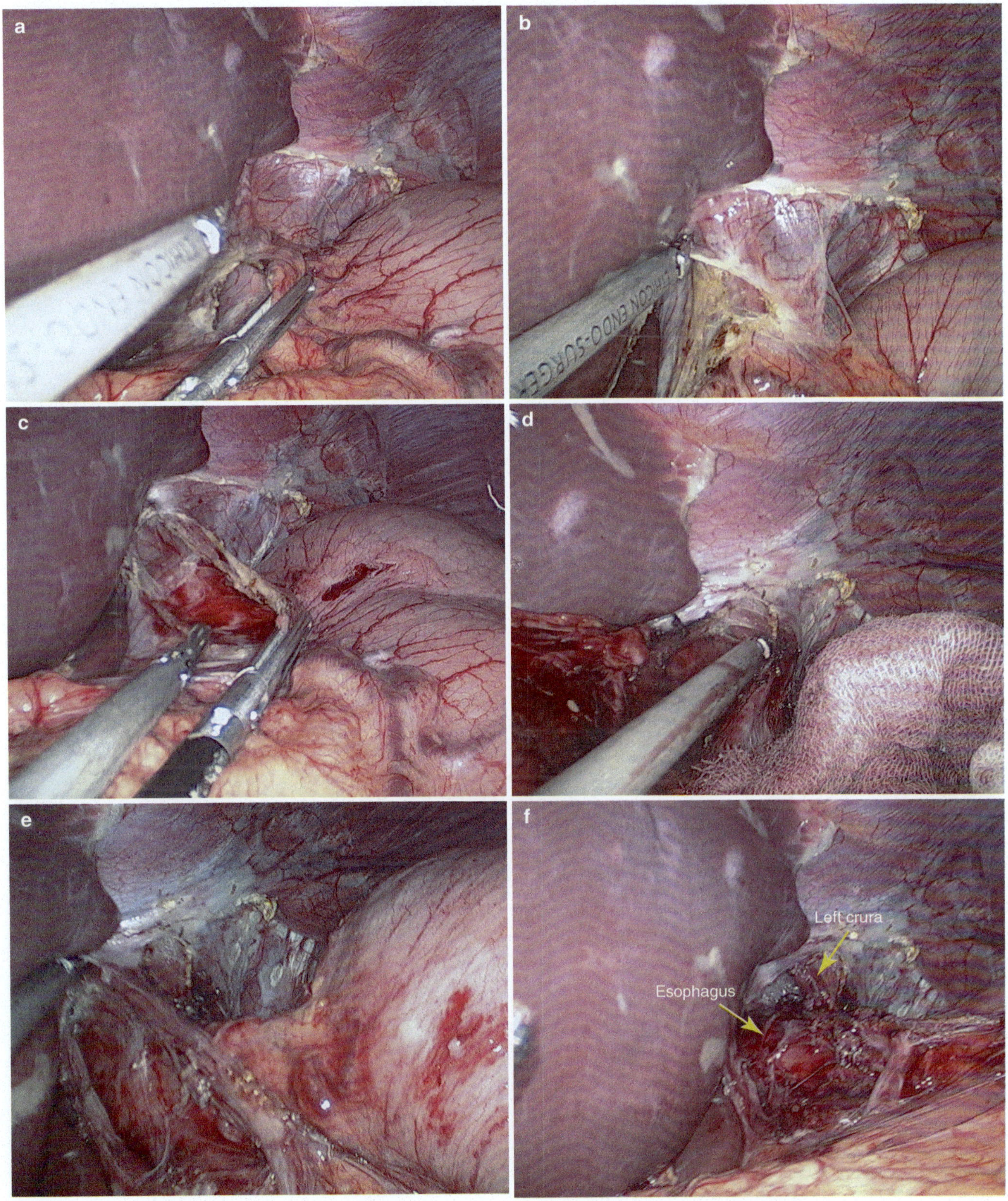

Fig. 2.9

The gastrocolic and gastrosplenic ligament were opened by using the harmonic scalpel to mobilize the fundus of the stomach until the fundus could be folded 180° in front of the esophagus. Continuous mobilization of the left crura was performed to fully free the abdominal segment of the esophagus (Fig. 2.10a–h).

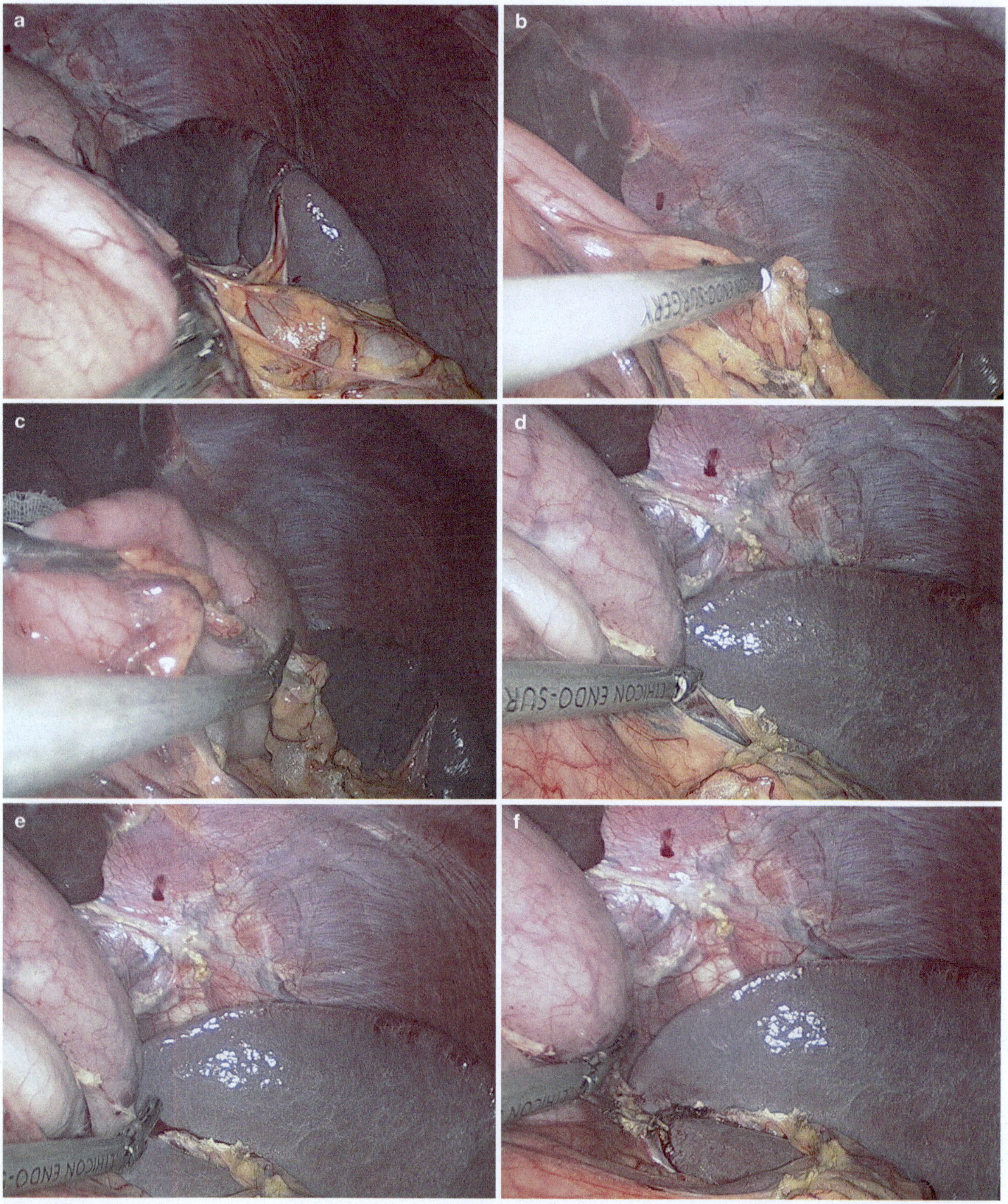

Fig. 2.10

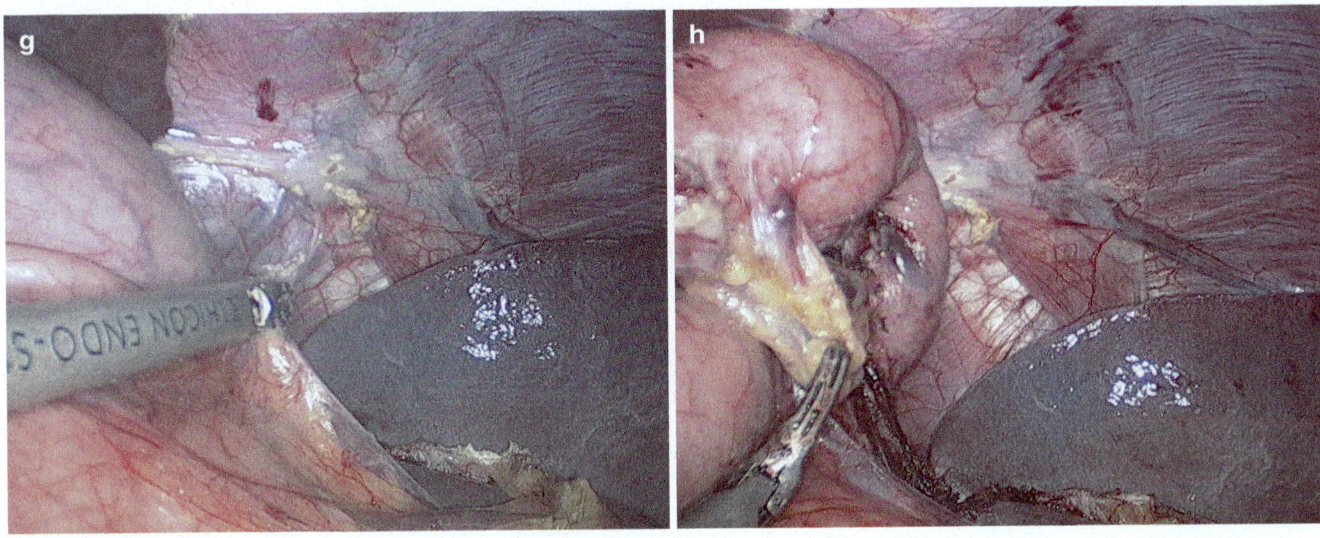

Fig. 2.10 (continued)

The stomach was retracted downward to expose the esophagus. The adipose tissues on the anterior wall of esophagus and cardia were cleared by using the harmonic scalpel (Fig. 2.11a–c).

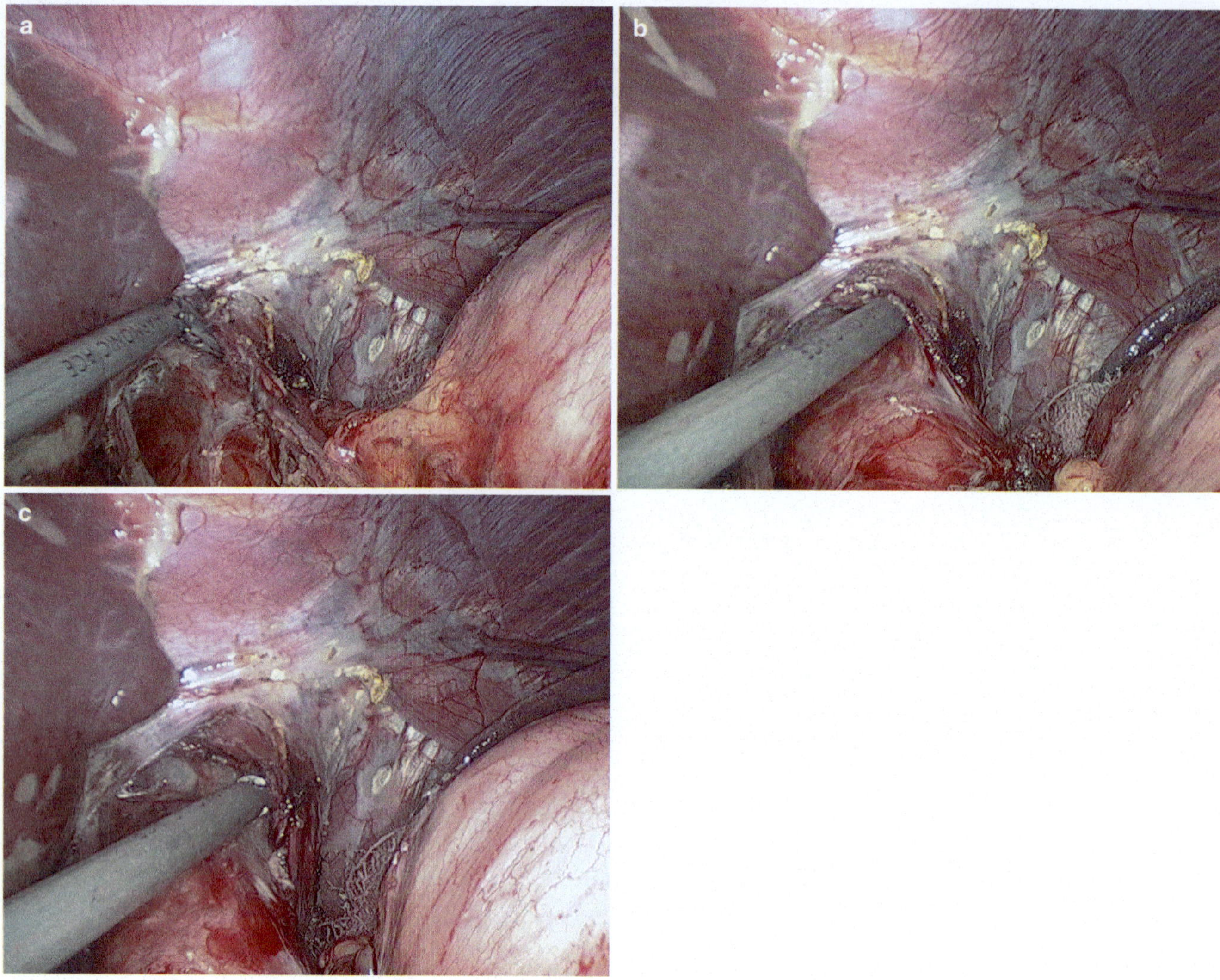

Fig. 2.11

4. Heller myotomy.

   The esophageal–gastric junction was identified by intraoperative gastroscope. The myotomy was to be 7 cm long, extending 2 cm to the gastric wall, using the Harmonic scalpel. Intraoperative gastroscope was used to assess the adequacy of the myotomy and to detect any esophageal mucosal tears (Fig. 2.12a–k).

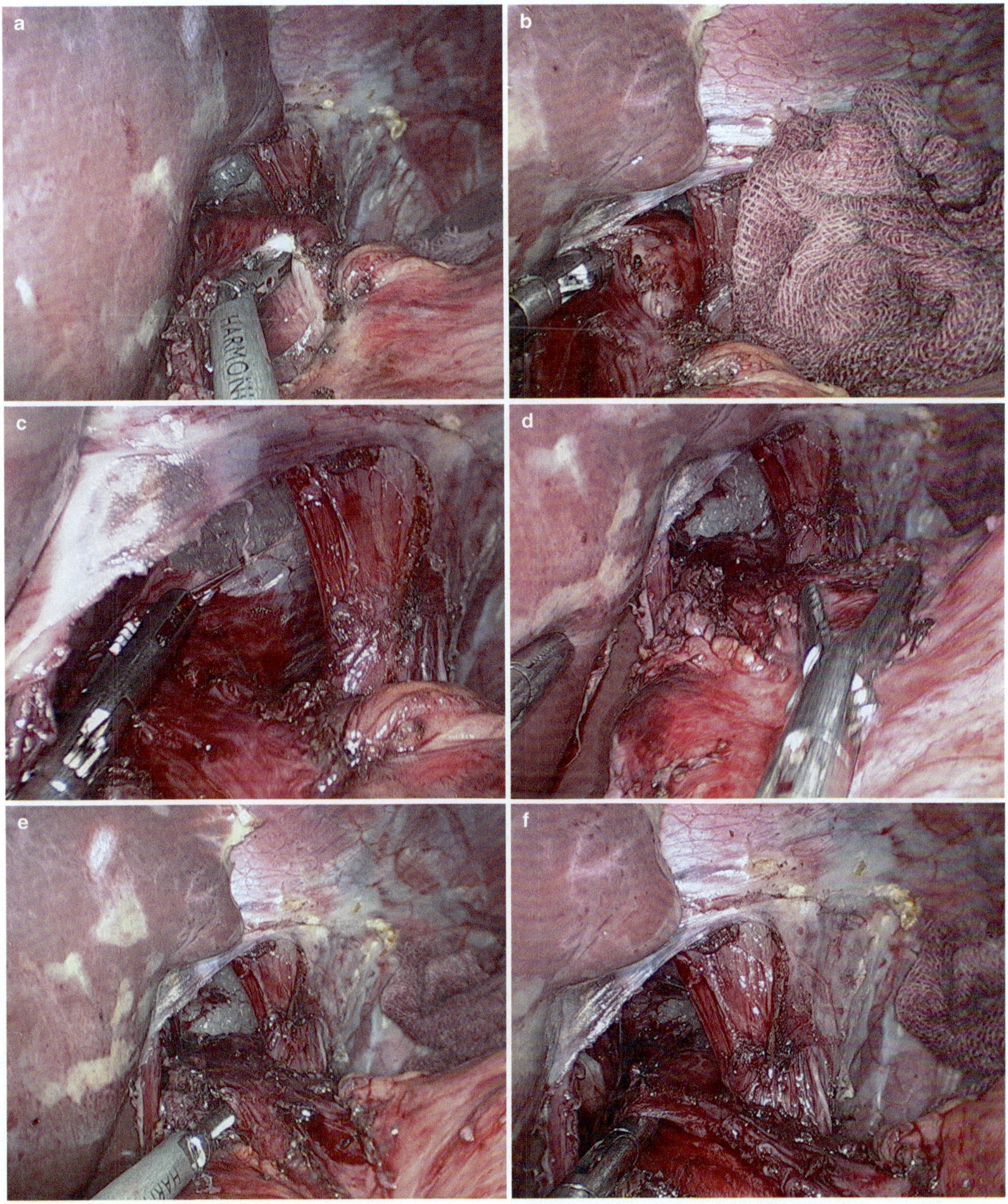

Fig. 2.12

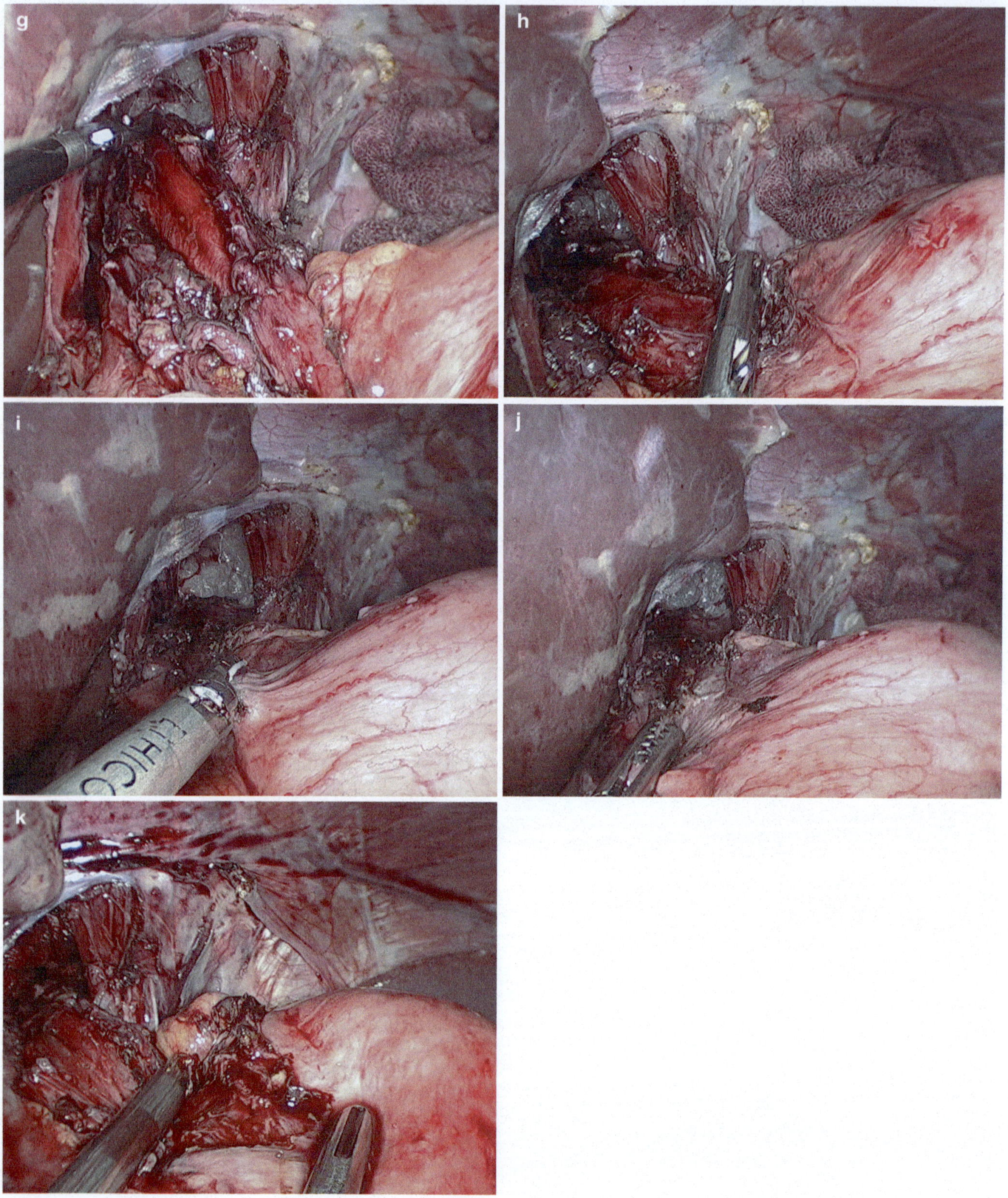

Fig. 2.12 (continued)

5. Dor fundoplication.
   The fundus was then brought in front of the esophagus creating a 180° wrap. Dor fundoplication was created the same as conventional laparoscopic multiple-incision procedure. The sutures were tied using the intracorporeal technique (Fig. 2.13a–p).

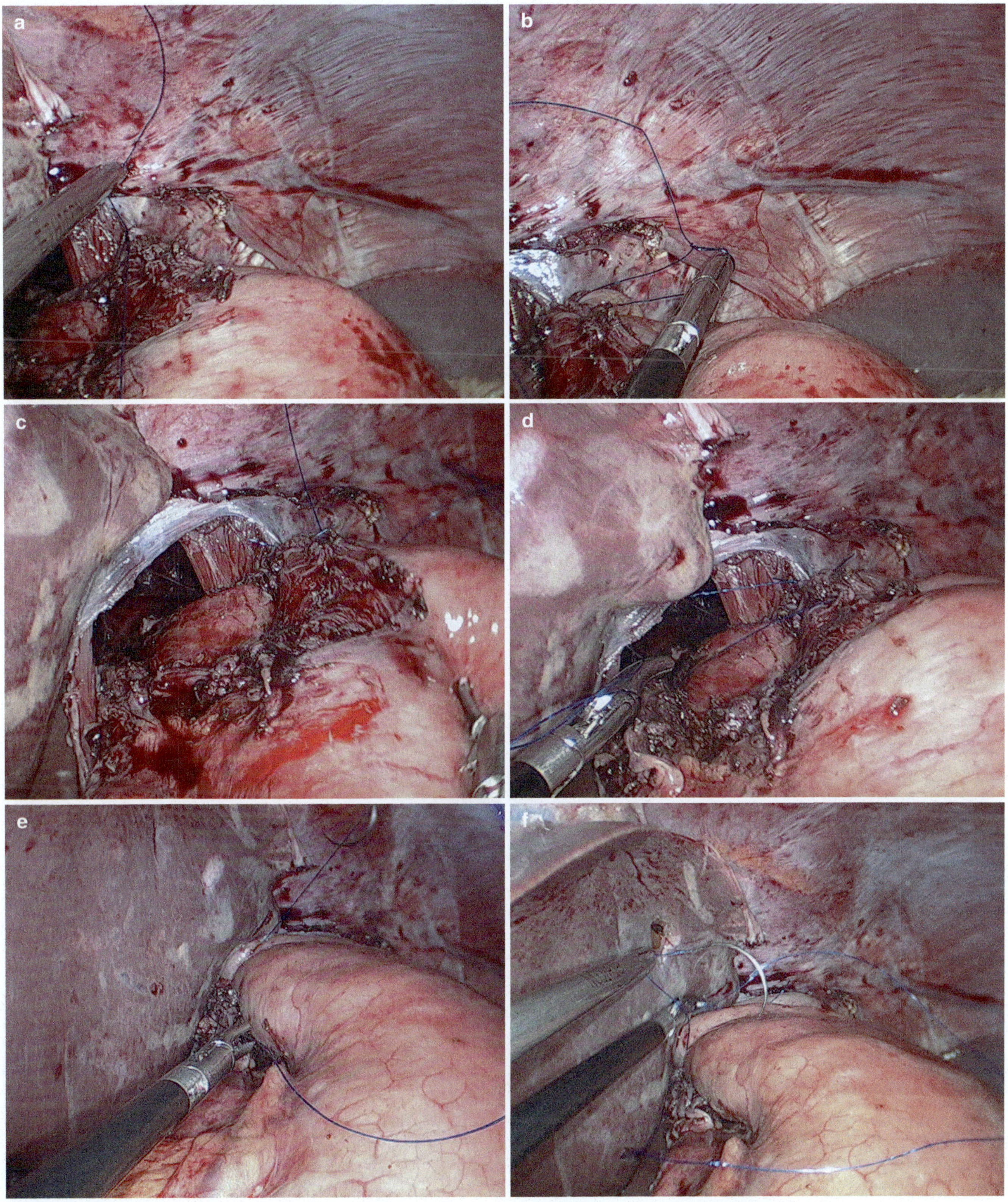

Fig. 2.13

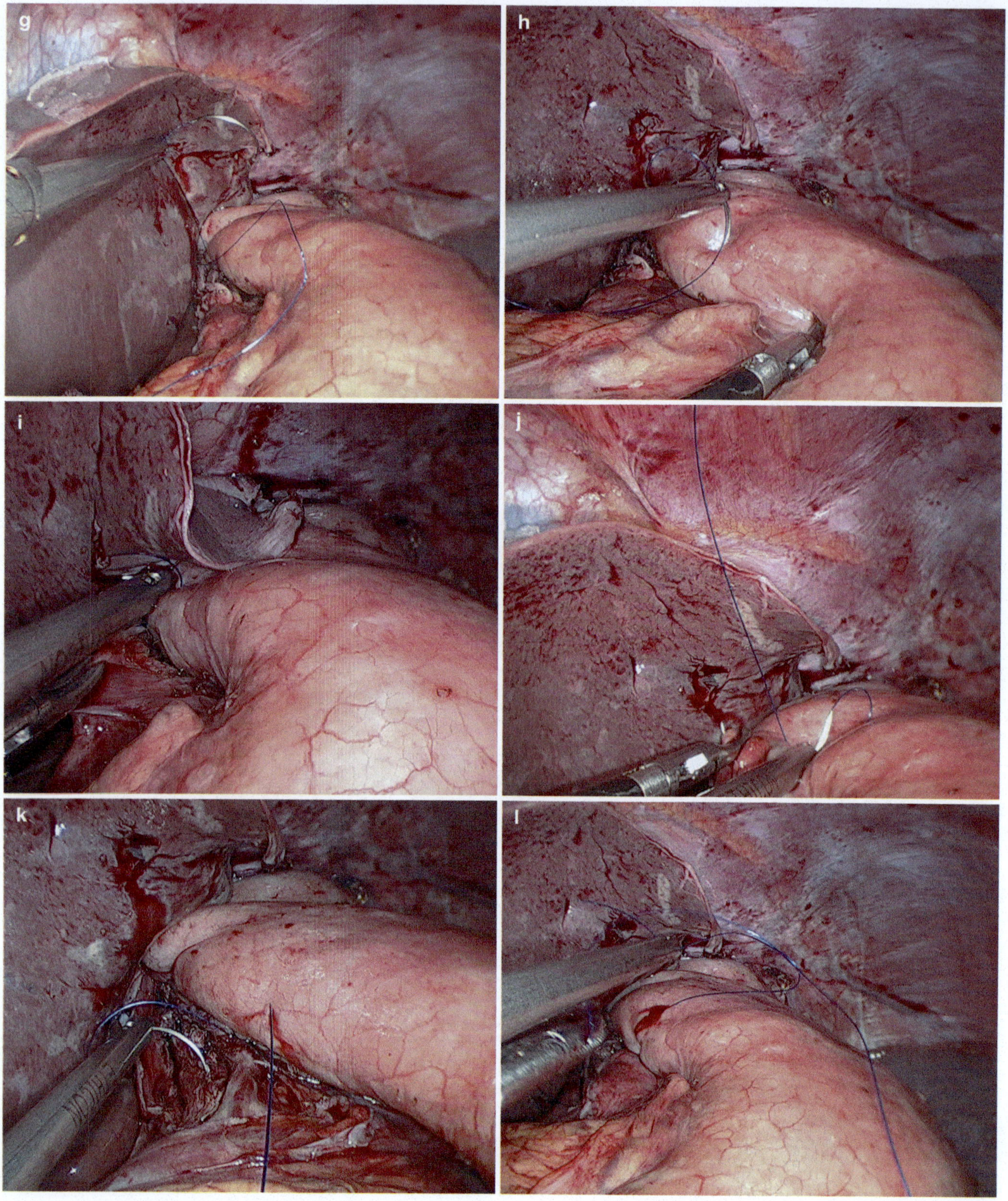

Fig. 2.13 (continued)

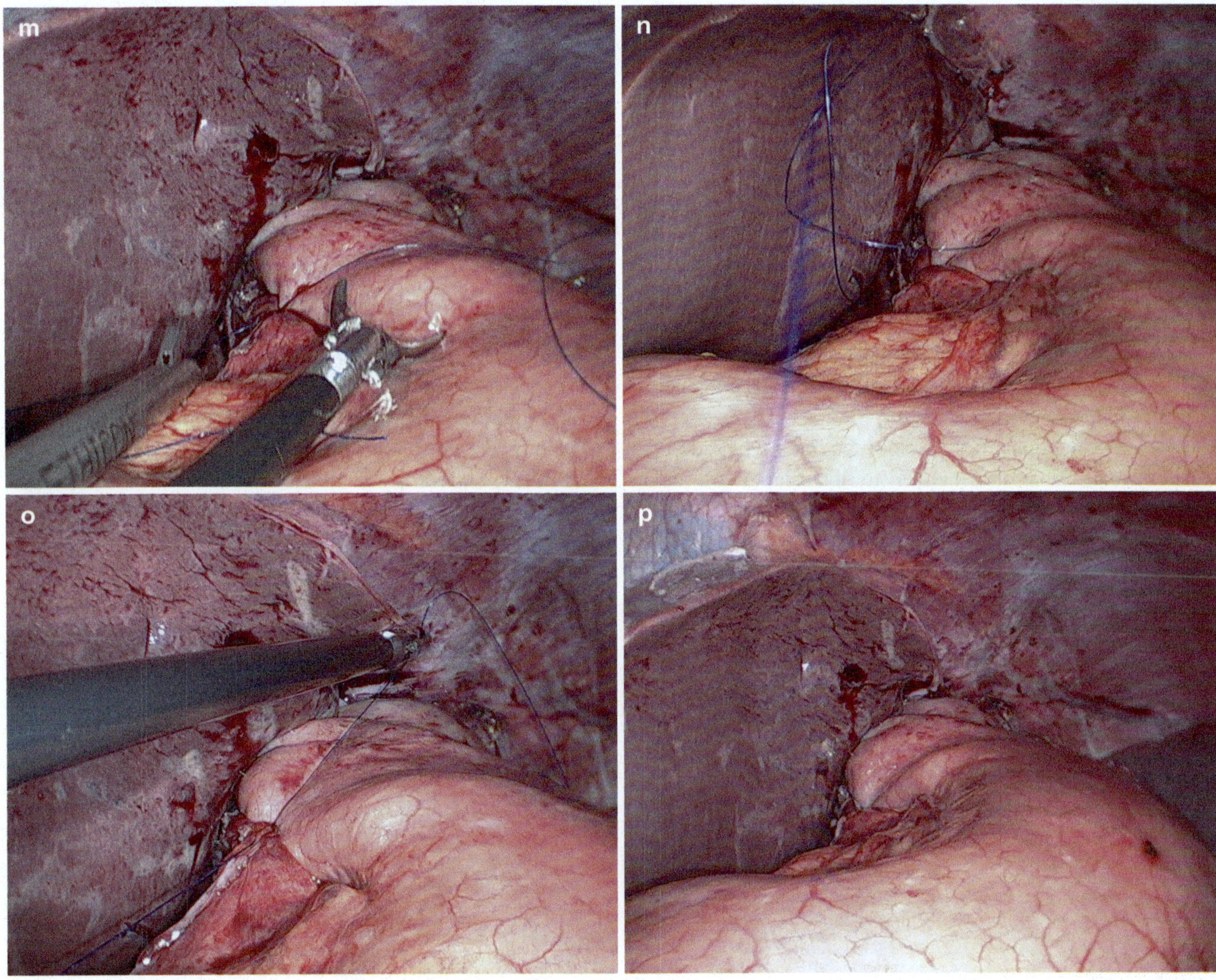

Fig. 2.13 (continued)

6. Placement of the suction drainage.
   After adequate flushing of the operative field, a closed suction drain was placed into the surgical field through the umbilical incision (Fig. 2.14a, b).

2.2.7 Tips and Tricks

1. The patient should be placed in the supine position with the legs straddled. The surgeon stood between the legs, and the first assistant and the cameraman (second assistant) stood on the right and left side of the patient, respectively.
2. The patient should be placed in an anti-Trendelenburg position and rotated to the right.
3. To achieve adequate retraction of the liver, we binded the lateral left lobe of the liver to the diaphragm using Cyanoacrylate glue as mentioned above.
4. All short gastric vessels were divided to relieve the tension from the wrap.
5. Heller myotomy was performed by incising approximately 6 cm of the abdominal esophagus and 2 cm of the gastric wall to relieve the obstruction.
6. After myotomy, endoscopy confirmed that the esophageal-gastric junction was sufficiently expanded, and the endoscope could be inserted into the stomach without resistance. Leakage of the endoscopic supply of air, which is a sign of mucosal tear, was not identified.
7. Dor fundoplication was subsequently performed. Several sutures with a polypropylene thread to cover the exposed submucosa were used to fix the edge of the esophageal sphincter and fundic wrap.
8. Finally, endoscopy confirmed the absence of large aperture and stenosis at the junction.

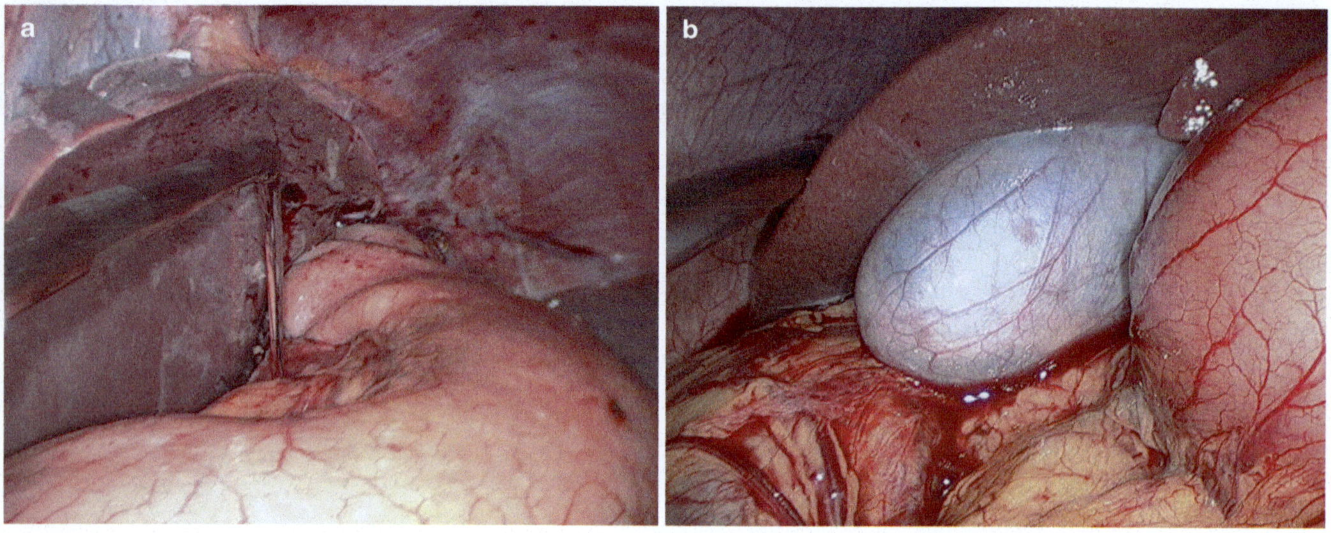

Fig. 2.14

2.3 Complications Analysis and Management

2.3.1 Haemorrhage

Bleeding in this procedure is rare and a greater risk of bleeding due to blunt dissection. The small arterial branches that feed the esophagus directly from the aorta or bronchial arteries are rarely the source of major haemorrhage. The greater risk is the violent tearing of venous structures, such as the azygous vein. Ultrasonic scalpel can directly cut off the vessels less than 1.5 mm in diameter. For the larger vessels, Ligasure or firing stapler is necessary for safe and effective hemostasis. Before the end of surgery, haemorrhage should be examined carefully, because there is also a risk of delayed bleeding from the short branches that feed the esophagus directly from the aorta, the short gastric vessels, or from an unrecognized splenic injury.

2.3.2 Esophageal Perforation

For the patient with severe esophagitis or obvious adhesions caused by huge hiatal hernias, esophagus can be damaged during the dissection of esophageal hiatus. Intraoperative repair under laparoscopy is feasible and the incidence of perforation is about 0.1 %. If the drainage is adequate and leak area is limited, fasting and persistent gastrointestinal decompression can be used for postoperative esophageal perforation. Surgery is used for invalid conservative treatment.

2.3.3 Spleen Damage

To avoid postoperative dysphagia caused by tight gastric fundus wrap, adequately dissection of gastric fundus is necessary. When dissecting the short gastric arteries, violently tearing or blindly cutting can induce capsular tears of the spleen. Most of these tears can be controlled with tamponade or electrocautery, but sometimes splenectomy is inevitable.

2.3.4 Esophageal Leak

Because only esophageal mucous layer of lower esophagus and anterior wall of cardia is kept in Heller myotomy, so this part is thin and breakable. Perforation can be induced by intraoperative ultrasonic scalpel thermal damage, which leads to delayed esophageal leak. The major manifestations are postoperative severe abdominal pain, fever and obvious peritonitis. An unrecognized, untreated esophageal perforation is deemed to be uniformly fatal. So, it is important to distinguish the muscular layer when using the ultrasonic scalpel to dissect the esophagus. It is necessary to put the clamping arm of ultrasonic scalpel into the inferior part of dissected muscular layer and keep the working (cutting) arm on the muscular layer surface, cut off the layer under direct vision. Intraoperative gastroscope is not only useful to verify the definite narrow part, but to distinguish perforation. The primary repair of a perforated esophagus without reinforcement is usually inadequate and prone to dehiscence. Therefore the gastric fundus wrap in the fundoplication is advocated to reinforce the primary repair.

2.3.5 Dysphagia

Postoperative dysphagia is the most common complication. The incidence is 17 % at the early stage and can decrease to 4 % after a period of training. Postoperative mucous layer edema may play an important part. If Nissen procedure makes a tight gastric fundus wrap, which may induce an esophageal stenosis, Toupet procedure is alternative. If the dysphagia is not released after 3–4 weeks postoperatively, balloon dilation is an advantage approach with the advantage of non-reoperation.

2.3.6 Postoperative Stenosis Does Not Alleviate

Most dysphagia can be alleviated postoperatively, but some will be not. Non-simple achalasia such as malignant esophageal lesion or diffuse esophageal spasm is not differentiated before the operation. Intraoperative cutting off area of muscular layer includes the entire stenosis part. Inadequate cutting off area can induce postoperative stenosis. Intraoperative gastroscope is significant to inspect the effects of incision and effectively avoid missing stenosis lesion. Postoperative cicatricial contraction and mucous layer edema also can induce dysphagia, and balloon dilation is recommended in these conditions with the advantage of a low rate of complication and non-reoperation.

2.3.7 Gastric Acid Reflux

Because the anti-reflux function of cardia and lower esophagus loses, gastric acid reflux is the most common postoperative complication. The introduction of gastric fundus wrap in the fundoplication can improve the manifestation caused by gastric acid reflux. But according to our observation, though the reflux symptoms can be released to a certain extent, but it can't be avoided completely.

2.3.8 Other Complications

Pyothorax, pneumothorax, subcutaneous emphysema and mediastinal emphysema are some rare complications of laparoscopic hiatus hernioplasty. But the incidence of these complications has no difference between laparoscopic and open procedure.

References

1. Campos G, Vittinghoff E, Rabl C, Takata M, Gadenstatter M, Lin F, Ciovica R. Endoscopic and surgical treatments of achalasia: a systemic review and meta-analysis. Ann Surg. 2009;249:45–57.
2. Rebecchi F, Giaccone C, Farinella E, Campaci R, Morino M. Randomized controlled trial of laparoscopic Heller myotomy plus Dor fundoplication versus Nissen fundoplication for achalasia: long-term results. Ann Surg. 2008;248:1023–30.
3. Tapper D, Morton C, Kraemer E, Villadolid D, Ross S, Cowgill S, Rosemurgy A. Does concomitant anterior fundoplication promote dysphasia after laparoscopic Heller myotomy? Am Surg. 2008;74:626–34.
4. Siddiqui MR, Abdulaal Y, Nisar A, Ali H, Hasan F. A meta-analysis of outcomes after open and laparoscopic Nissen's fundoplication for gastro-oesophageal reflux disease in children. Pediatr Surg Int. 2011;27:359–66.
5. Ostlie DJ, St Peter SD, Snyder CL, Sharp RJ, Andrews WS, Holcomb 3rd GW. A financial analysis of pediatric laparoscopic versus open fundoplication. J Laparoendosc Adv Surg Tech A. 2007;17:493–6.
6. Fan Y, Wu SD, Siwo EA. Emergency transumbilical single-incision laparoscopic splenectomy for the treatment of traumatic rupture of the spleen: report of the first case and literature review. Surg Innov. 2011;18:185–8.
7. Fan Y, Wu SD, Kong J. Single-port access transaxillary totally endoscopic thyroidectomy: a new approach for minimally invasive thyroid operation. J Laparoendosc Adv Surg Tech A. 2011;21:243–7.
8. Joseph M, Phillips M, Rupp CC. Single-incision laparoscopic cholecystectomy: a combined analysis of resident and attending learning curves at a single institution. Am Surg. 2012;78:119–24.
9. Huang CK, Houng JY, Chiang CJ, Chen YS, Lee PH. Single incision transumbilical laparoscopic Roux-en-Y gastric bypass: a first case report. Obes Surg. 2009;19:1711–5.
10. Sakaguchi Y, Ikeda O, Toh Y, Aoki Y, Harimoto N, Taomoto J, Masuda T, Ohga T, Adachi E, Okamura T. New technique for the retraction of the liver in laparoscopic gastrectomy. Surg Endosc. 2008;22:2532–4.
11. Gianni S, De Luca M, Oscar B, Andrea C, Luca B, David A, Franco F. Veress needle: a simple liver retraction technique for lap band positioning in (single incision laparoscopic technique) SILS. Obes Surg. 2012;22:190–1.
12. Fan Y, Wu SD, Kong J, Su Y, Tian Y. Transumbilical single-incision laparoscopic fundoplication: a new technique for liver retraction using cyanoacrylate. J Laparoendosc Adv Surg Tech A. 2013;23:356–60.

3 Gastrointestinal Surgery

Abstract

Since the introduction of laparoscopy in 1910, Nezhat et al. (J Reprod Med 34:127–134, 1989) the benefits of minimally invasive surgery have expanded its applicability to the treatment of benign and malignant gastric diseases (Liew et al., ANZ J Surg 77:787–791, 2007). But since the first publication about single incision laparoscopic sleeve gastrectomy reported by Saber (Obes Surg 18:1338–1342, 2008), only a few sporadic reports about single incision laparoscopic gastric surgery have appeared worldwide. These articles were always involved with laparoscopic sleeve gastrectomy in obese patients (Morales-Conde et al., Surg Innov [Epub ahead of print], 2011; Lakdawala et al., Obes Surg 21:1664–1670, 2011; Vilallonga et al., J Minim Access Surg 7:156–157, 2011). And in their opinion, this novel approach is feasible, but not always easily reproducible.

The first reported SILS partial resection of the stomach for the treatment of GIST was by Yasumitsu Hirano et al. in 2010 (Hirano et al., Surg Laparosc Endosc Percutan Tech 20:262–264, 2010). Then a few studies about SILS partial resection of the stomach or gastric wedge resection were reported (Na et al., J Gastric Cancer 11:225–229, 2011; Wu et al., Surg Innov [Epub ahead of print], 2012; Henckens et al., J Laparoendosc Adv Surg Tech A 20:469–471, 2010; Dapri et al., Ann Surg Oncol 18:191, 2011; Sasaki et al., Surg Today 41:133–136, 2011; Nonaka et al., Surg Laparosc Endosc Percutan Tech 22:e210–e213, 2012). In jin-UK's report, Na et al. (J Gastric Cancer 11:225–229, 2011) seven patients diagnosed with gastric submucosal tumor underwent the intragastric wedge resection. Though flexible laparoscope and curved or double-bended graspers were used frequently and made the SILS operation easier, conventional laparoscopic instruments can achieve the similar clinical outcomes (Wu et al., Surg Innov [Epub ahead of print], 2012). Also an extra mini-port for 2 mm Mini-loop was often used to retract the liver or gastric wall surrounding the tumor to facilitate the dissection and resection (Henckens et al., J Laparoendosc Adv Surg Tech A 20:469–471, 2010; Dapri et al., Ann Surg Oncol 18:191, 2011; Sasaki et al., Surg Today 41:133–136, 2011). Except wounding bleeding in one case, Na et al. (J Gastric Cancer 11:225–229, 2011) no intraoperative or other postoperative complications were experienced in all the patients including anastomotic leakage, bleeding or anastomotic stenosis.

A patient with an intractable gastric ulcer was treated by SILS gastrectomy with intracorporeal Roux-en-Y reconstruction in 2012 (Nonaka et al., Surg Laparosc Endosc Percutan Tech 22:e210–e213, 2012). The operative time was 412 min, with blood loss 90 ml. Also in 2012, another case about SILS perforated gastric ulcer repair was reported (Dapri et al., Surg Innov 19:130–133, 2012). The operation lasted 108 min. The blood loss was 86 ml.

S. Wu et al. (eds.), *Atlas of Single-Incision Laparoscopic Operations in General Surgery*,
DOI 10.1007/978-94-007-6955-7_3, © Springer Science+Business Media Dordrecht 2013

Ten patients underwent single-incision laparoscopic distal gastrectomy and lymph node D1α or D1β dissection in three reports (Omori et al., Surg Endosc 25:2400–2404, 2011; Park et al., Surg Laparosc Endosc Percutan Tech 22:e214–e216, 2012; Ozdemir et al., Surg Innov 18:NP1–NP4, 2011). The final pathology report showed that the tumor had invaded the submucosa or proper muscle with no seromuscular layer infiltration. A total of 172 lymph nodes were retrieved. Except one patient with 5 metastases among dissected 21 lymph nodes, Takahashi et al. (Am Surg 78:447–450, 2012) lymph nodes of other patients were identified with no tumor metastasis. In Lee JH's [19] report, the porcine model was used to compare the perioperative outcomes of SILS and conventional laparoscopic distal gastrectomy with D1+b lymph node dissection. The single-incision laparoscopic group was associated with a significantly longer operation time, but it had a similar mean number of resected lymph nodes and with similar inflammatory reaction and complication rates when compared with conventional laparoscopic.

Keywords

Partial gastrectomy • Subtotal gastrectomy • Billroth-II anastomosis • Gastroesophageal anastomosis • Proximal gastrectomy • Esophageal jejunum end-to-side anastomosis • Total gastrectomy

3.1 Laparoscopic Partial Gastrectomy

3.1.1 Indications and Case Selection

1. Patients with gastrointestinal stromal tumor.
2. Patients with adenomyxoma.
3. Patients with benign tumors.
   It is mainly indicated for patients with lesions located above the anterior wall and along the greater or smaller curvature of the stomach.

3.1.2 Contraindications

1. Absolute contraindications:
   (a) severe cardiorespiratory dysfunction,
   (b) inability to tolerate general anesthesia or pneumoperitoneum,
   (c) refractory coagulopathy.
   (d) complicated with gastric malignancies,
   (e) presence of metastatic disease.
2. Relative contraindications:
   (a) extensive previous surgery, or previous peritonitis leading to severe adhesion,
   (b) morbid obesity,
   (c) pregnancy.

3.1.3 Major Instruments or Energy Sources

1. Laparoscopy System.
2. Electrocautery.
3. Harmonic scalpel.
4. Endoscopic linear stapler.

3.1.4 Team Setup, Anesthesia and Position

Under general anesthesia, the patient was placed in supine position with the legs apart. The position of surgeon, assistants and nurses is shown in Fig. 3.1.

Fig. 3.1

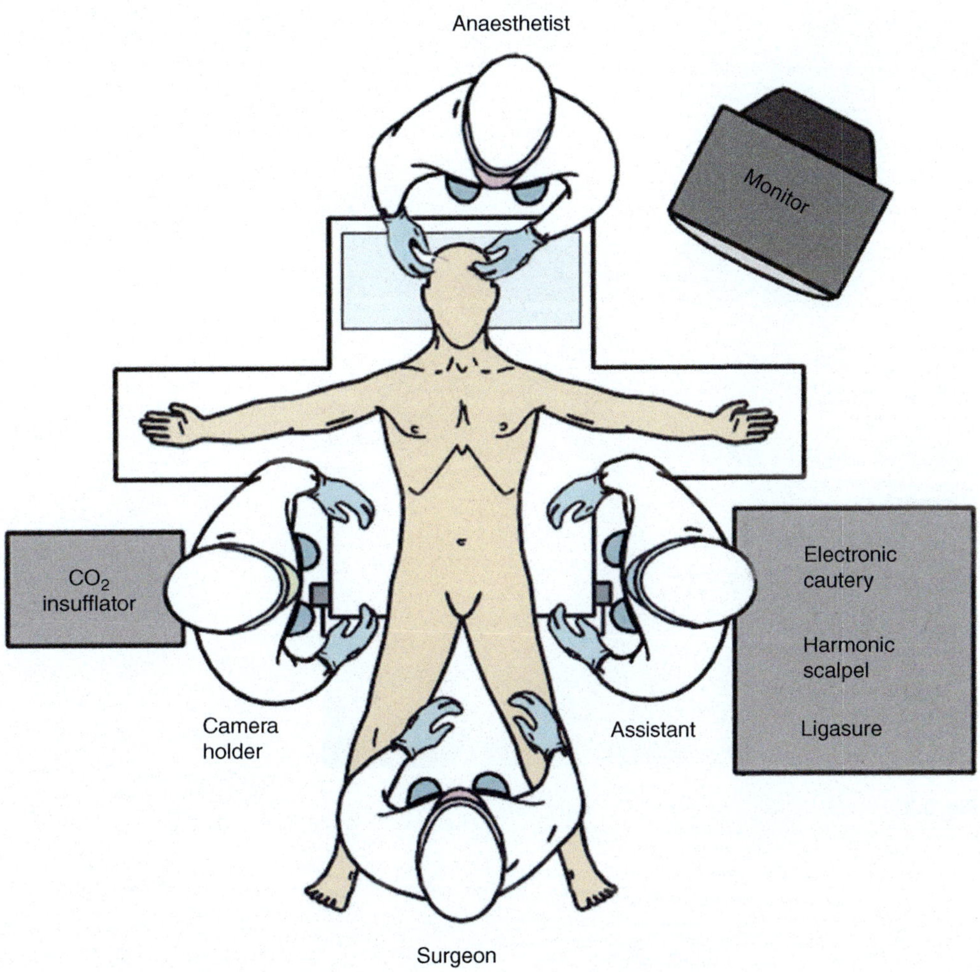

3.1.5 Key Steps

1. Establishment of Pneumoperitoneum and Placement of Trocars.
2. Abdominal Exploration.
3. Mobilization of the body of stomach and localization of the lesion.
4. Partial gastrectomy.

3.1.6 Surgical Techniques

1. Establishment of Pneumoperitoneum and Placement of Trocars.
2. Abdominal Exploration.
   First of all, a thorough exploration of the abdominal and pelvic cavity was performed to rule out the presence of ascites or nodules in the liver. The characteristics of the lesion of the stomach including its location, morphology, and relationship with surrounding organs such as the pancreas, gallbladder, bile duct or portal vein were determined (Fig. 3.2a–c).

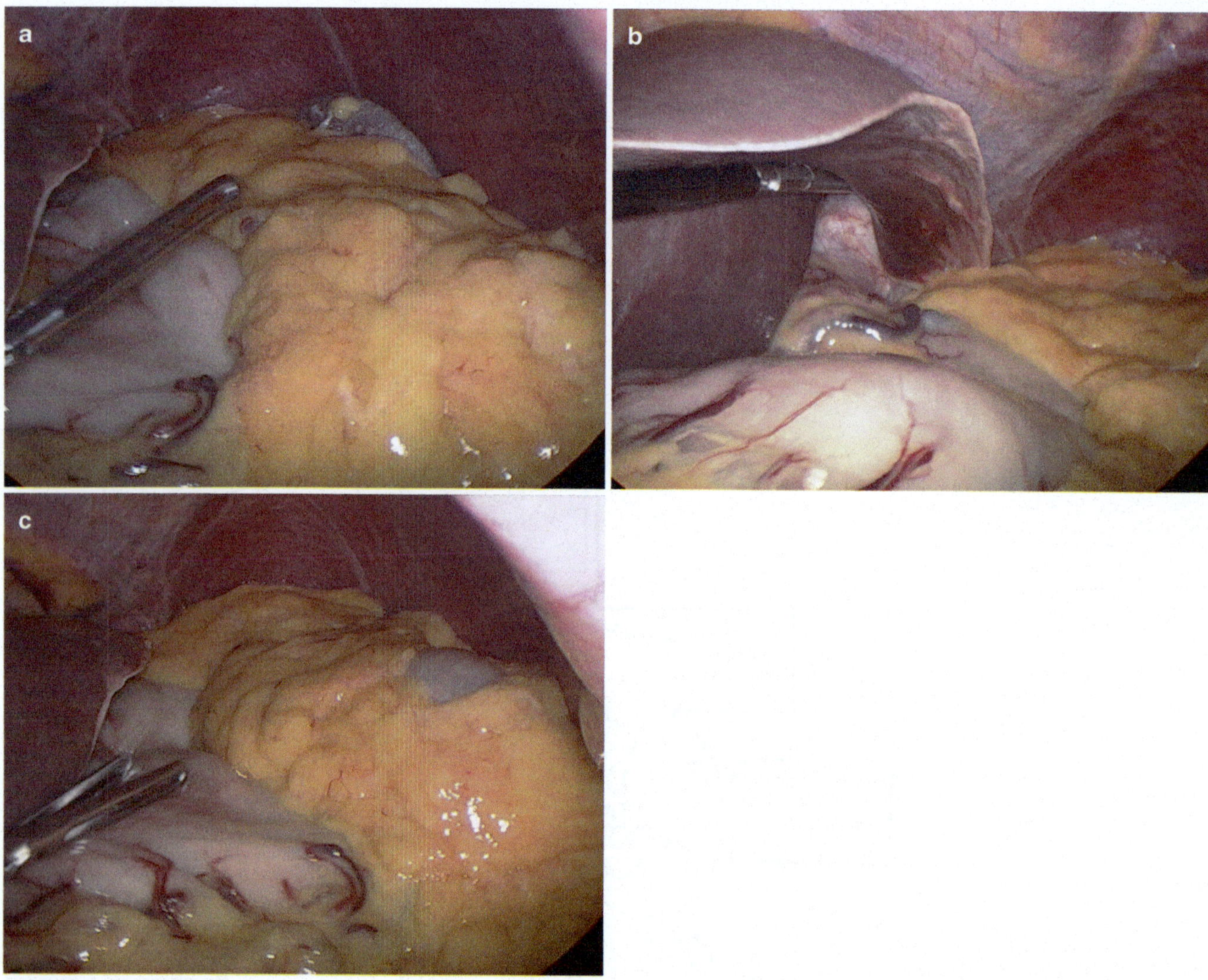

Fig. 3.2

3. Mobilization of the body of stomach and localization of the lesion.
   The greater curvature of stomach was elevated by using the atraumatic forcep in the left hand. Then, the gastrocolic ligament was opened outside the omental vascular arch by using the harmonic scalpel to expose the omental bursa and the posterior wall of the stomach (Fig. 3.3a–d).

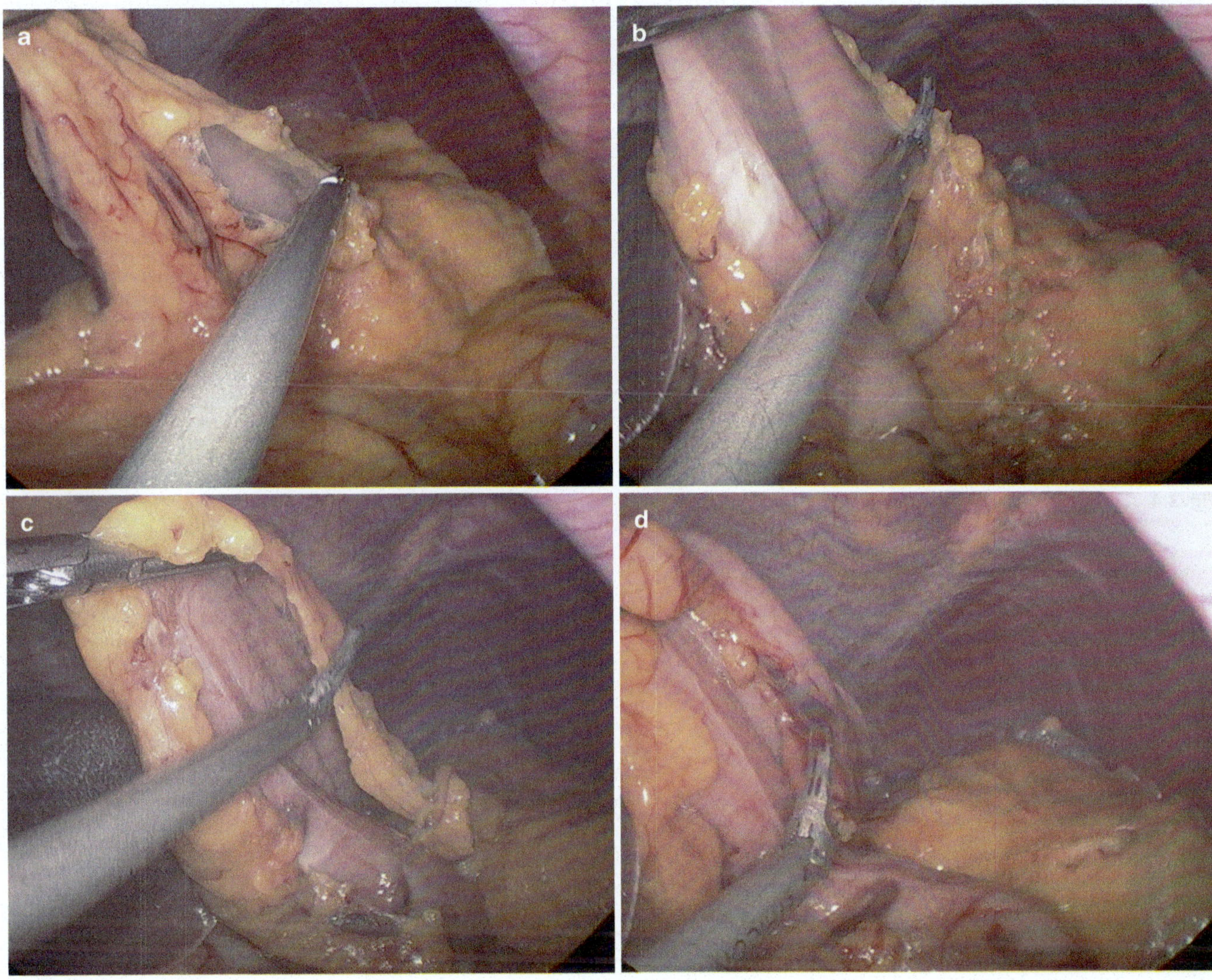

Fig. 3.3

The gastrosplenic ligament was dissected to mobilize the fundus of the stomach to further expose the lesion (Fig. 3.4a, b).

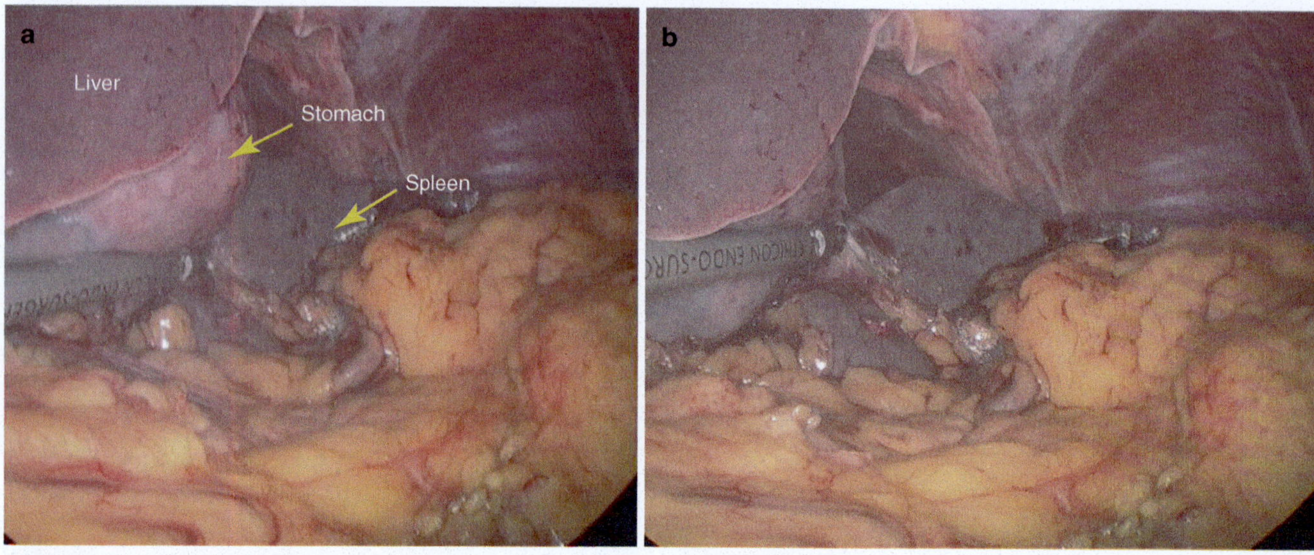

Fig. 3.4

4. Partial gastrectomy.
   The lesion was transected on the normal gastric wall at its base by using the 60 mm endoscopic linear stapler with a single bite. In the case of incomplete excision of the lesion with a single bite, the cartridge was replaced by a new one and the lesion was completely transected by continuous bite (Fig. 3.5a–d).

3.1.7 Tips and Tricks

1. Preoperative or intraoperative endoscopic assistance was necessary when small endoluminal tumors could not be easily detected by laparoscopic exploration. During the intraoperative endoscopic procedures, proximal jejunum below the Treitz ligament was gently clamped with laparoscopic instruments to minimize the gas insufflation into the small bowel.
2. The greater omentum and/or short gastric vessels were divided from the greater curvature with ultrasonic coagulating shears, as per requirement.
3. The tumor was elevated by retracting the normal gastric wall near the tumor with a laparoscopic grasper or by pulling the tagging suture on the gastric wall near the tumor.
4. After meticulous hemostasis was achieved along the stapled line, the specimen was placed in a laparoscopic specimen bag and extracted through the umbilicus.

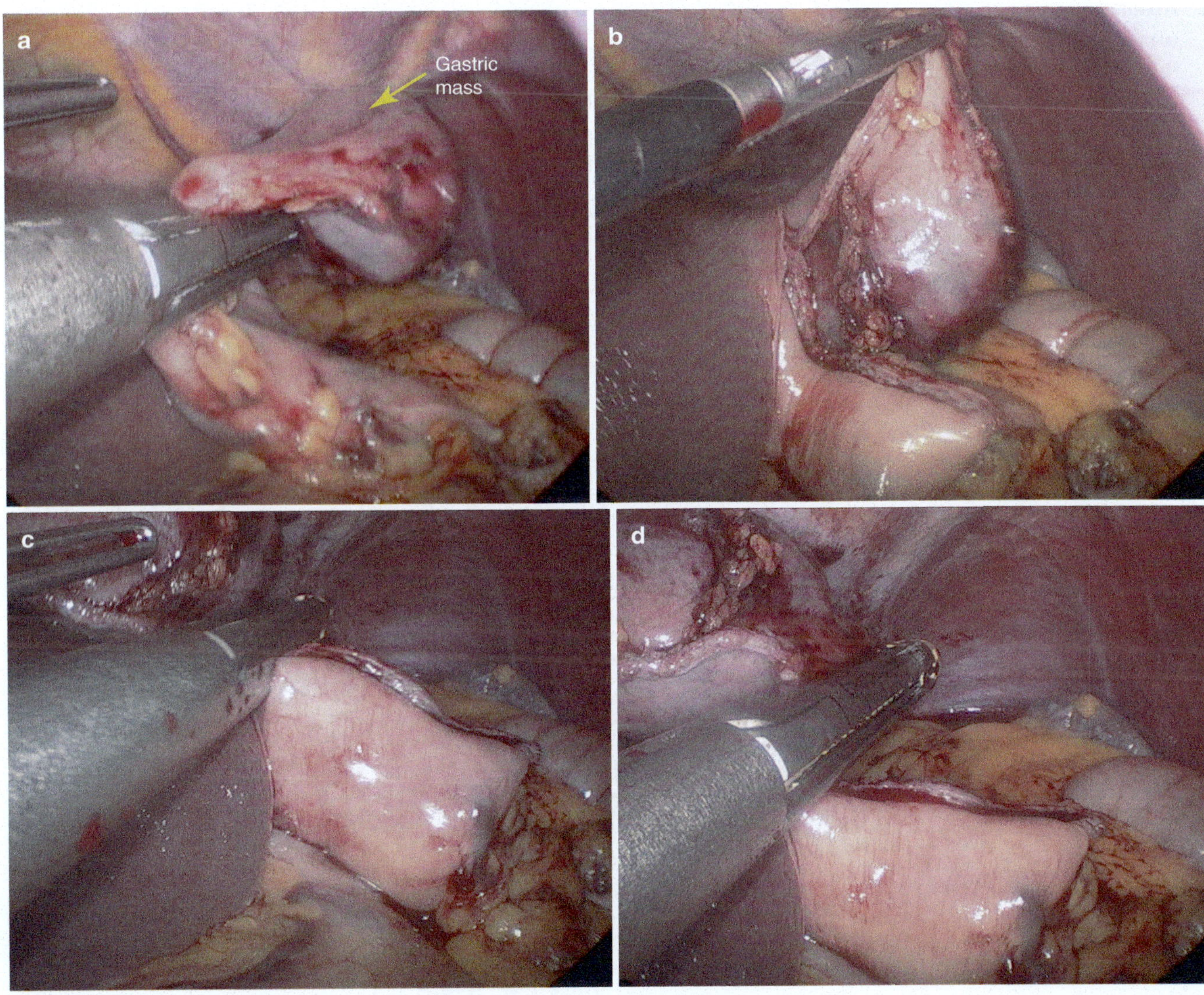

Fig. 3.5

3.2 Laparoscopic Subtotal Gastrectomy (Billroth-IIanastomosis)

3.2.1 Indications and Case Selection

1. Patients with peptic ulcer disease who undergo failure of medical therapy, obstruction, perforation and highly suspected for malignancy.
2. Patients with peptic ulcer who have over-secretion of gastric acid.
3. Patients with tumors in the distal gastric lesions.

3.2.2 Contraindications

1. Absolute contraindications:
   (a) severe cardiorespiratory dysfunction,
   (b) inability to tolerate general anesthesia or pneumoperitoneum,
   (c) refractory coagulopathy.
   (d) complicated with gastric malignancies,
   (e) presence of metastatic disease.
2. Relative contraindications:
   (a) large or acutely bleeding ulcers'
   (b) extensive previous surgery, or previous peritonitis leading to severe adhesion,
   (c) morbid obesity,
   (d) pregnancy.

3.2.3 Major Instruments or Energy Sources

1. Laparoscopy System.
2. Electrocautery.
3. Harmonic scalpel.
4. Endoscopic linear stapler.

3.2.4 Team Setup, Anesthesia and Position

Under general anesthesia, the patient was placed in supine position with the legs apart. The position of surgeon, assistants and nurses is shown in Fig. 3.6.

Fig. 3.6

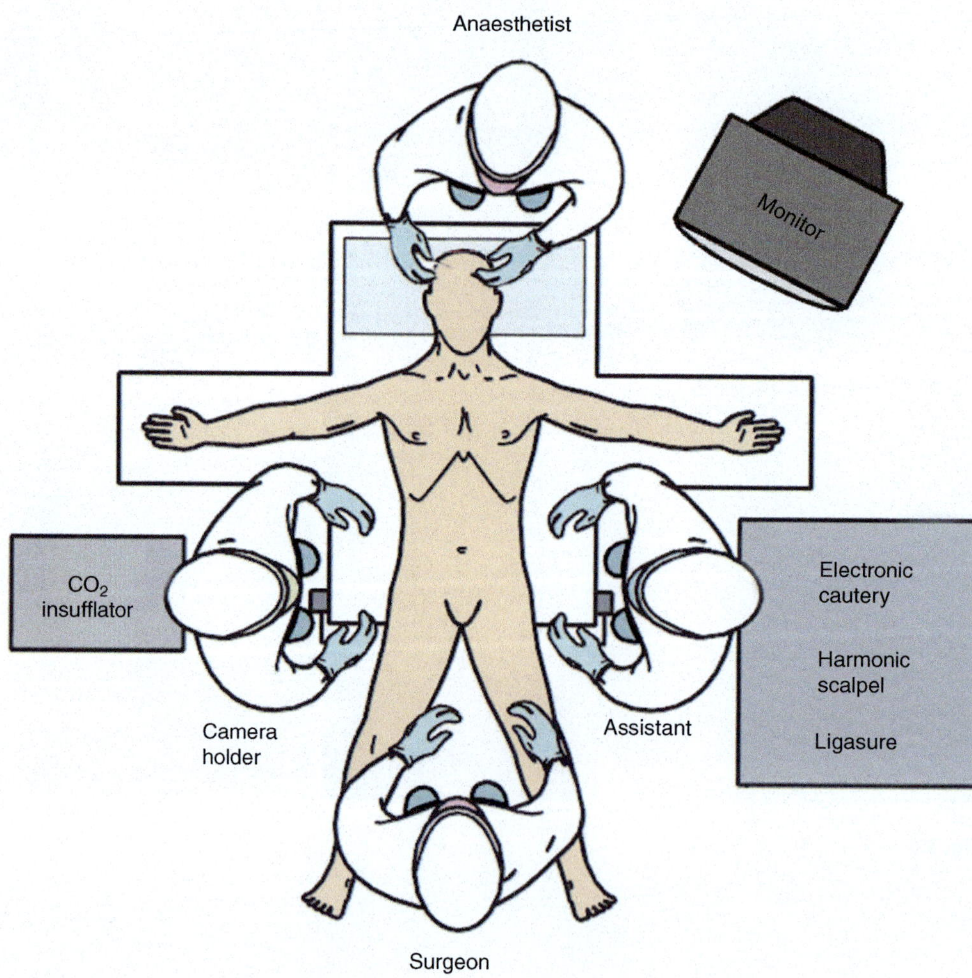

3.2.5 Key Steps

1. Establishment of Pneumoperitoneum and Placement of Trocars.
2. Mobilization of the gastrocolic ligament.
3. Mobilization of the hepatogastric ligament.
4. Mobilization of the hepatoduodenal ligament.
5. Mobilization of the left gastric vessels.
6. Transection of the duodenum.
7. Gastrojejunal anastomosis.
8. Subtotal gastrectomy.

3.2.6 Surgical Techniques

1. Establishment of Pneumoperitoneum and Placement of Trocars.
2. Mobilization of the gastrocolic ligament.
   The greater curvature of the stomach was lifted by using the atraumatic forcep in the left hand. The gastrocolic ligament was dissected from its avascular zone at the center by using the harmonic scalpel (Fig. 3.7a–f).

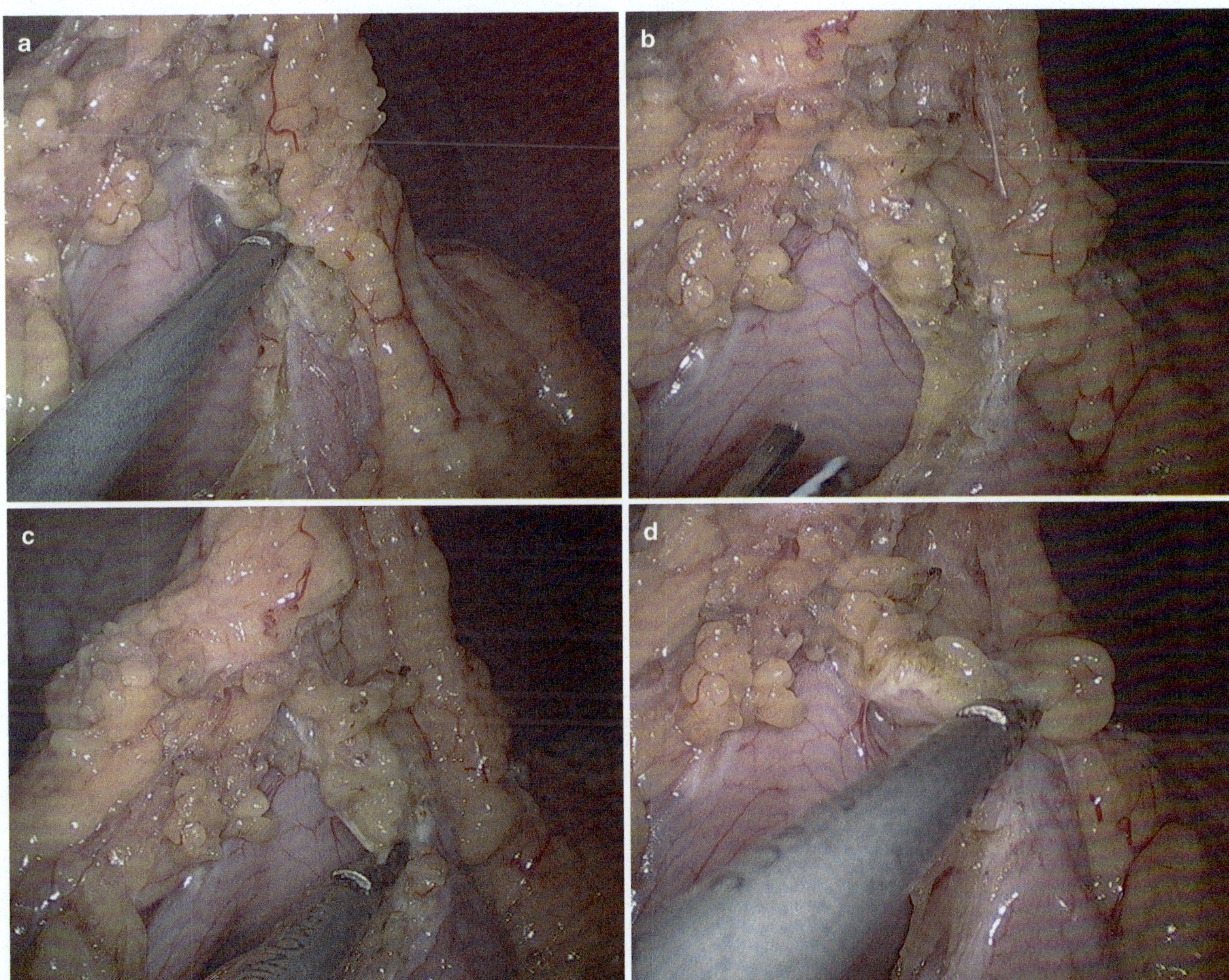

Fig. 3.7

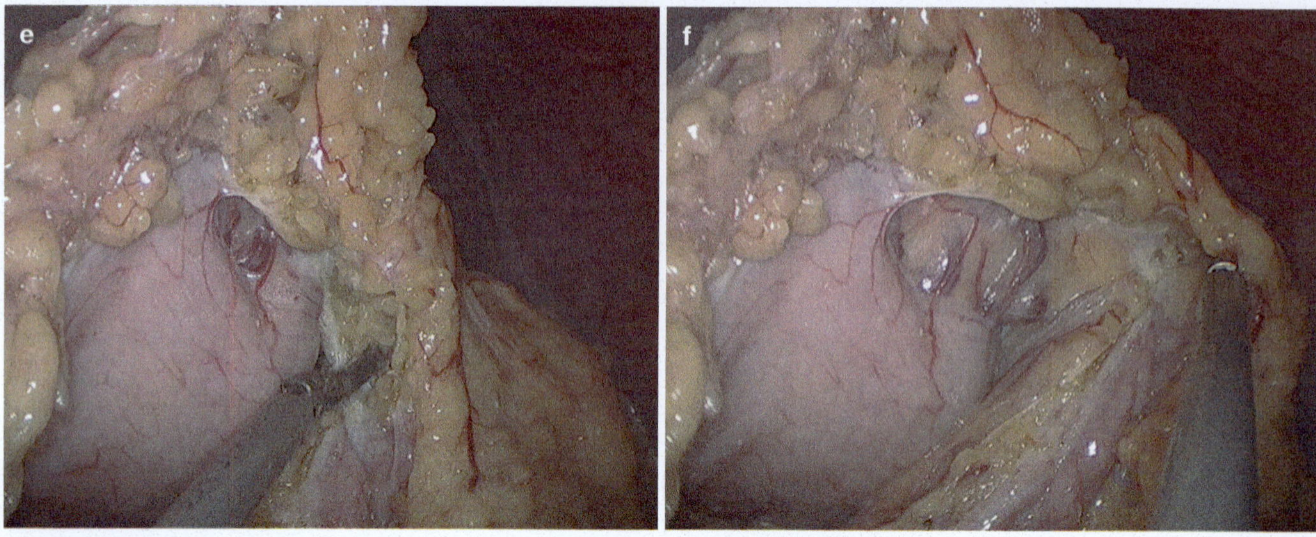

Fig. 3.7 (continued)

Continuous dissection to the left was done until the second terminal branch of the left gastroepiploic artery was reached (Fig. 3.8a, b).

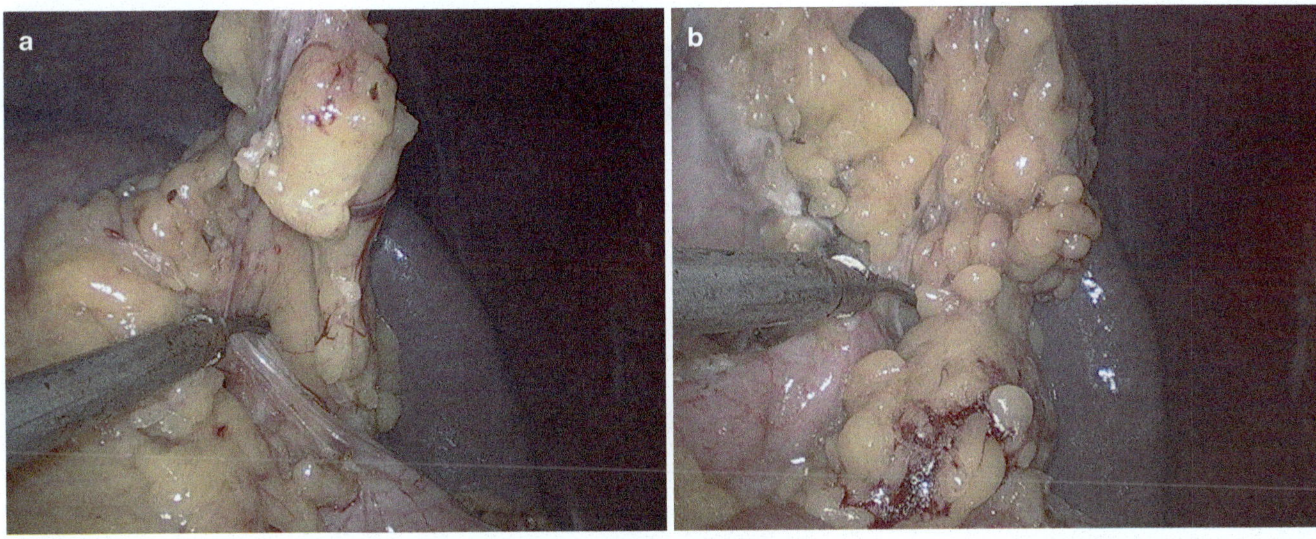

Fig. 3.8

After previous mobilization, the left part of the gastrocolic ligament was freed. To expose the right gastroepiploic vein, continuous dissection to the right was performed until the antrum was reached. At the lower margin of the pancreas, the right gastroepiploic vein was first encountered, dissected, clipped and cut. In this step, much attention must be paid to avoid injury to the vein, which is prone to tear (Fig. 3.9a–d).

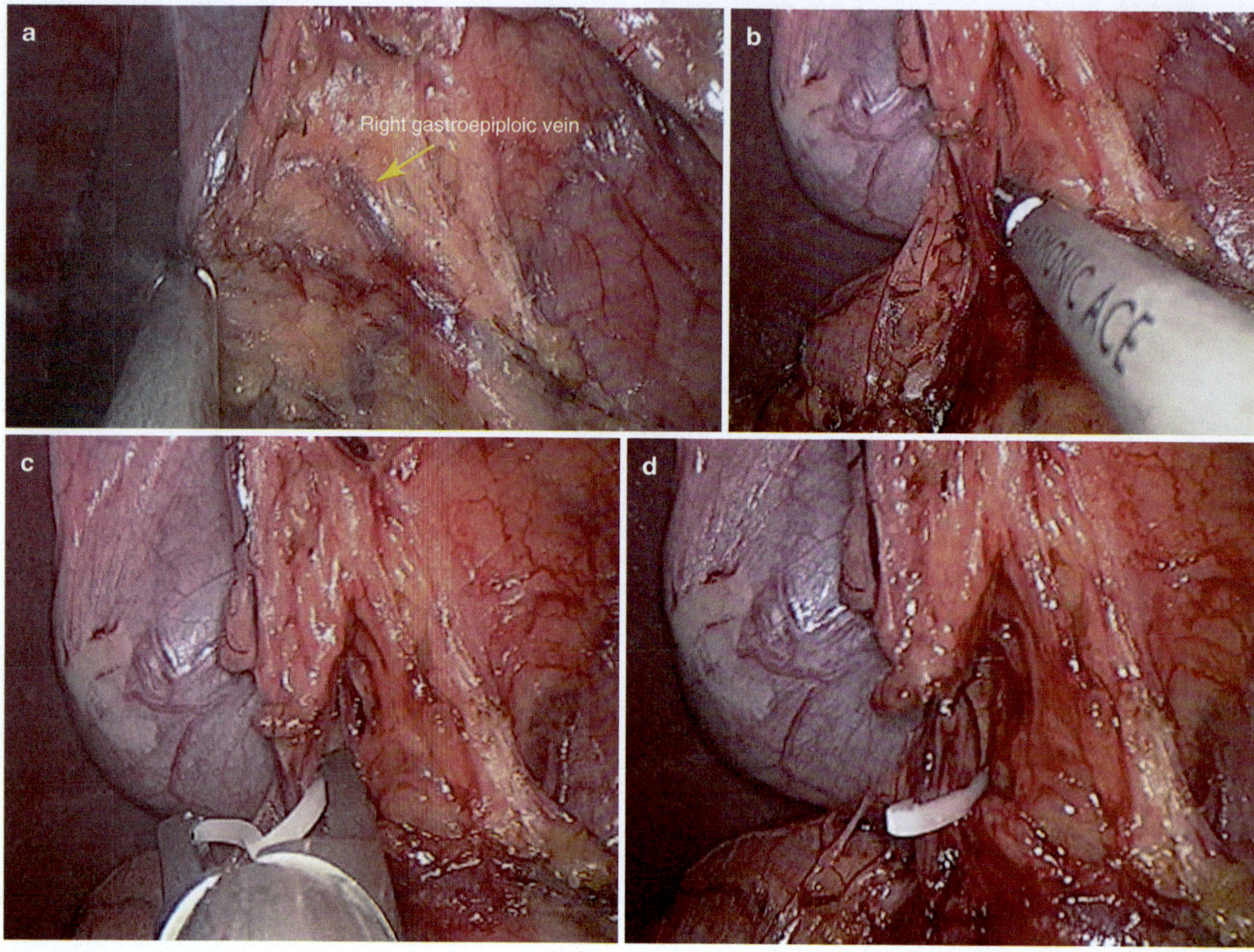

Fig. 3.9

Then, the right gastroepiploic artery was dissected, clipped and cut (Fig. 3.10a, b).

3. Mobilization of the hepatogastric ligament.
   The hepatogastric ligament was opened at its avascular zone by using the harmonic scalpel. Continuous dissection to the right was done until the superior margin of the duodenal bulb was reached (Fig. 3.11a, b).

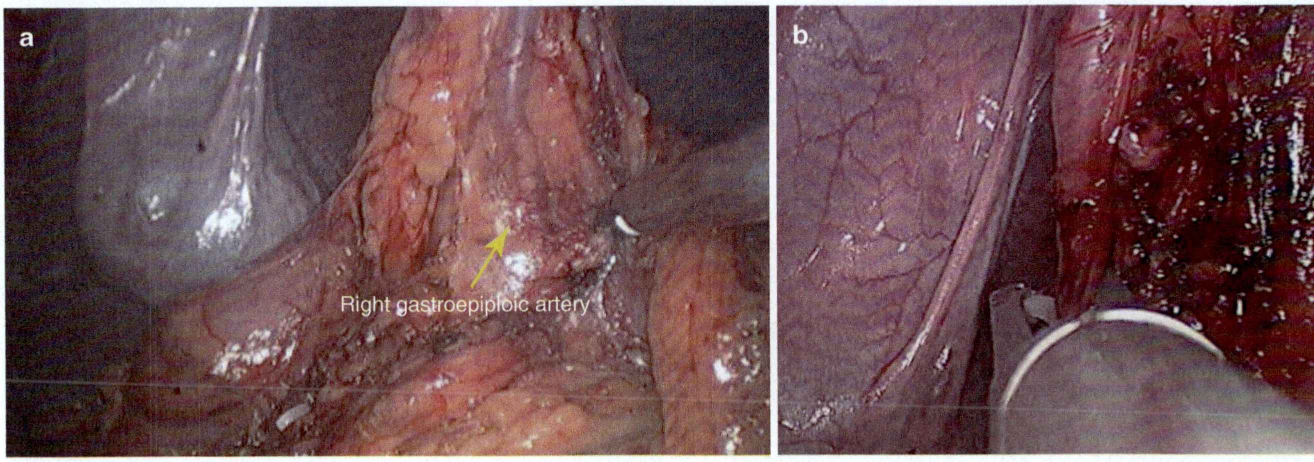

Fig. 3.10

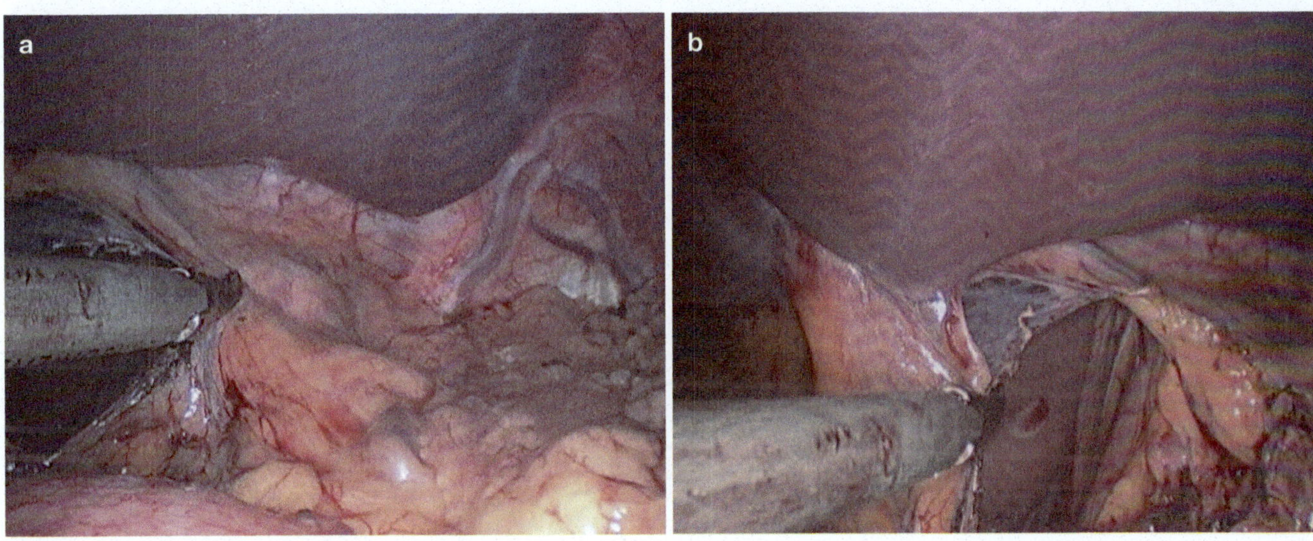

Fig. 3.11

4. Mobilization of the hepatoduodenal ligament.
   The right gastric artery in the hepatoduodenal ligament was dissected,clipped and cut (Fig. 3.12a–g).

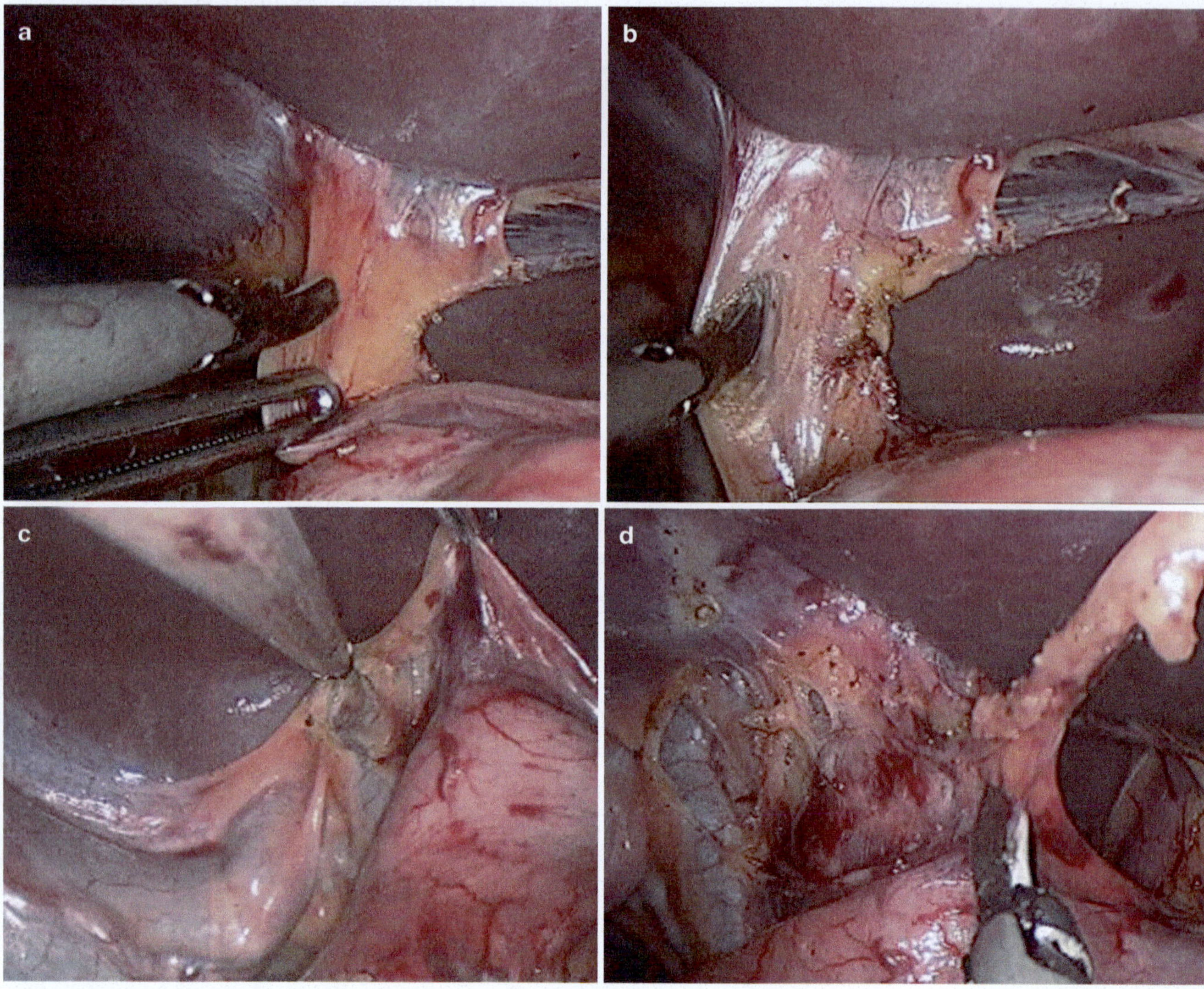

Fig. 3.12

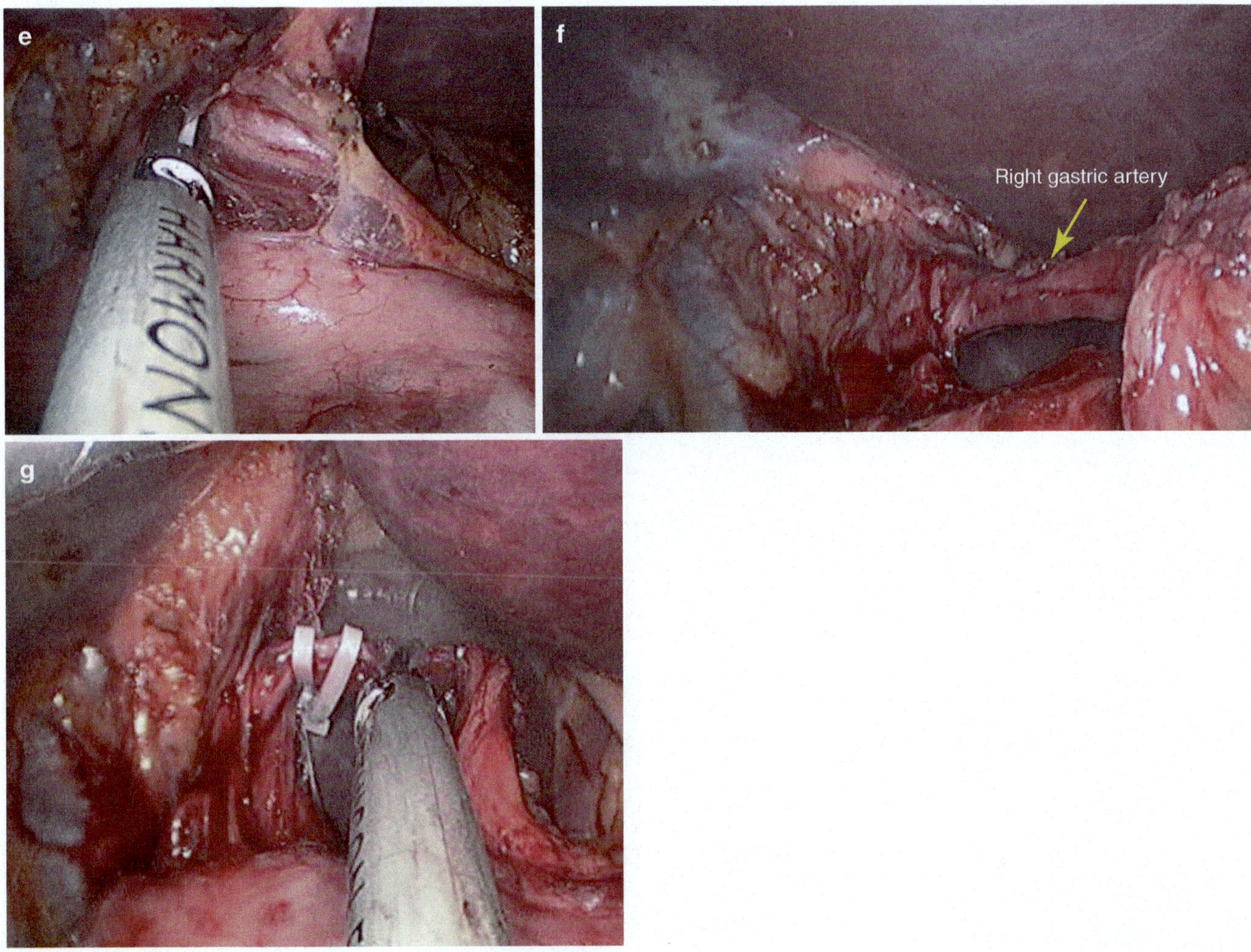

Fig. 3.12 (continued)

5. Mobilization of the left gastric vessels.
   With the stomach lifted posterior by the atraumatic grasper on the left hand, the pancreatiogastric fold was exposed. The left gastric vein and artery were clipped and cut at their origins (Fig. 3.13a–f).

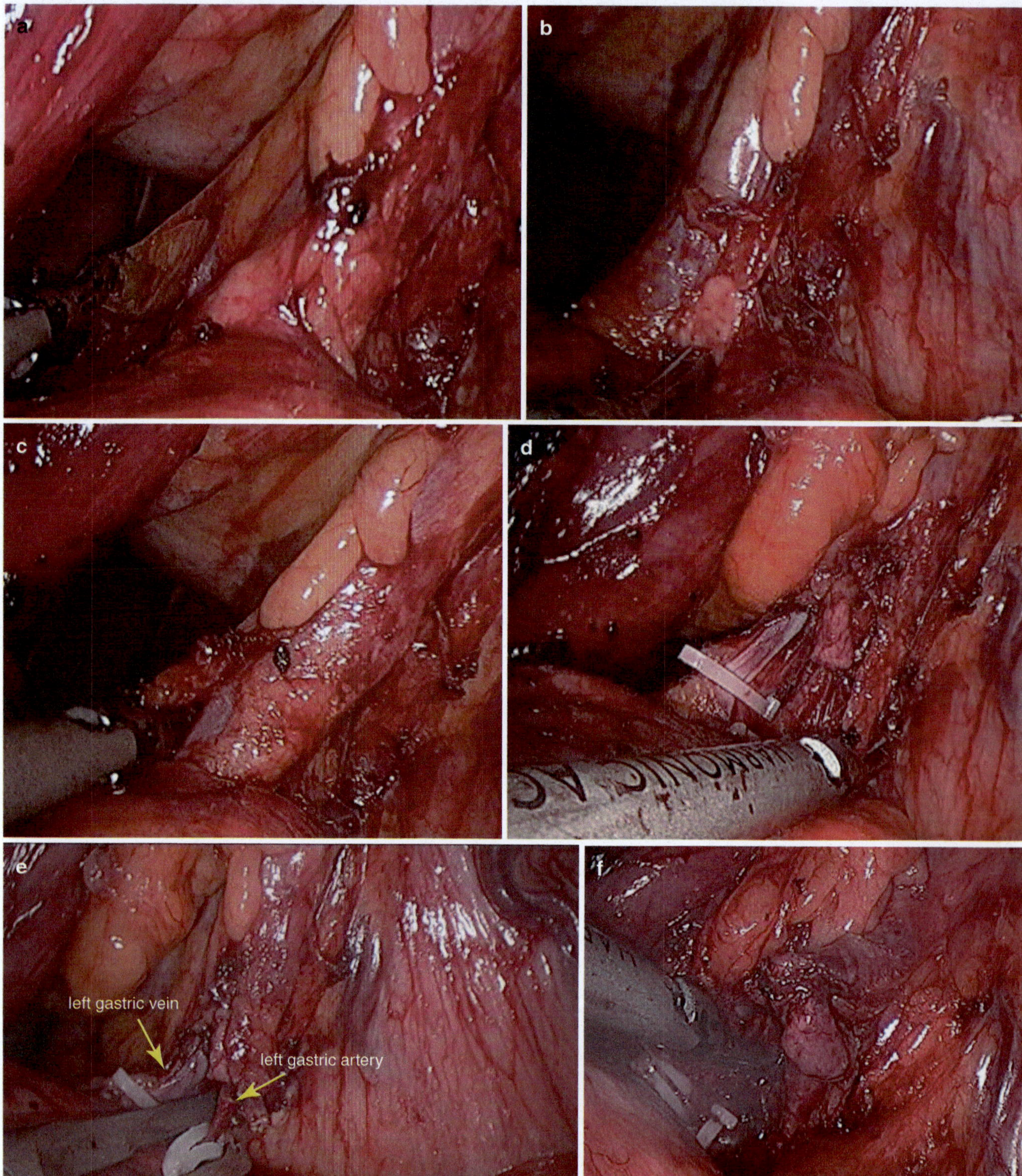

Fig. 3.13

6. Transection of the duodenum.

   The duodenum was transected just distal to the pyloric ring by using linear staplers (Fig. 3.14a–d).

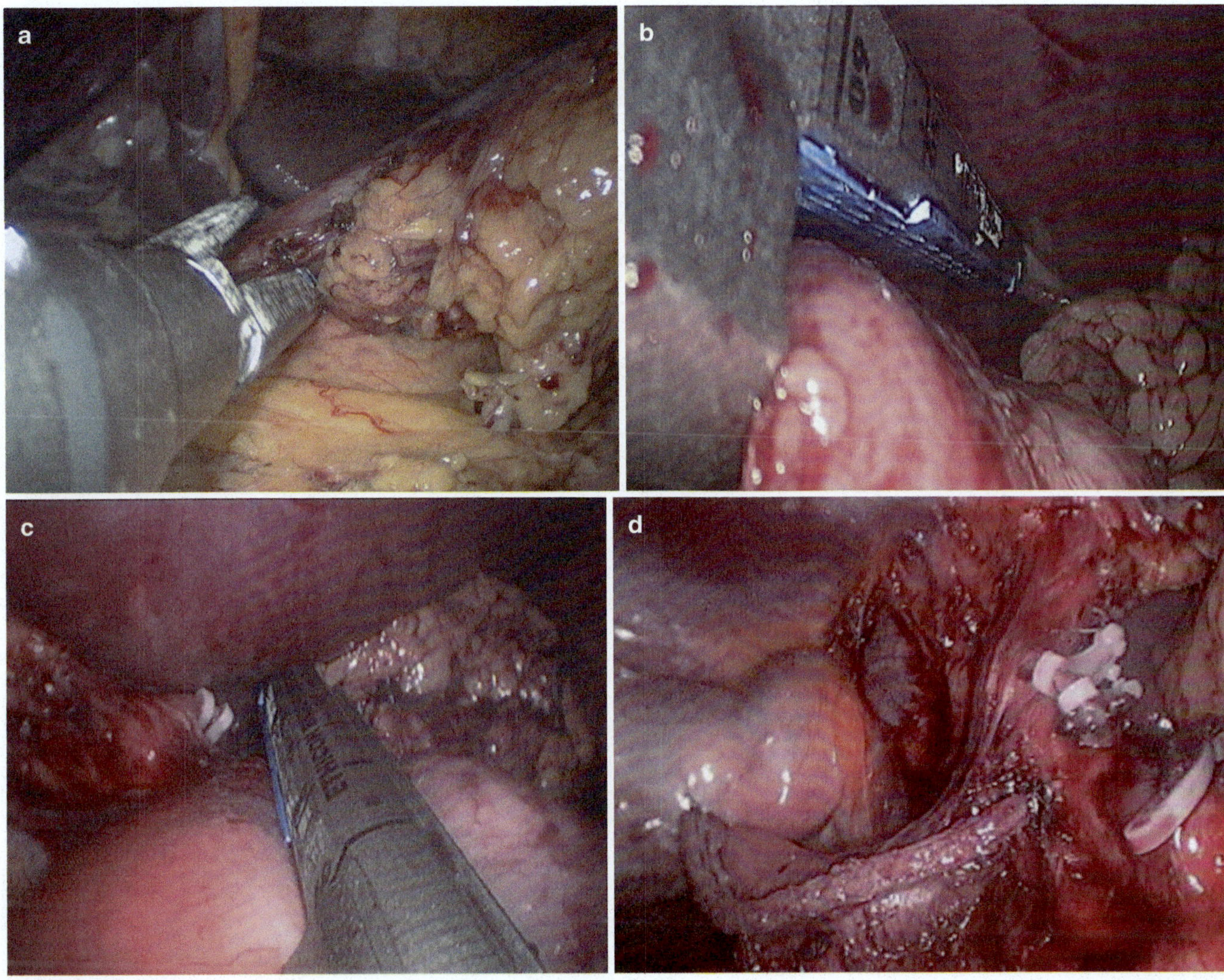

Fig. 3.14

7. Gastrojejunal anastomosis.

   The gastric antrum was lifted and 1 cm incision was made on the posterior wall of the stomach where the anastomosis was to made by using the harmonic scalpel (Fig. 3.15a–d).

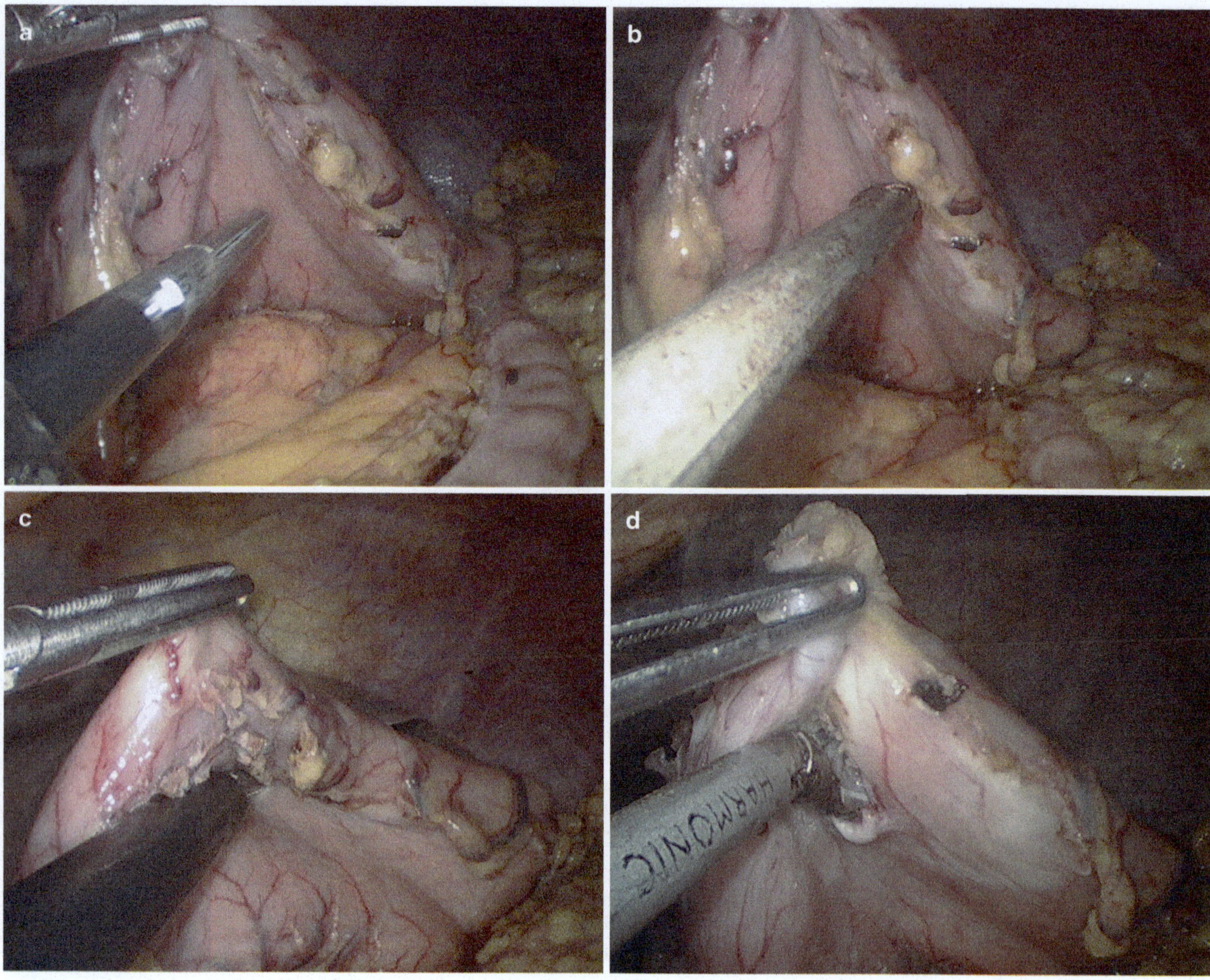

Fig. 3.15

A window was made on the transverse mesocolon through which the proximal jejunum was lifted to the upper transverse colon region. A small incision was made on the anti-mesenteric side of the jejunum, 10–12 cm from the duodenojejunal flexure (Fig. 3.16a, b).

After step-by-step insertion of the linear stapler forks, the posterior wall of the stomach and the anti-mesenteric side of the jejunum were put together, and an anastomosis was made with the linear stapler (Fig. 3.17a, b).

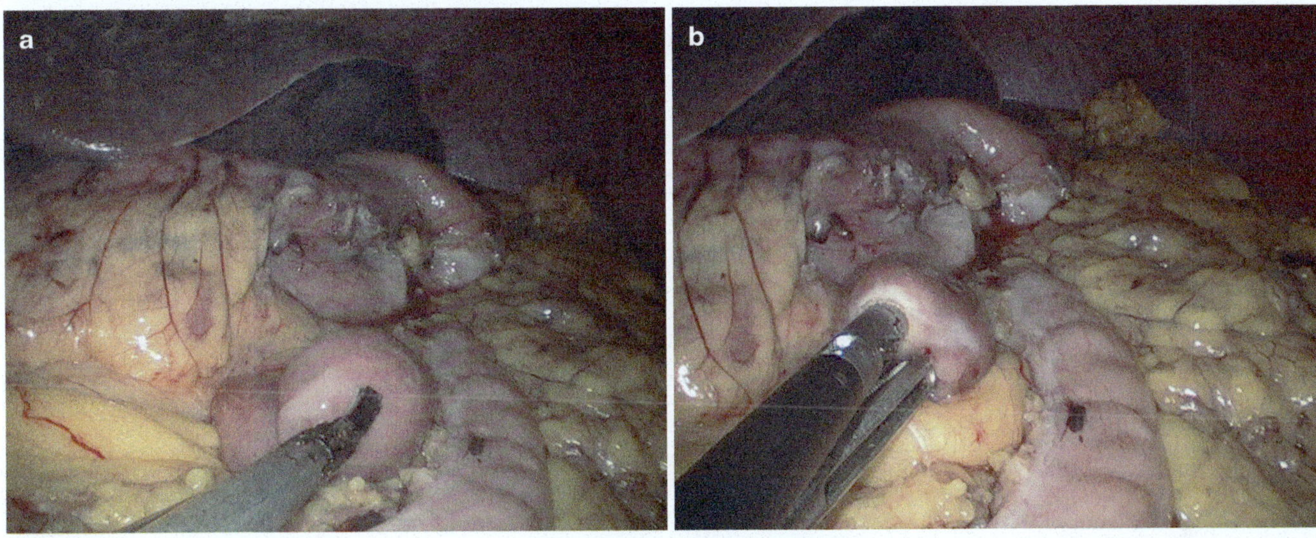

Fig. 3.16

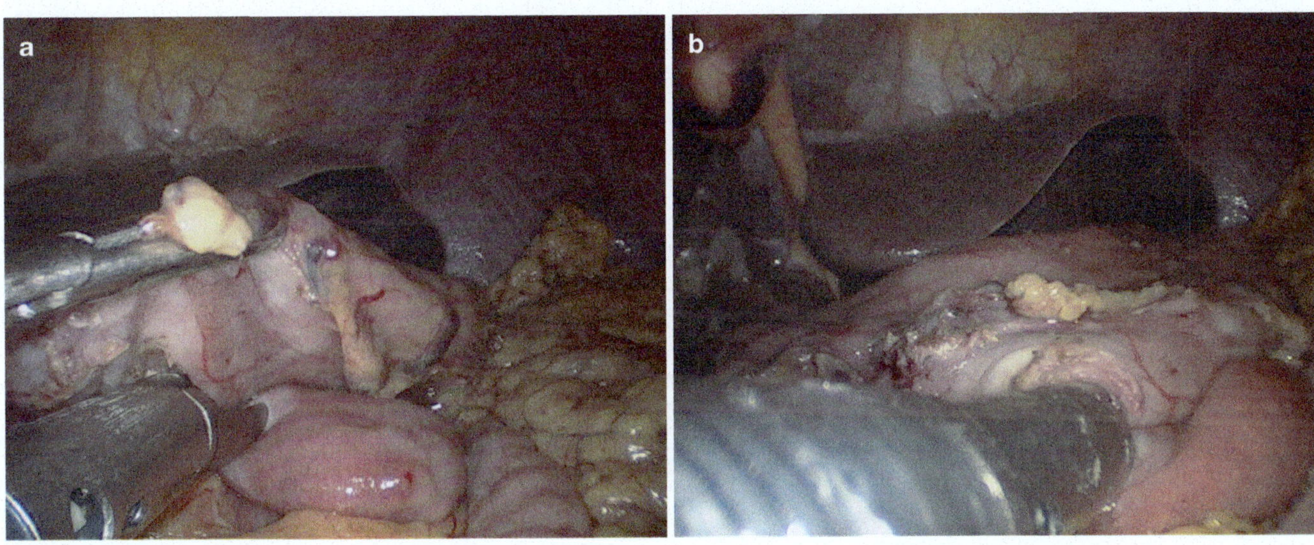

Fig. 3.17

The gastric suction tube was found through the anastomosis and put into the afferent loop (Fig. 3.18a–d).

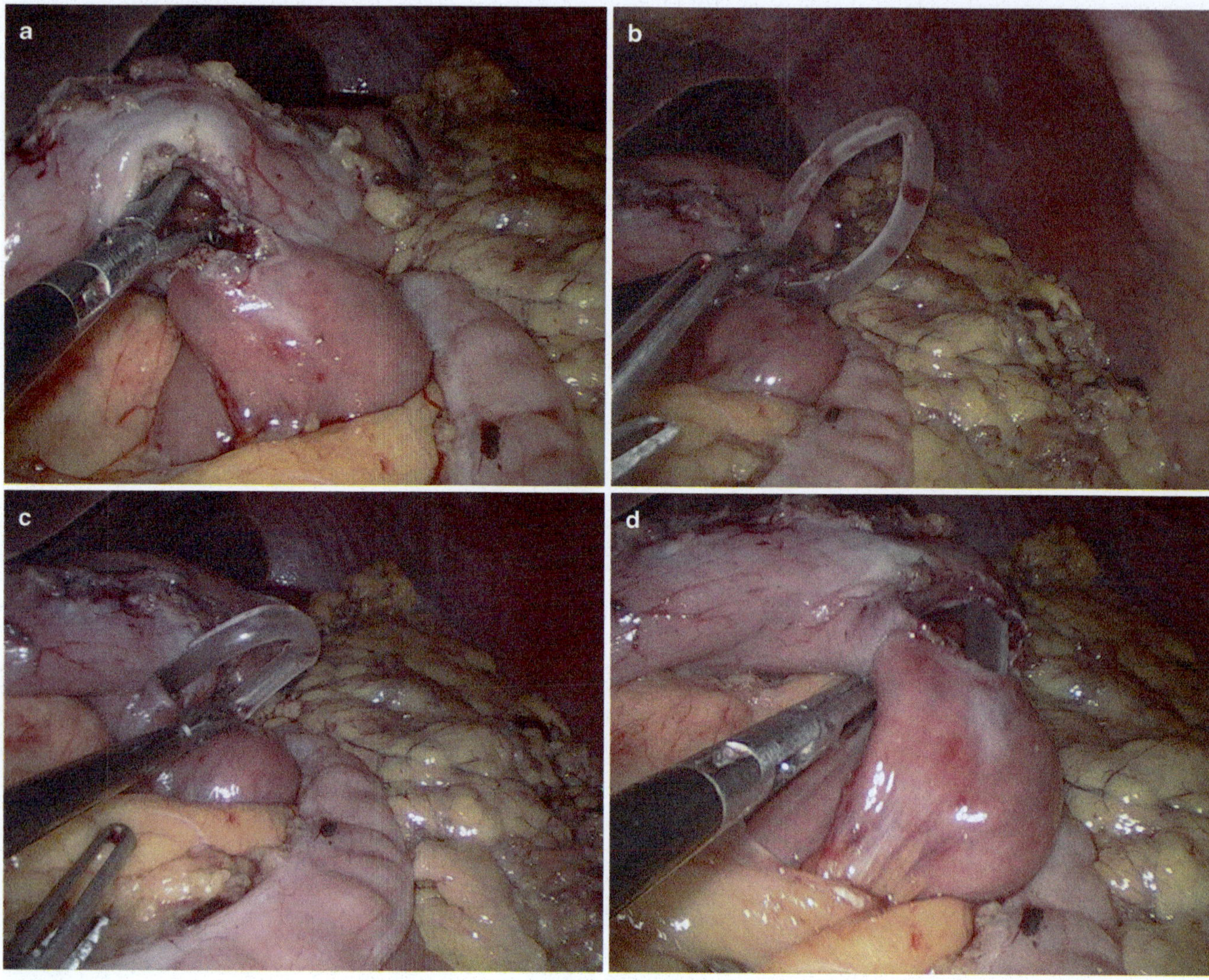

Fig. 3.18

The common incision was closed by running suture with 3/0 absorbable suture to complete the gastrojejunal anastomosis (Fig. 3.19a–h).

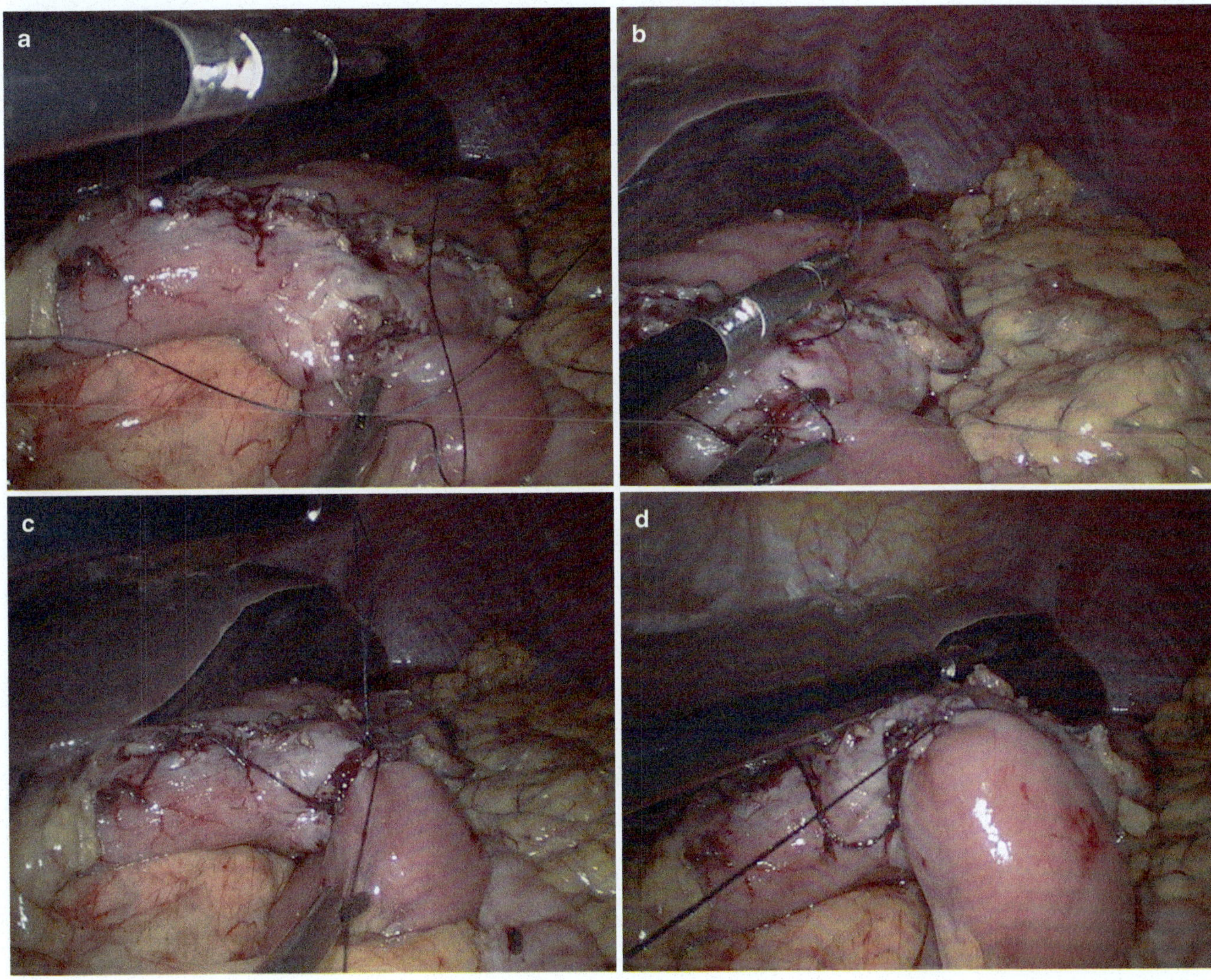

Fig. 3.19

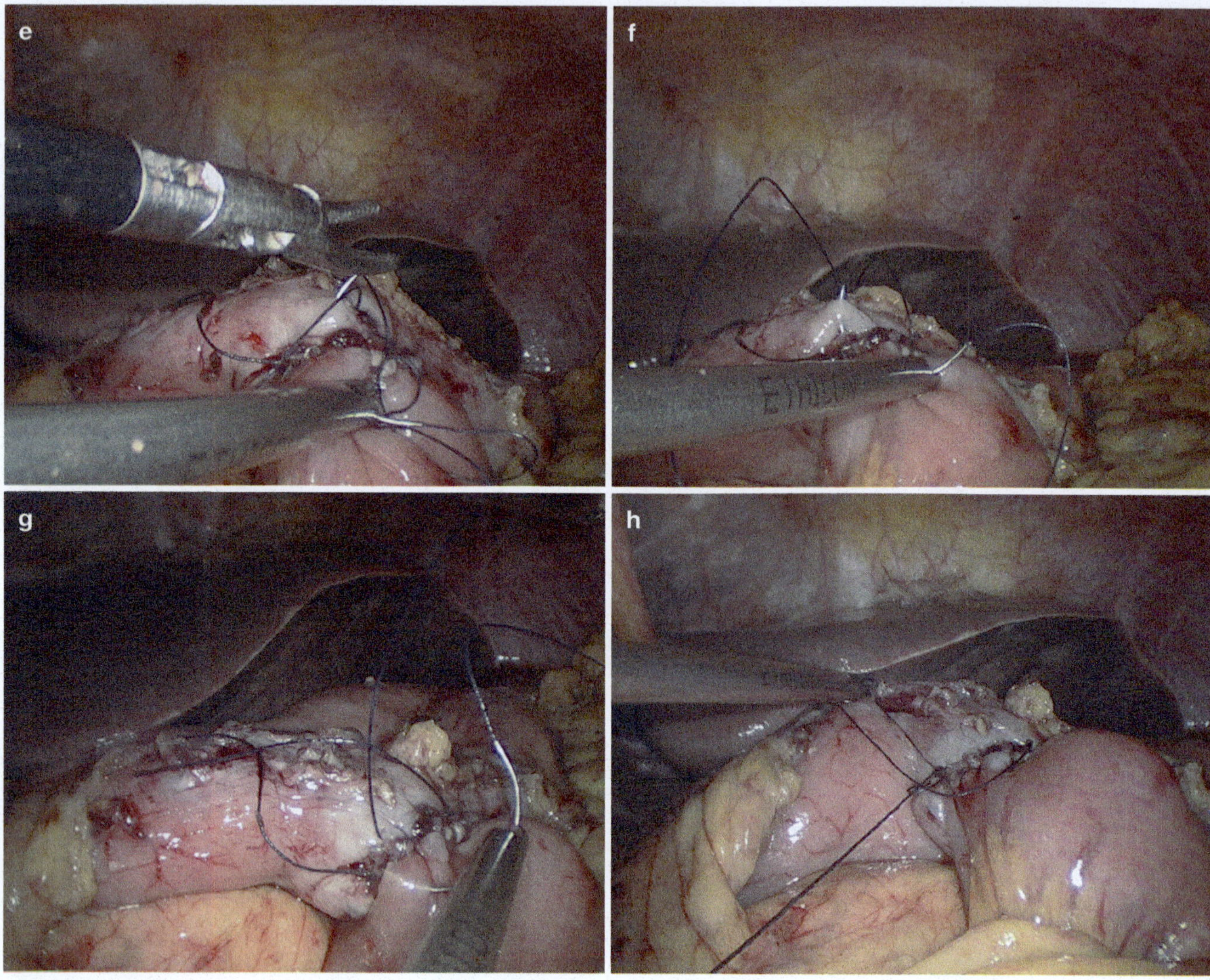

Fig. 3.19 (continued)

8. Subtotal gastrectomy.
   The stomach was transected at least 1 cm distal from the anastomosis by using linear staplers (Fig. 3.20a–f).

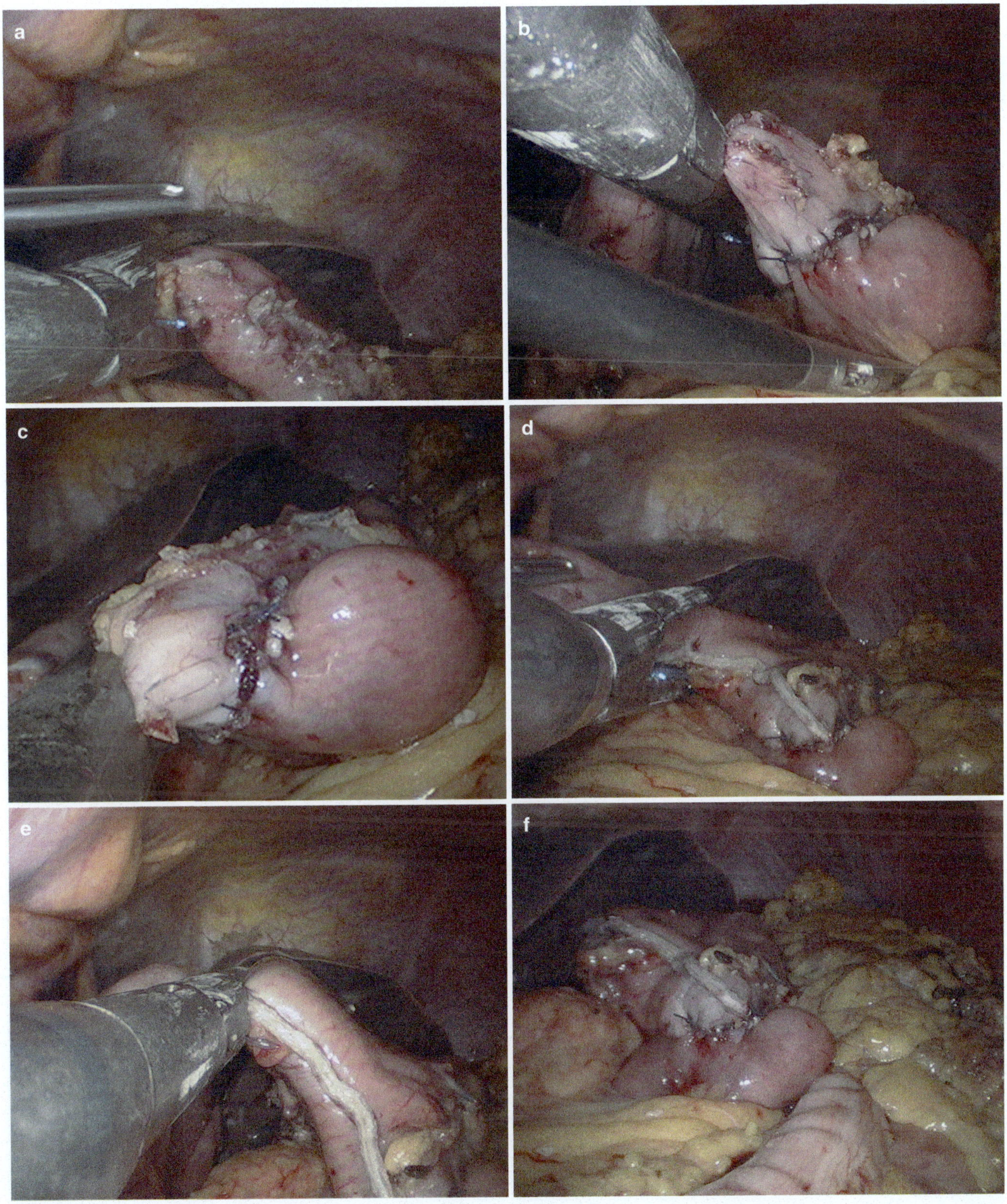

Fig. 3.20

The anastomosis was put downwards below the transverse mesocolon window. The margin of the window and the seromuscular layer of the stomach wall 2 cm distal from the anastomosis were sutured by interrupted suture technique (Fig. 3.21a–f).

The intact specimens were removed from the abdominal cavity by bag, and we often cut the connecting tissue between the 10 mm and the 12 mm-trocar to enlarge the incision for sample extracting.

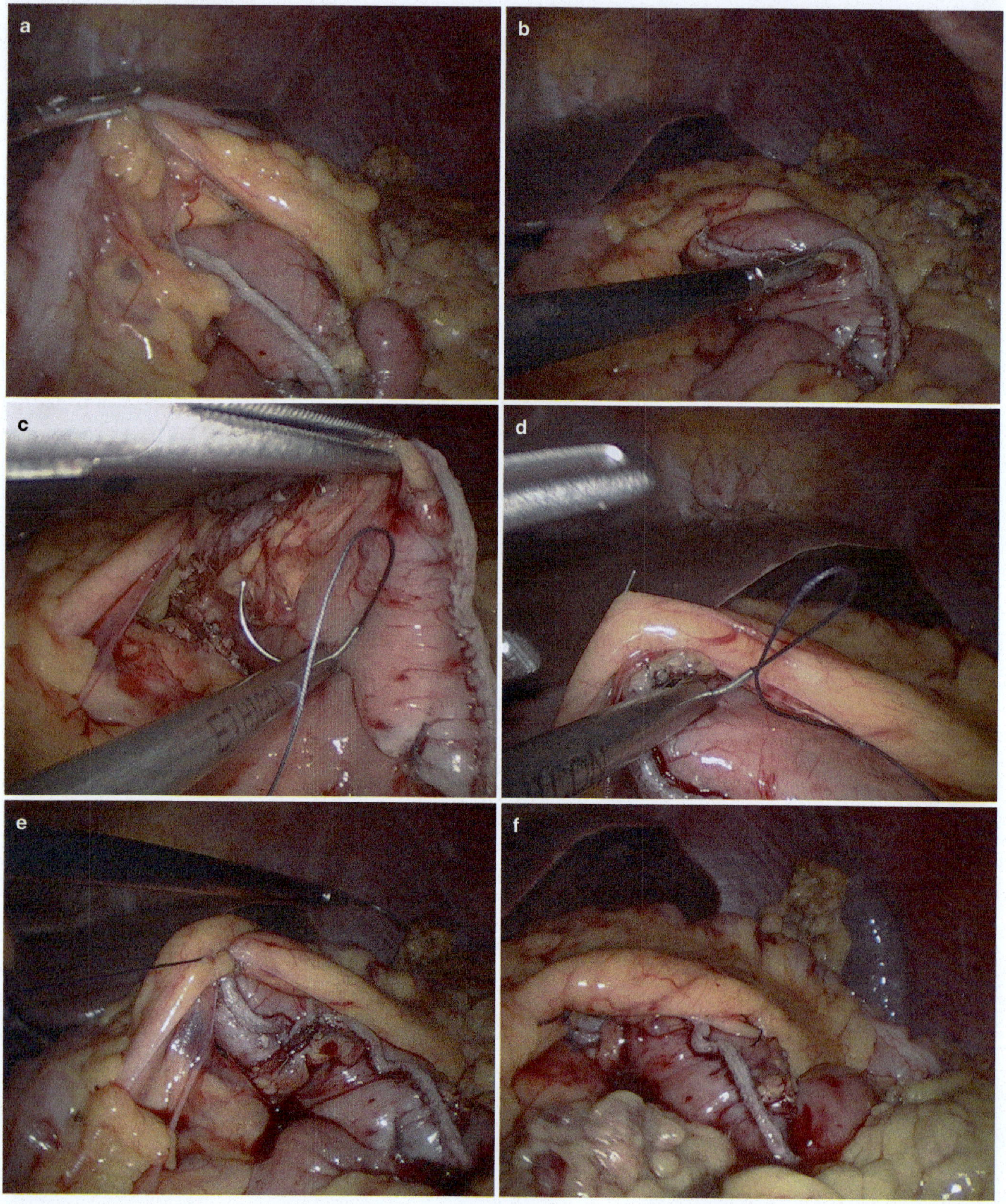

Fig. 3.21

After adequate flushing of the operative field and careful checking the anastomosis to exclude torsion or twist, a closed suction drain was placed into the surgical field through the umbilical incision (Fig. 3.22a–d).

3.2.7 Tips and Tricks

1. The patient was placed in the supine position with legs spread far apart. The surgeon was positioned between the patient's legs. Two assistants stood by the patient's side, one on the left and one on the right.
2. After the omental bursa had been opened, dissection of the omentum was advanced from side to side using ultrasonic coagulating shears to enable perigastric lymph node dissection.
3. The left gastroepiploic vessels were then divided, and the right gastroepiploic vein and artery were clipped and divided at the base to allow infra-pyloric lymph node dissection.
4. The right gastric vessels were identified and divided for supra-pyloric lymph node dissection.
5. The left gastric artery was lifted ventrally so that the supra-pancreatic lymph nodes could be dissected easily under optimal surgical exposure.
6. To achieve adequate retraction of the liver, we binded the lateral left lobe of the liver to the diaphragm using Cyanoacrylate glue as mentioned above.
7. For intracorporeal anastomosis, we used endoscopic flexible linear staplers (Echelon flex 60—3.5 and 4.5. Ethicon). To make a side-to-side anastomosis, two small holes were made on the posterior greater curvature wall of the stomach and the proximal part of jejunum, respectively. After step-by-step insertion of the linear stapler forks, the common opening in the stomach and jejunum was apposed and closed using the sutures.

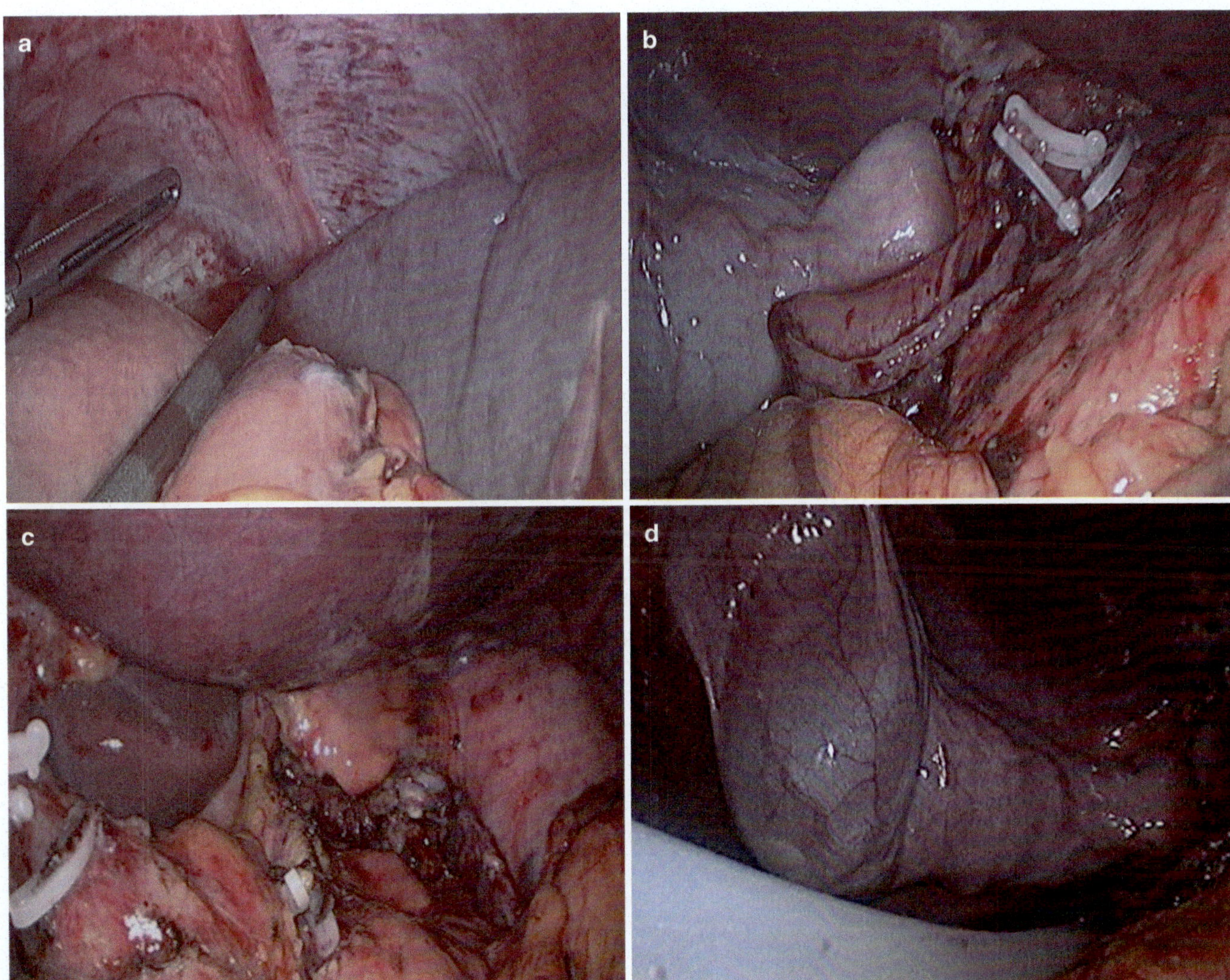

Fig. 3.22

3.3 Laparoscopic Proximal Gastrectomy

3.3.1 Indications and Case Selection

1. Patients with tumor in the proximal gastric or cardiac lesion, including carcinoma of gastric cardia or large benign tumor.
2. Patients with peptic ulcer in the body of stomach or cardiac lesion who undergo failure of medical therapy, obstruction, perforation.

3.3.2 Contraindications

1. Absolute contraindications:
   (a) severe cardiorespiratory dysfunction,
   (b) inability to tolerate general anesthesia or pneumoperitoneum,
   (c) refractory coagulopathy,
   (d) presence of metastatic disease.
2. Relative contraindications:
   (a) extensive previous surgery, or previous peritonitis leading to severe adhesion,
   (b) morbid obesity,
   (c) pregnancy.

3.3.3 Major Instruments or Energy Sources

1. Laparoscopy System.
2. Electrocautery.
3. Harmonic scalpel.
4. Endoscopic linear stapler.

3.3.4 Team Setup, Anesthesia and Position

Under general anesthesia, the patient was placed in supine position with the legs apart. The position of surgeon, assistants and nurses is shown in Fig. 3.23.

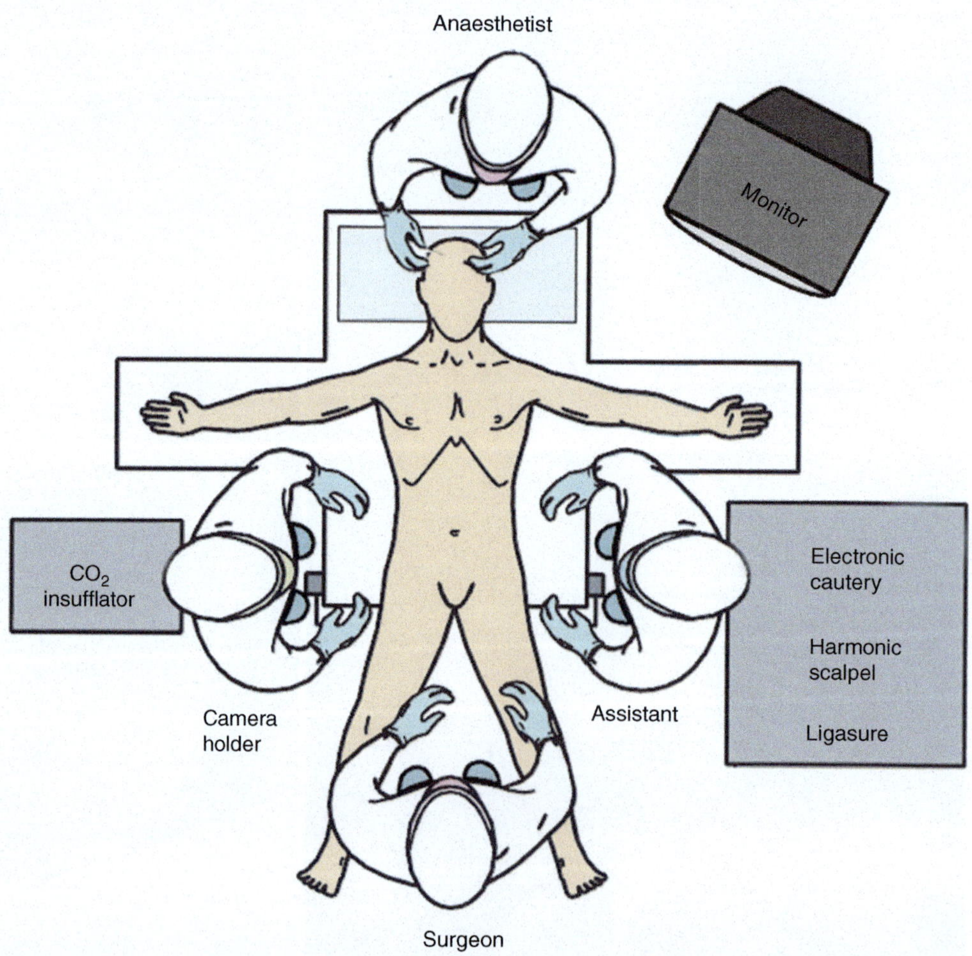

Fig. 3.23

3.3.5 Key Steps

1. Establishment of Pneumoperitoneum and Placement of Trocars.
2. Dissection of the greater omentum.
3. Mobilization of the gastrosplenic ligament and fundus of stomach.
4. Mobilization of the hepatogastric ligament.
5. Mobilization of the left gastric artery.
6. Mobilization of the lower segment of the esophagus.
7. Transection of the esophagus.
8. Gastroesophageal anastomosis.
9. Proximal gastrectomy.

3.3.6 Surgical Techniques

1. Establishment of Pneumoperitoneum and Placement of Trocars.
2. Dissection of the greater omentum.
   With an atraumatic grasper on the left hand and ultrasonic scalpel on the right, the omentum was dissected along the transverse colon firstly with the left side to the left flexure of colon, the left gastroepiploic vein were divided. The wall of the transverse colon should be protected from injury (Fig. 3.24a–h).

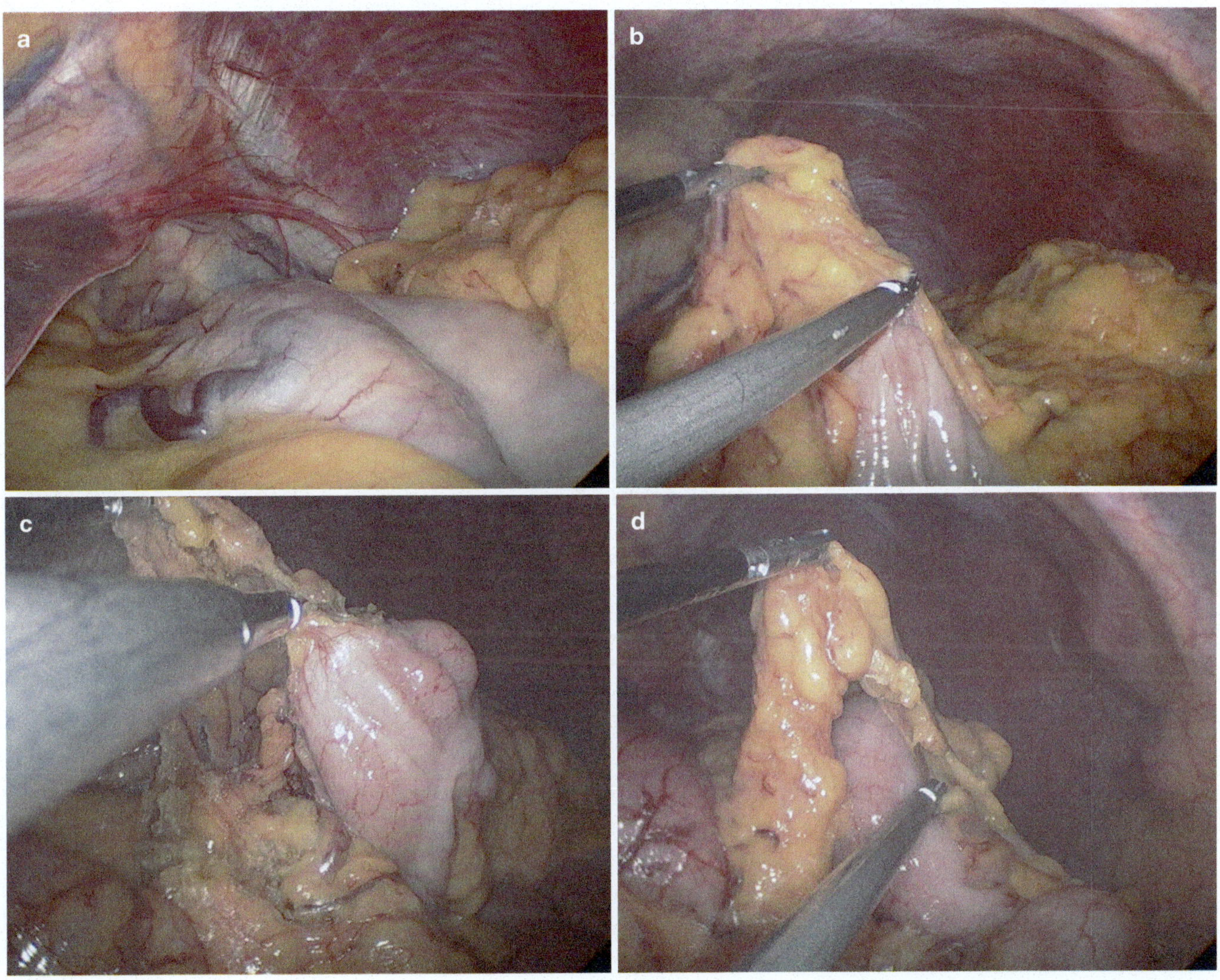

Fig. 3.24

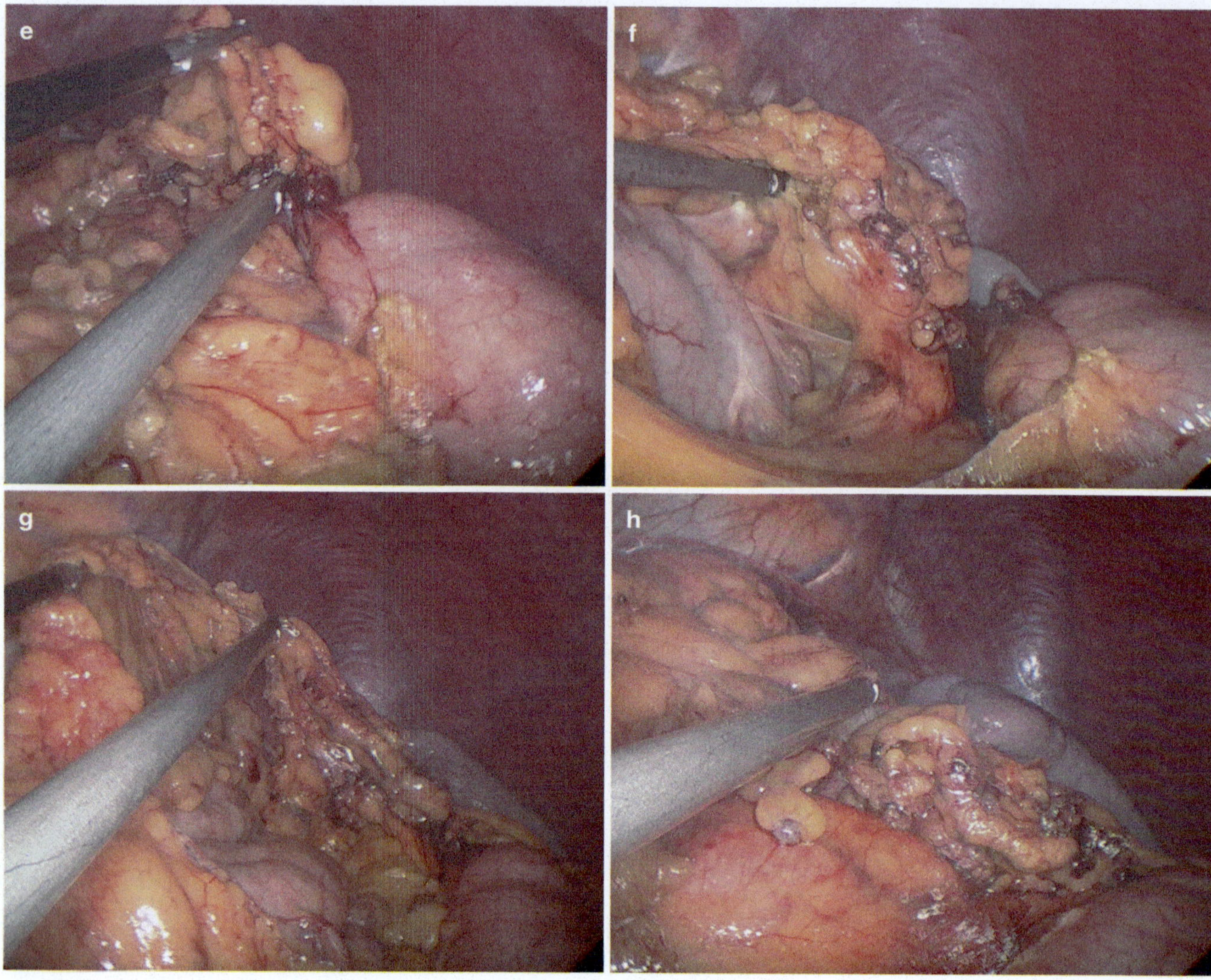

Fig. 3.24 (continued)

3. Mobilization of the gastrosplenic ligament and fundus of stomach.

   Continuous mobilization to the left was done and the short gastric vessels in the gastrosplenic ligament were dissected. The fundus of stomach was exposed and mobilized (Fig. 3.25a–d).

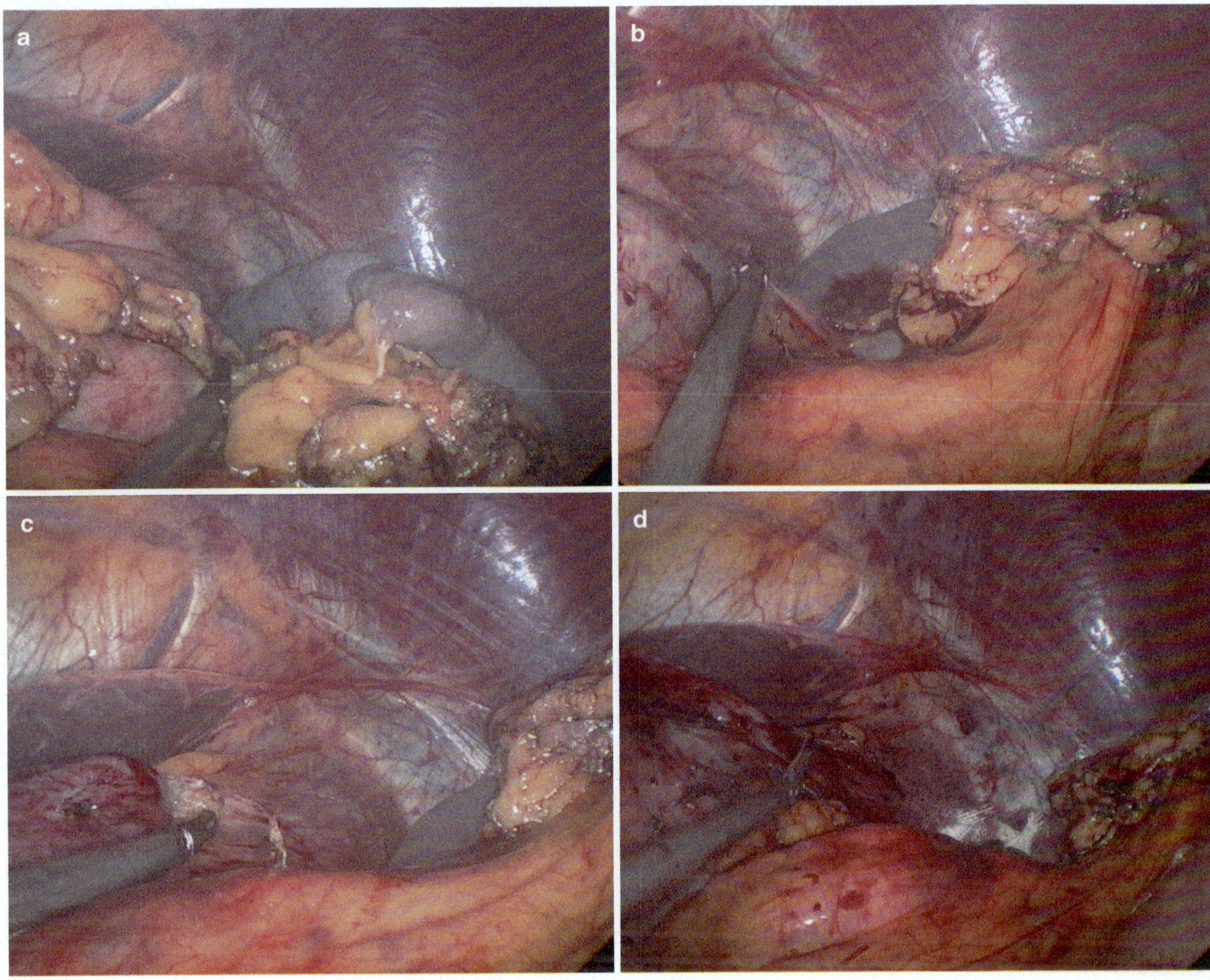

Fig. 3.25

4. Mobilization of the hepatogastric ligament.
   The left lateral of the liver was retracted to fully expose the lesser curvature of the stomach (Fig. 3.26a–d).

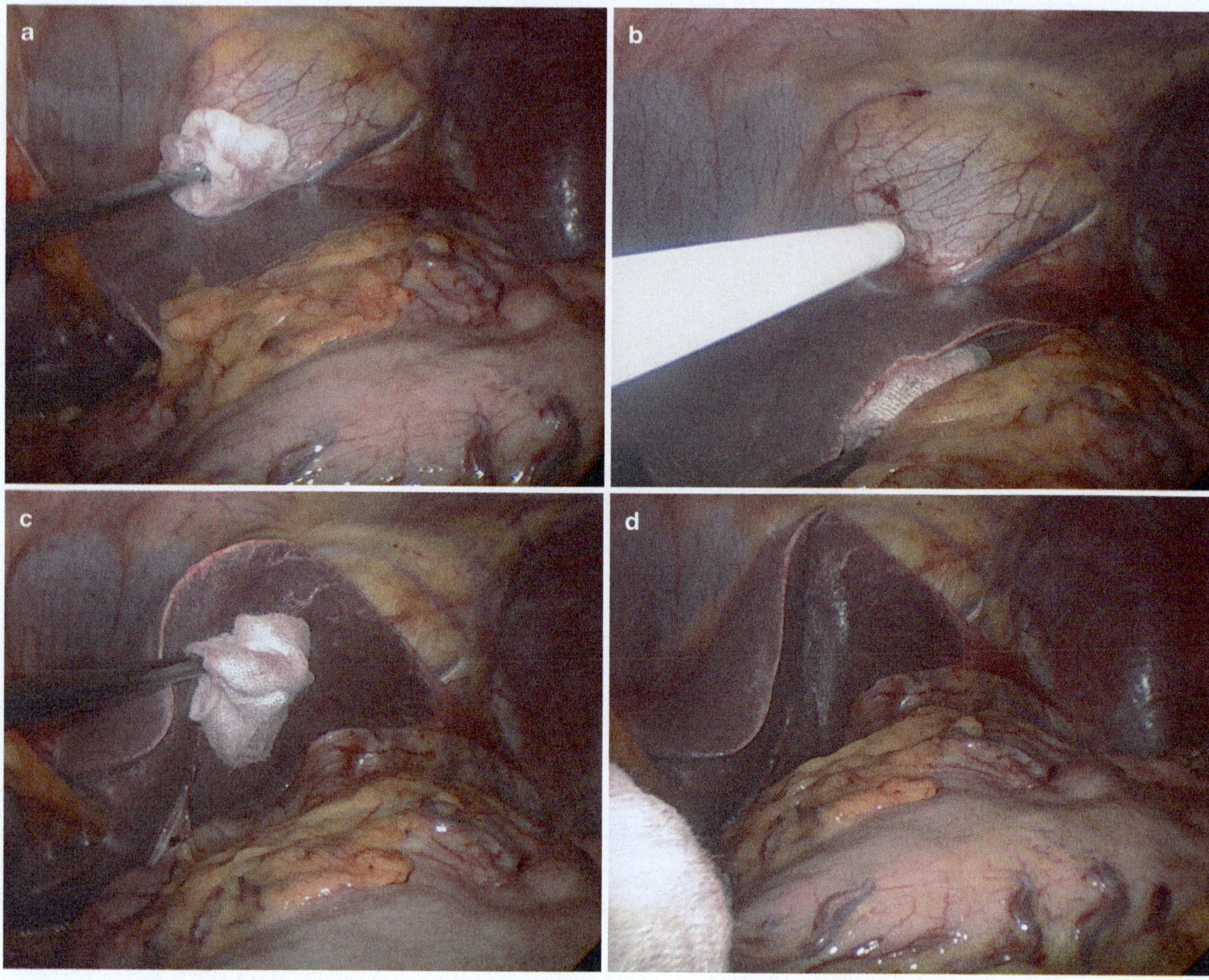

Fig. 3.26

Mobilization of the hepatogastric ligament was performed by using the harmonic scalpel (Fig. 3.27a, b).

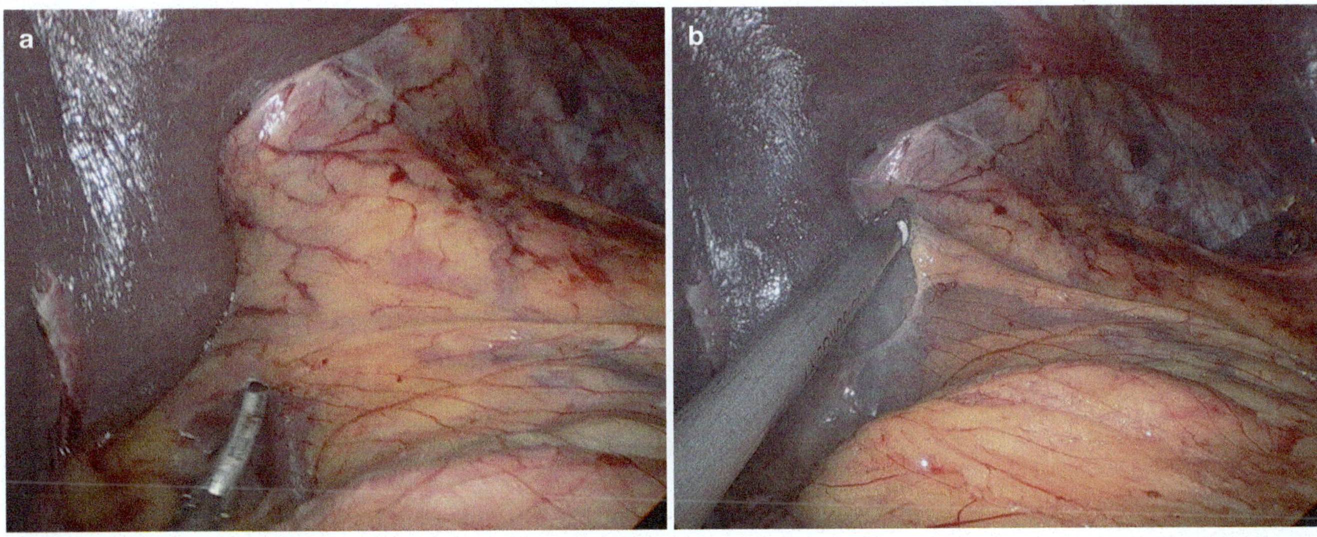

Fig. 3.27

Continuous dissection upwards was done to expose the right margin of the esophagus and the anterior peritoneum of the esophagus was cleared (Fig. 3.28a–d).

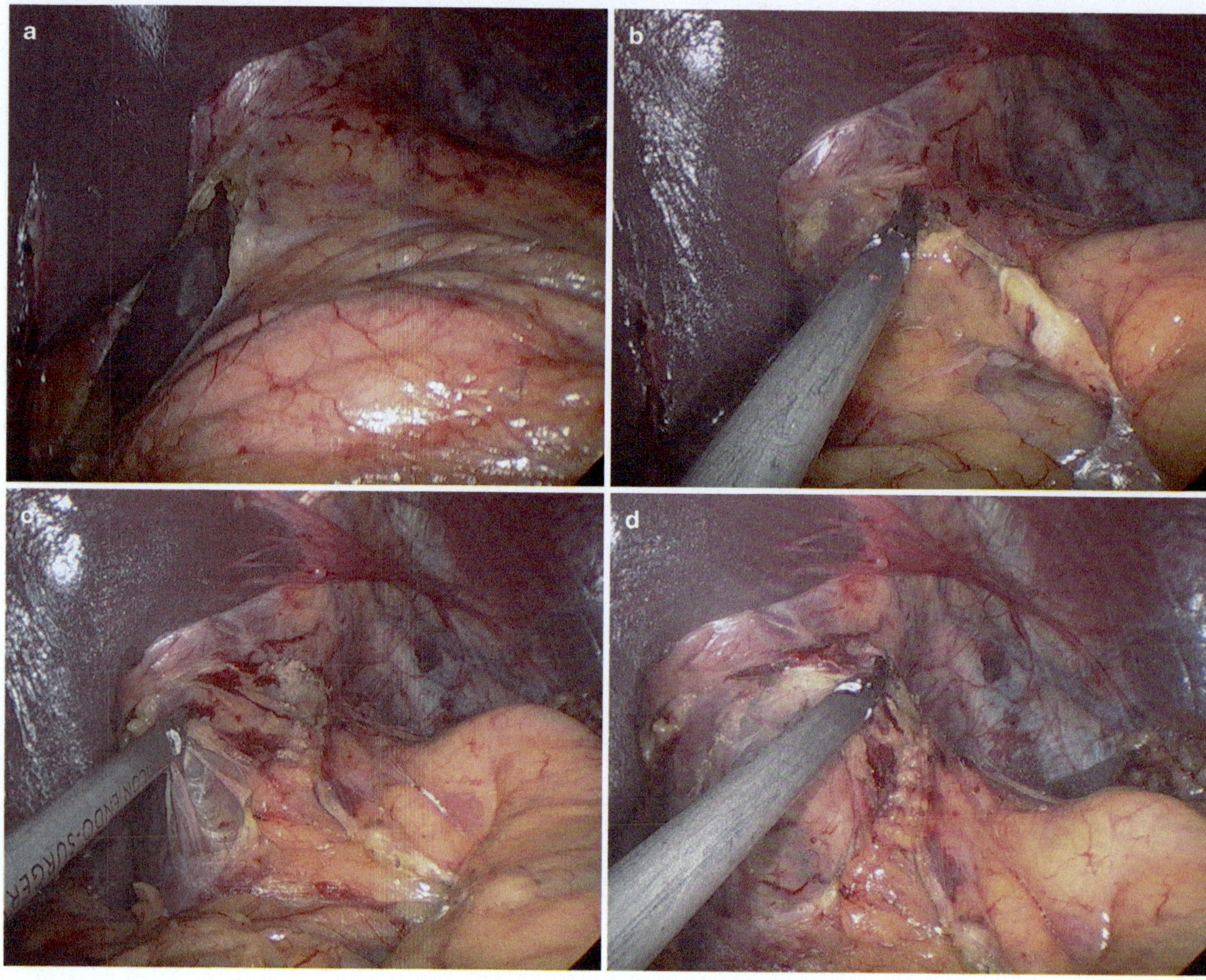

Fig. 3.28

5. Mobilization of the left gastric artery.
   With the stomach lifted posterior by the atraumatic grasper on the left hand, the pancreatiogastric fold was exposed. The left gastric vein and artery were clipped and cut at their origins (Fig. 3.29a–h).

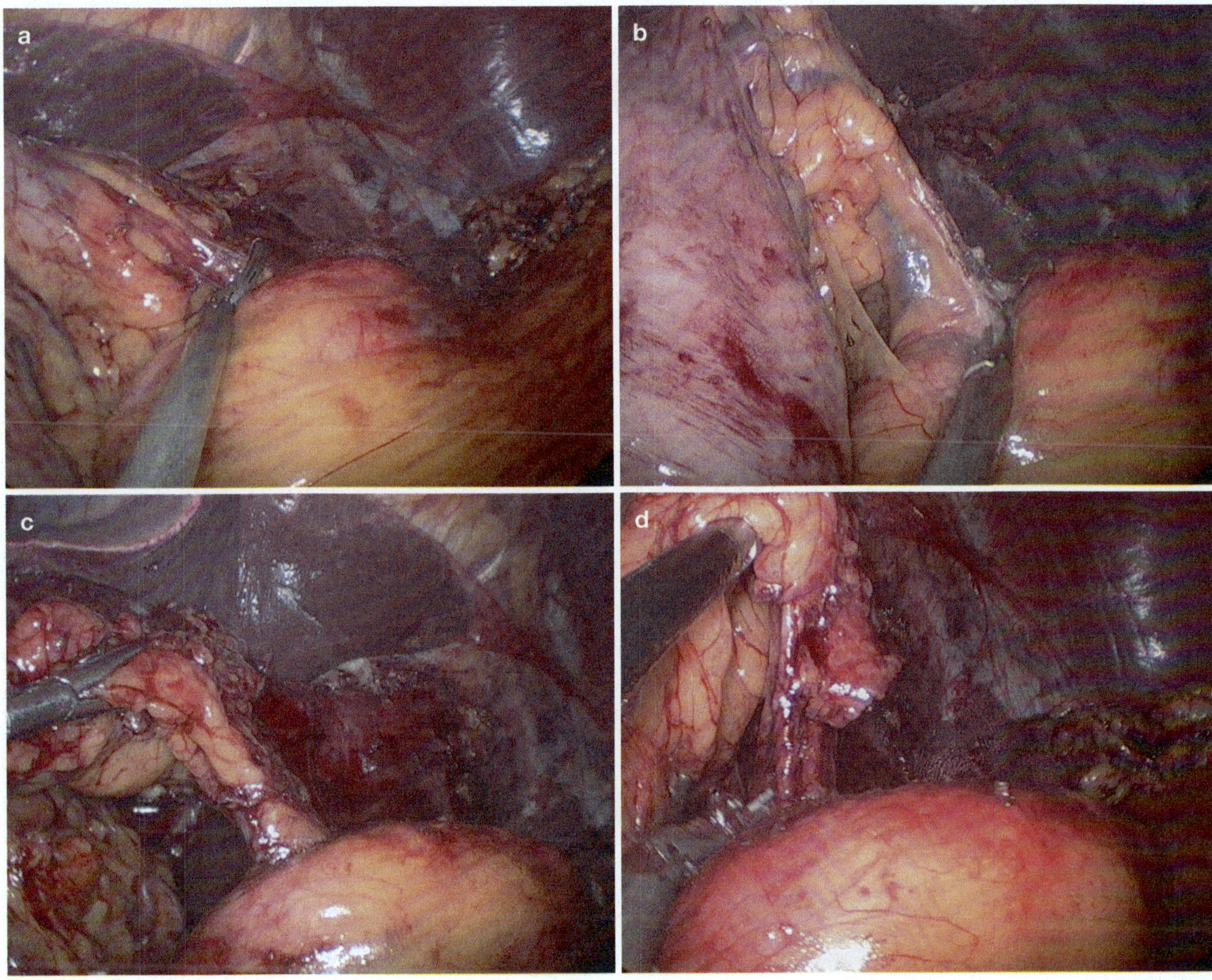

Fig. 3.29

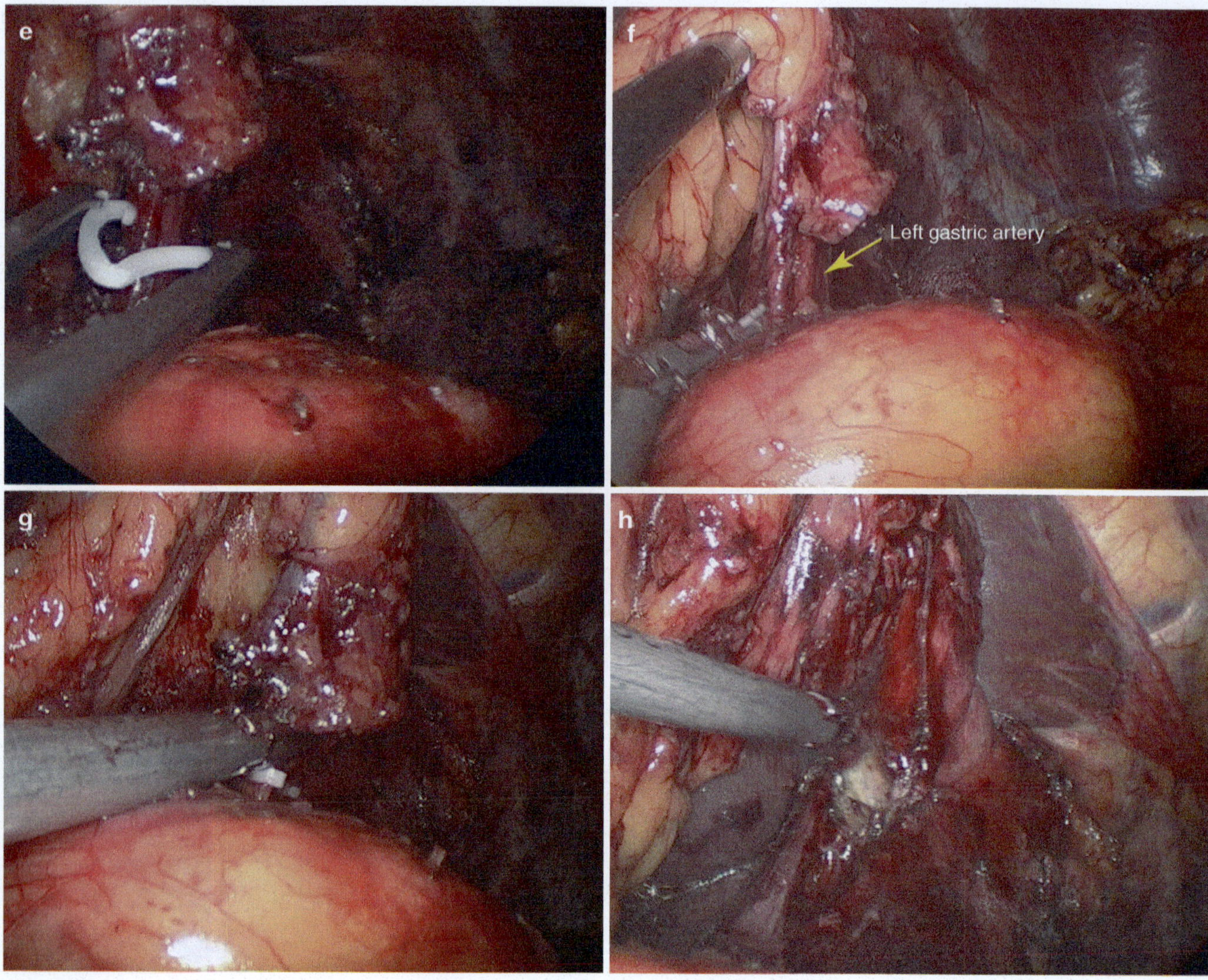

Fig. 3.29 (continued)

6. Mobilization of the lower segment of the esophagus.
   The bilateral crura were exposed and retracted laterally with a roticulated grasper, and peritoneum was incised with harmonic scalpel. The cardia and the lower esophagus 4 cm distal to the cardia were dissected and fully mobilized (Fig. 3.30a, b).

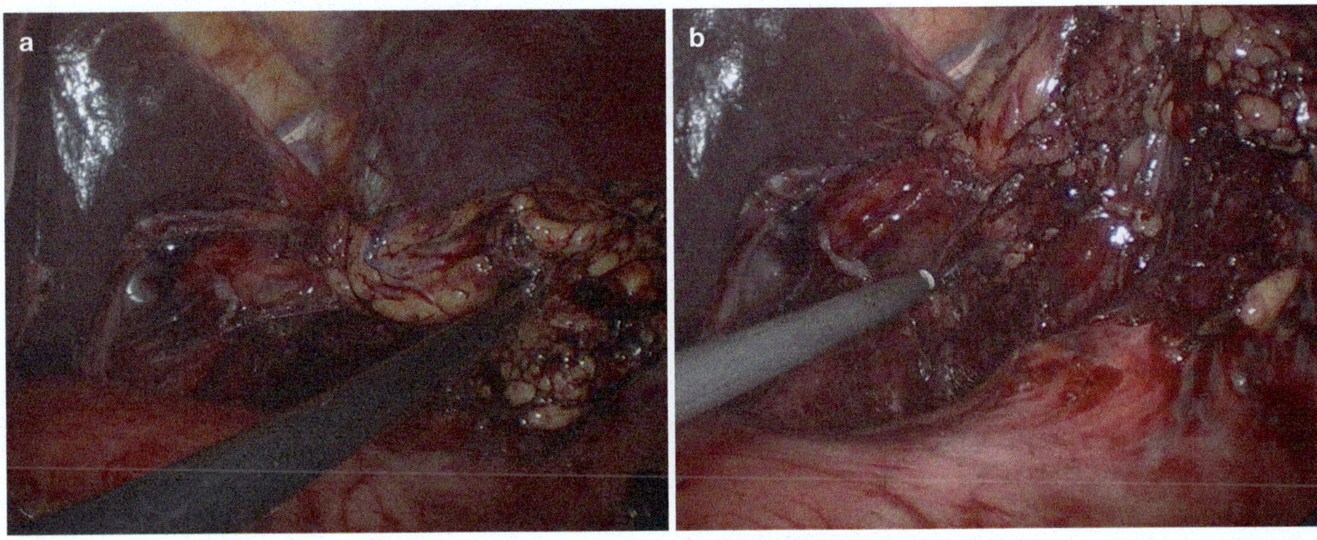

Fig. 3.30

7. Transection of the esophagus.
   The esophagus was transected by using flexible endoscopic linear staplers (Fig. 3.31a–c).

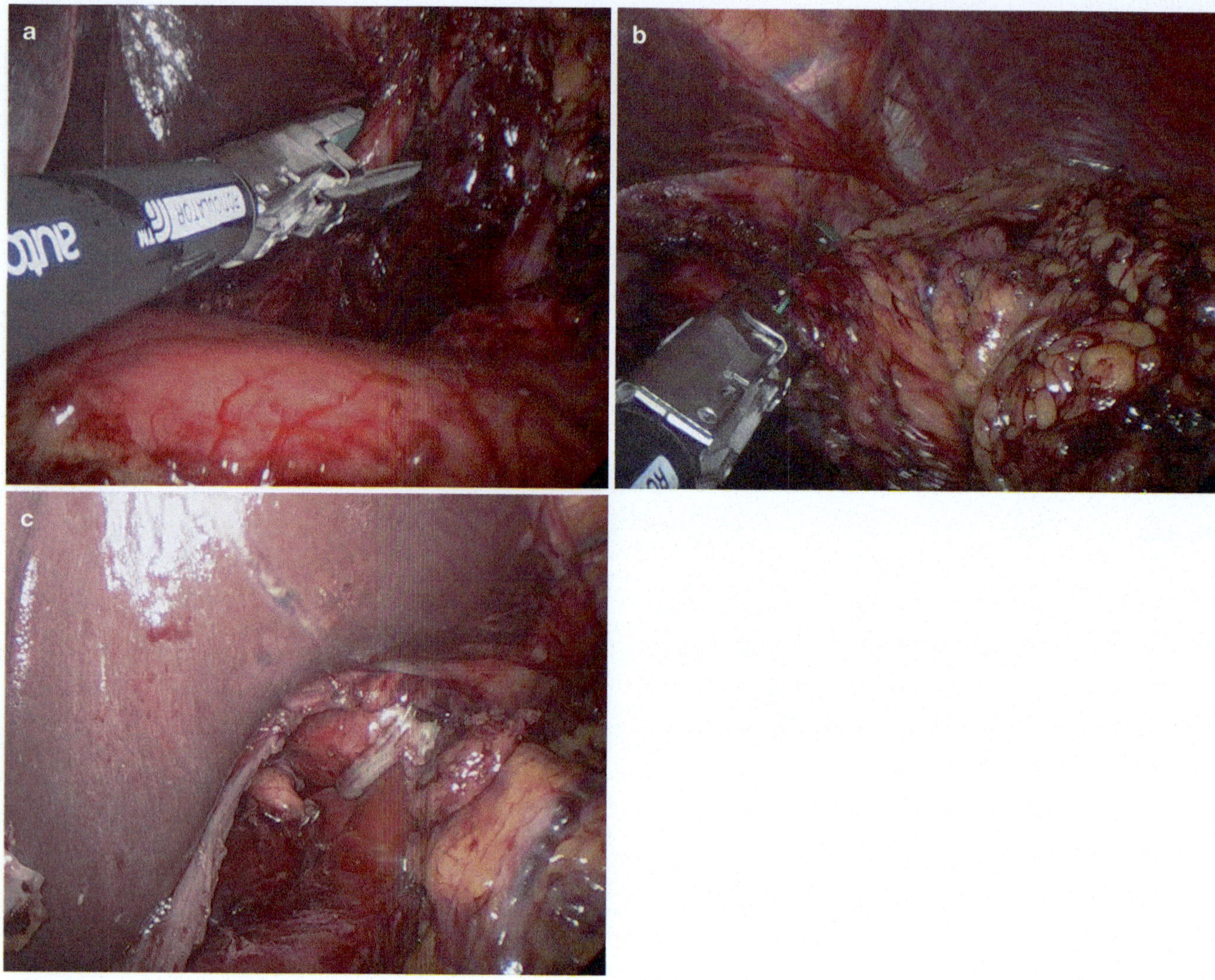

Fig. 3.31

8. Gastroesophageal anastomosis.

   A 25 mm Orvil anvil with a guiding tube was inserted into the esophagus through the oral cavity. A small incision was made on the central part of the esophageal stump, through which the guiding tube was pulled out to pull and fix the anvil to the esophageal stump. The fixed line on the guiding tube was cut off and the tube was removed (Fig. 3.32a–f).

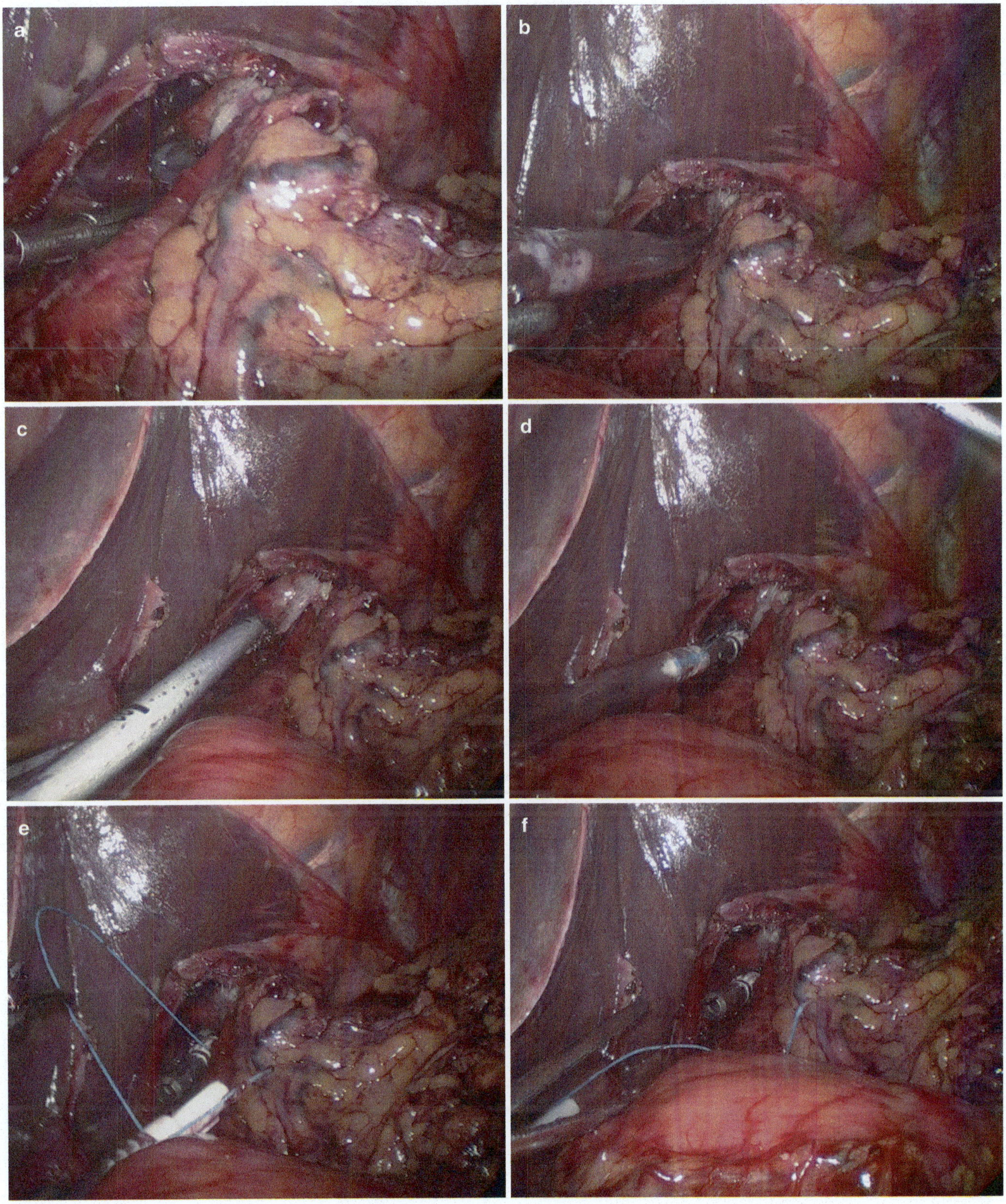

Fig. 3.32

An incision was made on the anterior wall of the stomach and the handle lever of the Orvil stapler was implanted into the gastric cavity through this incision and punctured out through the posterior wall of the stomach where the anastomosis was to made (Fig. 3.33a–d).

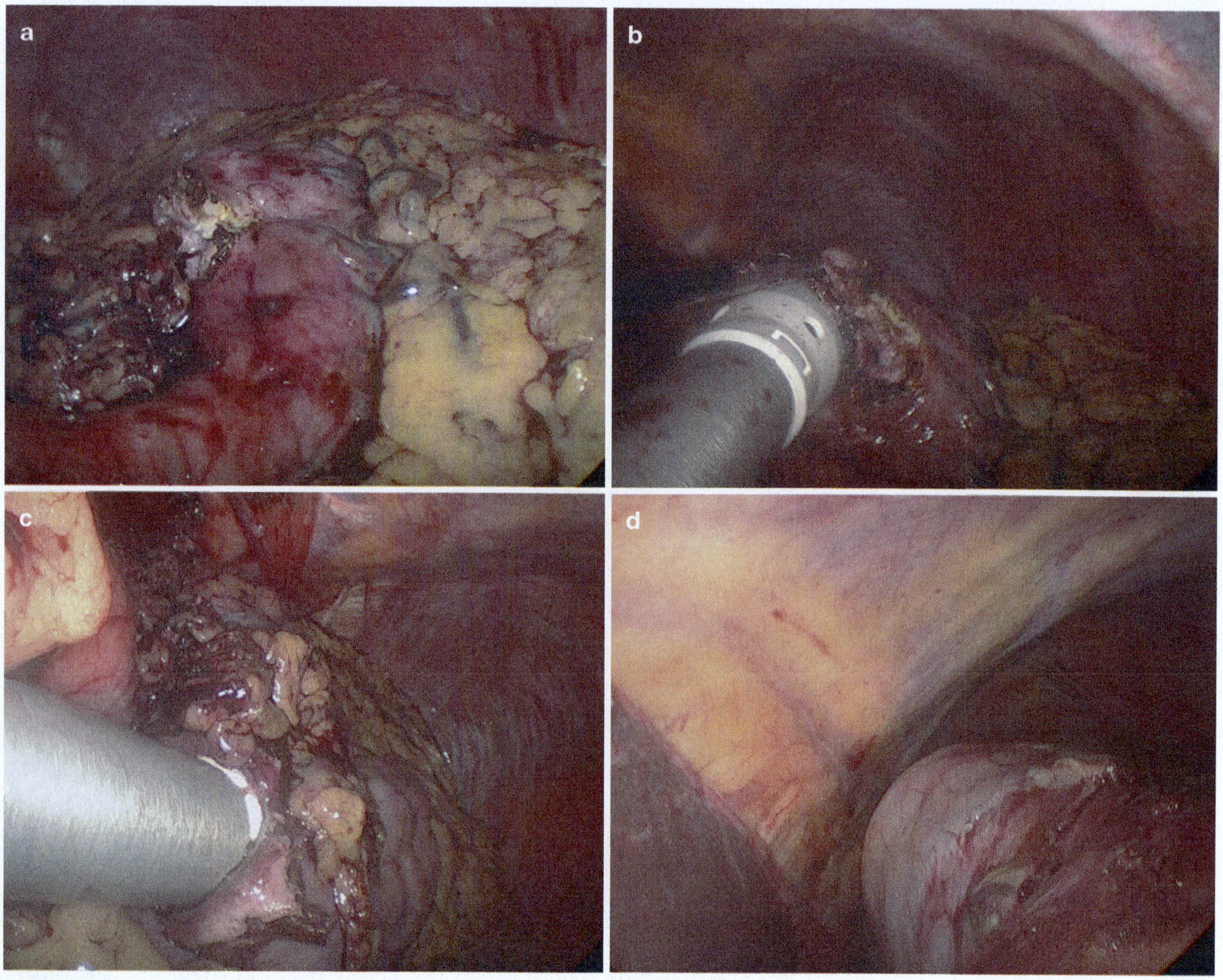

Fig. 3.33

The handle lever and anvil of the Orvil stapler were connected, screwed and firmly locked. After careful checking the connection part, the stapler was fired to complete the gastroesophageal anastomosis. Careful examination of the anastomosis was done to be sure of devoid of torsion, twist or bleeding (Fig. 3.34a–j).

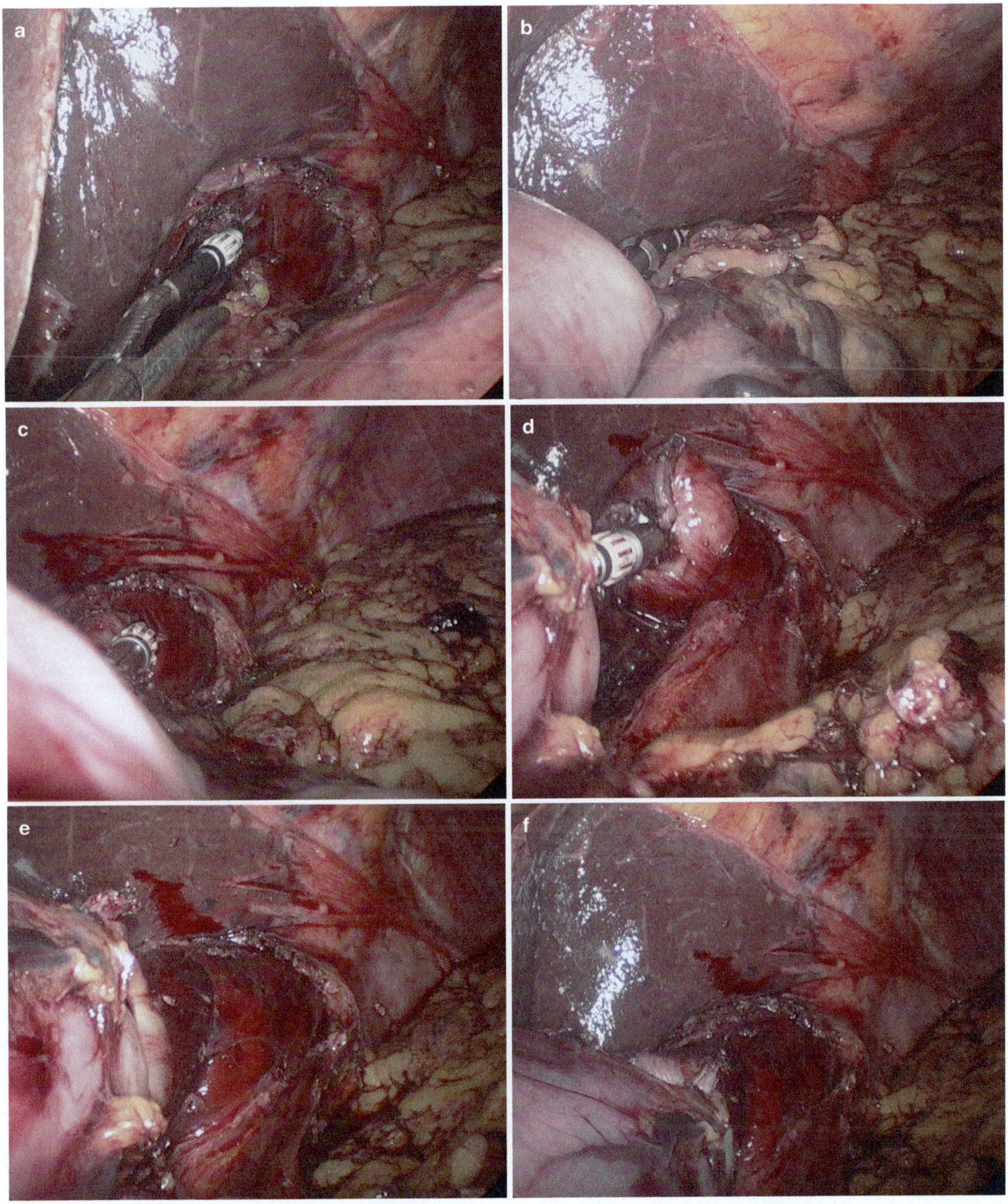

Fig. 3.34

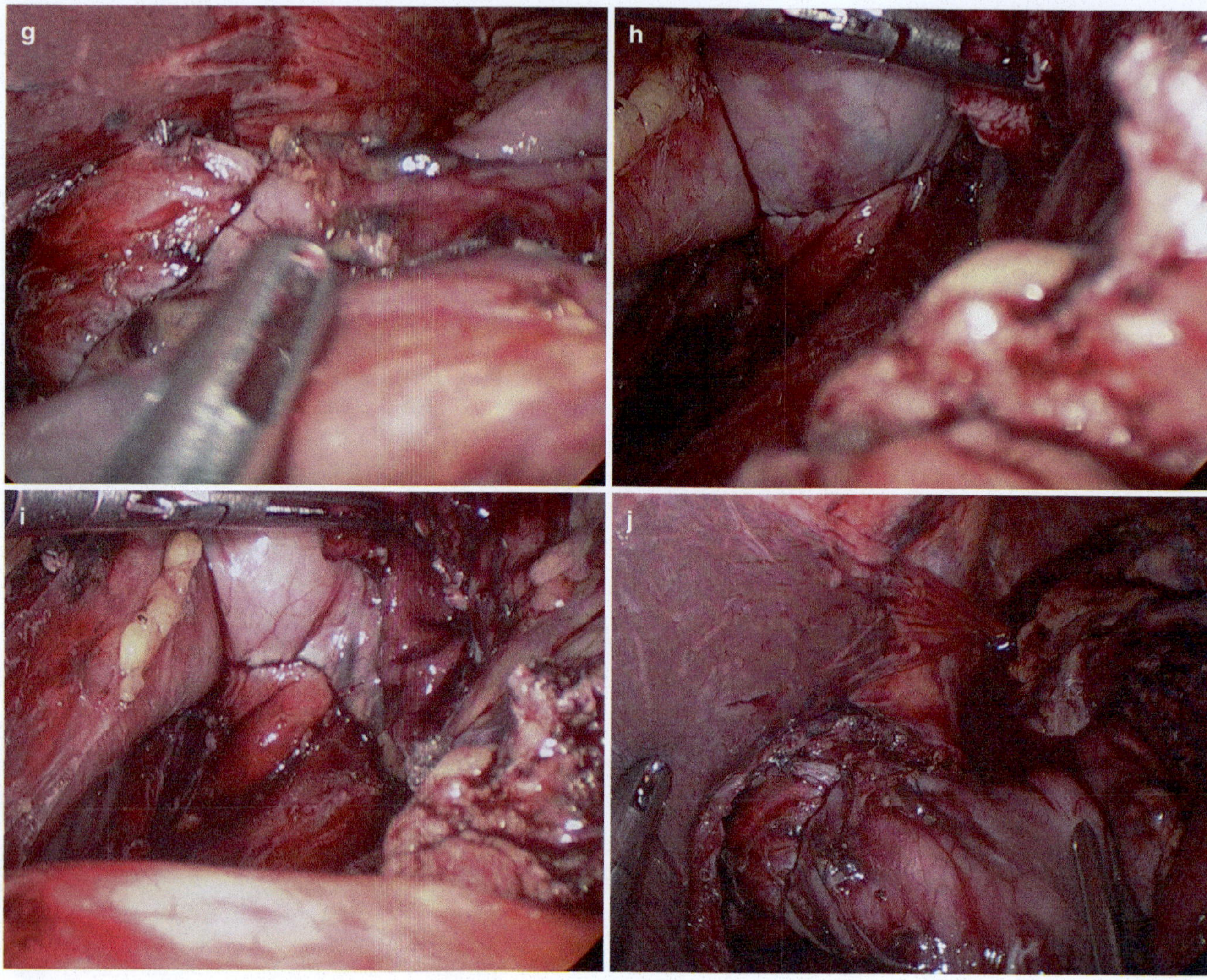

Fig. 3.34 (continued)

9. Proximal gastrectomy.
   The proximal stomach was transected 2 cm distal from the anastomosis by using the linear stapler with single or multiple bites (Fig. 3.35a–f).

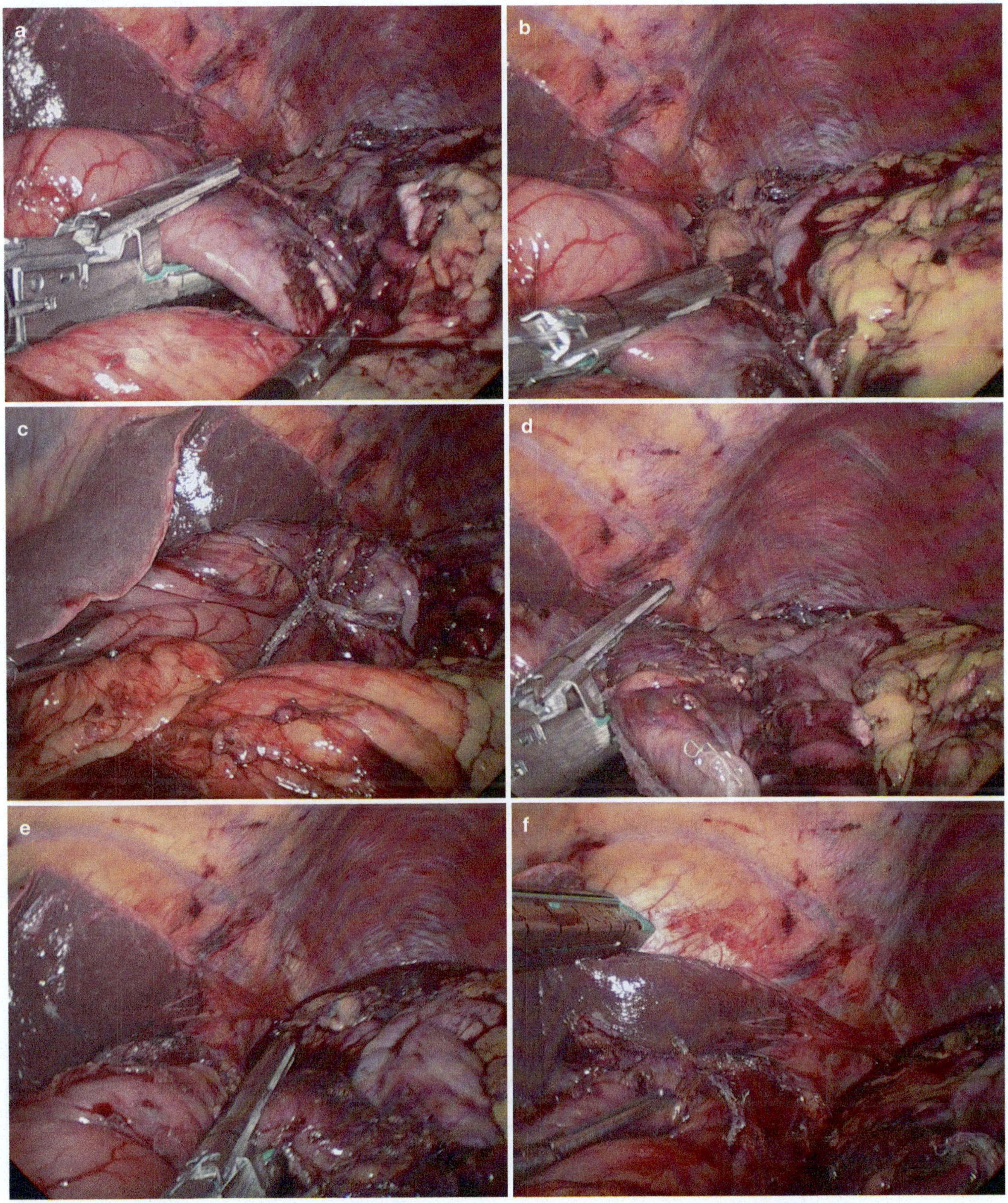

Fig. 3.35

The anastomosis was reinforced by seromuscular layer suture (Fig. 3.36a, b).

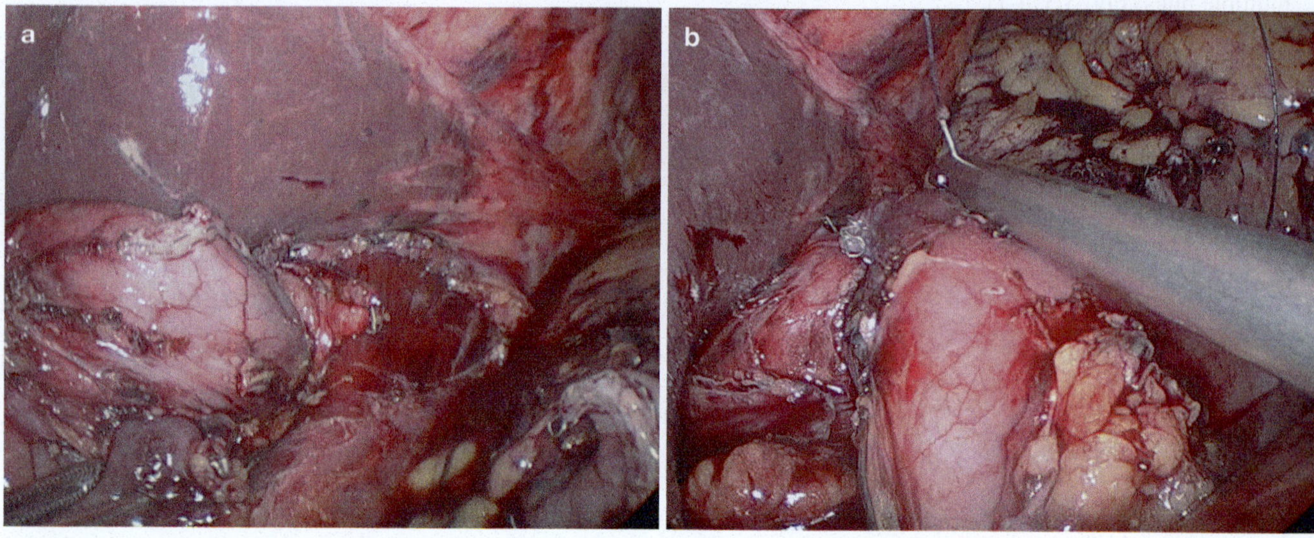

Fig. 3.36

The intact specimens were removed from the abdominal cavity by bag, and we often cut the connecting tissue between the 10 mm and the 12 mm-trocar to enlarge the incision for sample extracting. After adequate flushing of the operative field and careful checking the anastomosis to exclude torsion or twist, a closed suction drain was placed behind the anastomosis through the umbilical incision (Fig. 3.37a, b).

3.3.7 Tips and Tricks

1. Reconstruction of the esophagogastrostomy by double stapling method using EEA™ OrVil™
2. EEA™. OrVil™ is a device that permits mechanical purse-string suture. An anvil head with a diameter of 21 or 25 mm is fastened in a tilted state at about 170° to a tube as long as about 95 mm via No. 1 polyester yarn with a white plastic connector. The tube is calibrated in 5-cm increments starting with the anvil head. The tip of the tube is called a valve tip. Purse-string suture is enabled by connecting the center rod of the anvil head and the main unit of the automated stapler, and conducting firing.
3. Placement of an anvil head within the esophagus: EEA™ OrVil™ was orally inserted slowly from the valve tip until the valve tip reached the end of the esophagus. A small hole was created with harmonic ace at the tensed site while tension was confirmed. The valve tip was made to pass through. Grasping forceps were inserted via a trocar. A tube was led outside the abdominal cavity while the valve tip at a small hole at the end of the esophagus was being grasped. The cuffs of the endotracheal intubation tube tend to cause resistance during transit. To alleviate this resistance, the throat cavity was widened during transit through the larynx, and the cuffs were deflated. When the tube was pulled further, the anvil was led from the open end of the esophagus into the abdominal cavity. Then, the grasping notch of the center rod was securely grasped with grasping forceps. The anvil head and the tube were connected with two pieces of No. 1 polyester yarn, which were cut to disconnect the anvil and place the anvil head within the esophagus.
4. Preparation of residual stomach: An automated stapler was led into abdominal cavity through umbilical incision and inserted from the anterior wall of the stomach. Then, the main unit of the automated stapler and the posterior wall of the stomach were fastened to prevent dropout of the stomach wall from the automated stapler.
5. Connection with anvil, and anastomosis: The anvil and the main unit were connected after it was confirmed that an automated stapler and the center rod were made fully linear. Firing then completed the anastomosis.

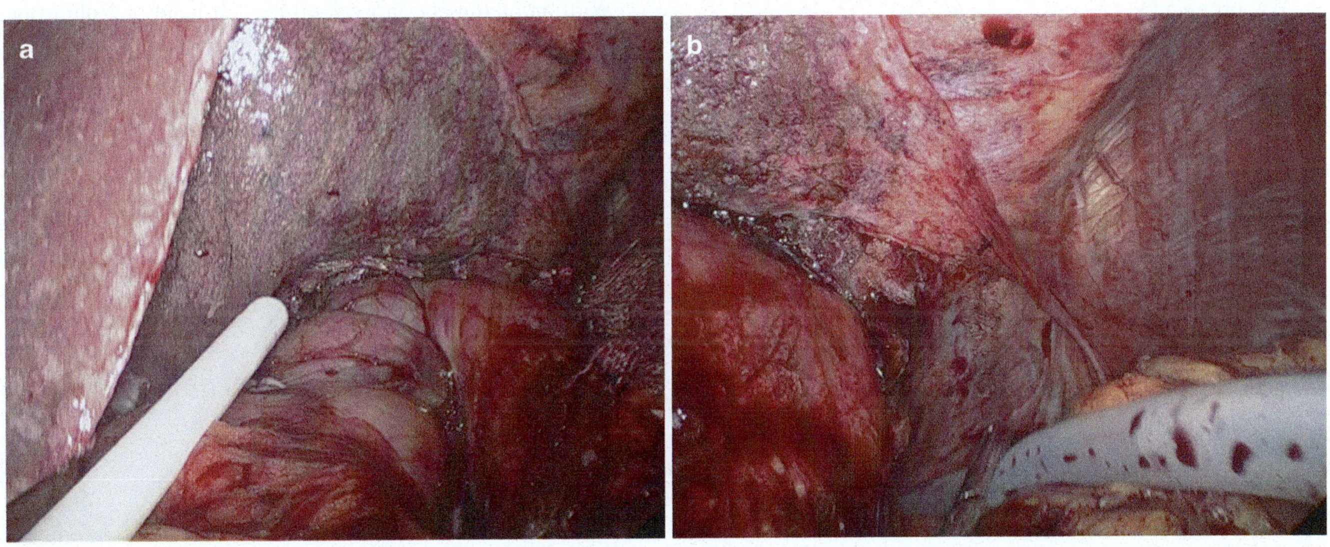

Fig. 3.37

3.4 Laparoscopic Total Gastrectomy

3.4.1 Indications and Case Selection

1. Patients with peptic ulcer disease who undergo failure of medical therapy, obstruction, perforation and highly suspected for malignancy.
2. Patients with peptic ulcer who have over-secretion of gastric acid.
3. Patients with early gastric cancer, or palliative operation for late gastric cancer.
4. Patients with gastric cancer in the body or fundus of the stomach.

3.4.2 Contraindications

1. Absolute contraindications:
   (a) severe cardiorespiratory dysfunction,
   (b) inability to tolerate general anesthesia or pneumoperitoneum,
   (c) refractory coagulopathy,
   (d) presence of metastatic disease.
2. Relative contraindications:
   (a) extensive previous surgery, or previous peritonitis leading to severe adhesion,
   (b) morbid obesity,
   (c) pregnancy.

3.4.3 Major Instruments or Energy Sources

1. Laparoscopy System.
2. Electrocautery.
3. Harmonic scalpel.
4. Endoscopic linear stapler.

3.4.4 Team Setup, Anesthesia and Position

The same as Sect. 3.3.4.

3.4.5 Key Steps

1. Establishment of Pneumoperitoneum and Placement of Trocars.
2. Mobilization of the gastrocolic ligament.
3. Mobilization of the hepatogastric ligament.
4. Transection of the duodenum.
5. Transection of the esophagus.
6. Esophageal jejunum end-to-side anastomosis.
7. Jejunal side-to-side anastomosis.
8. Operative field flushing and placement of drainage tube.

3.4.6 Surgical Techniques

1. Establishment of Pneumoperitoneum and Placement of Trocars.
2. Mobilization of the gastrocolic ligament.
   With an atraumatic grasper on the left hand and ultrasonic scalpel on the right, the omentum was dissected along the transverse colon firstly with the left side to the left flexure of colon, the left gastroepiploic vein were divided. Continuous mobilization to the left was done and the short gastric vessels in the gastrosplenic ligament were dissected. The fundus of stomach was exposed and mobilized (Fig. 3.38a–j).

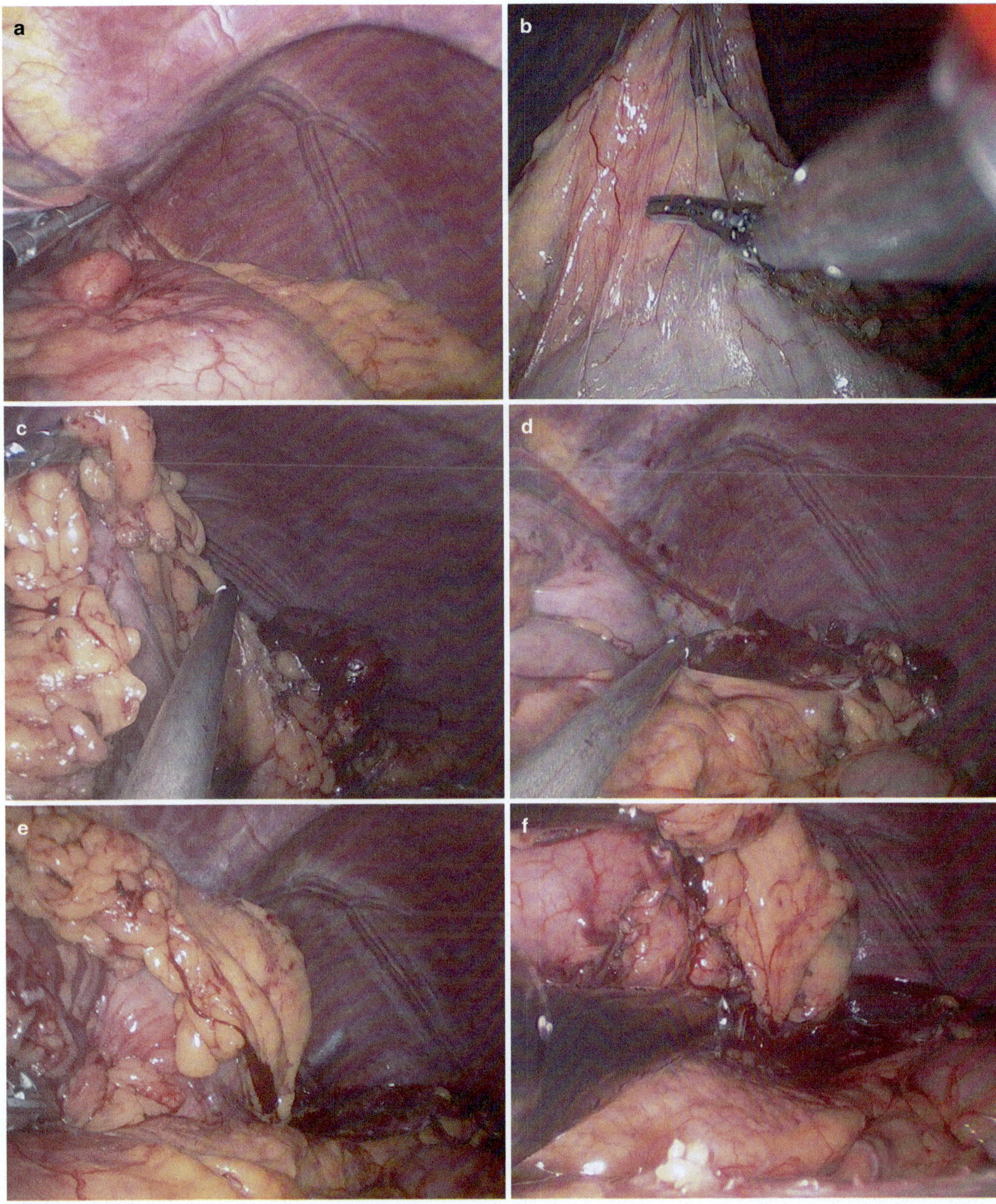

Fig. 3.38

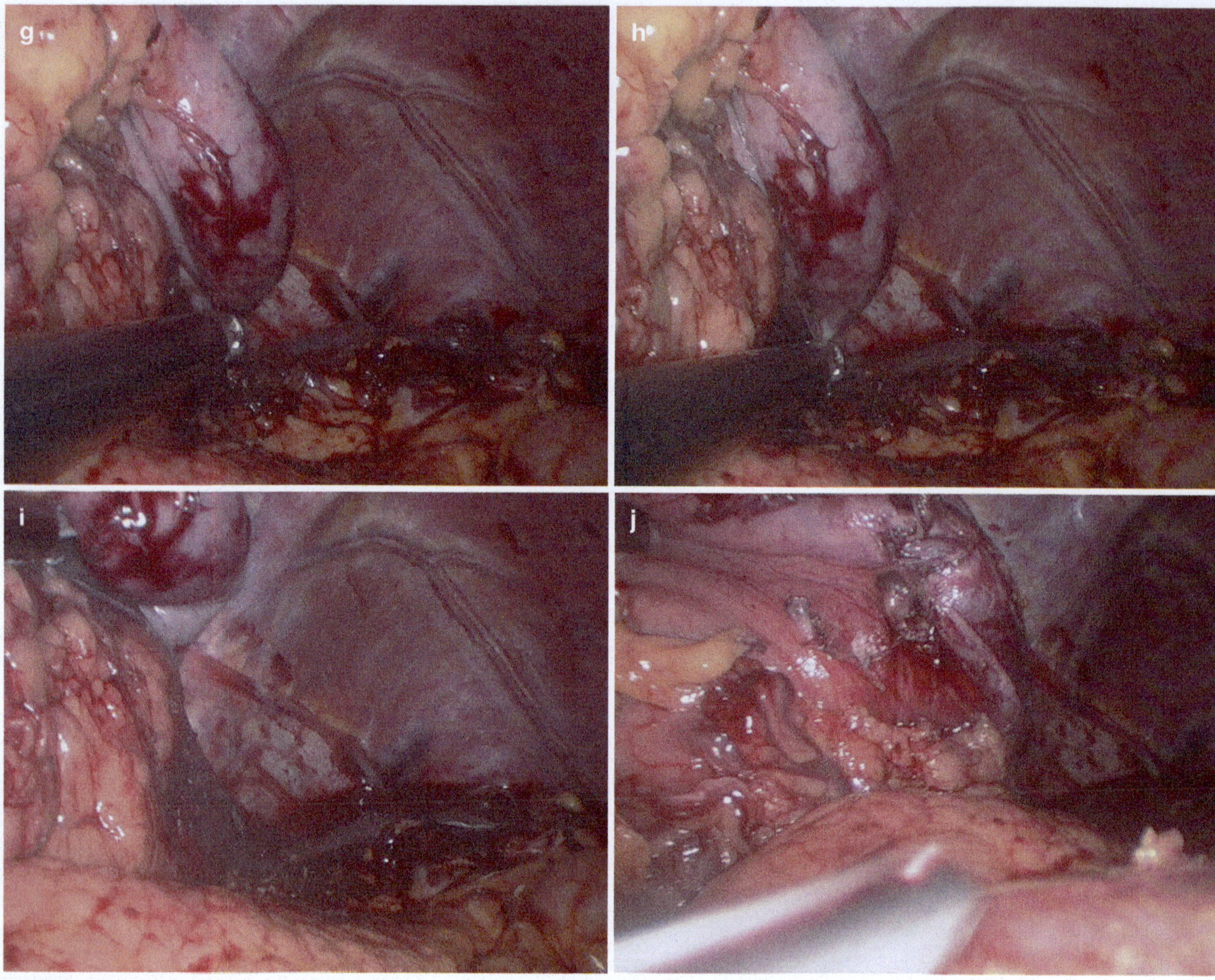

Fig. 3.38 (continued)

Continuous dissection to the hepatic flexure of colon was performed until 2-3 cm distal to the pylorus. The right gastroepiploic vein and artery were clipped and divided (Fig. 3.39a–j).

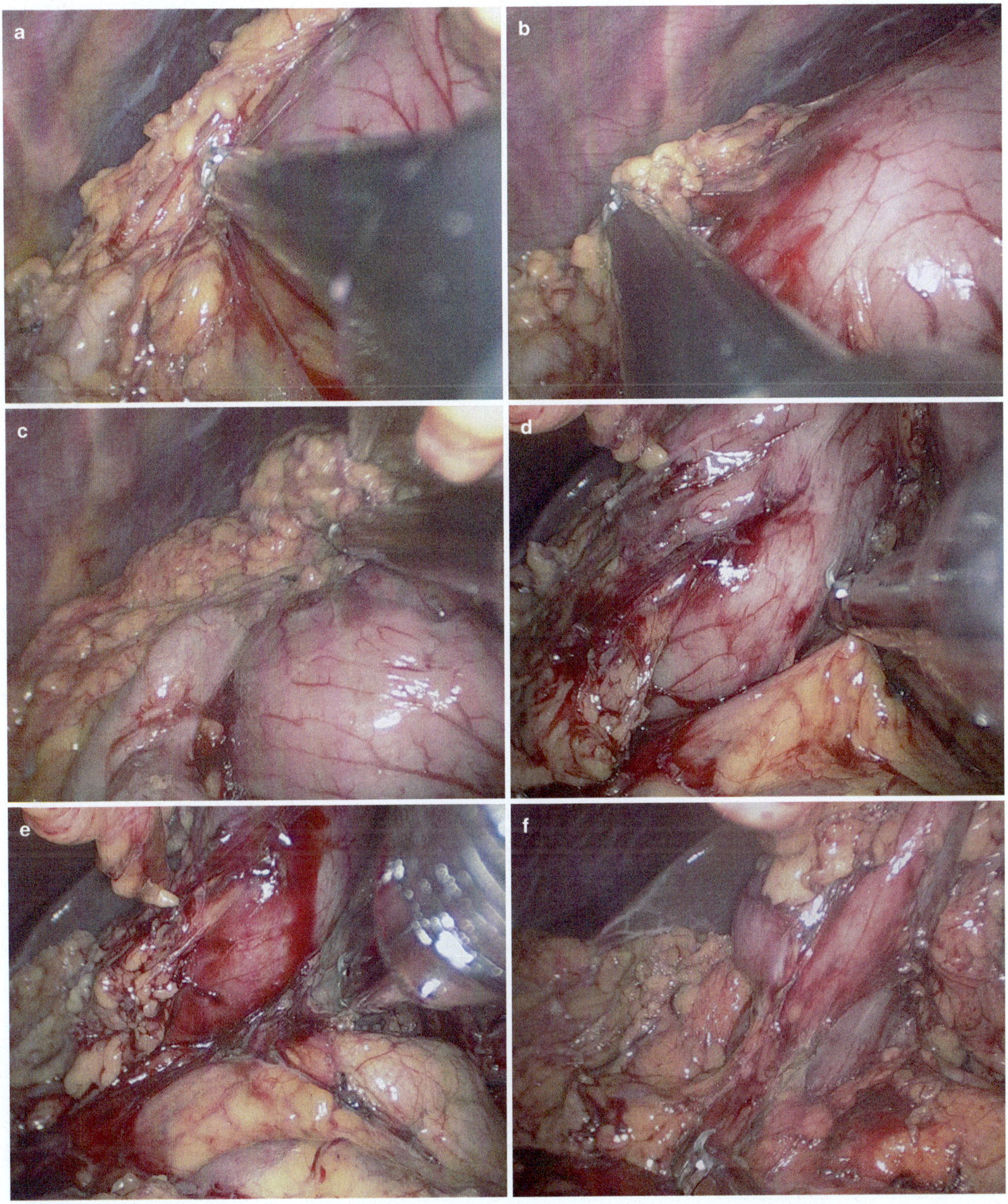

Fig. 3.39

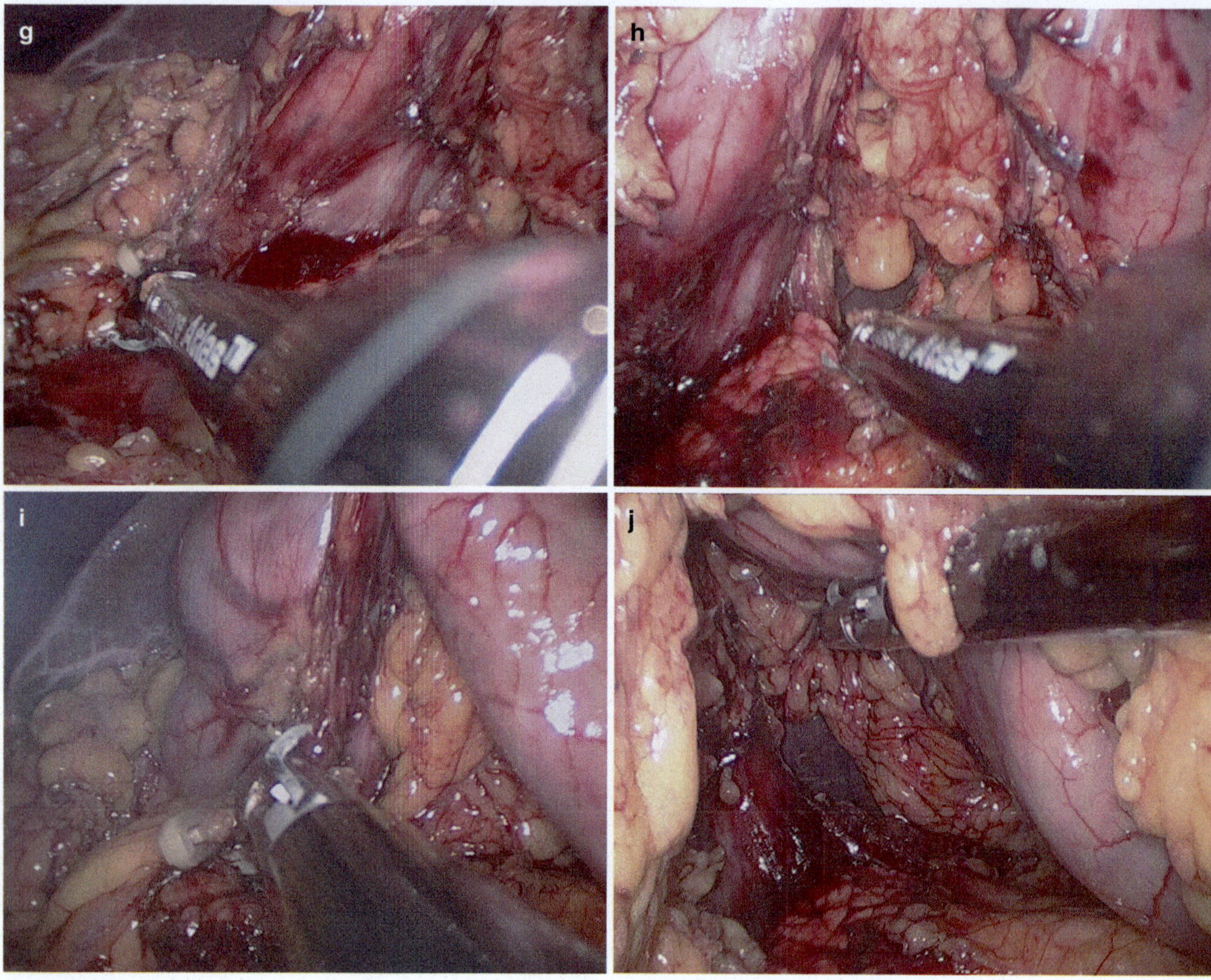

Fig. 3.39 (continued)

3. Mobilization of the hepatogastric ligament.

   The omentum of the gastric lesser curvature was lifted. With a harmonic scalpel in the right hand, the lesser omentum was opened at its avascular zone to expose the omental bursa. Mobilization to the gastric cardia and pylorus side along the lesser curvature was performed respectively. Upwards, the bilateral crura were exposed to mobilize the lower esophagus 4 cm above the cardia (Fig. 3.40a–d). Mobilizations of the hepatogastric and hepatoduodenal ligaments near the pylorus were the same as mentioned in the previous section.

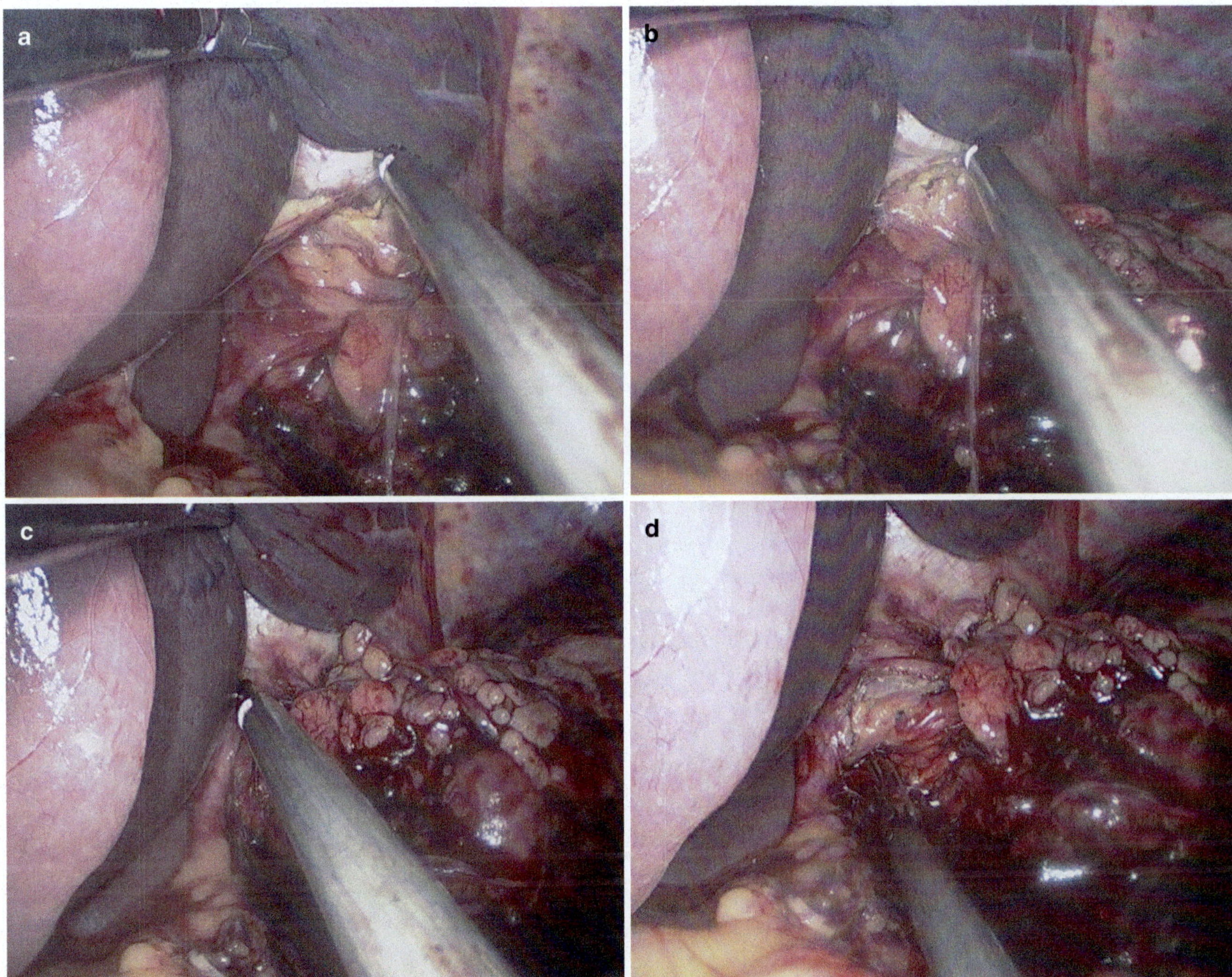

Fig. 3.40

4. Transection of the duodenum.
   The duodenum was transected just distal to the pyloric ring by using 45 mm linear staplers (Fig. 3.41a–f).

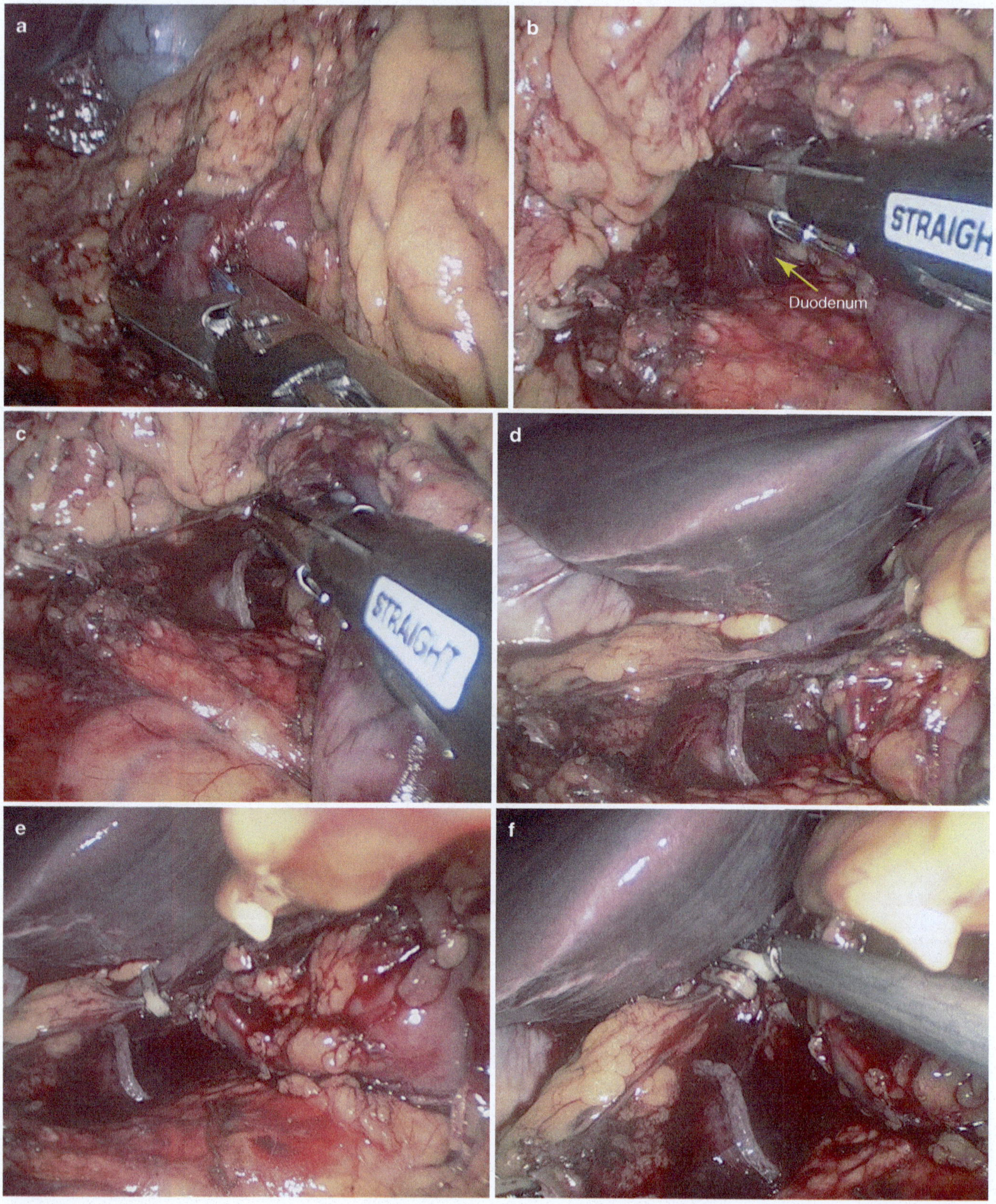

Fig. 3.41

5. Transection of the esophagus.
   The esophagus was transected by using flexible endoscopic linear staplers 2 cm above the cardia. The intact specimens were removed from the abdominal cavity by bag, and we often cut the connecting tissue between the 10 mm and the 12 mm-trocar to enlarge the incision for sample extracting (Fig. 3.42a–h).

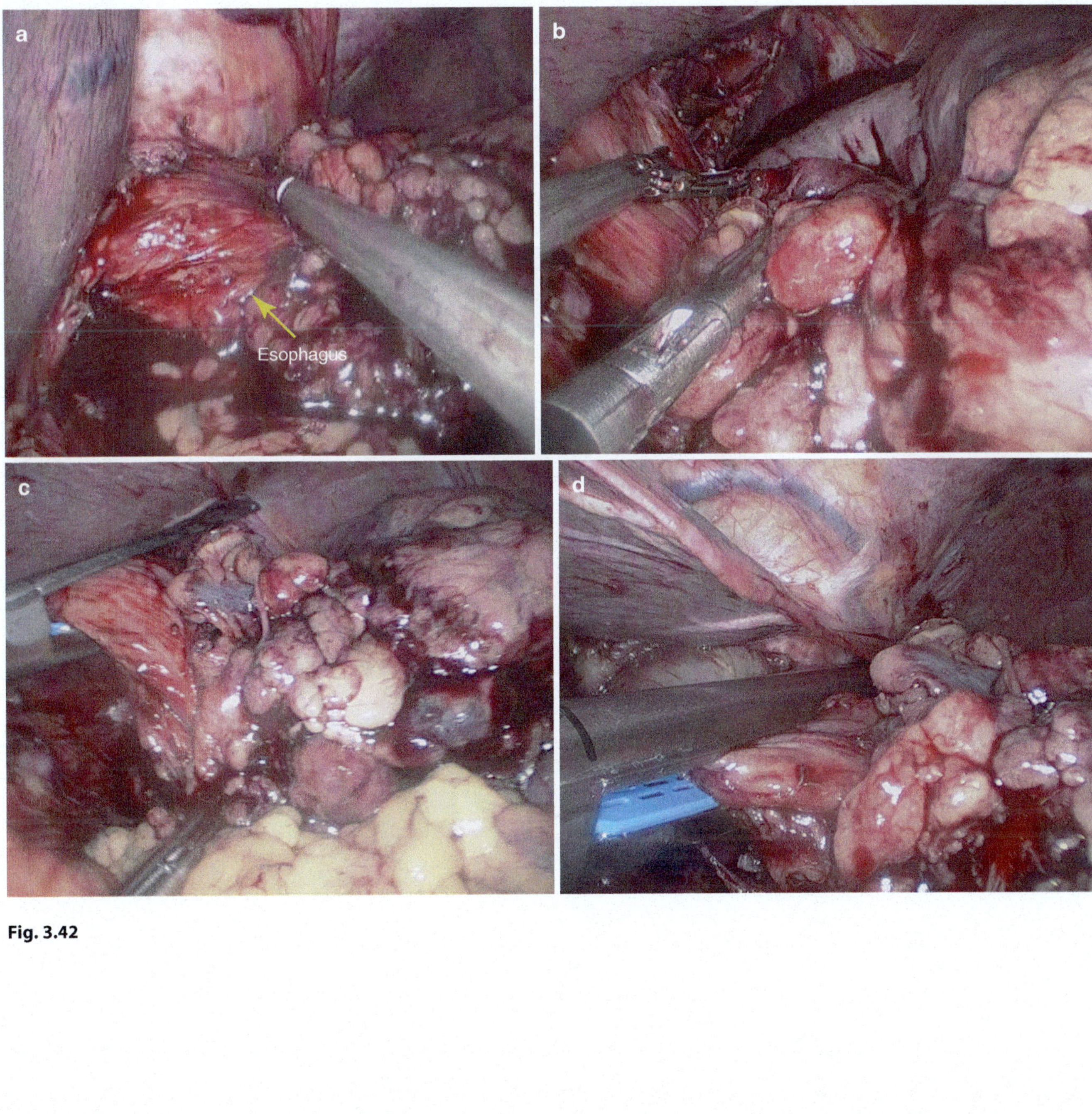

Fig. 3.42

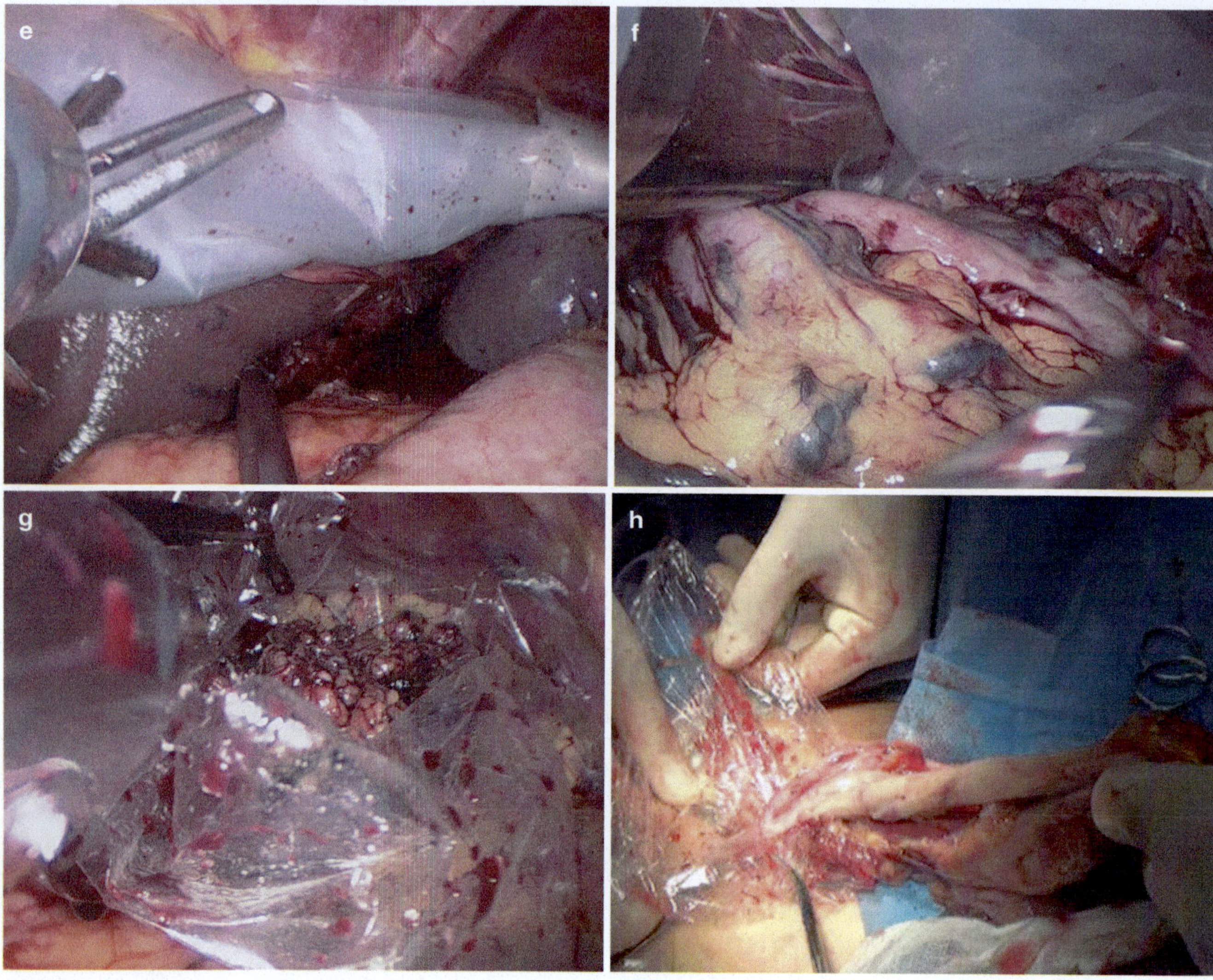

Fig. 3.42 (continued)

6. Esophageal jejunum end-to-side anastomosis.
   A 25 mm Orvil anvil with a guiding tube was inserted into the esophagus through the oral cavity. A small incision was made on the central part of the esophageal stump, through which the guiding tube was pulled out to pull and fix the anvil to the esophageal stump. The fixed line on the guiding tube was cut off and the tube was removed (Fig. 3.43a–f).

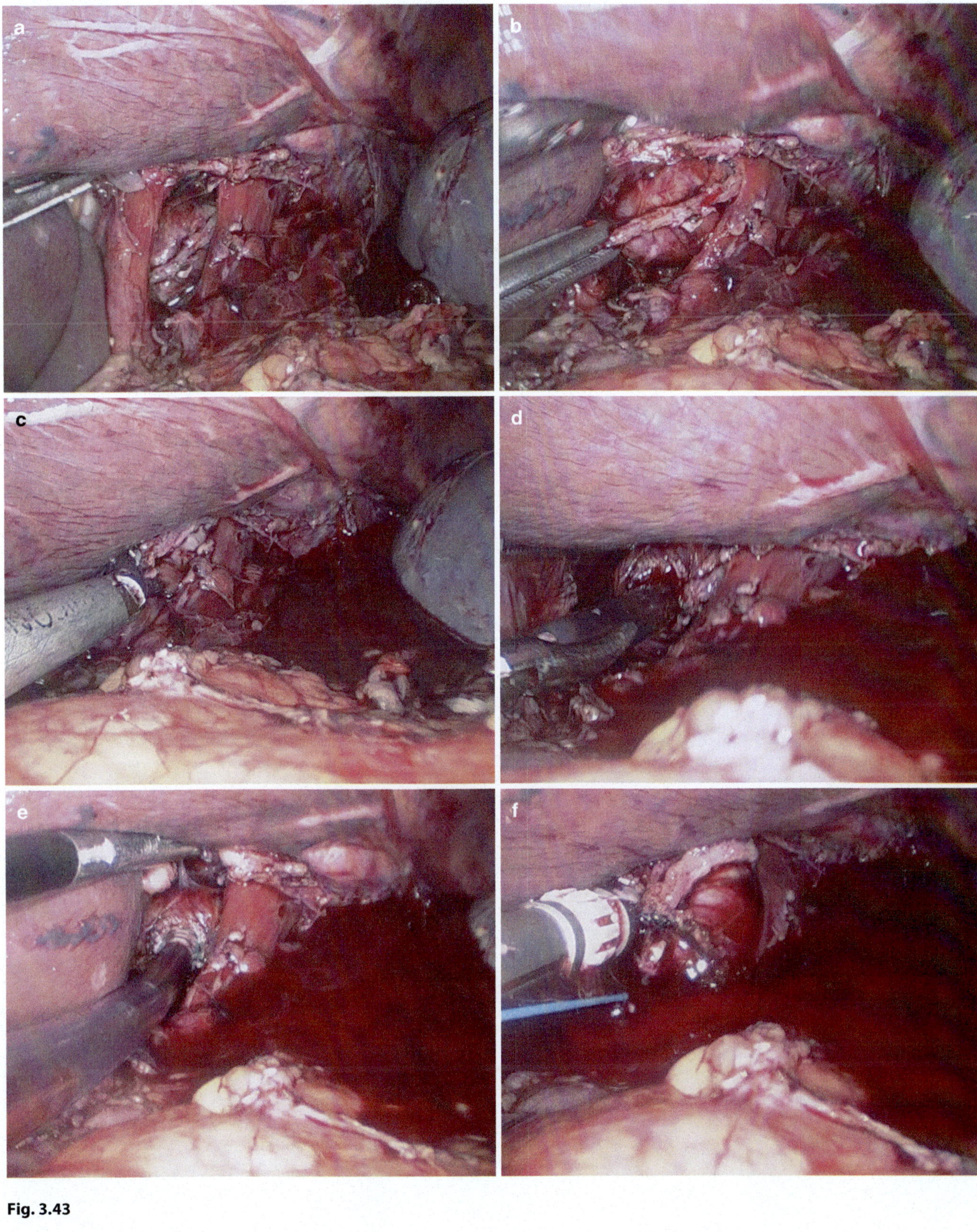

Fig. 3.43

The transverse colon was lifted and the initial proximal jejunum was found along the Treitz ligament. The jejunum was lifted upwards to the subdiaphragmatic area. The suitable length of the jejunum for esophageal anastomosis was designed and the mobility of the mesentery was checked to avoid excessive tension (Fig. 3.44a, b).

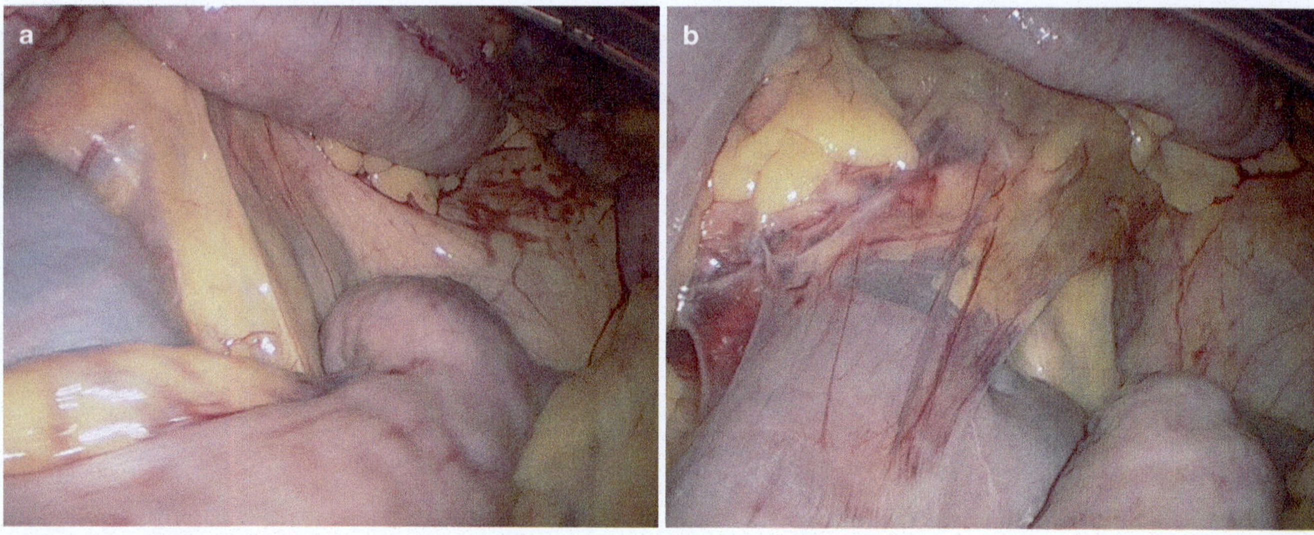

Fig. 3.44

The mesentery of the jejunum to be anastomosed was mobilized by using the harmonic scalpel. The umbilical incision was expanded to 3 cm, through which the jejunum was pulled out of the abdominal cavity and transected under direct vision (Fig. 3.45a–d).

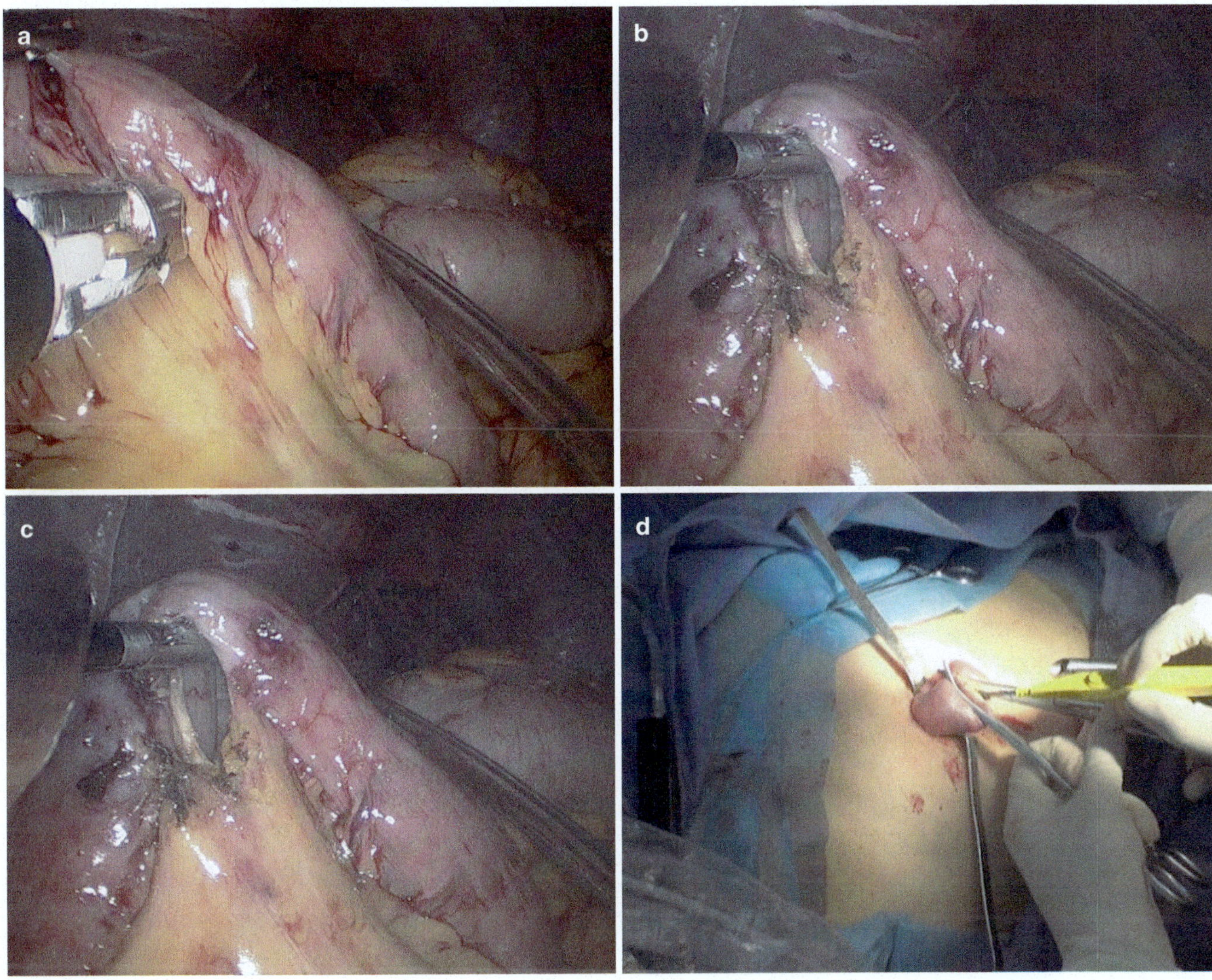

Fig. 3.45

The proximal jejunum was ligated with a 7# silk suture. The stay suture was retained extracorporeally for future searching of the broken end of the jejunum, while the proximal jejunum was put back into the abdominal cavity. The handle lever of the 25 mm circular stapler was implanted into the distal jejunum about 6 cm in depth (Fig. 3.46a, b).

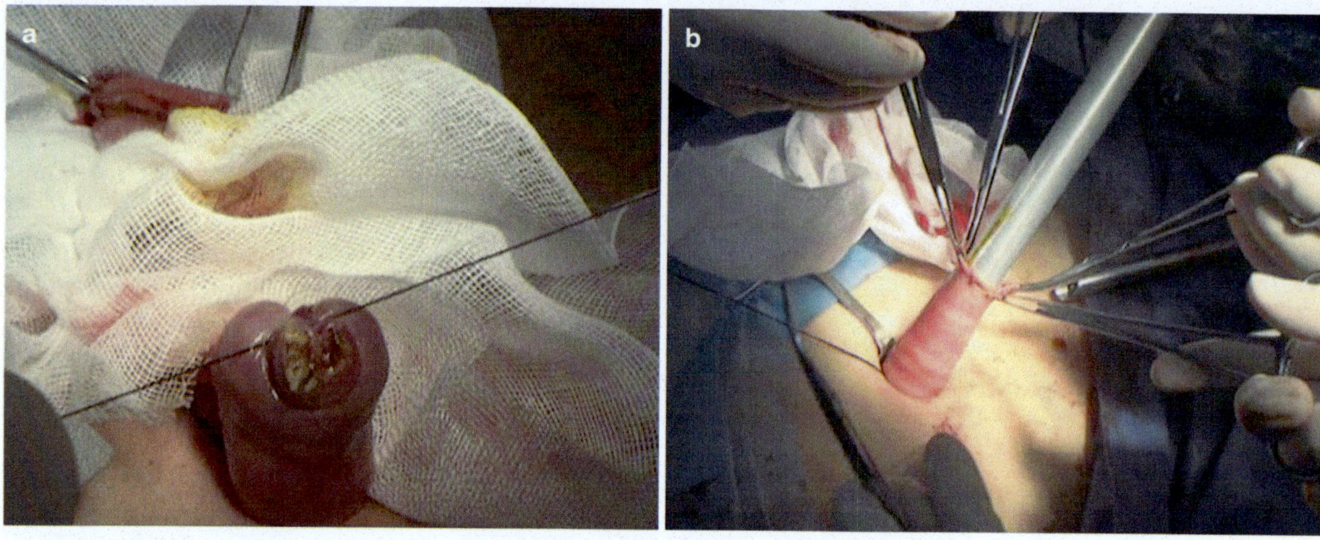

Fig. 3.46

The broken edge of the distal jejunum was fixed on the stapler by using the silk thread ligation. The stapler was introduced into the abdominal cavity and the pneumoperitoneum was re-established (Fig. 3.47a, b).

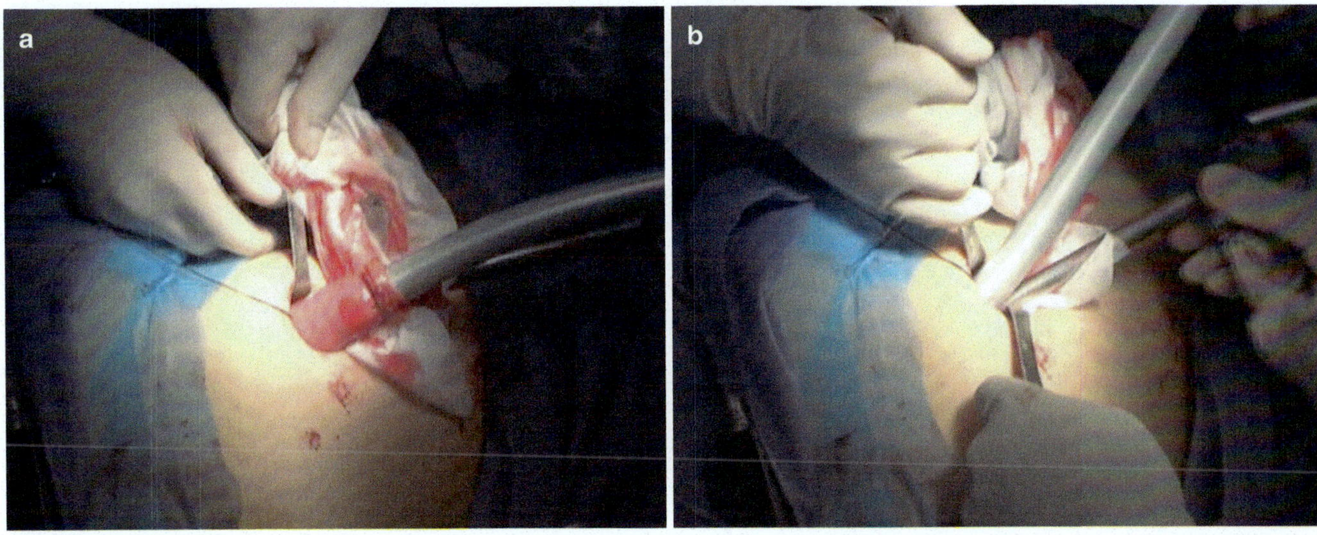

Fig. 3.47

Under the surveillance of the laparoscope, the stapler was screwed out of the lateral wall of the jejunum about 6 cm apart from the broken end of the distal jejunum. The handle lever and anvil of the Orvil stapler were connected, screwed and firmly locked (Fig. 3.48a–n).

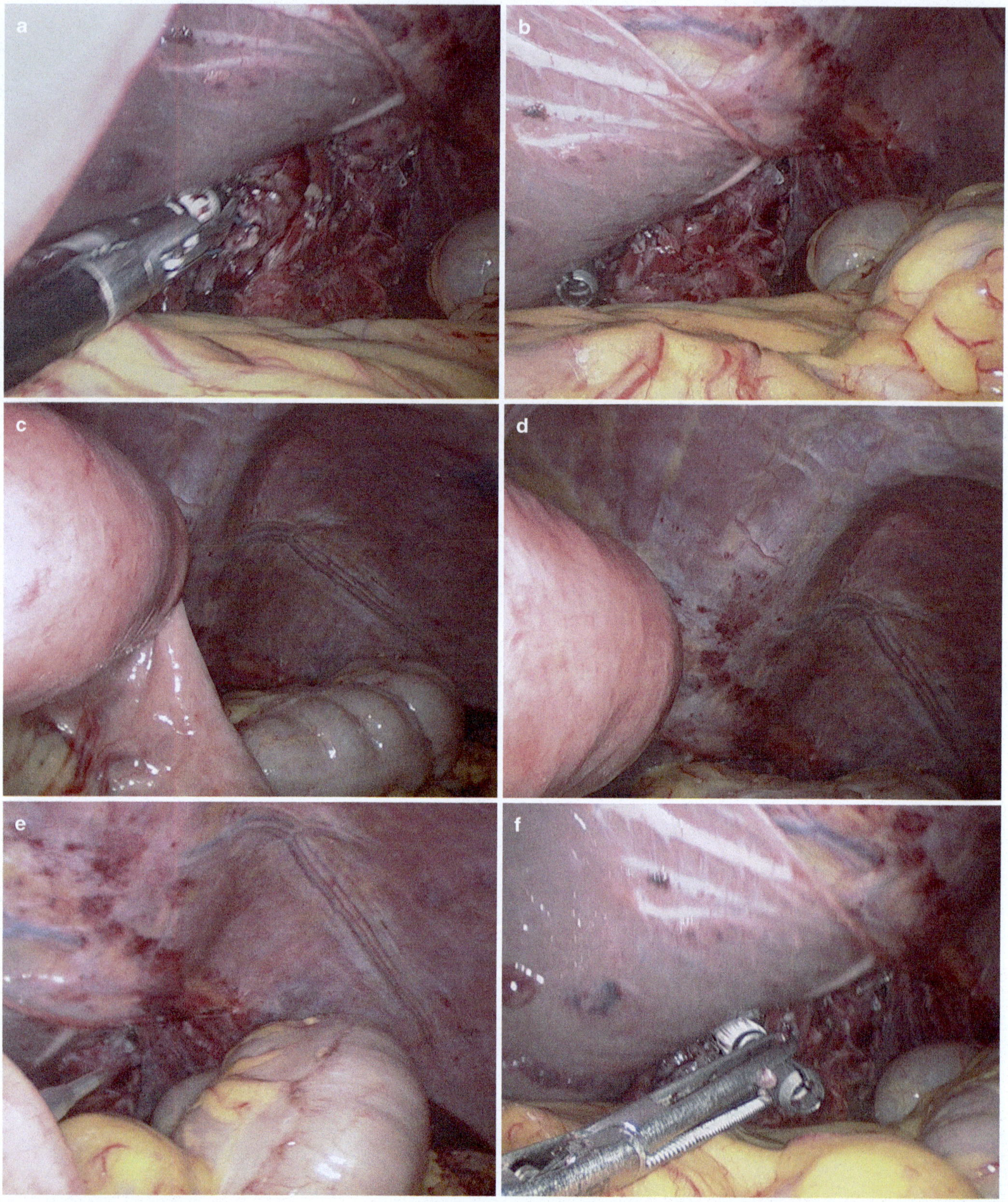

Fig. 3.48

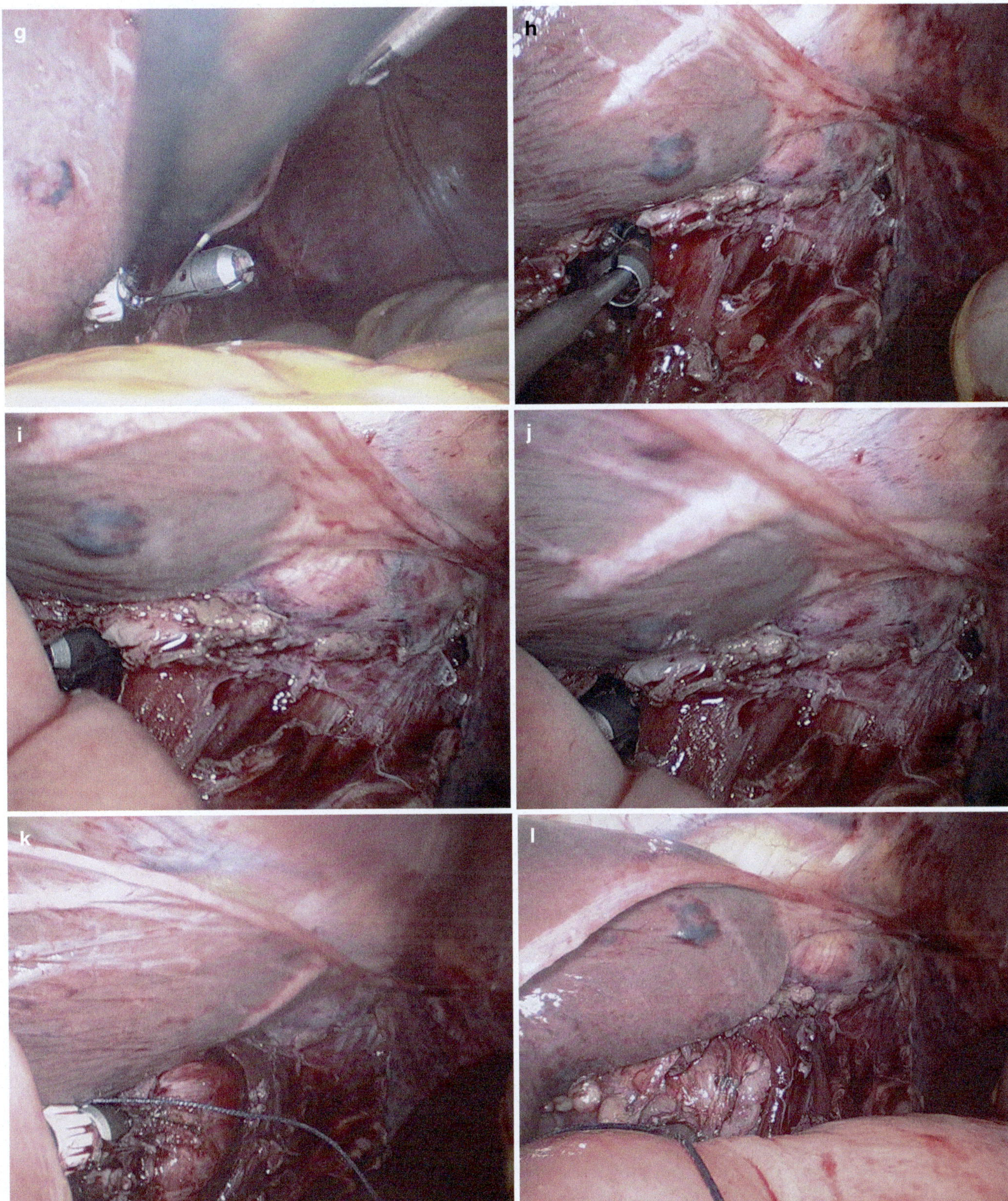

Fig. 3.48 (continued)

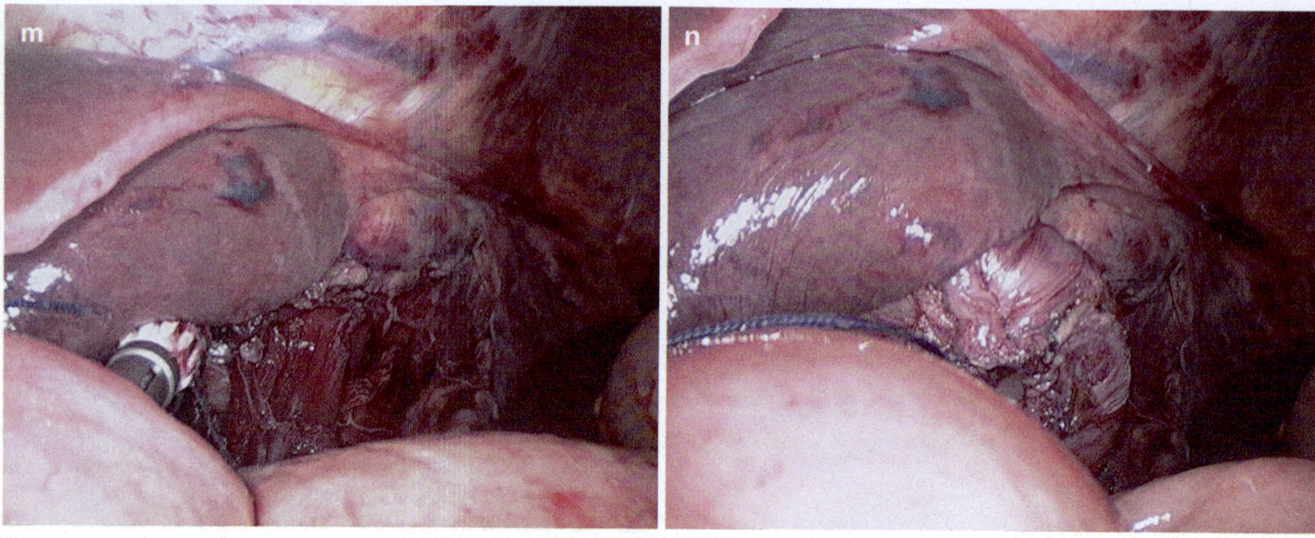

Fig. 3.48 (continued)

After careful checking the connection part, the stapler was fired to complete the esophageal jejunum end-to-side anastomosis. Careful examination of the anastomosis was done to ensure the devoid of torsion, twist or bleeding. The ligation thread on the stapler handle was cut off and the stapler was carefully pulled out of the jejunum (Fig. 3.49a–d).

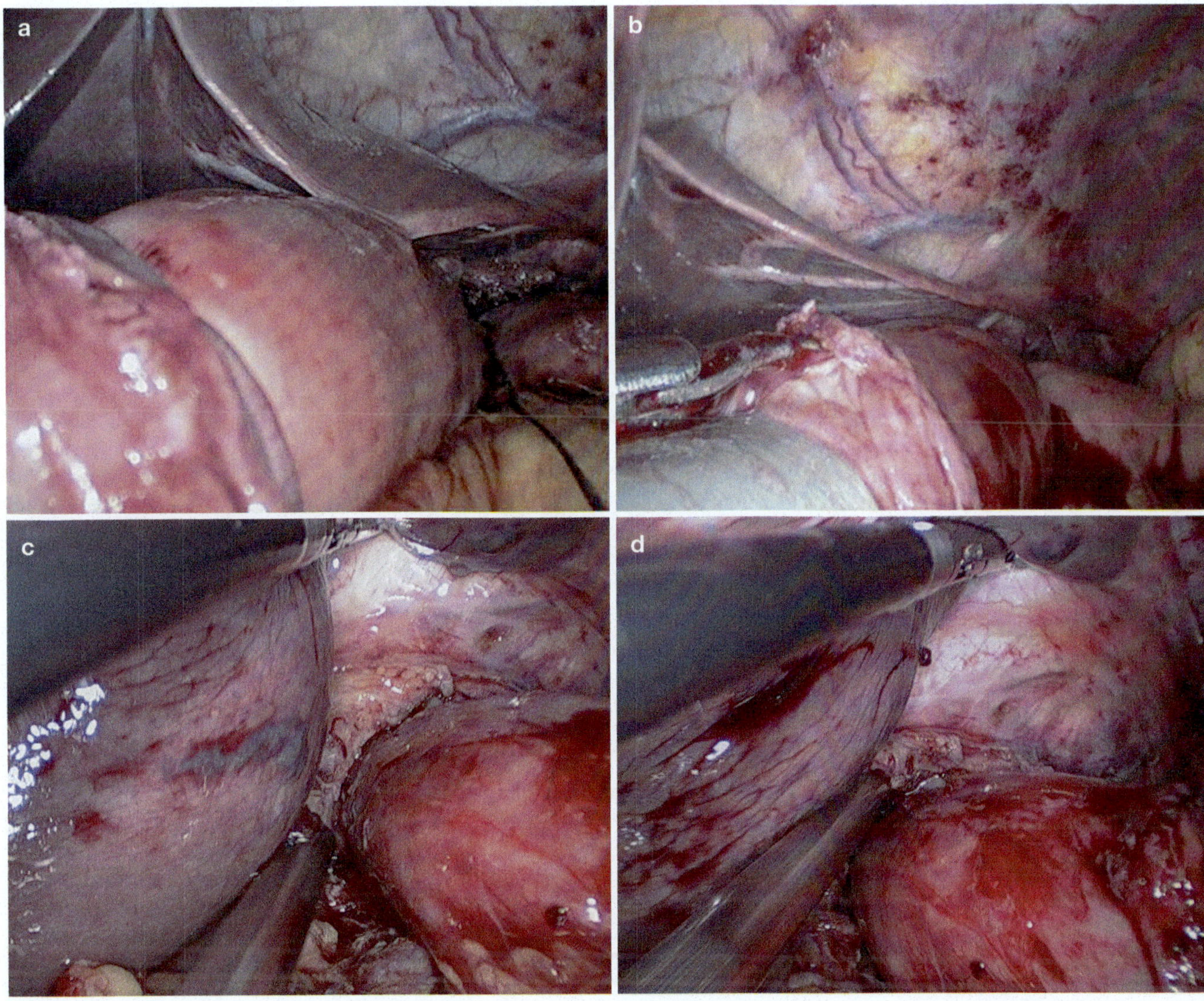

Fig. 3.49

The stump of the distal jejunum was transected by using the flexible linear stapler, then check the anastomosis to avoid leakage or bleeding (Fig. 3.50a–f).

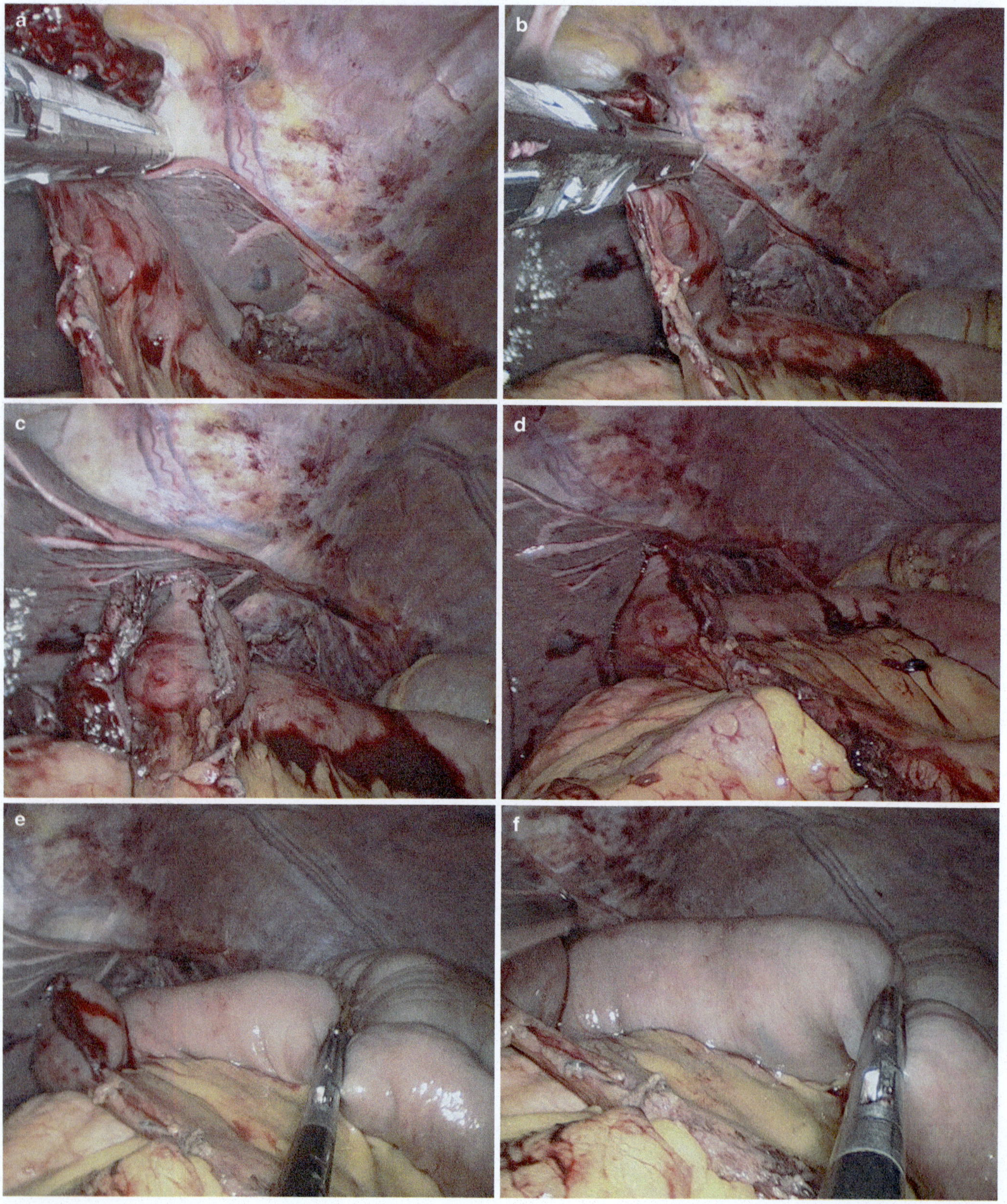

Fig. 3.50

7. Jejunal side-to-side anastomosis.
   The jejunal side-to-side anastomosis was completed extracorporeally under direct vision (Fig. 3.51a, b).

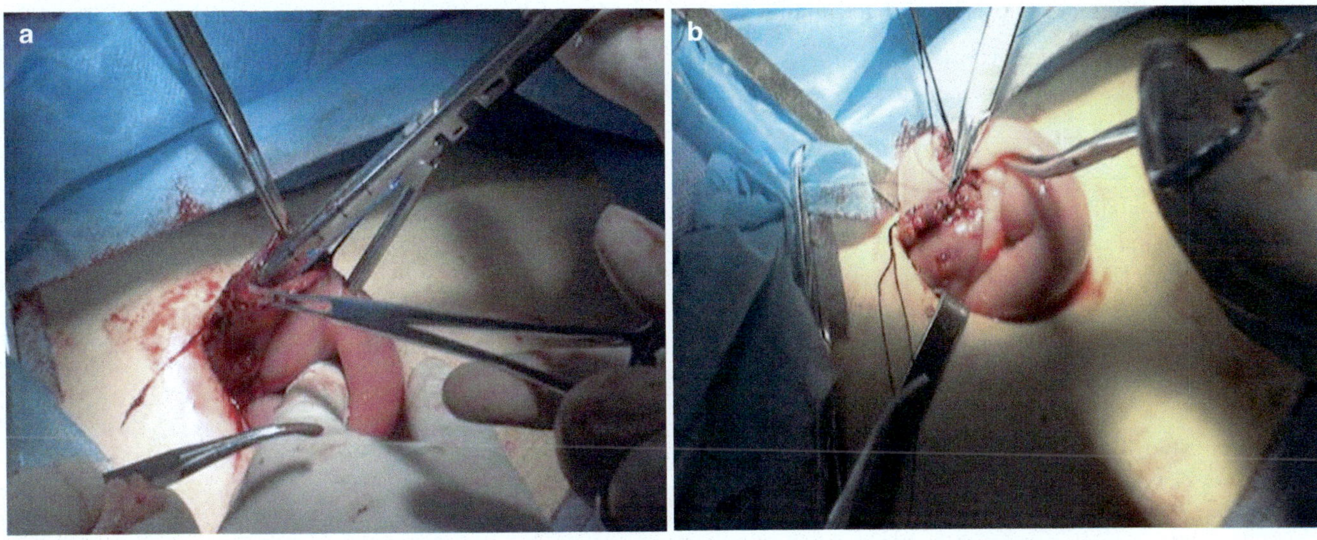

Fig. 3.51

8. Operative field flushing and placement of drainage tube.

   The umbilical incision was sutured and the pneumoperitoneum was re-established. After adequate flushing of the operative field and careful checking of the anastomosis to exclude torsion or twist, a closed suction drain was placed behind the anastomosis through the umbilical incision (Fig. 3.52a–c).

3.4.7 Tips and Tricks

1. Reconstruction of the esophagojejunostomy by double stapling method using EEA™ OrVil™.
2. Placement of an anvil head within the esophagus: As mentioned above.
3. Preparation of lifted jejunum: The jejunum 20 cm away from the ligament of Treitz was led from umbilical incision to outside the abdominal cavity and also cut off with an automated stapler. An automated stapler was inserted from the open end of the lifted jejunum. Then, the main unit of the automated stapler and the lifted jejunum were fastened with silk thread to prevent dropout of the small intestines from the automated stapler. The abdomen was again inflated and the lifted jejunum was led into the abdominal cavity.
4. Connection with anvil, and anastomosis: The anvil and the main unit were connected after it was confirmed that an automated stapler and the center rod were fully made linear. Firing then completed the anastomosis. The inlet of the automated stapler at the open end of the lifted jejunum was closed with an automated stapler inserted via a trocar of the umbilicus. Then, anastomosis between the esophagus and jejunum was completed.

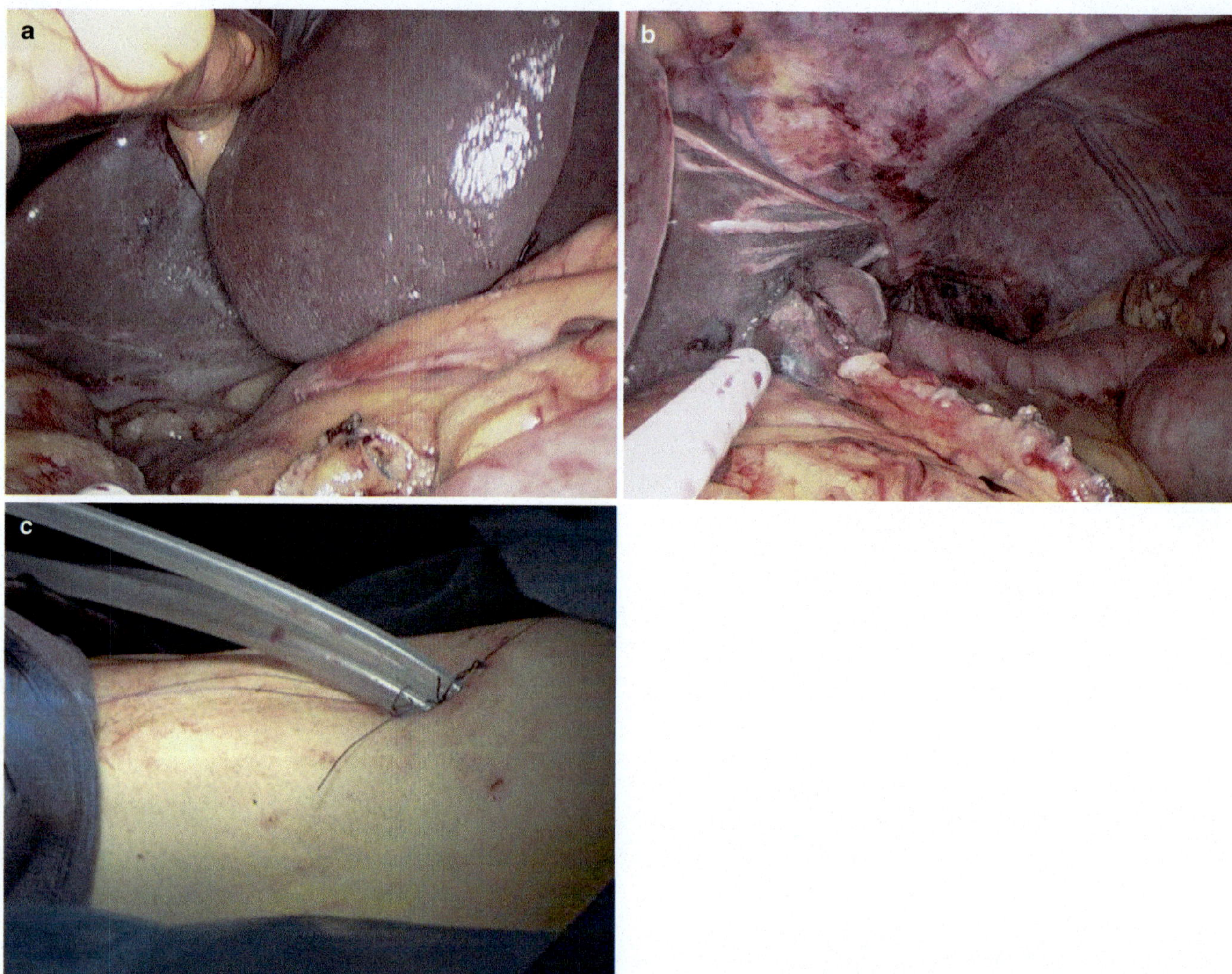

Fig. 3.52

3.5 Complications Analysis and Management

3.5.1 Haemorrhage

The exact hemostasis plays an important role in laparoscopic gastrectomy. Large amount of bleeding may lead to an obscure surgical field, which makes it difficult to identify anatomical structure and affect the surgeon's emotion. Blood can absorb light, therefore making the image on monitor look darkened and vague. Intraoperative haemorrhage is always due to incorrect dissected layer or inadequate hemostatic techniuqe. Excessive dependence on endoscopic stapler is another important reason.

Tearing of short gastric blood vessels, incorrect ligation of left/right gastric vessels and gastroepiploic vessels, falling off clamps and unstable stapling are the primary reasons of postoperative haemorrhage.

The greater risk is the violent tearing of venous structures. Appropriate hemostatic way should be used in unambiguous distinguished artery and veins. Ultrasonic scalpel can directly cut off the vessels less than 1.5 mm in diameter. For the larger vessels, Ligasure or firing stapler is necessary for safe and effective hemostasis. Double ligation by biological clamps is appropriate for larger vessels such as left gastric artery. Though endoscopic linear stapler can staple the gastric wall well, anastomotic stoma of stapler bleeds if the gastric wall is thicker. In this case, hemostatic suture is absolutely essential.

3.5.2 Anastomotic Leak and Duodenal Stump Dehiscence

Patients with anastomotic leaks usually present with abdominal pain, tachycardia, fever, distension and leukocytosis after the fifth postoperative day. With open surgery, laparoscopic gastrectomy also faces anastomotic leak and duodenal stump dehiscence. In the majority of cases, the leak is due to a technical error and failure of the stapler. Because laparoscopic anastomosis depends on different kinds of staplers, reasonable choice and skilled application of staplers are particularly important to avoid anastomotic leak. The model of stapler is just based on the thickness of anastomotic tissue. When the stapler is fired, the surgeon should make sure that no peripheral tissue is tied to stapler. Anastomotic tension and hemodynamic disorder should be avoided. Correct gastrointestinal anastomotic angle can avoid input and output section obstruction. Laparoscopic reinforced suture is necessary to unsatisfied instrumental anastomosis. Injection of methylene blue by stomach tube is an effective method to distinguish the existence of anastomotic leak. Small leaks may be managed non-operatively if they are adequately drained, and may heal spontaneously while the patient is supported using total parenteral nutrition (TPN).

3.5.3 Anastomotic Obstruction

Anastomosis of laparoscopic surgery is always completed by stapler, so the selection criteria and principles of circular stapler are the same with open surgery. Anastomotic site decided the model of stapler. The length of linear stapler determines the length of anastomosis, so shorter stapler always makes smaller anastomosis. Twice fired stapler can form a larger anastomotic stoma. The angle of stapler should be in parallel with vertical axis of jejunum, which can guarantee a free-flowing anastomotic stoma. For additional plasma muscle layer suture, too much tissue should not be involved in the suture part and contralateral should not be sewed.

3.5.4 Intraoperative Failing Anastomosis

It may be due to unsuccessful firing of the stapler or insufficient nailing. Large leaks can be found easily, but small leaks are always observed by injecting methylene blue from stomach tube. In this case, further treatment and even switching to open surgery is always needed.

References

1. Nezhat C, Winer WK, Cooper JD, Nezhat F, Nezhat C. Endoscopic infertility surgery. J Reprod Med. 1989;34:127–34.
2. Liew V, Taylor C, Ghusn M, Jamnagerwalla M, Layani L. Laparoscopic gastric resection research for benign and malignant conditions: lessons learned from 35 consecutive caese. ANZ J Surg. 2007;77:787–91.
3. Saber AA, Elgamal MH, Rao AJ. Single incision laparoscopic sleeve gastrectomy: a novel technique. Obes Surg. 2008;18:1338–42.
4. Morales-Conde S, Dominguez G, Cañete Gomez J, Socas M, Barranco A, García Moreno J, Padillo FJ. Magnetic-assisted single-port sleeve gastrectomy. Surg Innov. 2011. [Epub ahead of print].
5. Lakdawala MA, Muda NH, Goel S, Bhasker A. Single-incision sleeve gastrectomy versus conventional laparoscopic sleeve gastrectomy – a randomised pilot study. Obes Surg. 2011;21:1664–70.
6. Vilallonga R, Rius J, Fort JM, Armengol M. Single port access sleeve gastrectomy: is it reasonable? J Minim Access Surg. 2011;7:156–7.
7. Hirano Y, Watanabe T, Uchida T, Yoshida S, Kato H, Hosokawa O. Laparoendoscopic single site partial resection of the stomach for gastrointestinal stromal tumor. Surg Laparosc Endosc Percutan Tech. 2010;20:262–4.
8. Na J-U, Lee S-IL, Noh S-M. The single incision laparoscopic intragastric wedge resection of gastric submucosal tumor. J Gastric Cancer. 2011;11:225–9.
9. Wu S-D, Kong J, Su Y, Fan Y. Safety and application of transumbilical single-incision laparoscopic gastrectomy for GIST: SILS in Benign Gastric Disease. Surg Innov. 2012. [Epub ahead of print].

10. Henckens T, Van de Putte D, Van Renterghem K, Ceelen W, Pattyn P, Van Nieuwenhove Y. Laparoendoscopic single-site gastrectomy for a gastric GIST using double-bended instruments. J Laparoendosc Adv Surg Tech A. 2010;20:469–71.
11. Dapri G, Ntounda R, Himpens J, Carnevali P, Scomersi S, Cadière GB. Single-incision transumbilical laparo-endoscopic gastric benign tumor resection. Ann Surg Oncol. 2011;18:191.
12. Sasaki A, Koeda K, Nakajima J, Obuchi T, Baba S, Wakabayashi G. Single-incision laparoscopic gastric resection for submucosal tumors: report of three cases. Surg Today. 2011;41:133–6.
13. Nonaka T, Hidaka S, Takafumi A, Fukuoka H, Takeshita H, Atsushi N, Sawai T, Yasutake T, Nagayasu T. Single-incision laparoscopy-assisted subtotal gastrectomy for intractable gastric ulcer: a case report. Surg Laparosc Endosc Percutan Tech. 2012;22:e210–3.
14. Dapri G, El Mourad H, Himpens J, Evola G, Marsili L, Cadière GB. Transumbilical single-access laparoscopic perforated gastric ulcer repair. Surg Innov. 2012;19:130–3.
15. Omori T, Oyama T, Akamatsu H, Tori M, Ueshima S, Nishida T. Transumbilical single-incision laparoscopic distal gastrectomy for early gastric cancer. Surg Endosc. 2011;25:2400–4.
16. Park do J, Lee JH, Ahn SH, Eng AK, Kim HH. Single-port laparoscopic distal gastrectomy with D1 + β lymph node dissection for gastric cancers: report of 2 cases. Surg Laparosc Endosc Percutan Tech. 2012;22:e214–6.
17. Ozdemir BA, Thomas RL, Soon Y. Single-port laparoscopic subtotal gastrectomy with DIα lymphadenectomy. Surg Innov. 2011;18:NP1–4.
18. Takahashi T, Takeuchi H, Kawakubo H, Saikawa Y, Wada N, Kitagawa Y. Single-incision laparoscopic surgery for partial gastrectomy in patients with a gastric submucosal tumor. Am Surg. 2012;78:447–50.
19. Lee JH, Lee MS, Kim HH, et al. Comparison of single-incision laparoscopic distal gastrectomy and laparoscopic distal gastrectomy for gastric cancer in a porcine model. J Laparoendosc Adv Surg Tech A. 2011;21:935–940.

Colorectal Surgery

4

Abstract

Since a case series on laparoscopic colectomy was firstly published in 1991 (Jacobs et al., Surg Laparosc Endosc 1:144–150, 1991), various randomized controlled trials (RCTs), non-RCTs and other types of studies had been performed, focusing on the evaluation of feasibility and safety of laparoscopic colorectal surgeries. Several meta-analyses and systematic reviews basing on RCTs and non-RCTs related to the comparison of laparoscopic and laparotomic colorectal surgeries have been established, finding out that laparoscopic surgery for colorectal cancer was non-inferior to laparotomy in terms of overall survival (Martel et al., PLoS One 7:e35292, 2012), short-term and long-term of oncological outcomes (Huang et al., Int J Colorectal Dis 26:415–421, 2011; Ma et al., Med Oncol 28:925–933, 2011), and also with shorter post-operative hospital stay (Lourenco et al., Surg Endosc 22:1146–1160, 2008). No significant differences were identified in the occurrence of major surgical complications but were associated with lower overall morbidity and minor complication rate in the management of diverticulitis (Siddiqui et al., Am J Surg 200:144–161, 2010; Cirocchi et al., Colorectal Dis 14:671–683, 2012) in the laparoscopic groups.

Substantially, laparoendoscopic single-site colorectal surgery (SILSC) is an evaluation of traditional multiport laparoscopic colorectal surgery (MLC), offering the minimally invasive advantages and cosmetic advantages over MLC with a single incision typically hidden in the umbilicus (Lu et al., Colorectal Dis 14:e171–e176, 2012). It has been applied to several colorectal procedures successfully, including right hemicolectomy, total colectomy, proctocolectomy with ileal pouch anal anastomosis, and left colectomy (Lu et al., Colorectal Dis 14:e171–e176, 2012; Chen et al., Surg Endosc 25:1887–1892, 2011; Kim et al., Ann Surg 254:933–940, 2011; Lai et al., Colorectal Dis 14:1138–1144, 2012; Papaconstantinou and Thomas, Surgery 150:820–827, 2011; Fujii et al., Surg Endosc 26:1403–1411, 2012; Poon et al., Surg Endosc 26:2729–2734, 2012; Ramos-Valadez et al., Surg Endosc 26:96–102, 2012; Rijcken et al., Dis Colon Rectum 55:140–146, 2012; Huscher et al., Am J Surg 204:115–120, 2012; Lee et al., Dis Colon Rectum 54:1355–1361, 2011; Waters et al., Dis Colon Rectum 53:1467–1472, 2010; Champagne et al., Dis Colon Rectum 54:183–186, 2011; Champagne et al., Ann Surg 255:66–69, 2012; Adair et al., Dis Colon Rectum 53:1549–1554, 2010; Gaujoux et al., J Gastrointest Surg 16:629–634, 2012; Kanakala et al., Tech Coloproctol 16:423–428, 2012; McNally et al., Surg Endosc 25:3559–3565, 2011; Wolthuis et al., Colorectal Dis 14:634–641, 2012; Papaconstantinou et al., J Am Coll Surg 213:72–80, 2011). A deceased post-operative pain score was reported, which might be due to the reduced number of lateral ports, thus decreasing post-operative discomfort (Champagne et al., Dis Colon Rectum 54:183–186, 2011; Chambers et al., Colorectal Dis 13:393–398, 2011). Additionally, the lower cost

S. Wu et al. (eds.), *Atlas of Single-Incision Laparoscopic Operations in General Surgery*,
DOI 10.1007/978-94-007-6955-7_4, © Springer Science+Business Media Dordrecht 2013

(McNally et al., Surg Endosc 25:3559–3565, 2011; Chambers et al., Colorectal Dis 13:393–398, 2011), faster recovery (Chambers et al., Colorectal Dis 13:393–398, 2011), decreased length of the largest incision (Lu et al., Colorectal Dis 14:e171–e176, 2012; Fujii et al., Surg Endosc 26:1403–1411, 2012; Lee et al., Dis Colon Rectum 54:1355–1361, 2011; Zhou et al., Dig Dis Sci 57:2103–2112, 2012), and diminished risk of incisional hernias (Ramos-Valadez et al., Surg Endosc 26:96–102, 2012) were also reviewed.

Though no criteria of contraindications for SILSC has been created, emergent condition, T4 tumors, history of abdominal surgery, morbid obesity, poor American Society of Anesthesiologists class or large size of malignant disease may act as risk factors for the performance of SILSC (Chen et al., Surg Endosc 25:1887–1892, 2011; Kim et al., Ann Surg 254:933–940, 2011; Ramos-Valadez et al., Surg Endosc 26:96–102, 2012; Huscher et al., Am J Surg 204:115–120, 2012; Waters et al., Dis Colon Rectum 53:1467–1472, 2010).

Though with potentially higher overall conversion rate, SILSC may be more feasible and safe in experienced hands if the patients are carefully selected, especially for malignancies. SILSC will benefit the patients more with its superiority over MLC.

Keywords

Cecectomy • Terminal ileum resection • Ileocolic anastomosis • Line of Toldt • Right hemicolectomy • Gerota's fascia • Toldt's fascia • Tranverse colectomy • Sigmoidectomy • Colorectal anastomosis • Rectal Carcinoma • Dixon Technique • Miles Technique • Artificial anus • Pancolectomy • Ileosigmoid anastomosis • Appendectomy

4.1 Laparoscopic Cecectomy and Terminal Ileum Resection

4.1.1 Indications and Case Selection

Laparoscopic cecectomy and terminal ileectomy is most frequently indicated in patients with benign disease located in the ileocecal regions, including.

1. Crohn's disease.
2. Cecal diverticulitis.
3. Intestinal tuberculosis.
4. Enteric Behcet's disease.
5. Submucosal tumors: including lipoma, gastrointestinal stromal tumor, lymphoma, carcinoid, etc.
6. Giant villous adenoma.
7. Polyps.

4.1.2 Contraindications

1. Patients with nonlocalized intraabdominal abscesses.
2. Patients underwent multiple previous bowel operations with possible dense adhesions.
3. Patients having fixed mass with multiple fistulas.
4. Patients with acute intestinal obstruction.
5. Patients underwent perforation of cecum or terminal ileum.

4.1.3 Major Instruments or Energy Sources

1. Laparoscopy System.
2. Electrocautery.
3. Harmonic scalpel.
4. Endoscopic linear and circular stapler.

4.1.4 Team Setup, Anesthesia and Position

Under general anesthesia, the patient was placed in supine position with the arms adducted along the side. The position of surgeon, assistants and nurses is shown in Fig. 4.1.

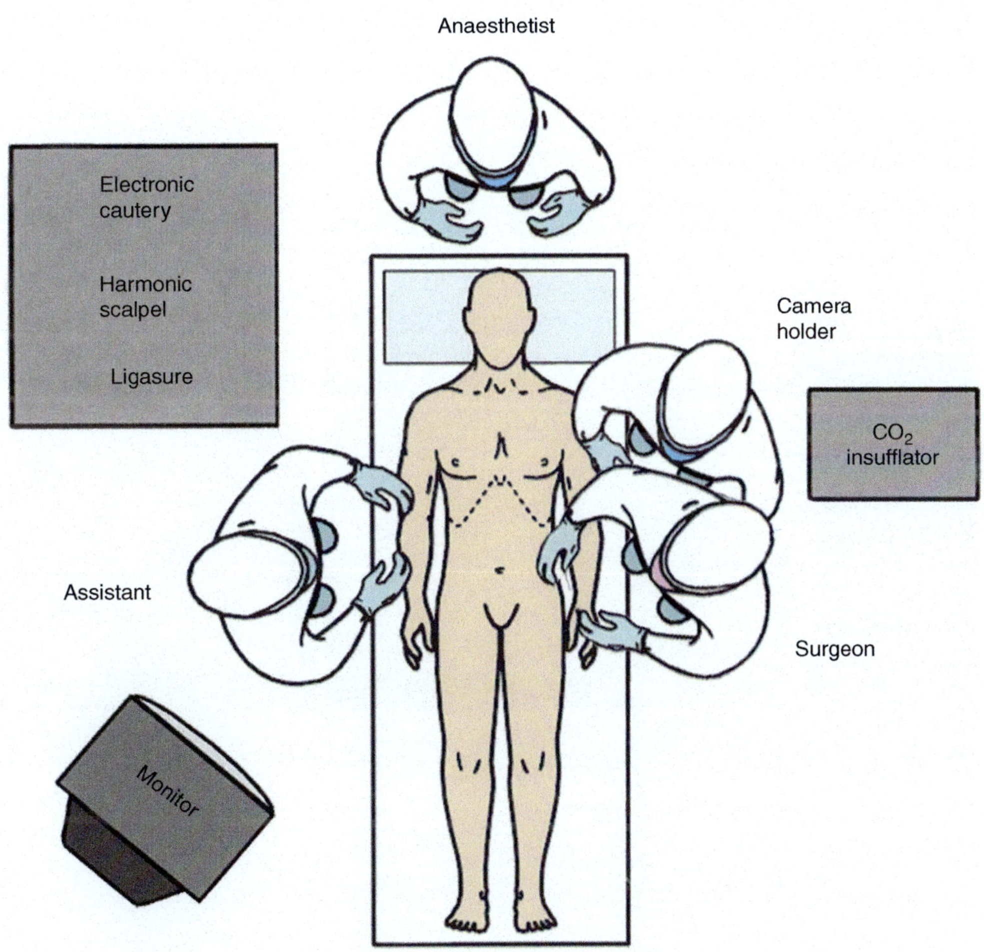

Fig. 4.1

4.1.5 Key Steps

1. Establishment of Pneumoperitoneum and Placement of Trocars.
2. Mobilization of the ascending colon.
3. Mobilization of the terminal ileum.
4. Ileal resection and purse-string suture.
5. Ileocolic end-to-side anastomosis.
6. Cecectomy and Terminal Ileum Resection.
7. Flushing and suturing the incision.

4.1.6 Surgical Techniques

1. Establishment of Pneumoperitoneum and Placement of Trocars.
2. Mobilization of the ascending colon.
   A lateral to medial technique was used by the surgeon. The ascending colon was retracted medially by using an atraumatic forceps in the left hand. The terminal ileum, cecum, and ascending colon were mobilized from the line of Toldt to the midline by using the harmonic scalpel. Small bleeders encountered were cauterized. The right ureter was identified and preserved (Fig. 4.2a–h).

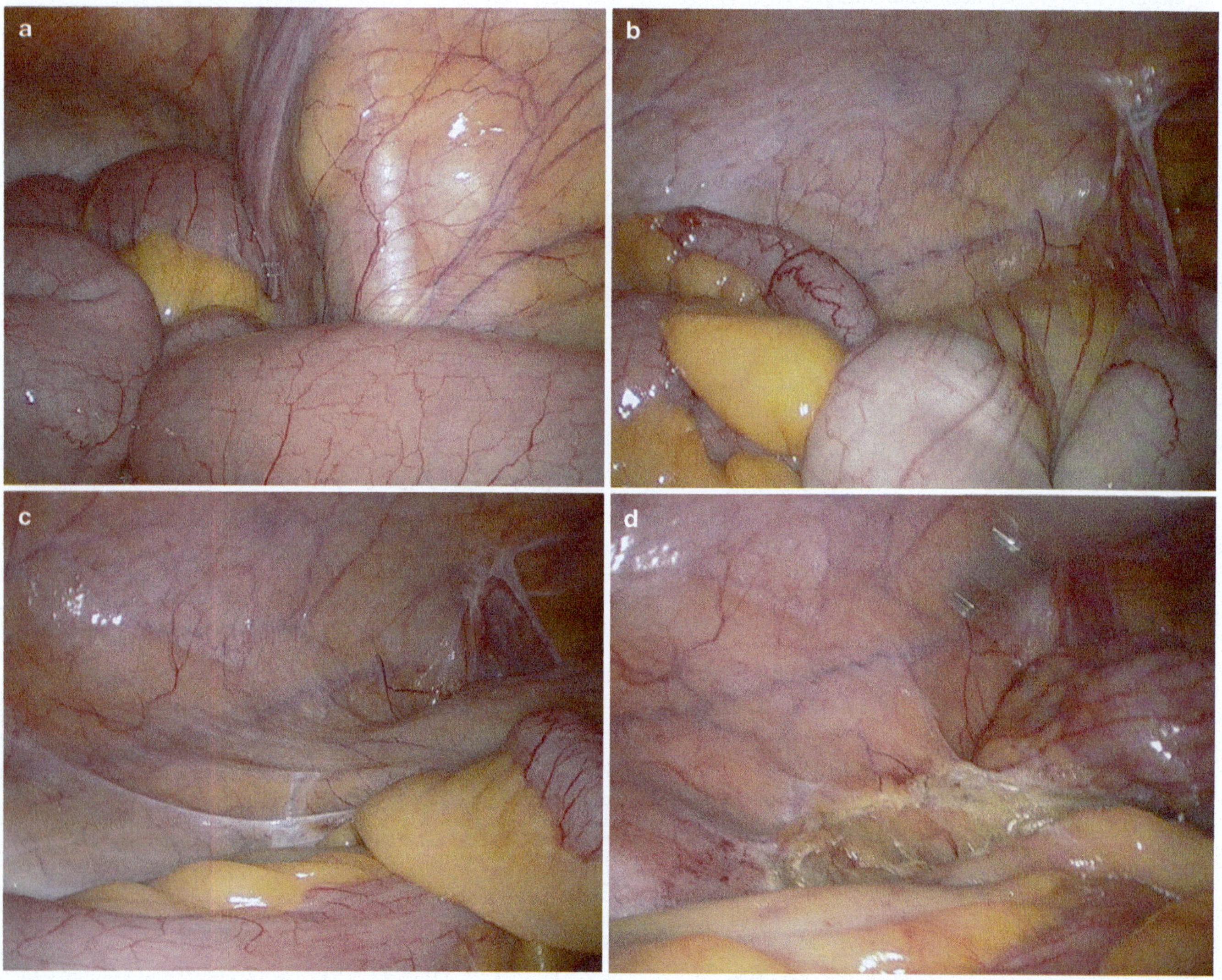

Fig. 4.2

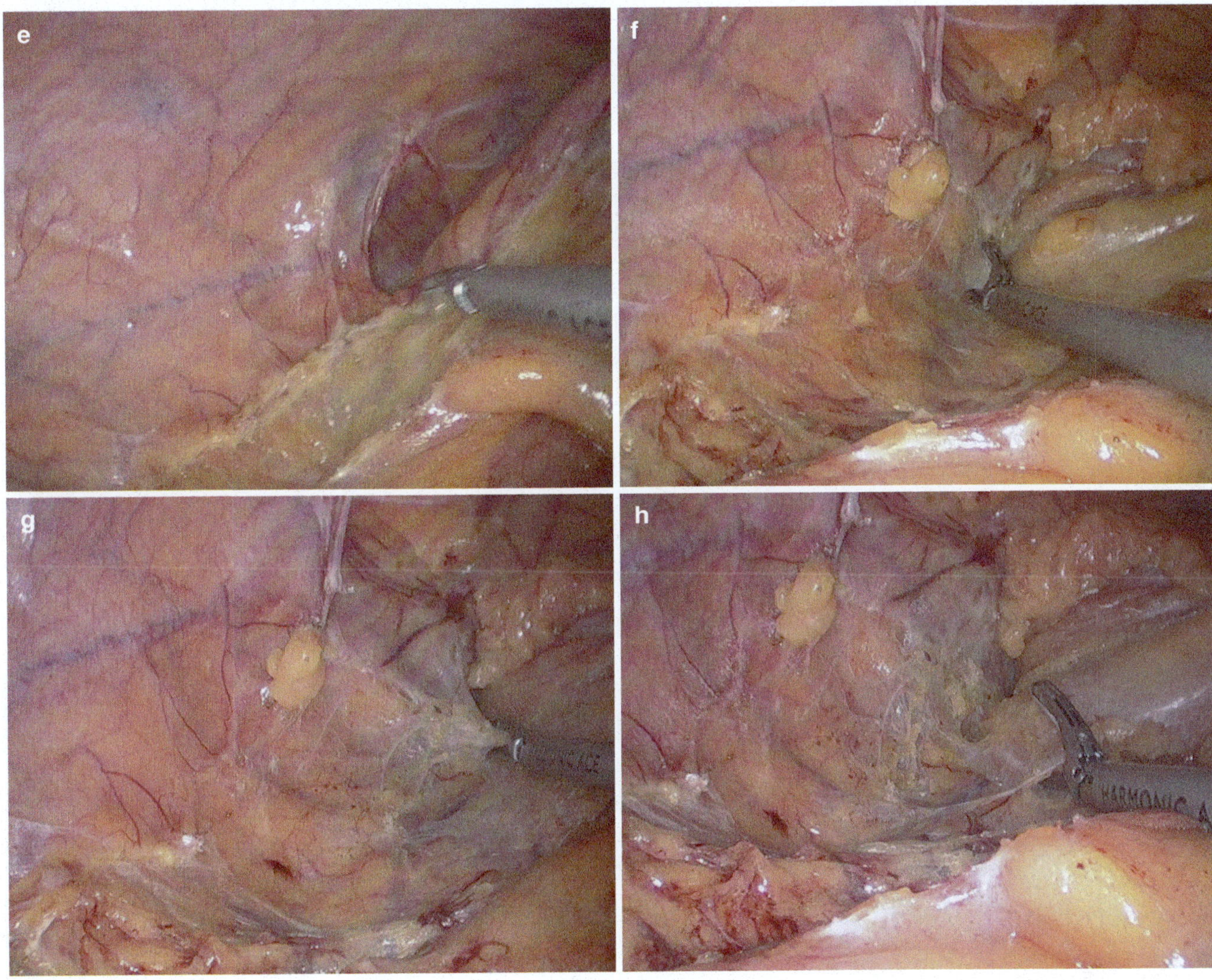

Fig. 4.2 (continued)

3. Mobilization of the terminal ileum.
   The terminal ileum was lifted superiorly and laterally to expose the mesentery of the ileum. The mesentery was mobilized by using the harmonic scalpel and the ileocolic vessels were ligated and amputated until the terminal ileum, cecum and ascending colon were completely mobilized from their posterior attachment (Fig. 4.3a–f).

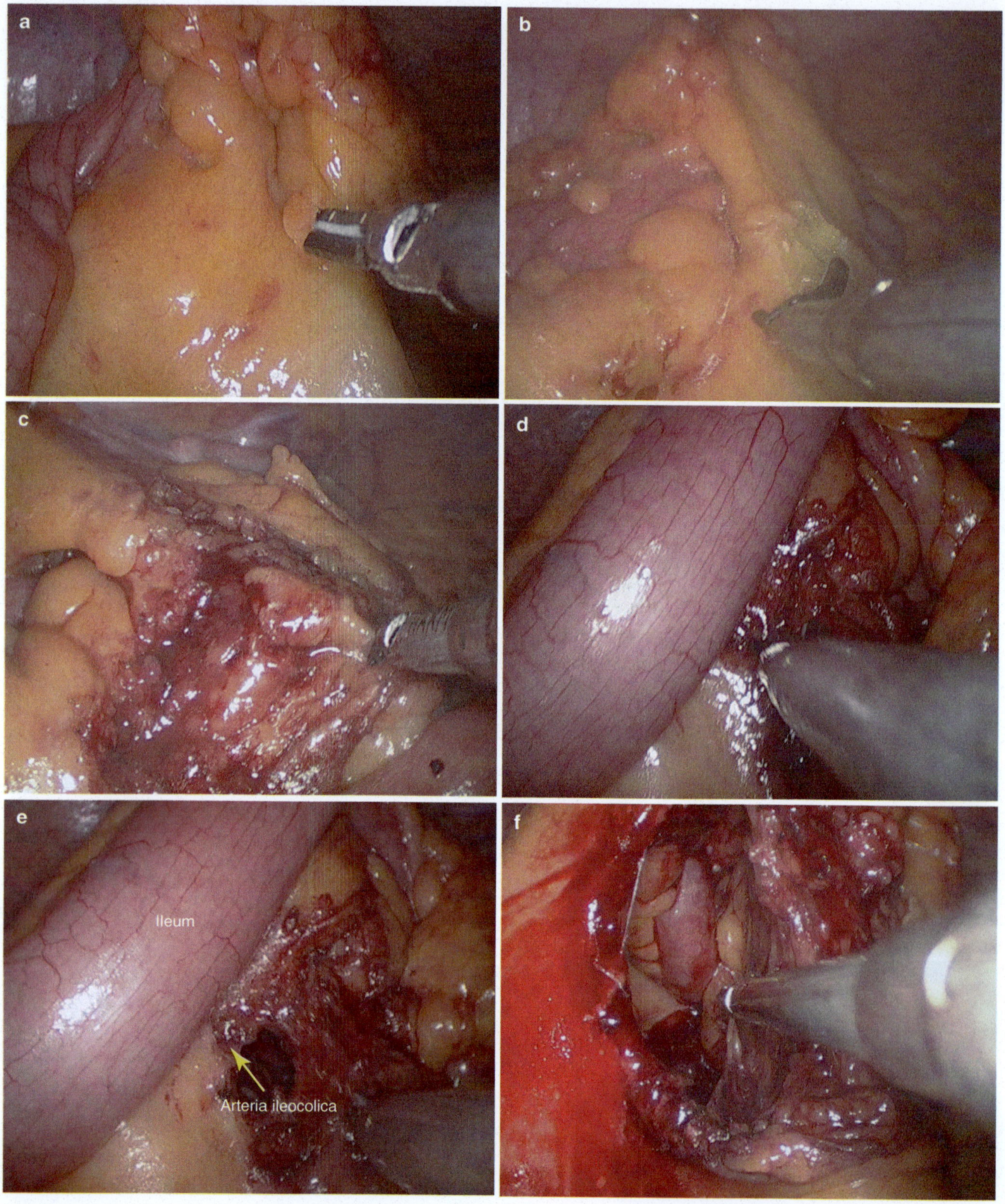

Fig. 4.3

4. Ileal resection and purse-string suture.
   Once mobilization was complete, the ports were removed and the incision was extended to 3 cm total in length to facilitate exteriorization of the specimen. The terminal ileum, cecum, and ascending colon were then brought outside the abdomen. A purse-string stapler was used to divide the terminal 10 cm ileum. The anvil of the circular stapler was put into the proximal stump of the ileum and embedded (Fig. 4.4a–h).

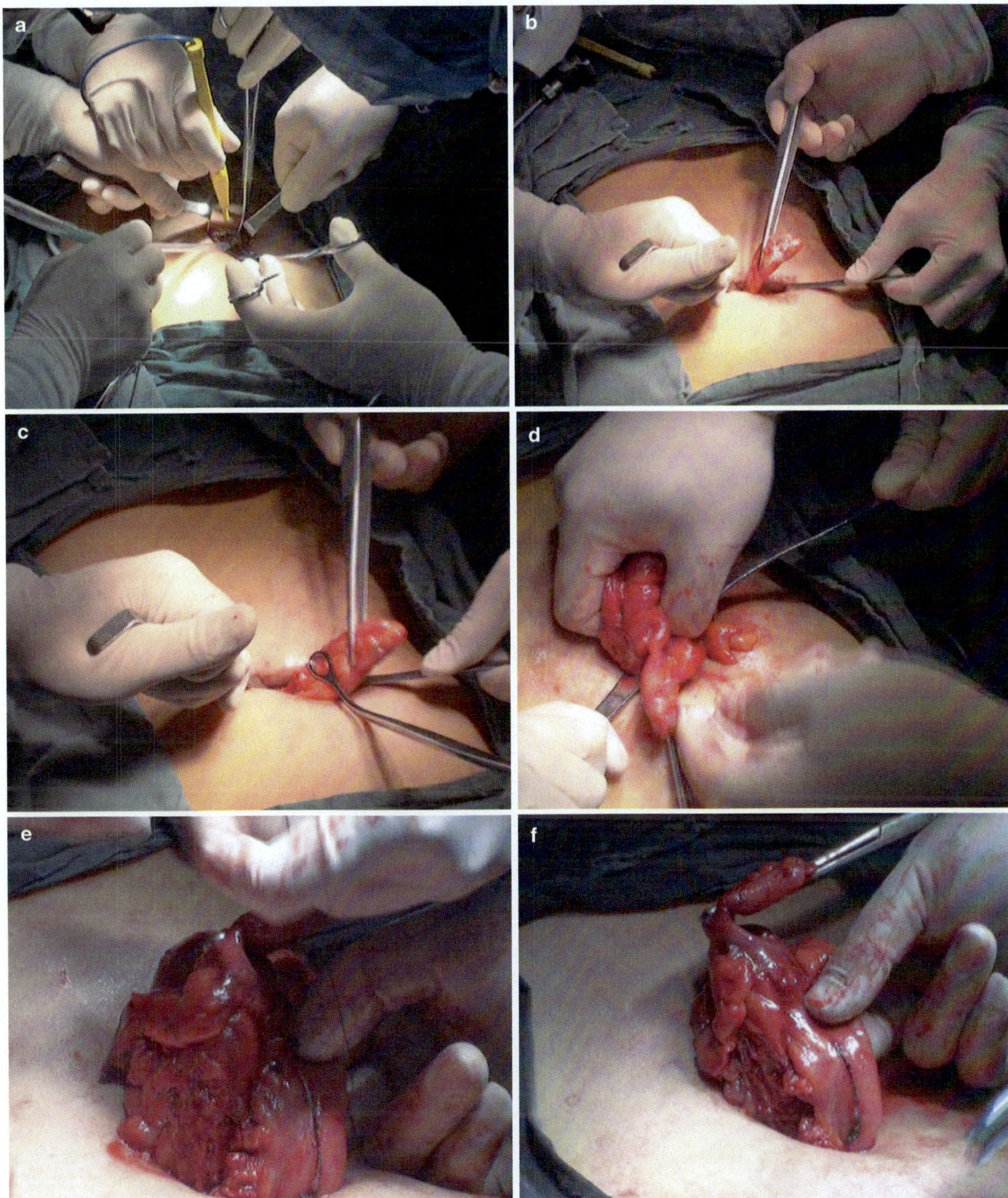

Fig. 4.4

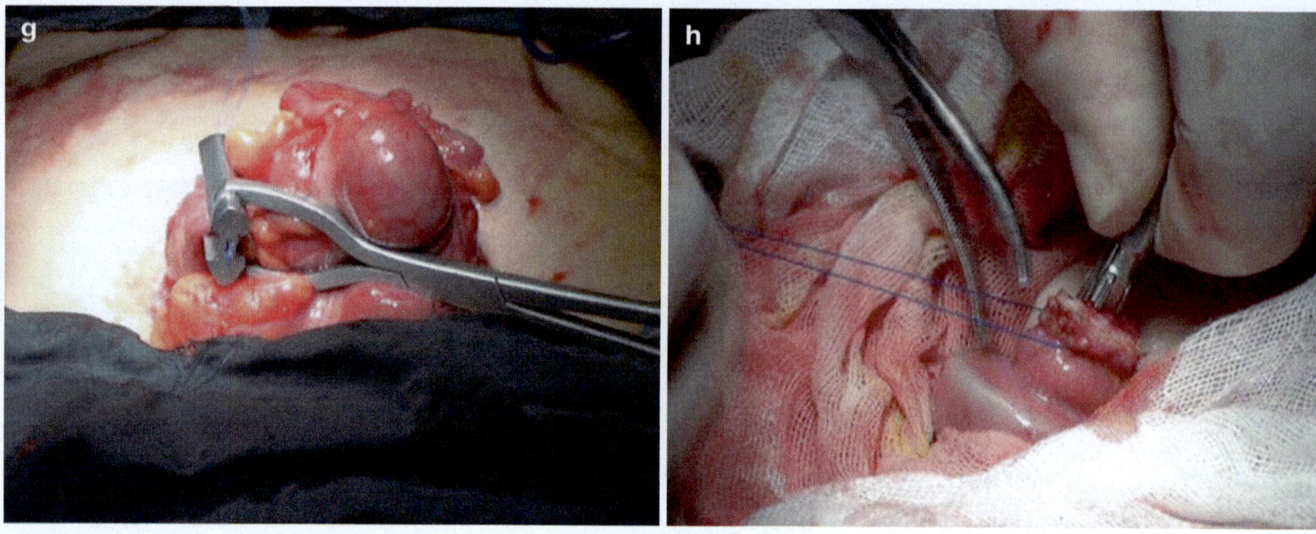

Fig. 4.4 (continued)

5. Ileocolic end-to-side anastomosis.
   An incision was made on the anterior wall of the cecum and the handle lever of the circular stapler was implanted into the colic lumen through this incision and punctured out through the lateral wall of the ascending colon where the anastomosis was to be made. The handle lever and anvil of the stapler were connected, screwed and firmly locked. After careful checking the connection part, the stapler was fired to complete the ileocolic end-to-side anastomosis. Careful examination of the anastomosis was done ensure the devoid of torsion, twist or bleeding (Fig. 4.5a–f).

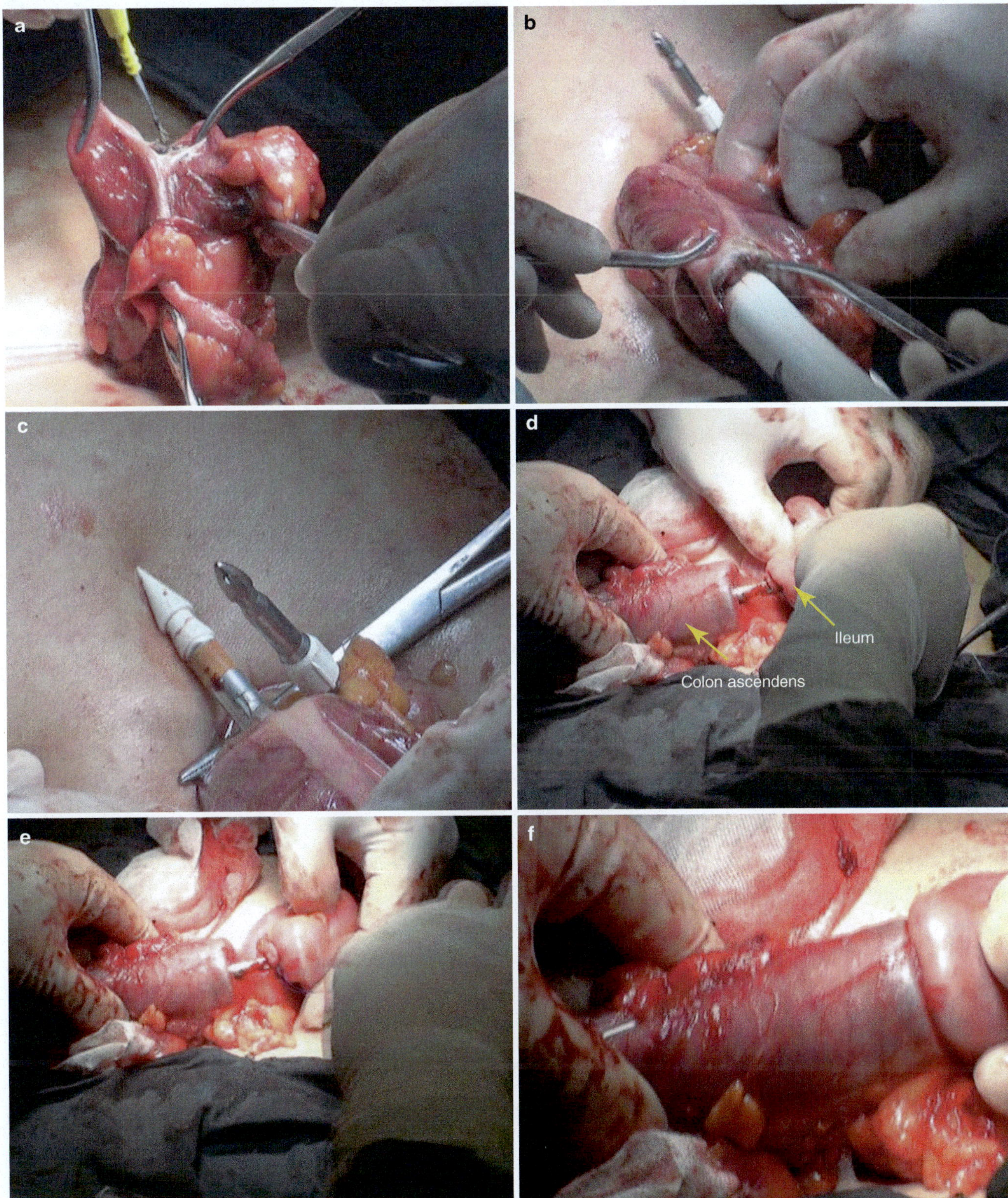

Fig. 4.5

6. Cecectomy and Terminal Ileum Resection.
The colectomy was closed with a liner stapler 2–3 cm distal to the anastomosis. The whole specimen including the cecum and terminal ileum were removed. We closed the mesentery by using 2-0 silk figure-of-eight sutures. The stump of the ascending colon was embedded by using continuous seromuscular layer suture with absorbable thread (Fig. 4.6a, b).

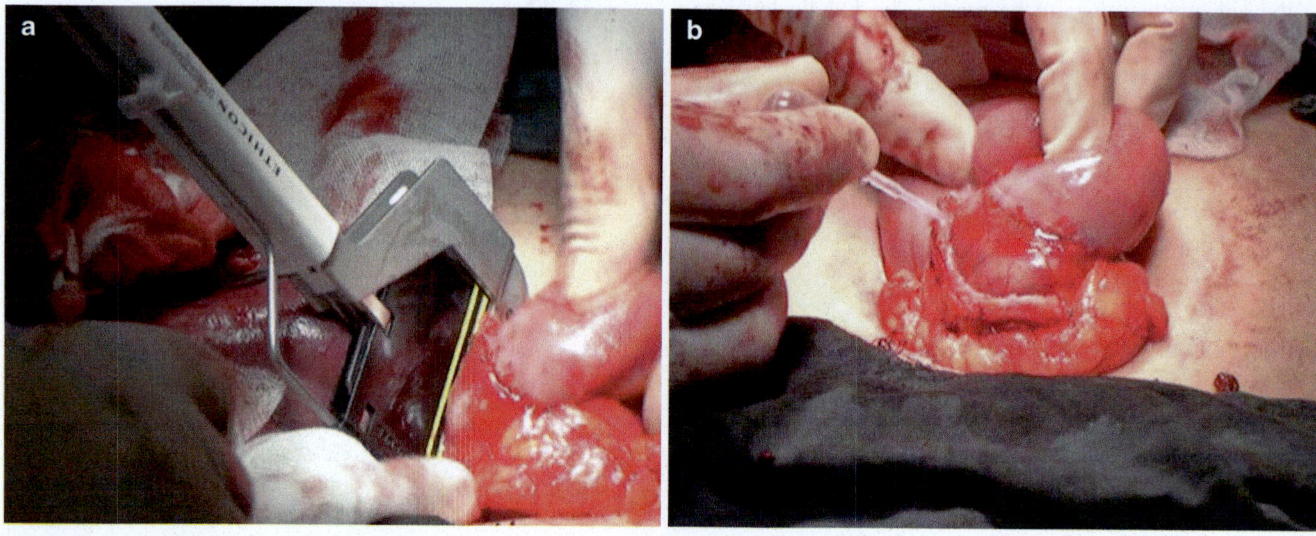

Fig. 4.6

7. Flushing and suturing the incision.
   The anastomosis was then pushed back into the abdominal cavity. Three trocars were reinserted and routine inspection and washing were performed. After carefully checking the anastomosis to exclude torsion or twist, a closed suction drain was placed near the anastomosis through the umbilical incision (Fig. 4.7a–d).

4.1.7 Tips and Tricks

1. Ileocolic resection involves mobilizing the right colon and terminal ileum with extracorporeal vessel transection and anastomosis.
2. The patient should be prepared and secured to the table the same way as any laparoscopic procedure. Split-leg extenders can be beneficial for the camera driver to stay out of the field of motion of the operating surgeon in the procedures.

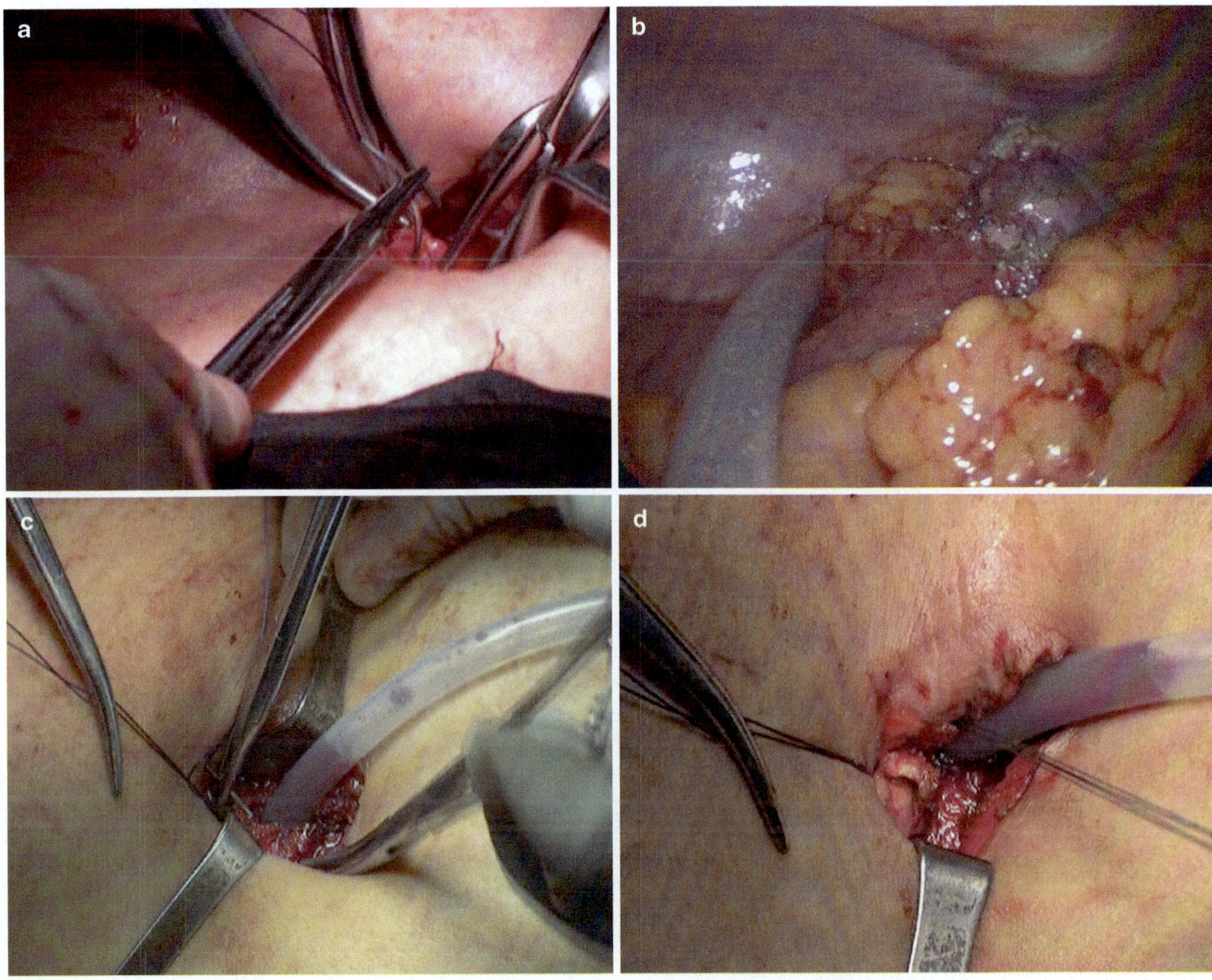

Fig. 4.7

4.2 Laparoscopic Right Hemicolectomy

4.2.1 Indications and Case Selection

1. Patients with severe damages of the cecum or ascending colon.
2. Patients with malignancies in the cecum, ascending colon, or hepatic flexure of colon, but with no remote metastasis.
3. Patients with ileocecal tuberculosis complicated with partial intestinal obstruction.
4. Patients with ileocolic intussusception complicated with intestinal necrosis.
5. Others, including cecal volvulus, inflammatory granuloma in the ileocecal junction, chronic and localized enteritis.

4.2.2 Contraindications

It's the same as Sect. 4.1.2.

4.2.3 Major Instruments or Energy Sources

1. Laparoscopy System.
2. Electrocautery.
3. Harmonic scalpel.
4. Endoscopic linear and circular stapler.

4.2.4 Team Setup, Anesthesia and Position

Under general anesthesia, the patient was placed in supine position with the arms adducted along the side. The position of surgeon, assistants and nurses is shown in Fig. 4.8.

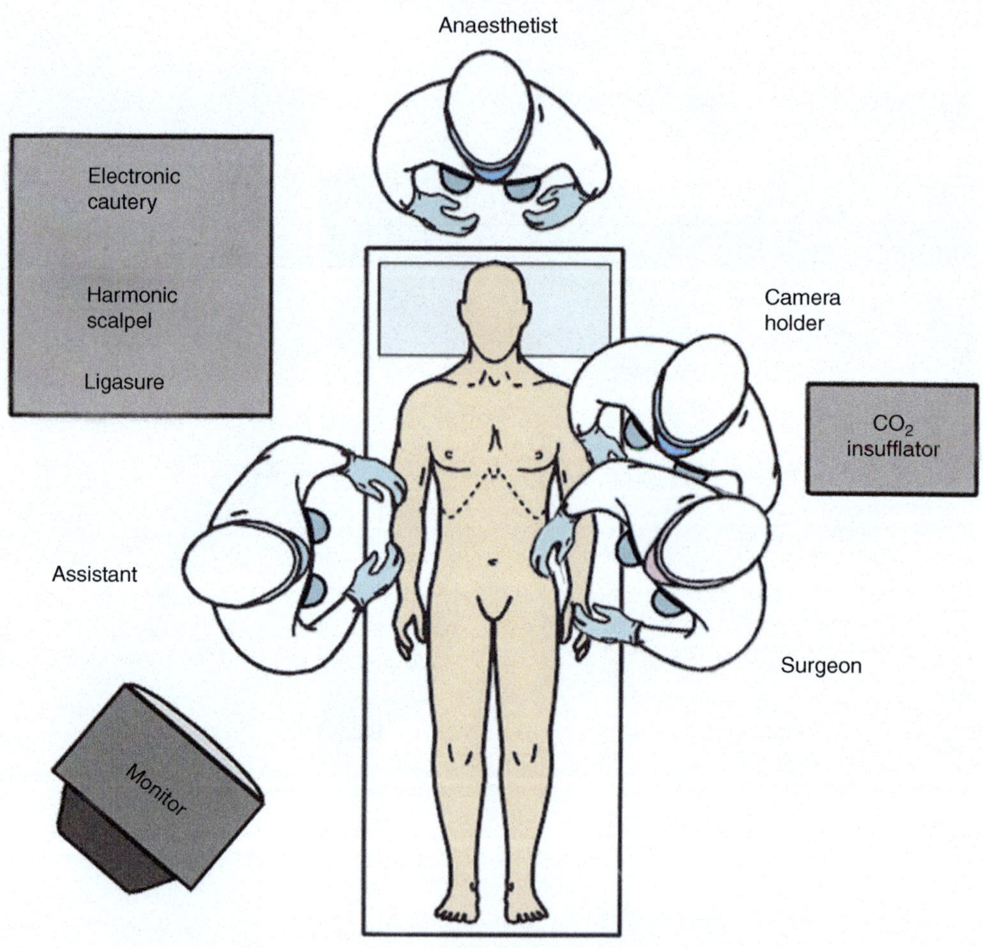

Fig. 4.8

4.2.5 Key Steps

1. Establishment of Pneumoperitoneum and Placement of Trocars.
2. Mobilization of the ascending colon.
3. Mobilization of the hepatic flexure of the colon.
4. Mobilization of the gastrocolic ligament.
5. Mobilization of the ileocolic mesentery.
6. Transection of the transverse colon.
7. Right hemicolectomy.
8. Ileocolic anastomosis.
9. Flushing and suturing the incision.

4.2.6 Surgical Techniques

1. Establishment of Pneumoperitoneum and Placement of Trocars.
2. Mobilization of the ascending colon.
   A lateral to medial technique was used by the surgeon. The ascending colon was retracted medially by using an atraumatic forceps in the left hand. The terminal ileum, cecum, and ascending colon were mobilized from the line of Toldt to the midline by using the harmonic scalpel. Small bleeders encountered were cauterized. The right ureter was identified and preserved (Fig. 4.9a–j).

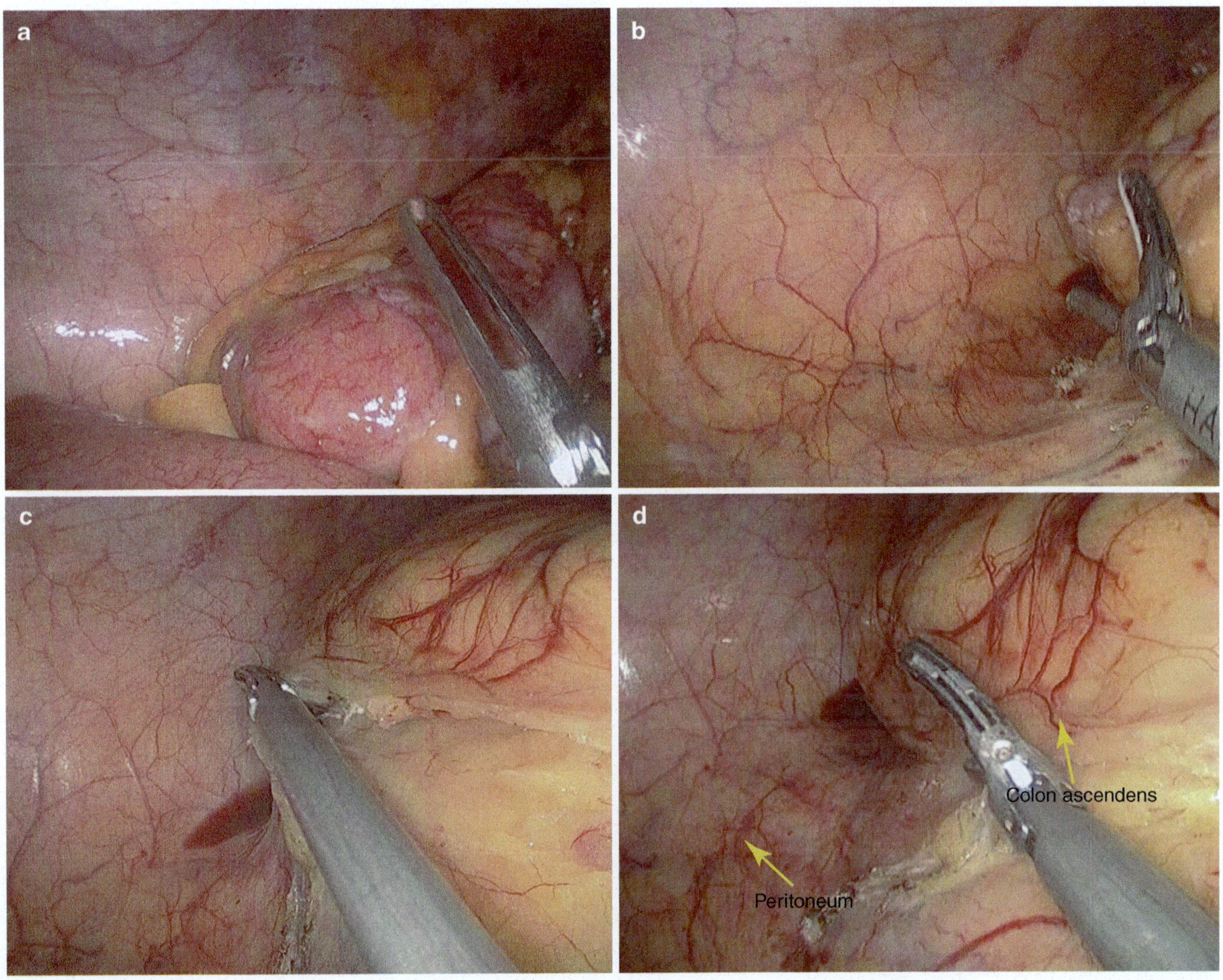

Fig. 4.9

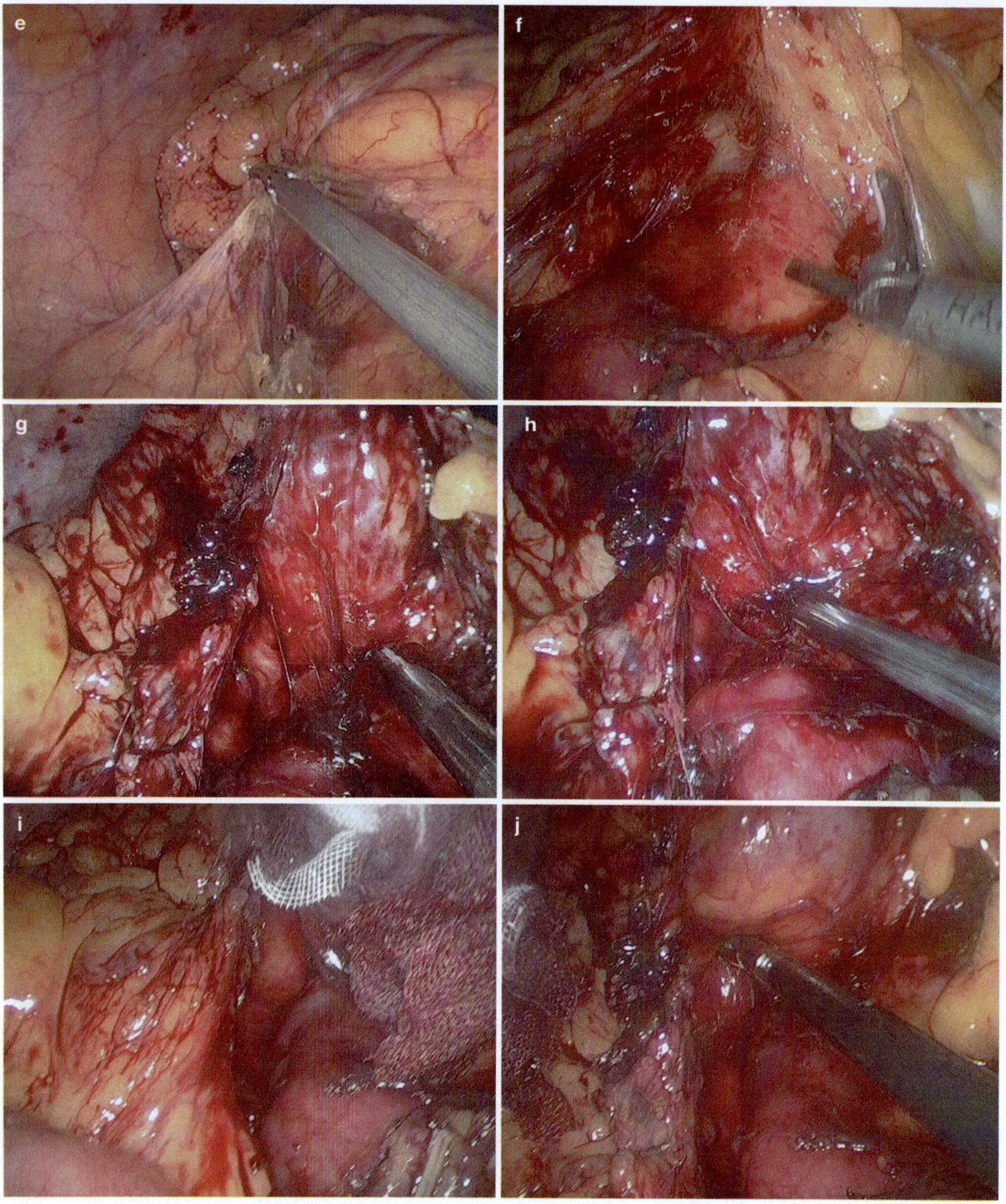

Fig. 4.9 (continued)

3. Mobilization of the hepatic flexure of the colon.
   Continuous mobilization upward was performed until the hepatic flexure of colon was fully freed from its attachment. The right part of transverse mesocolon was mobilized by using the harmonic scalpel. The duodenum was recognized and protected (Fig. 4.10a–d).

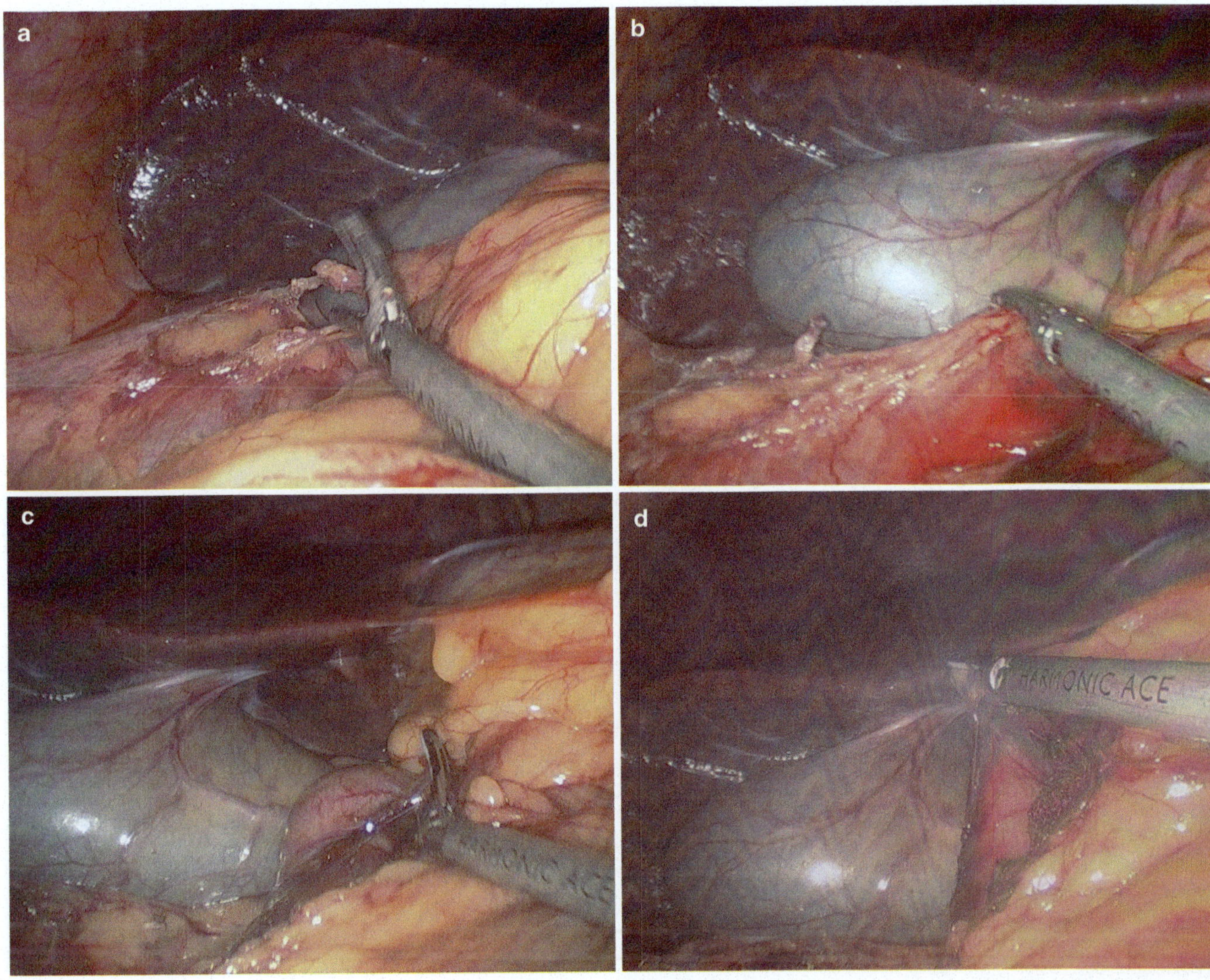

Fig. 4.10

4. Mobilization of the gastrocolic ligament.
   The hepatic flexure was retracted downward. The right part of the gastrocolic ligament was mobilized by using the harmonic scalpel (Fig. 4.11a–e).
5. Mobilization of the ileocolic mesentery.
   Mobilization of the ileocolic mesentery was carried out from the inferior to the superior direction in the avascular plane between Gerota's fascia and Toldt's fascia. During

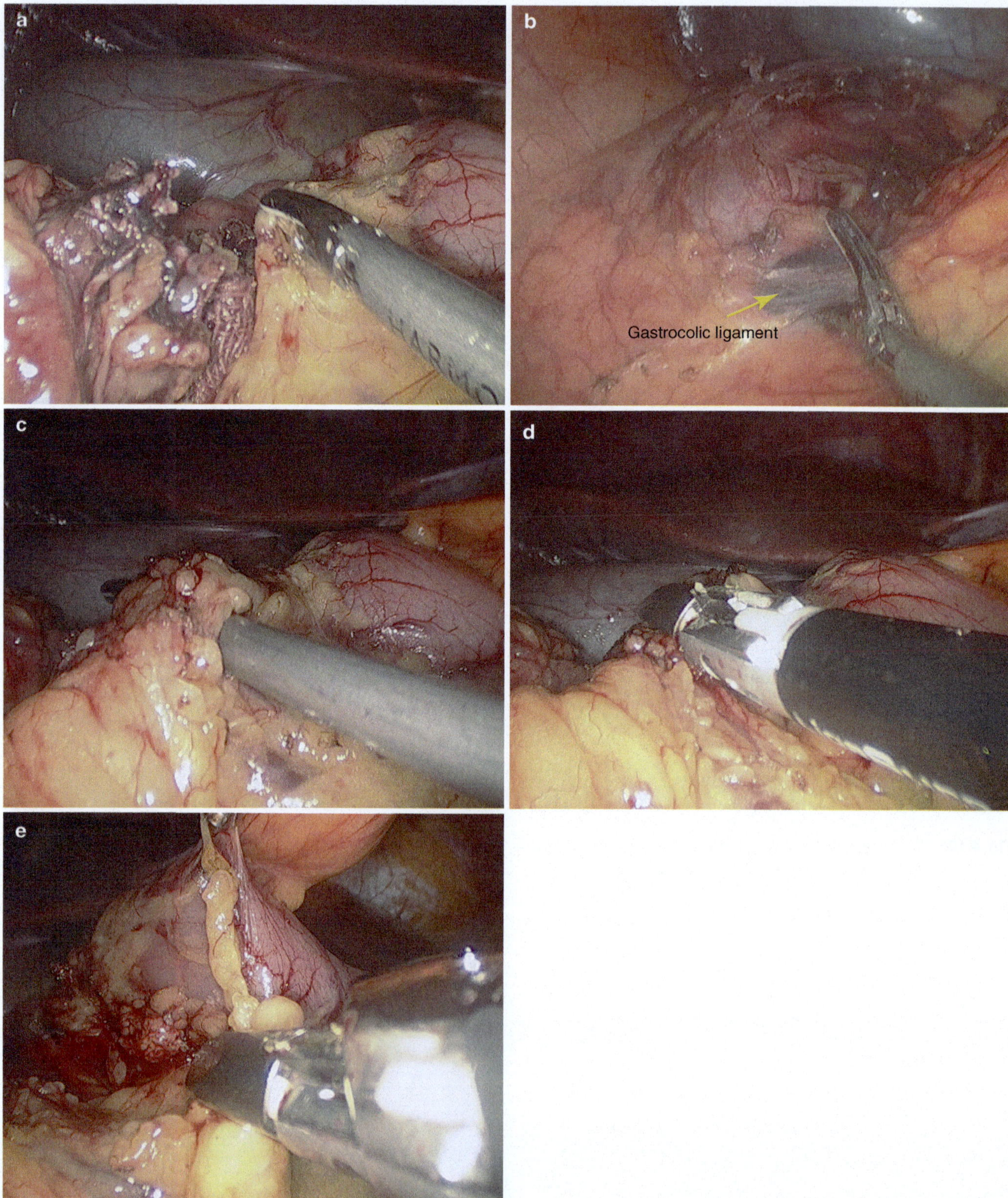

Fig. 4.11

this procedure, the duodenum was used as a landmark for safe upward dissection. The ileocolic vessel was then isolated and separately ligated near the superior mesenteric vessel with Hemolock. Thereafter, using a dissection along the lateral part of the middle colic vessel, the right branch of the middle colic vessel was severed. The gastrocolic trunk from the superior mesenteric vein was then exposed (Fig. 4.12a–j).

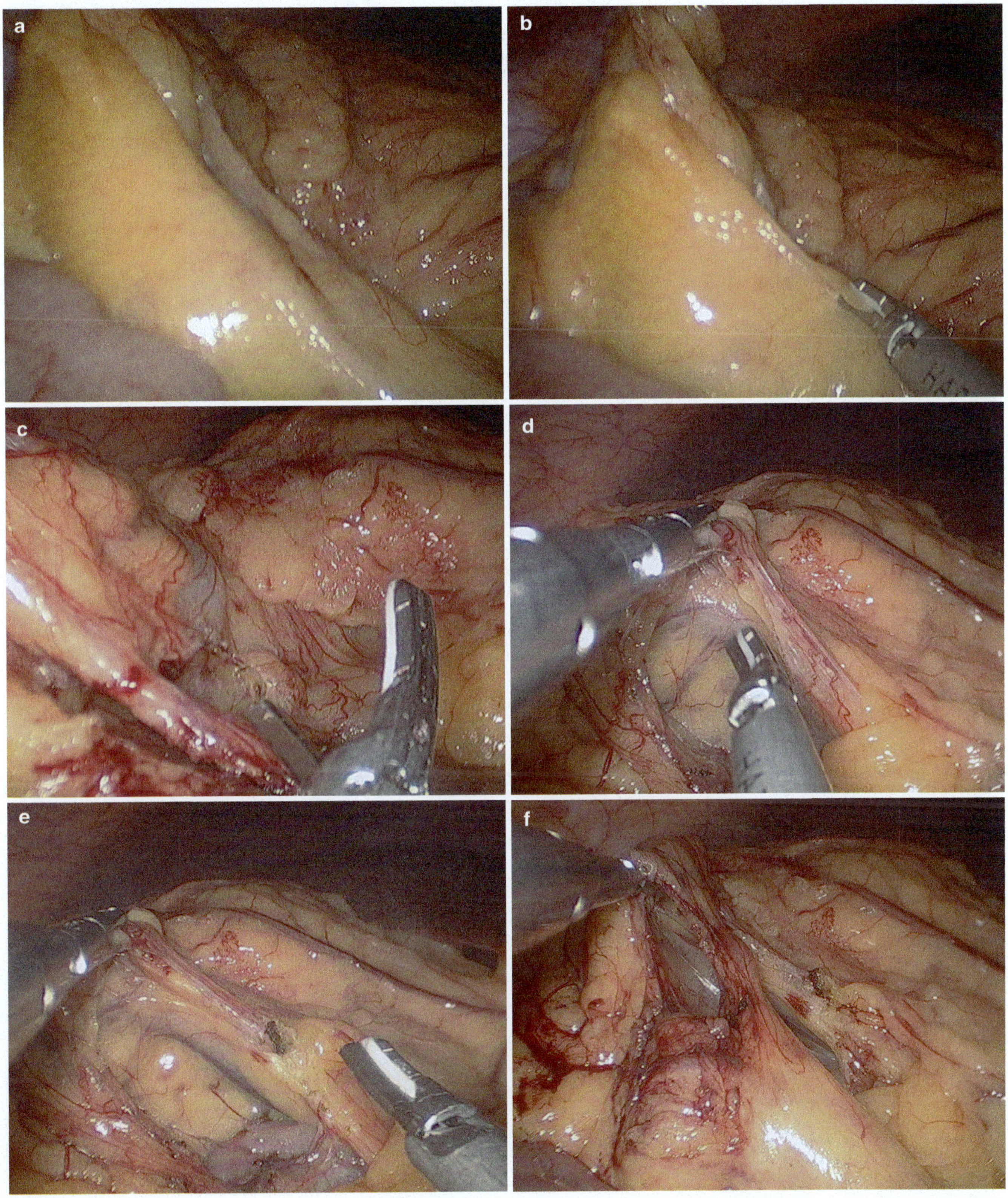

Fig. 4.12

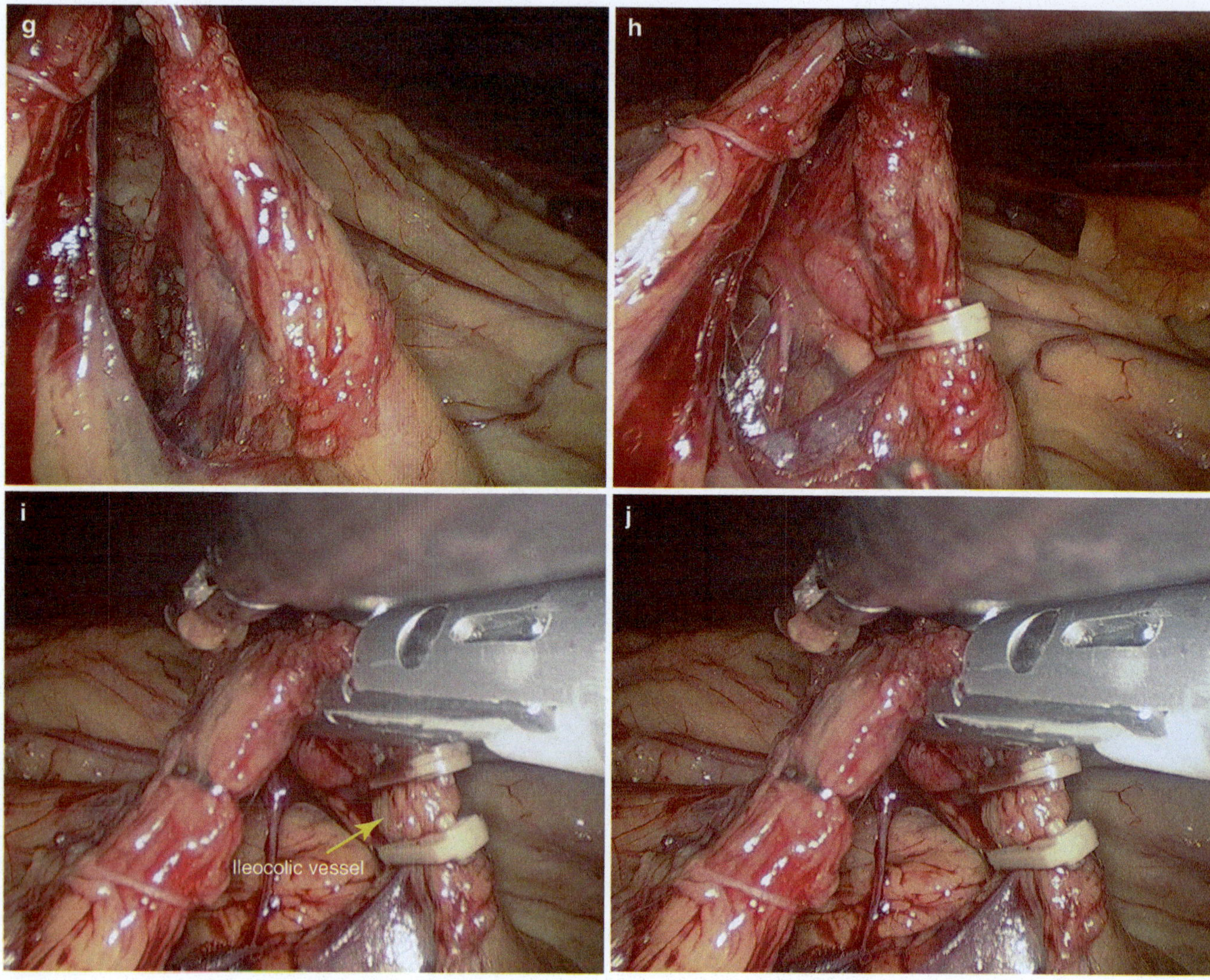

Fig. 4.12 (continued)

6. Transection of the transverse colon.

   The transverse colon was transected on the right side of the middle colic vessel. The ports were removed and the incision was extended to 3 cm total in length to facilitate exteriorization of the specimen. The terminal ileum, cecum, ascending colon and right part of the transverse colon were then brought outside the abdomen (Fig. 4.13a–f).

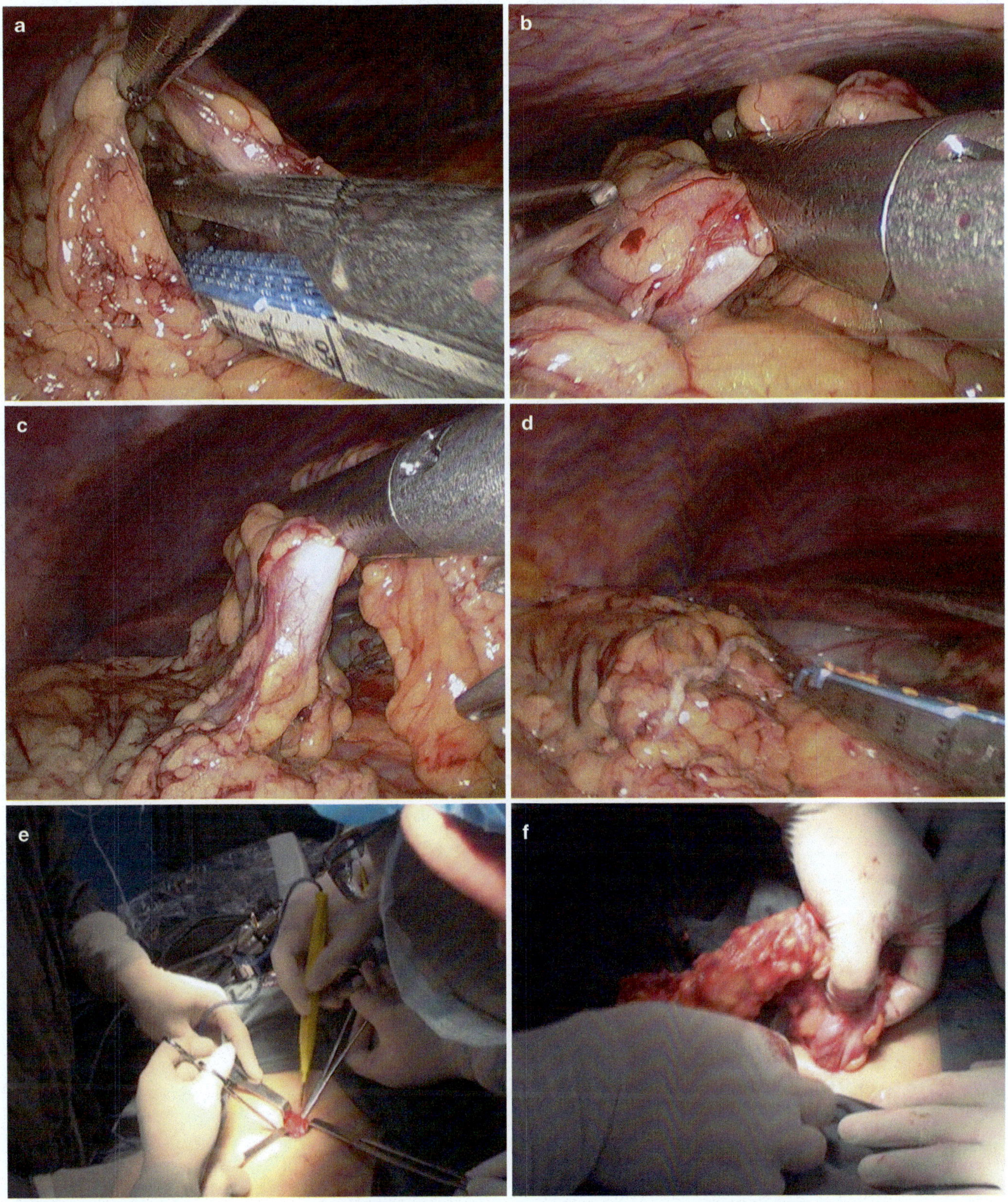

Fig. 4.13

7. Right hemicolectomy.
   A purse-string stapler was used to divide the terminal 15 cm ileum. The anvil of the circular stapler was put into the proximal stump of the ileum and embedded. Then, the stump of the ileum was put back into the abdominal cavity (Fig. 4.14a–d).

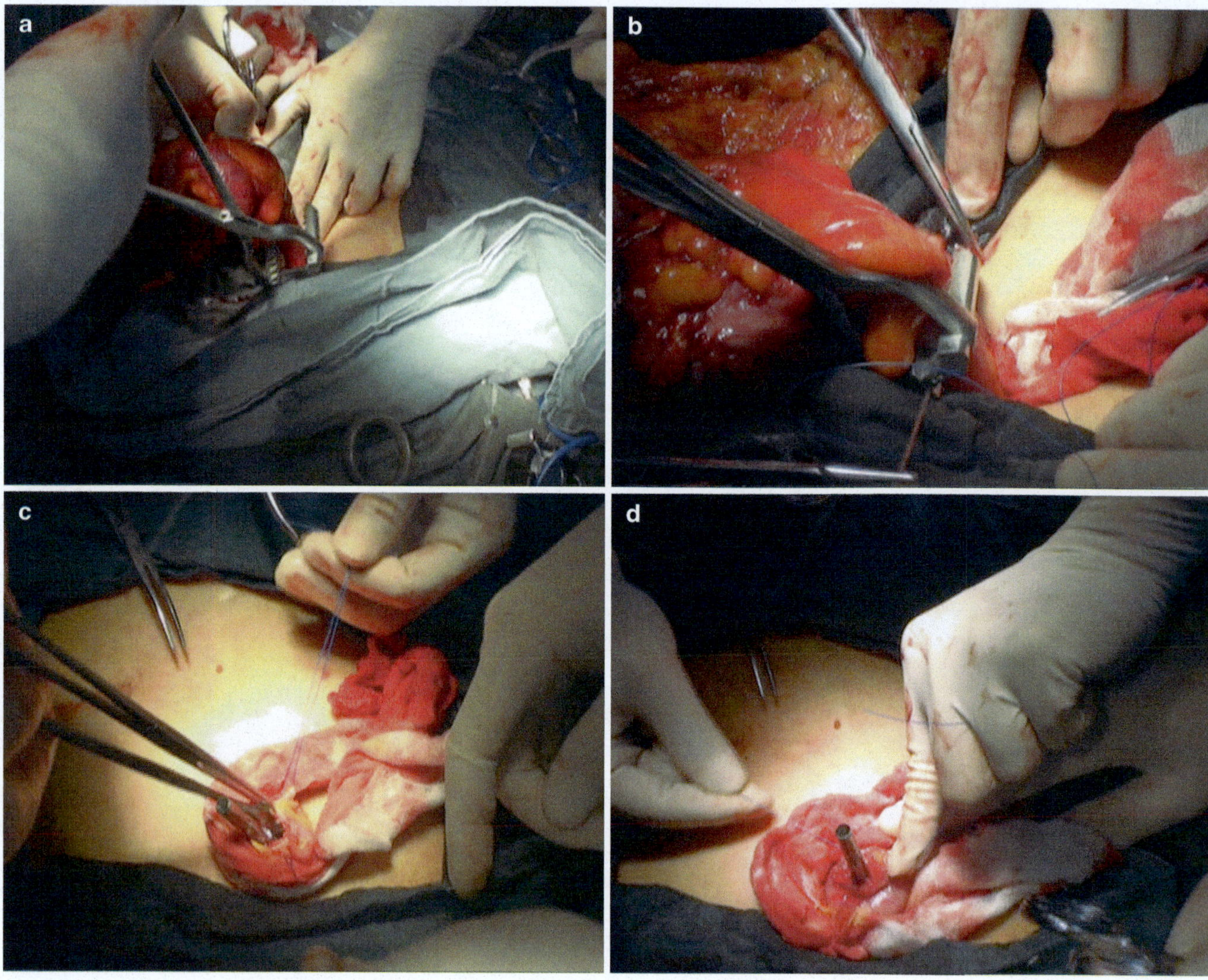

Fig. 4.14

8. Ileocolic anastomosis.
   The distal stump of the transverse colon was brought outside the abdomen. The stump was opened and the handle lever of the circular stapler was implanted into the colic lumen through the stump and punctured out through the lateral wall of the transverse colon where the anastomosis was to be made. The handle lever and anvil of the stapler were connected, screwed and firmly locked. After careful checking the connection part, the stapler was fired to complete the ileocolic end-to-side anastomosis. Careful examination of the anastomosis was done to ensure the devoid of torsion, twist or bleeding. The stump of the transverse colon was then transected by using liner stapler (Fig. 4.15a–d).

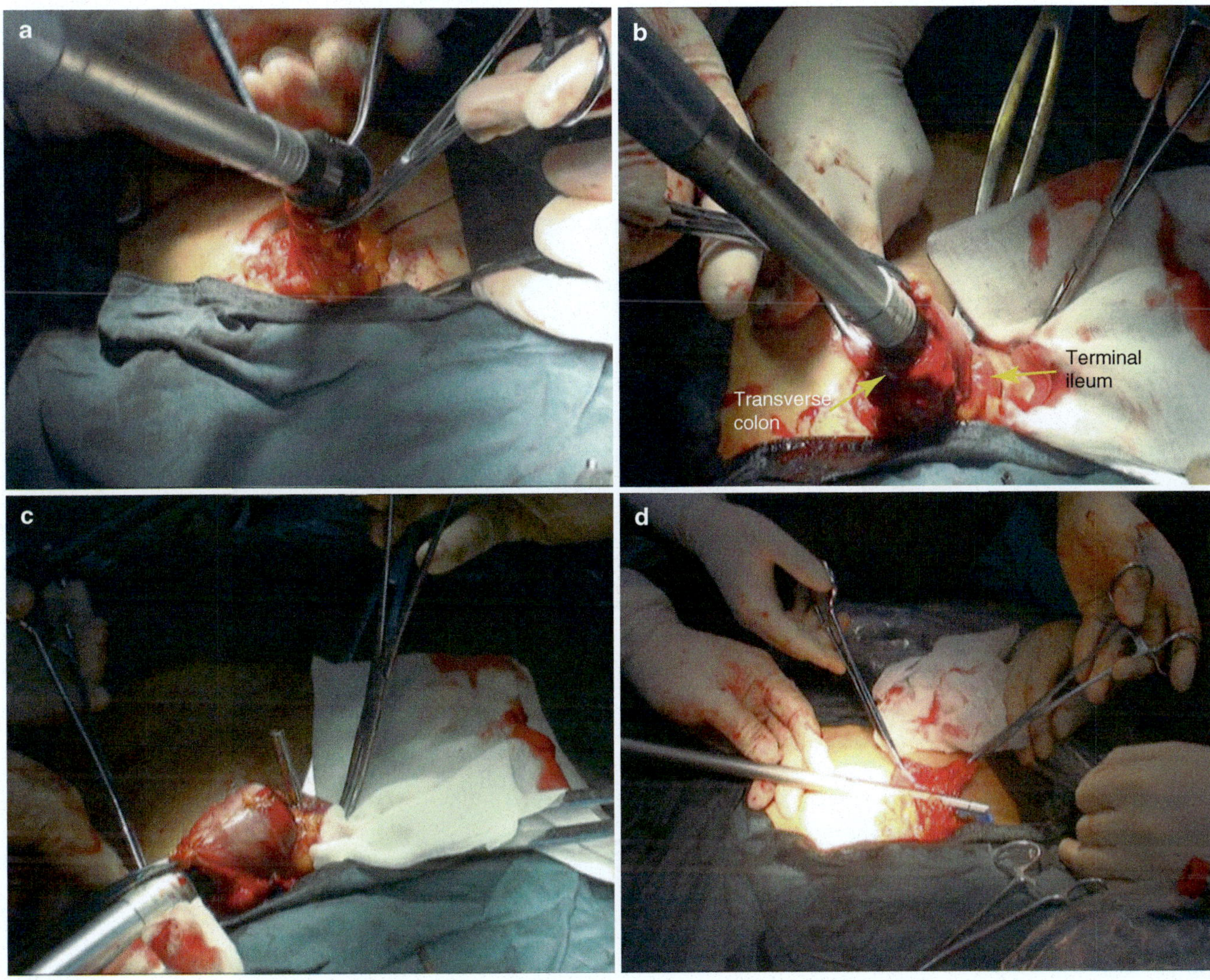

Fig. 4.15

9. Flushing and suturing the incision.
   The anastomosis was then pushed back into the abdominal cavity. Three trocars were reinserted and routine inspection and washing were performed. After careful checking the anastomosis to exclude torsion or twist, a closed suction drain was placed near the anastomosis through the umbilical incision (Fig. 4.16a–f).

4.2.7 Tips and Tricks

1. In the case of a right hemicolectomy, a high ligation of the ileocolic vessels can be performed using this vascular sealing device.
2. Visualization of the hepatic flexure can be a challenge, requiring practice retracting with only 1 instrument. It is helpful to move the table to the reverse Trendelenburg position and, with a bowel grasper, sweep the right colon medially and anteriorly, which will display the hepatocolic attachments in reference to the duodenum. This procedure can be executed with lateral retraction on the colonic wall alone without the need to grasp the colon itself, potentially minimizing injury.
3. Once the right colon is adequately mobilized and the mesentery is dissected free from the retroperitoneum, the bowel is grasped and brought out through the wound protector of umbilicus and conducted the anastomosis.

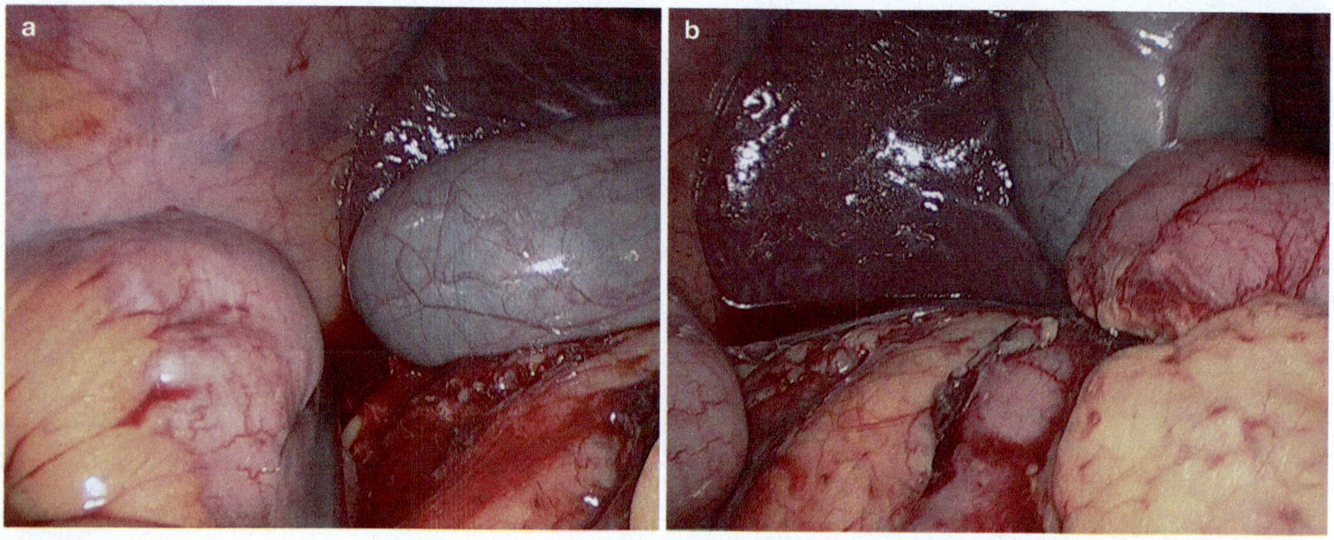

Fig. 4.16

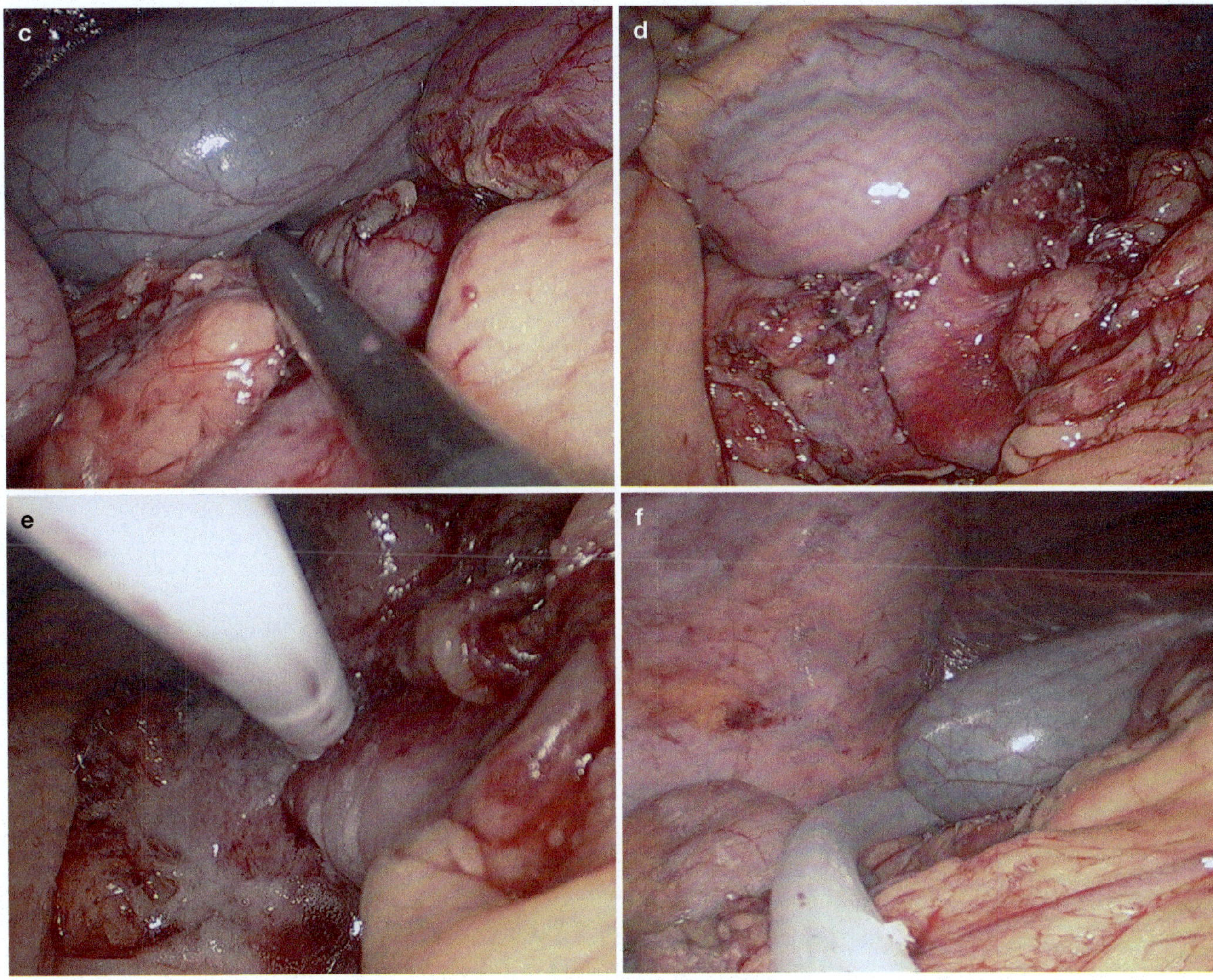

Fig. 4.16 (continued)

4.3 Laparoscopic Transverse Colectomy

4.3.1 Indications and Case Selection

1. Patients with malignancies in the middle of transverse colon, hepatic or splenic flexure of colon, but with no remote metastasis.
2. Patients with adenomatosis of the transverse colon.
3. Patients with damages, or torsion with infarction of the transverse colon.

4.3.2 Contraindications

It's the same as Sect. 4.1.2.

4.3.3 Major Instruments or Energy Sources

1. Laparoscopy System.
2. Electrocautery.
3. Harmonic scalpel.
4. Endoscopic linear and circular stapler.

4.3.4 Team Setup, Anesthesia and Position

Under general anesthesia, the patient was placed in supine position with the legs apart. The position of surgeon, assistants and nurses is shown in Fig. 4.17.

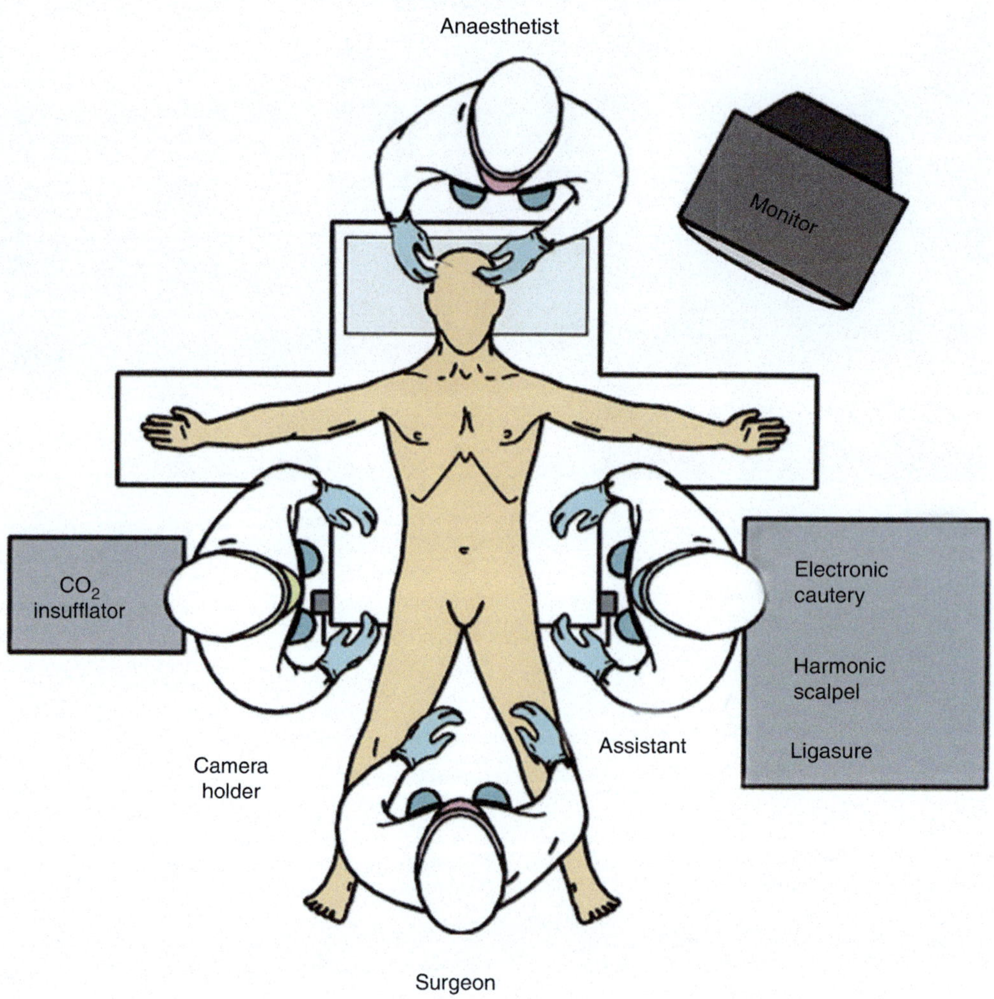

Fig. 4.17

4.3.5 Key Steps

1. Establishment of Pneumoperitoneum and Placement of Trocars.
2. Mobilization of the gastrocolic ligament.
3. Mobilization of the transverse mesocolon.
4. Mobilization of the ascending colon.
5. Transection of the transverse colon.
6. Flushing and suturing the incision.

4.3.6 Surgical Techniques

1. Establishment of Pneumoperitoneum and Placement of Trocars.
2. Mobilization of the gastrocolic ligament.
   With an atraumatic grasper on the left hand and ultrasonic scalpel on the right, the gastrocolic ligament was mobilized below the vascular arch with the left side to the left flexure of colon and the right to the hepatic flexure of colon (Fig. 4.18a–f).

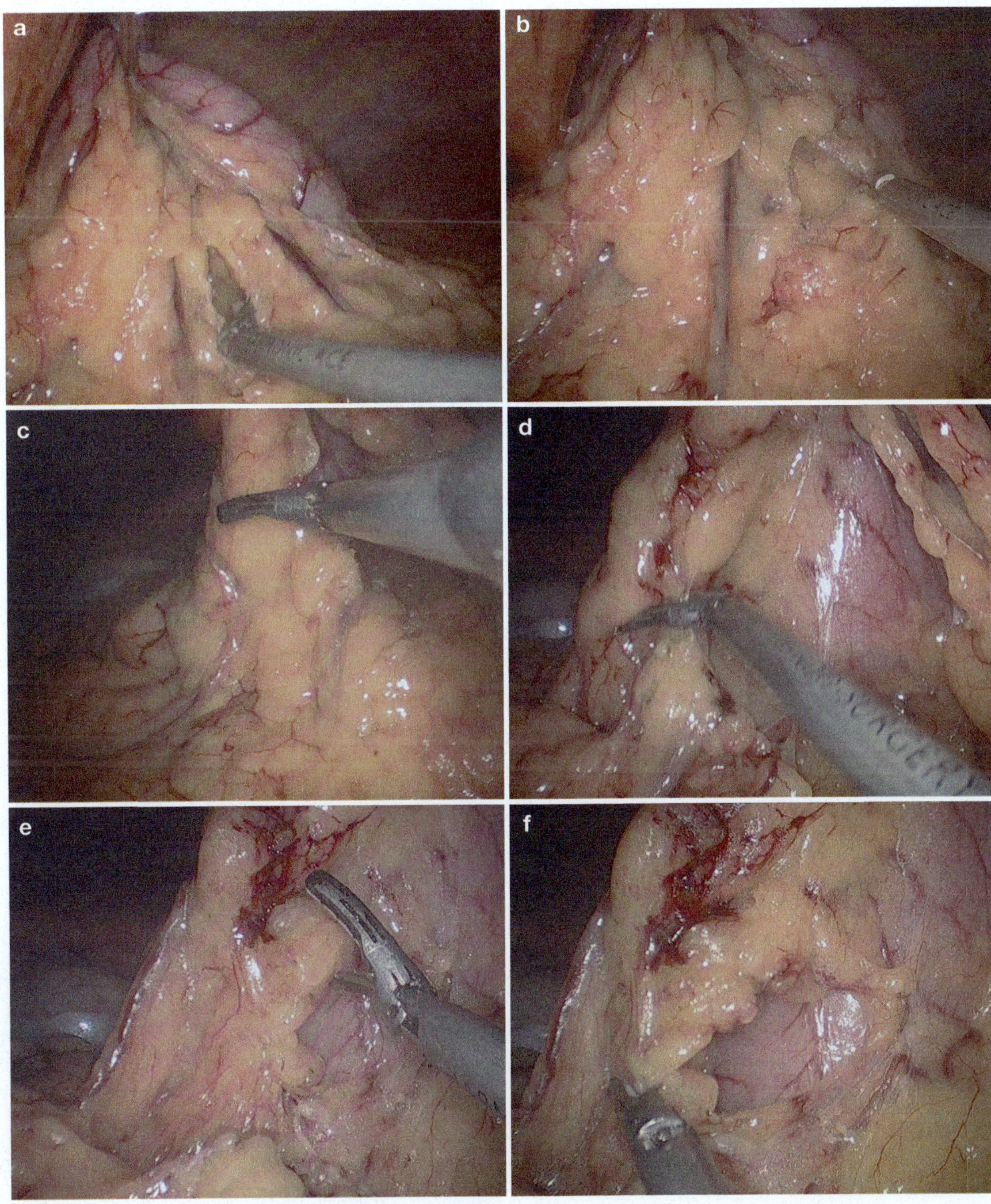

Fig. 4.18

3. Mobilization of the transverse mesocolon.
   Mobilization of the transverse mesocolon was carried out from the medial to lateral direction in the avascular plane between Gerota's fascia and Toldt's fascia. During this procedure, the duodenum and pancreas were used as a landmark for safe dissection. The middle colic vessels were severed (Fig. 4.19a–g).

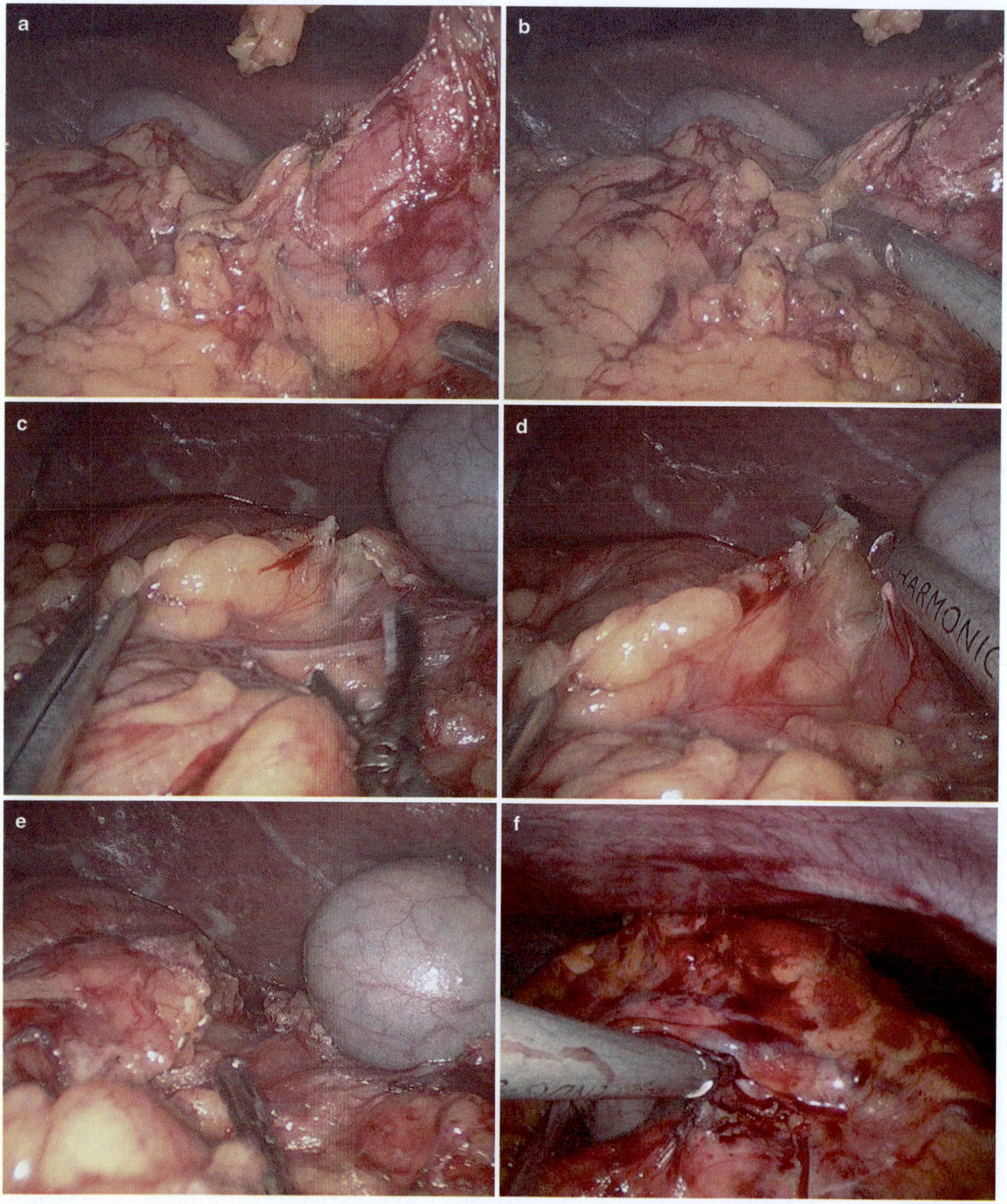

Fig. 4.19

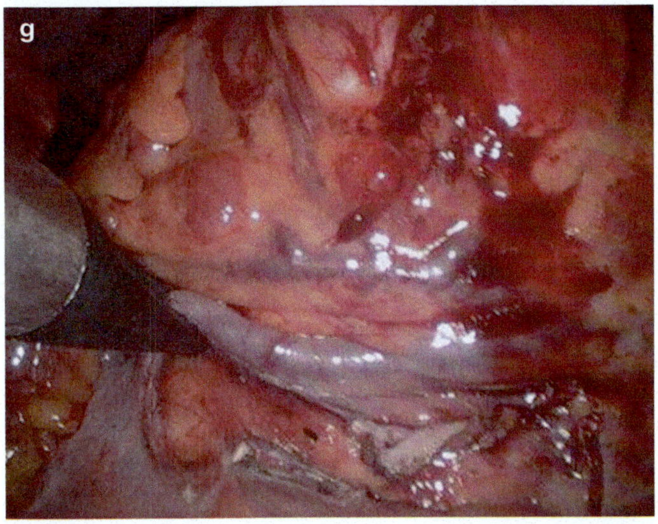

Fig. 4.19 (continued)

4. Mobilization of the ascending colon.
   The ascending colon was retracted medially by using an atraumatic forceps in the left hand. The cecum and ascending colon were mobilized from the line of Toldt by using the harmonic scalpel. Small bleeders encountered were cauterized (Fig. 4.20a–j).

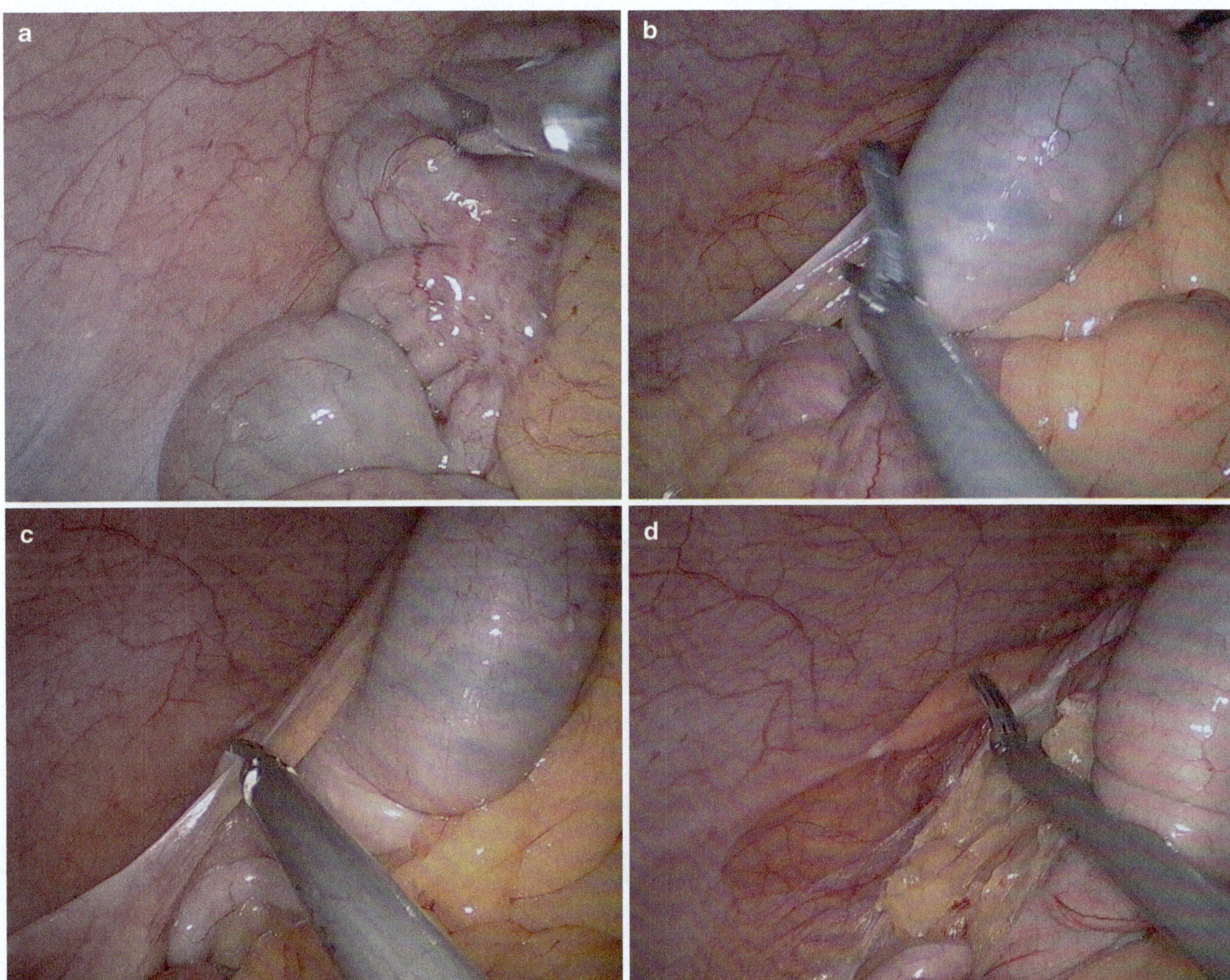

Fig. 4.20

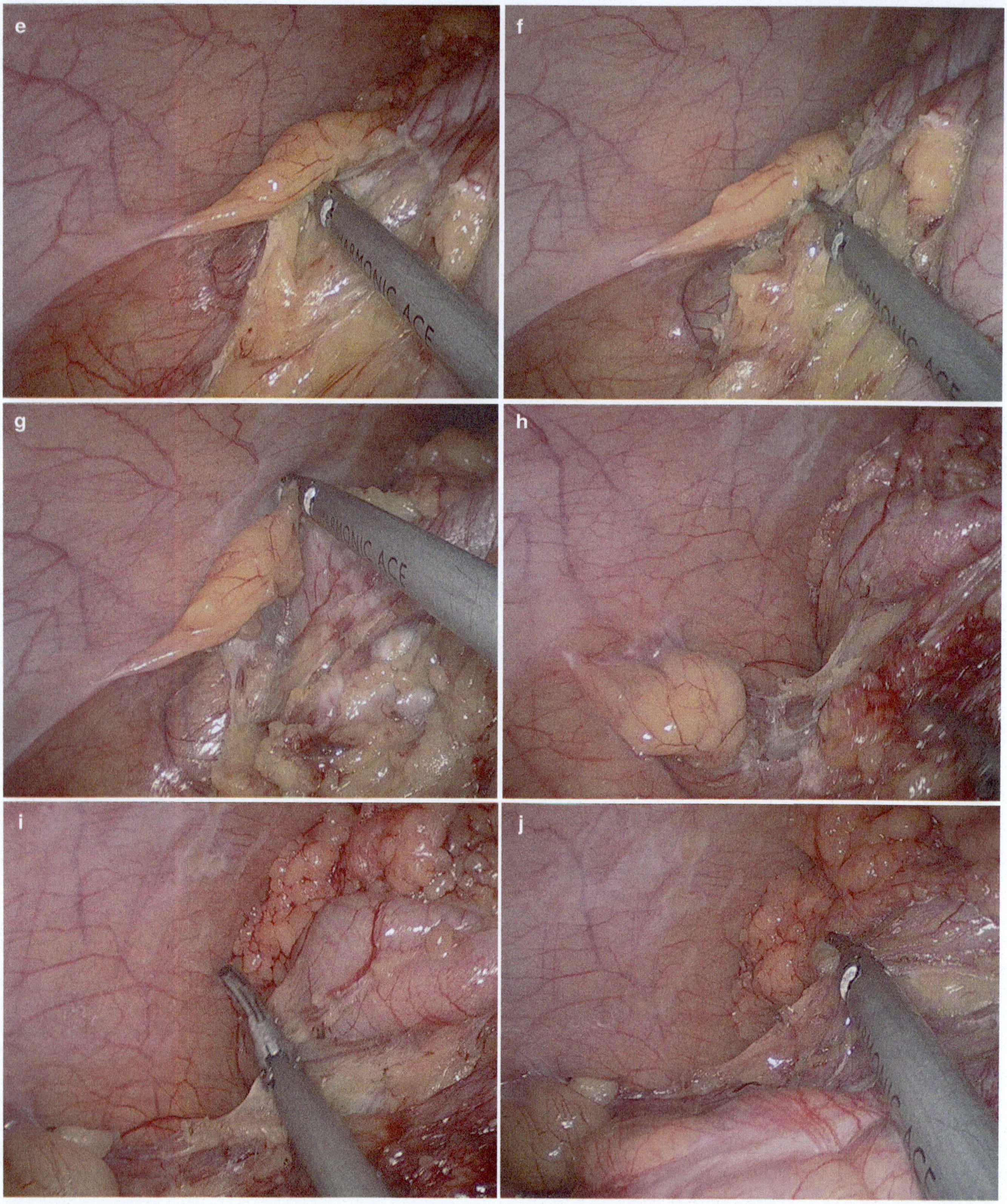

Fig. 4.20 (continued)

5. Transection of the transverse colon.
   The transverse colon was transected on its left side by using the liner stapler. The ports were removed and the incision was extended to 3 cm total in length to facilitate exteriorization of the specimen. Transverse colon resection and end-to-end anastomosis were performed under direct vision (Fig. 4.21a, b).

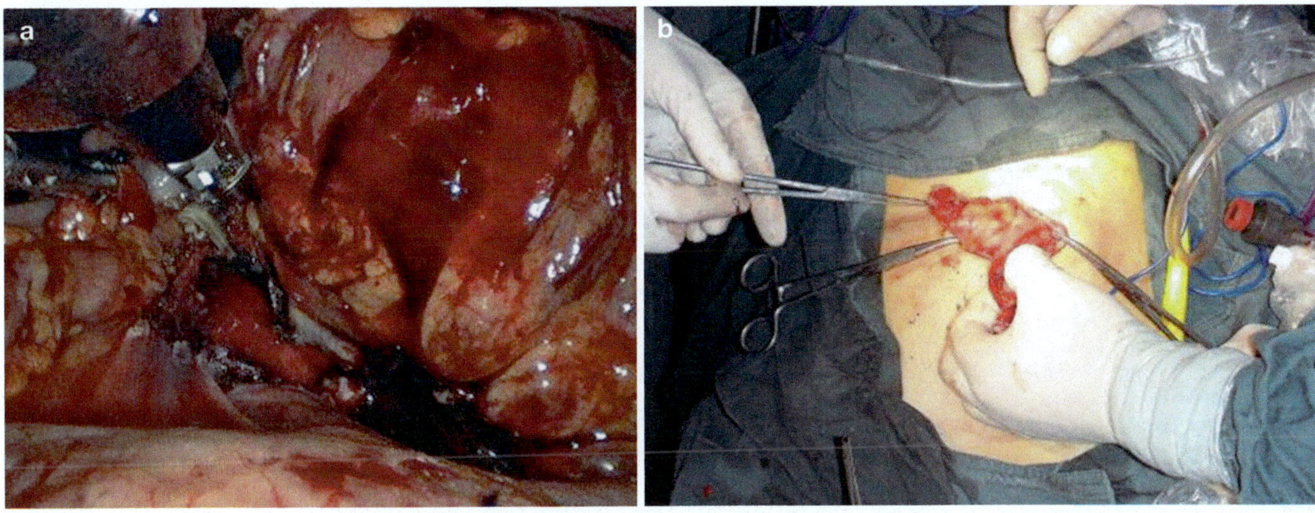

Fig. 4.21

6. Flushing and suturing the incision.
   The anastomosis was then pushed back into the abdominal cavity. Three trocars were reinserted and routine inspection and washing were performed. After careful checking the anastomosis to exclude torsion or twist, a closed suction drain was placed near the anastomosis through the umbilical incision (Fig. 4.22a–c).

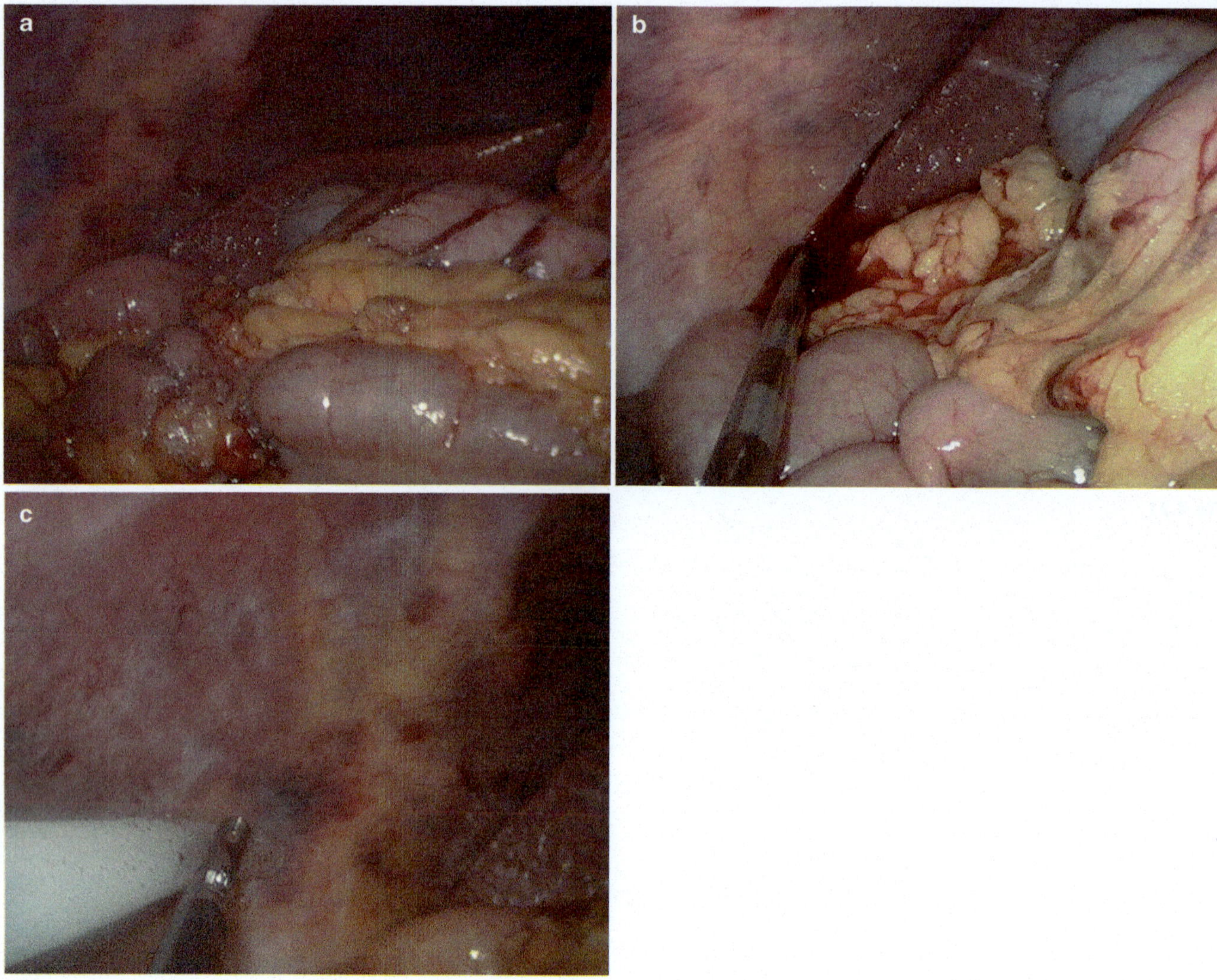

Fig. 4.22

4.4 Laparoscopic Sigmoidectomy

4.4.1 Indications and Case Selection

Indications for laparoscopic sigmoid colectomy are identical to the indications for open colectomy. Benign disease or malignant tumors in the juncture of descending colon and sigmoid colon, or in the sigmoid colon are all indicated.

4.4.2 Contraindications

Factors that may hinder a laparoscopic approach include severe adhesions from prior abdominal or pelvic operations or inflammatory processes, cardiopulmonary insufficiency, morbid obesity, and cancer invading other structures.

4.4.3 Major Instruments or Energy Sources

1. Laparoscopy System.
2. Electrocautery.
3. Harmonic scalpel.
4. Endoscopic linear and circular stapler.

4.4.4 Team Setup, Anesthesia and Position

The patient was positioned lithotomy under general anesthesia. The position of surgeon, assistants and nurses is shown in Fig. 4.23.

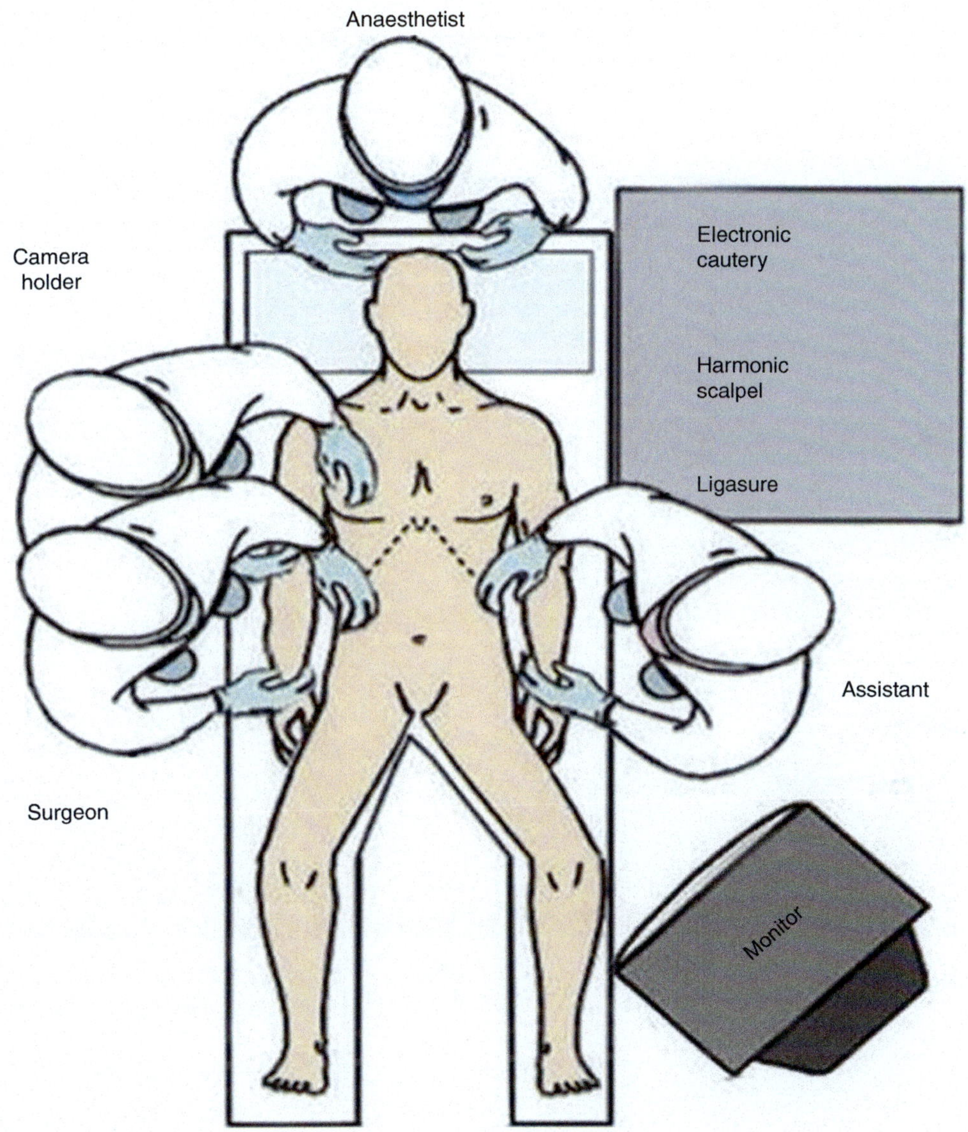

Fig. 4.23

4.4.5 Key Steps

1. Establishment of Pneumoperitoneum and Placement of Trocars.
2. Mobilization of the sigmoid colon.
3. Mobilization of the sigmoid mesocolon.
4. Ligation of the inferior mesenteric vessels.
5. Transection of the rectum.
6. Removal of the sigmoid colon.
7. Colorectal anastomosis.
8. Flushing and suturing the incision.

4.4.6 Surgical Techniques

1. Establishment of Pneumoperitoneum and Placement of Trocars.
2. Mobilization of the sigmoid colon.
   The surgeon used a lateral to medial technique. The sigmoid colon was retracted medially by using an atraumatic forceps in the left hand and was mobilized from the line of Toldt to the midline by using harmonic scalpel. Small bleeders encountered were cauterized (Fig. 4.24a–h).

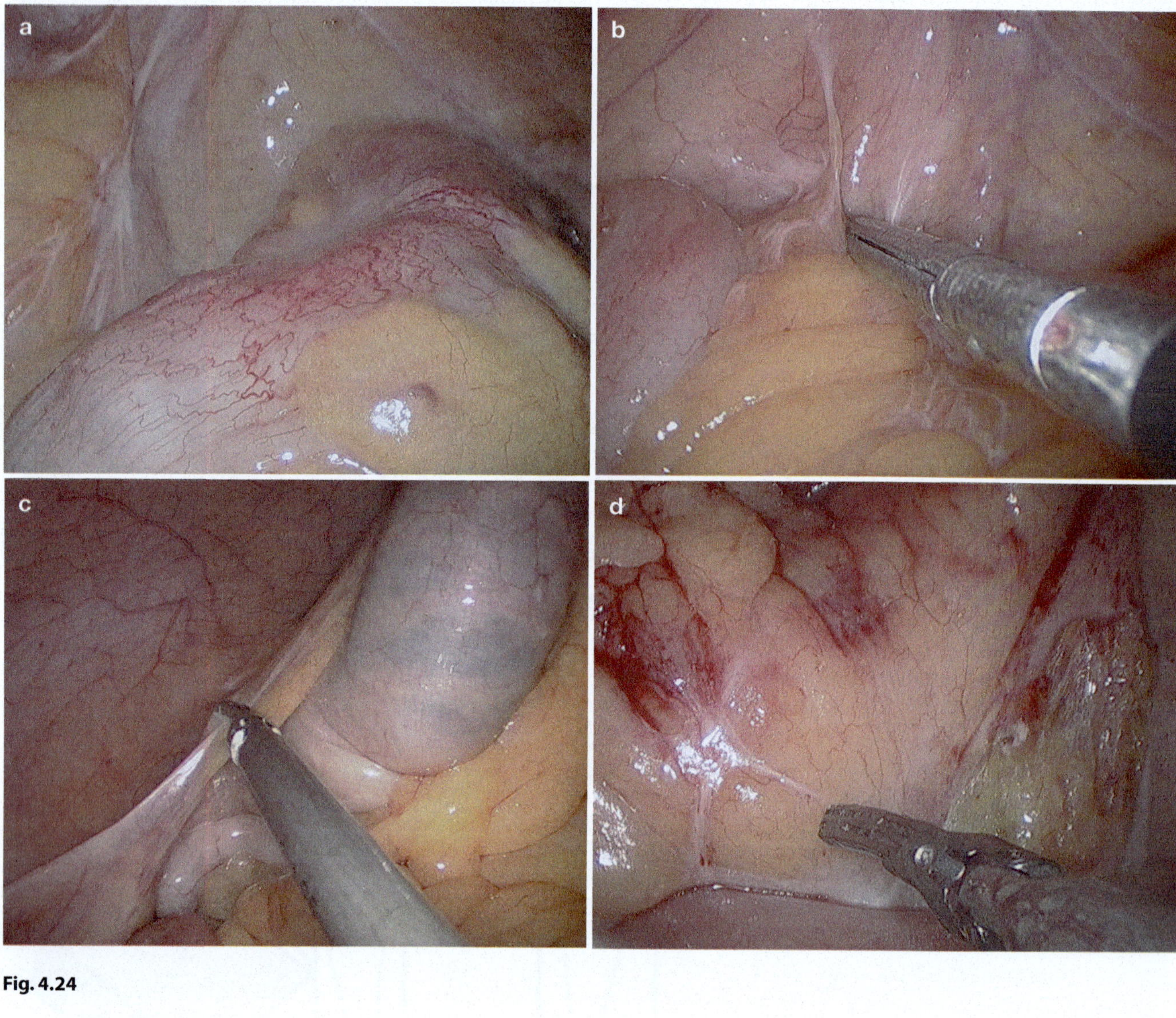

Fig. 4.24

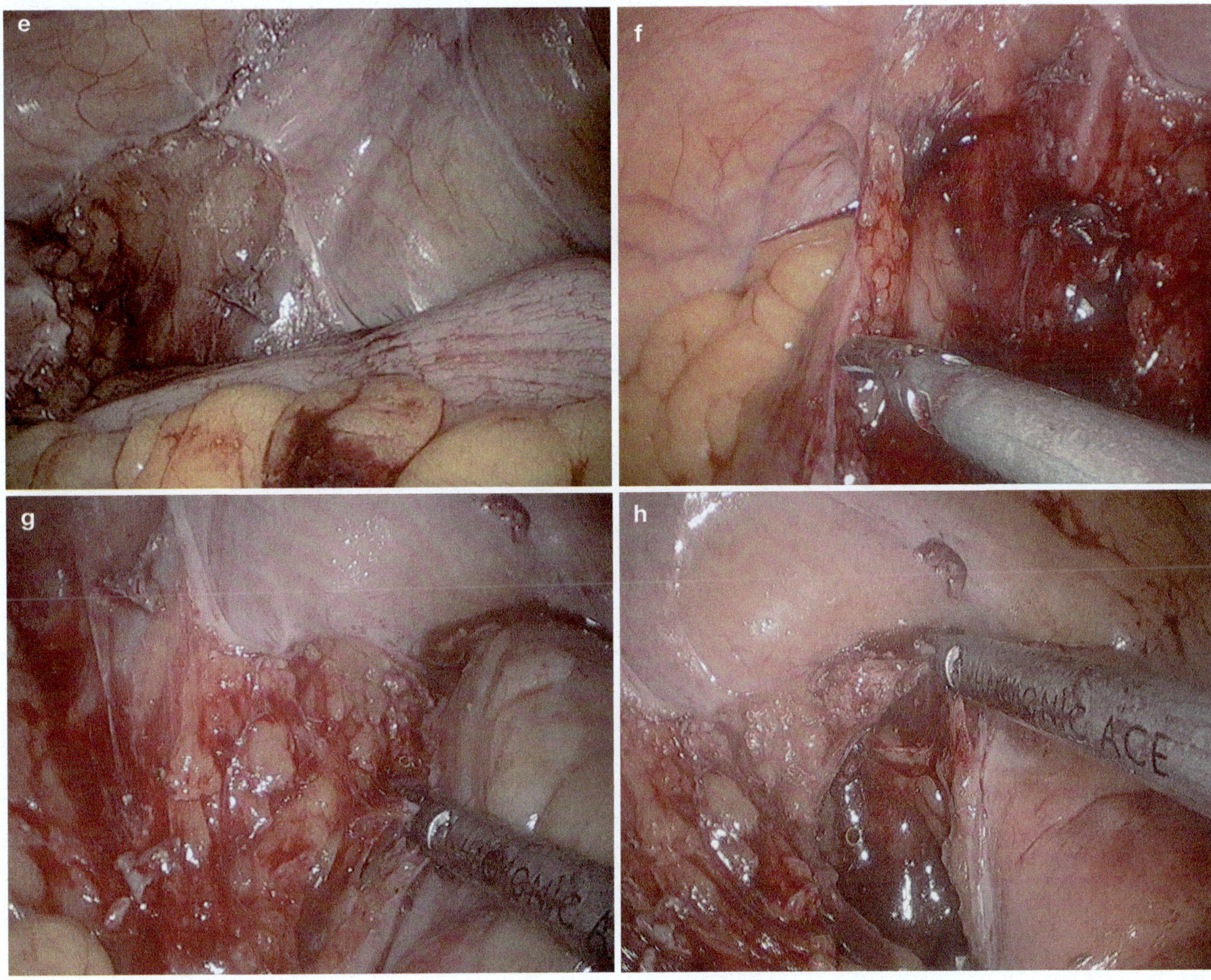

Fig. 4.24 (continued)

3. Mobilization of the sigmoid mesocolon.

   Mobilization of the sigmoid mesocolon was carried out from the inferior to superior direction in the avascular plane between Gerota's fascia and Toldt's fascia. The medial-to-lateral dissection was continued until the left-sided colon was separated from the retroperitoneum. the left ureter and gonadal vessels were then identified and preserved (Fig. 4.25a–f).

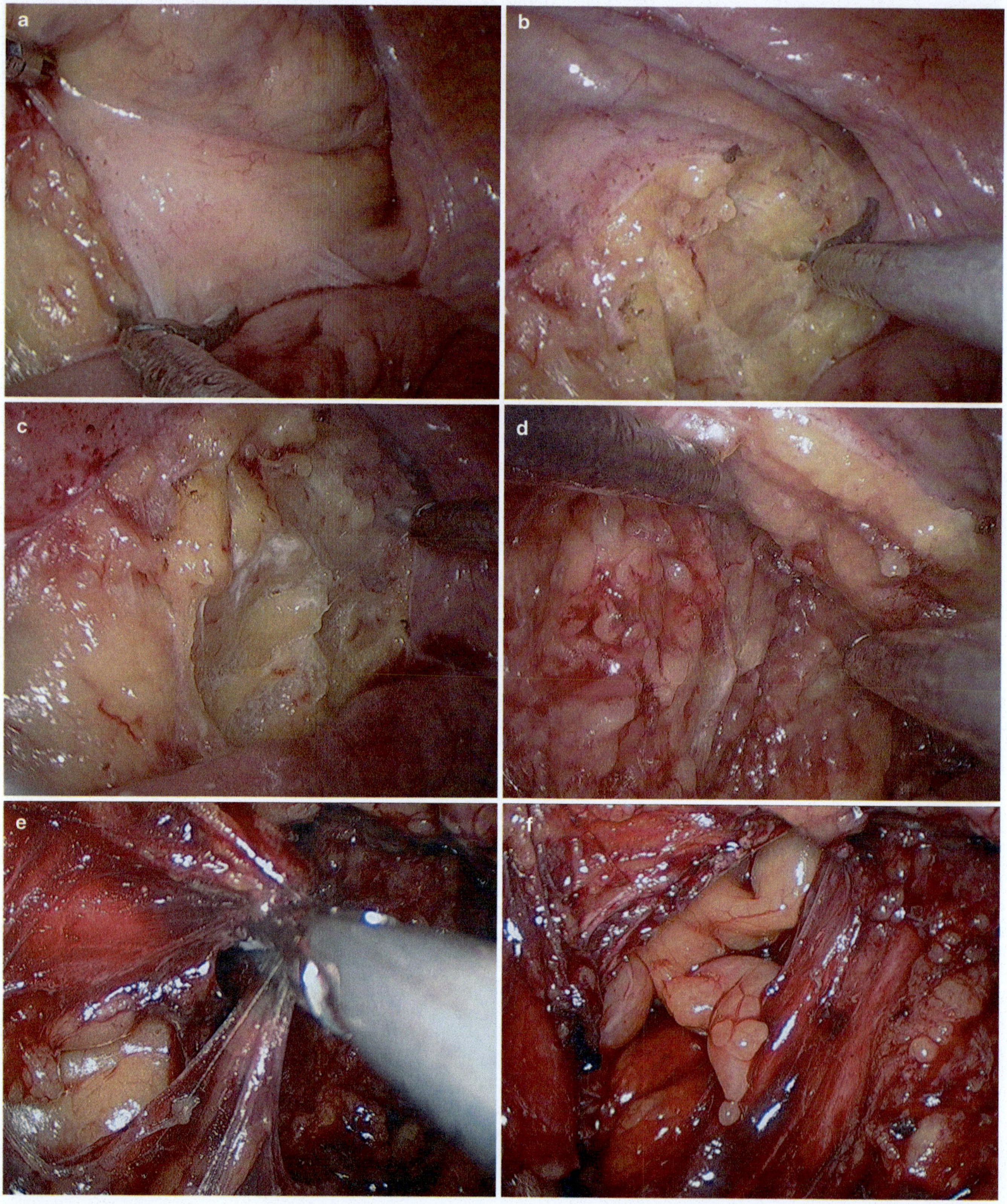

Fig. 4.25

4. Ligation of the inferior mesenteric vessels.
   Initially, the inferior mesenteric artery (IMA) was retracted with the double fenestrated forceps, and the IMA was ligated near the origin by using clip placement or linear stapler. Thereafter, division of the inferior mesenteric vein was performed close to the Treitz ligament (Fig. 4.26a–d).

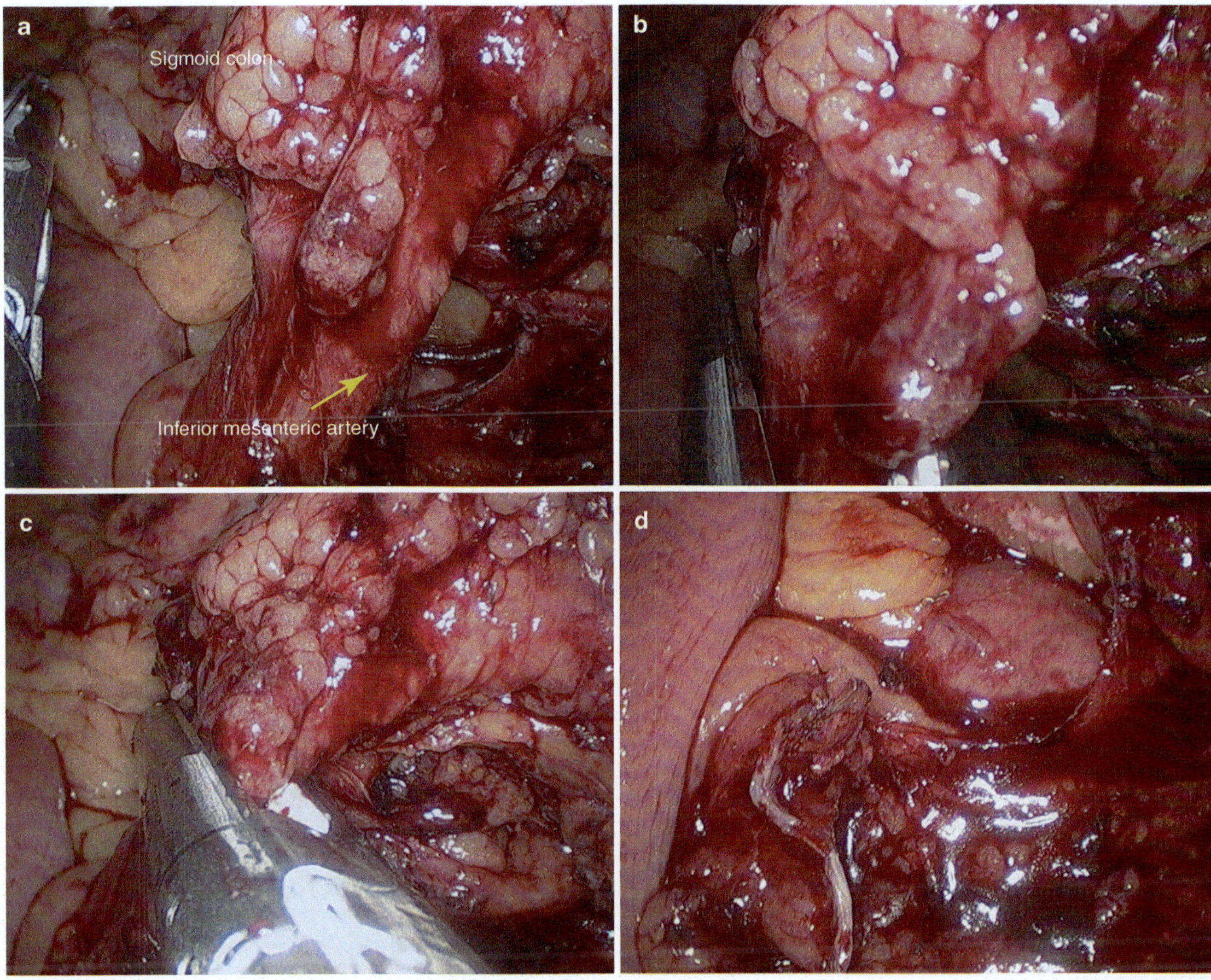

Fig. 4.26

5. Transection of the rectum.
   The rectum was retracted upward and was transected 10 cm distal to the lesion by using a 12 mm flexible linear stapler which was introduced through the 12 mm port (Fig. 4.27a–f).

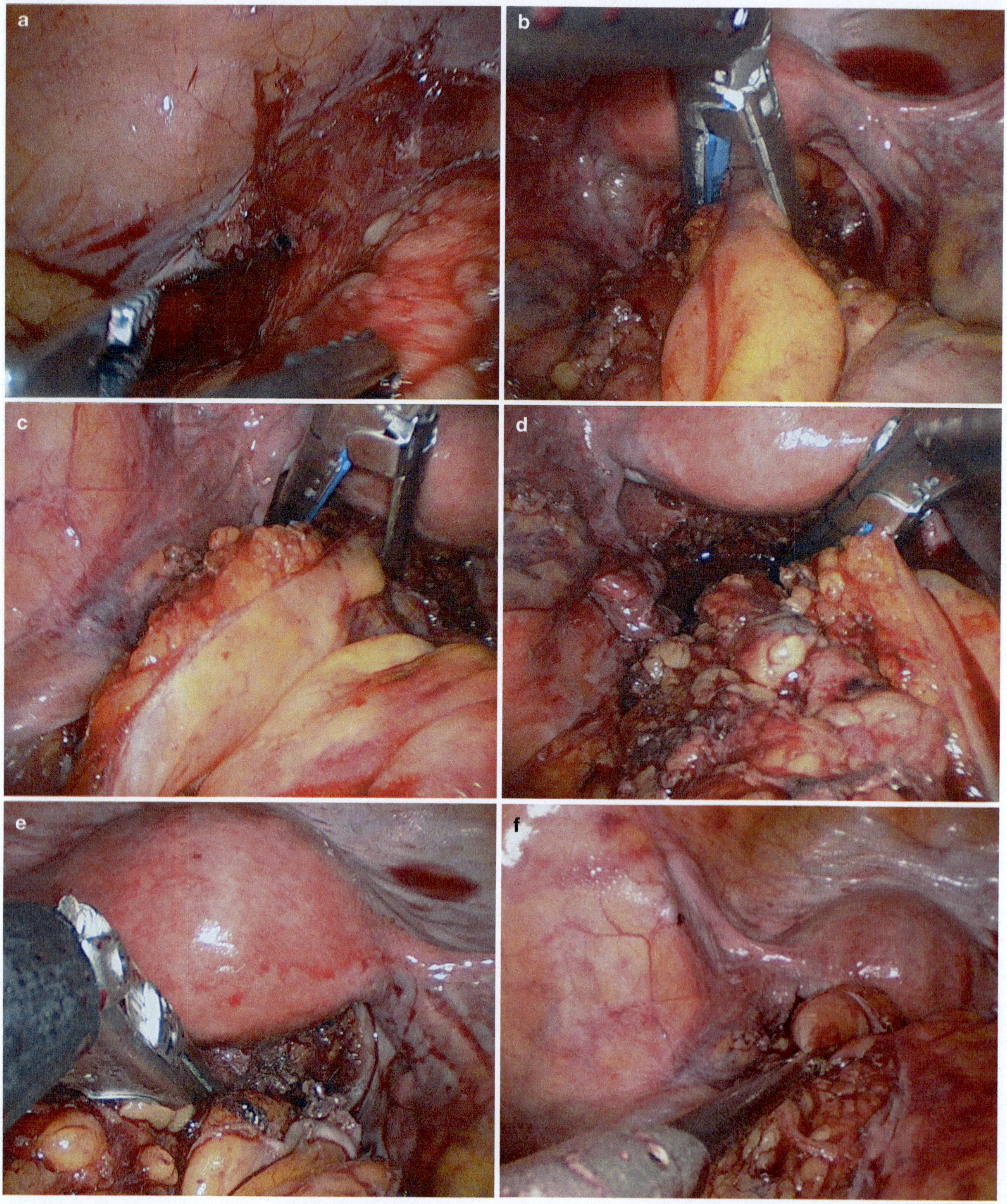

Fig. 4.27

6. Removal of the sigmoid colon.
   The ports were removed and the incision was extended to 3 cm total in length to facilitate exteriorization of the specimen. The sigmoid was then brought outside the abdomen. A purse-string stapler was used to divide the proximal 10 cm sigmoid colon. The anvil of the circular stapler was put into the proximal stump of the colon and embedded. Then, the stump of the colon was put back into the abdominal cavity (Fig. 4.28a–d).

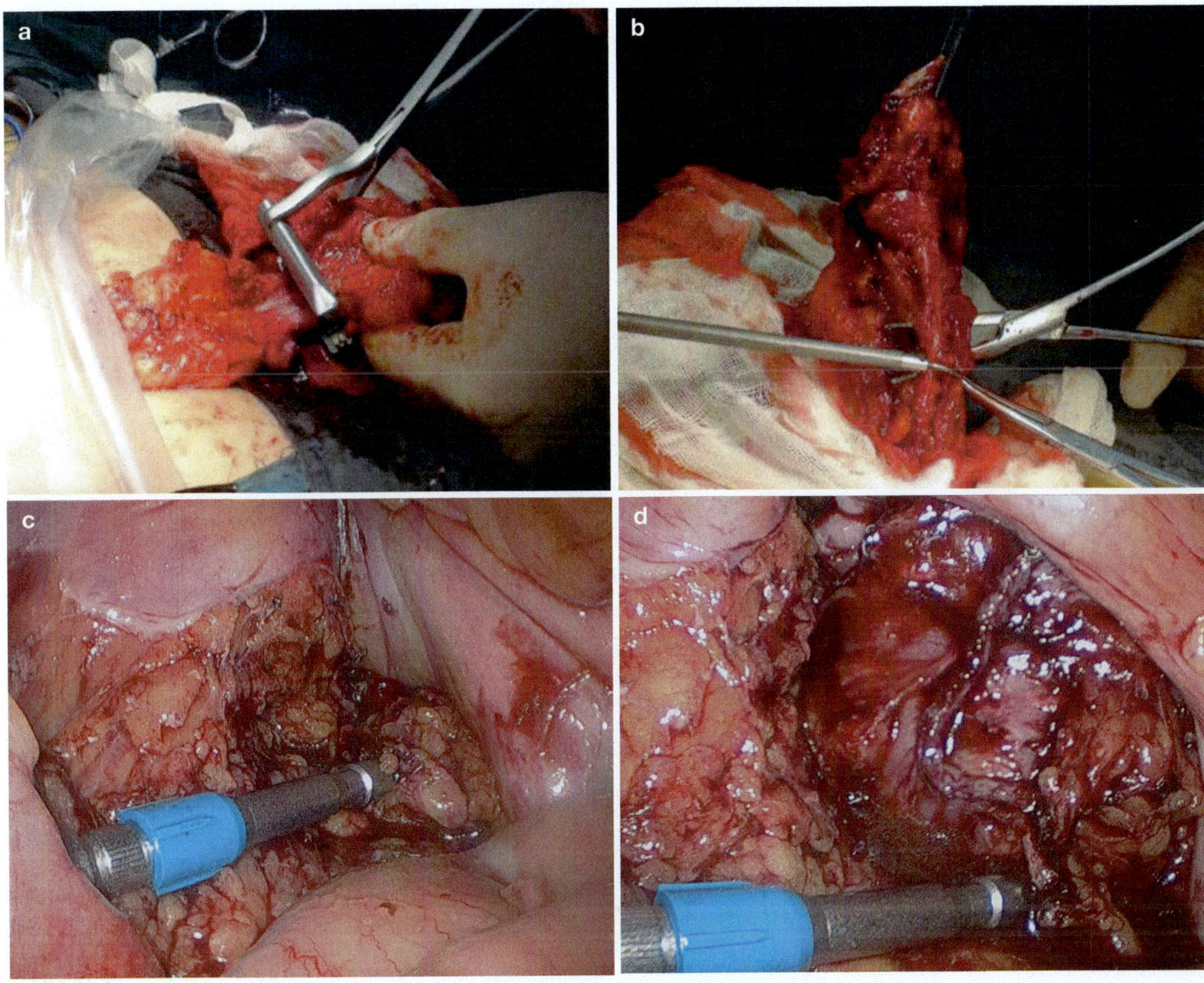

Fig. 4.28

7. Colorectal anastomosis.

   The handle lever of the circular stapler was implanted into the rectal lumen through the anus and punctured out through the middle point of the rectal stump where the anastomosis was to be made. The handle lever and anvil of the stapler were connected, screwed and firmly locked. After careful checking the connection part, the stapler was fired to complete the colorectal end-to-end anastomosis. Careful examination of the anastomosis was done to ensure the devoid of torsion, twist or bleeding (Fig. 4.29a–j).

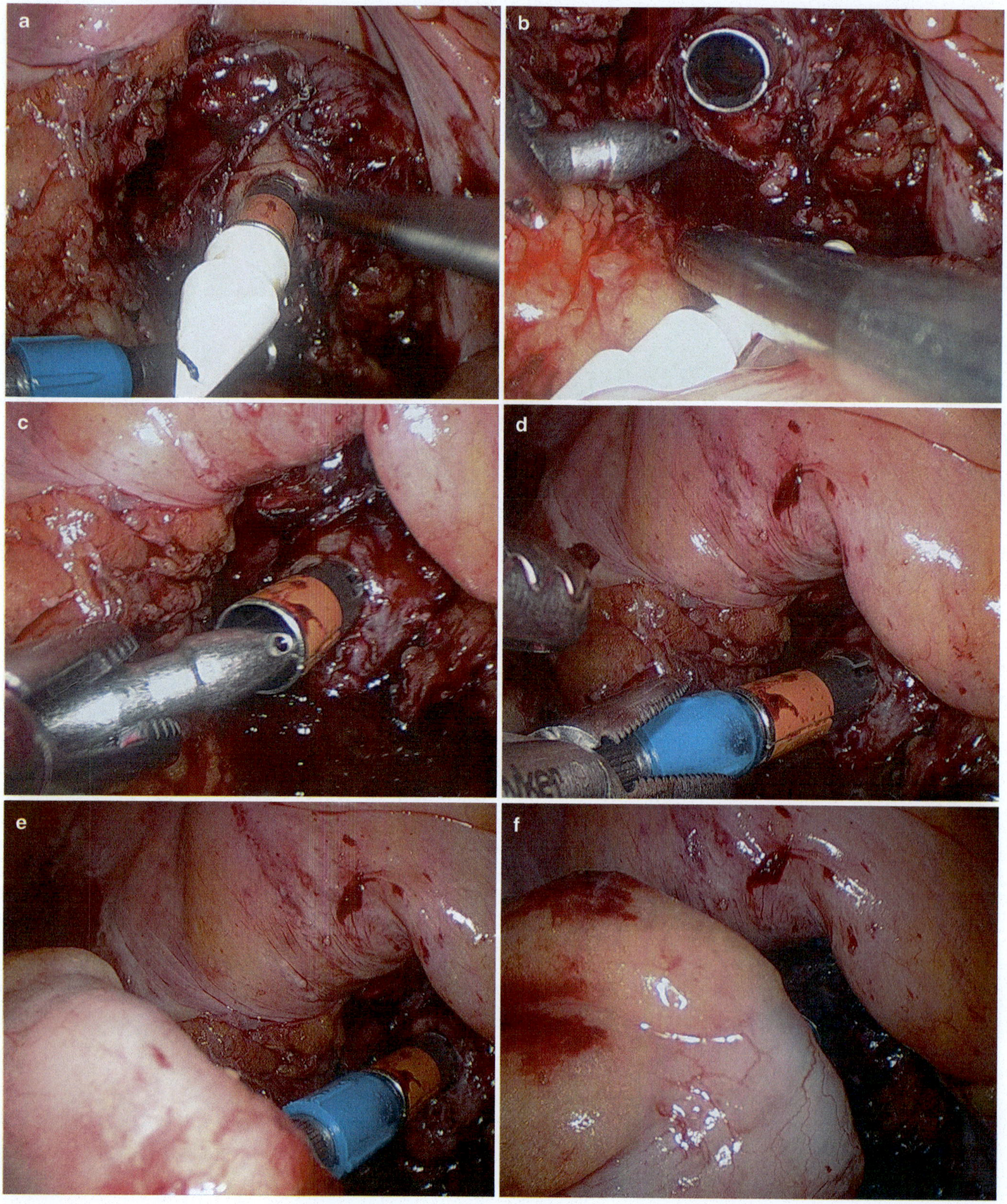

Fig. 4.29

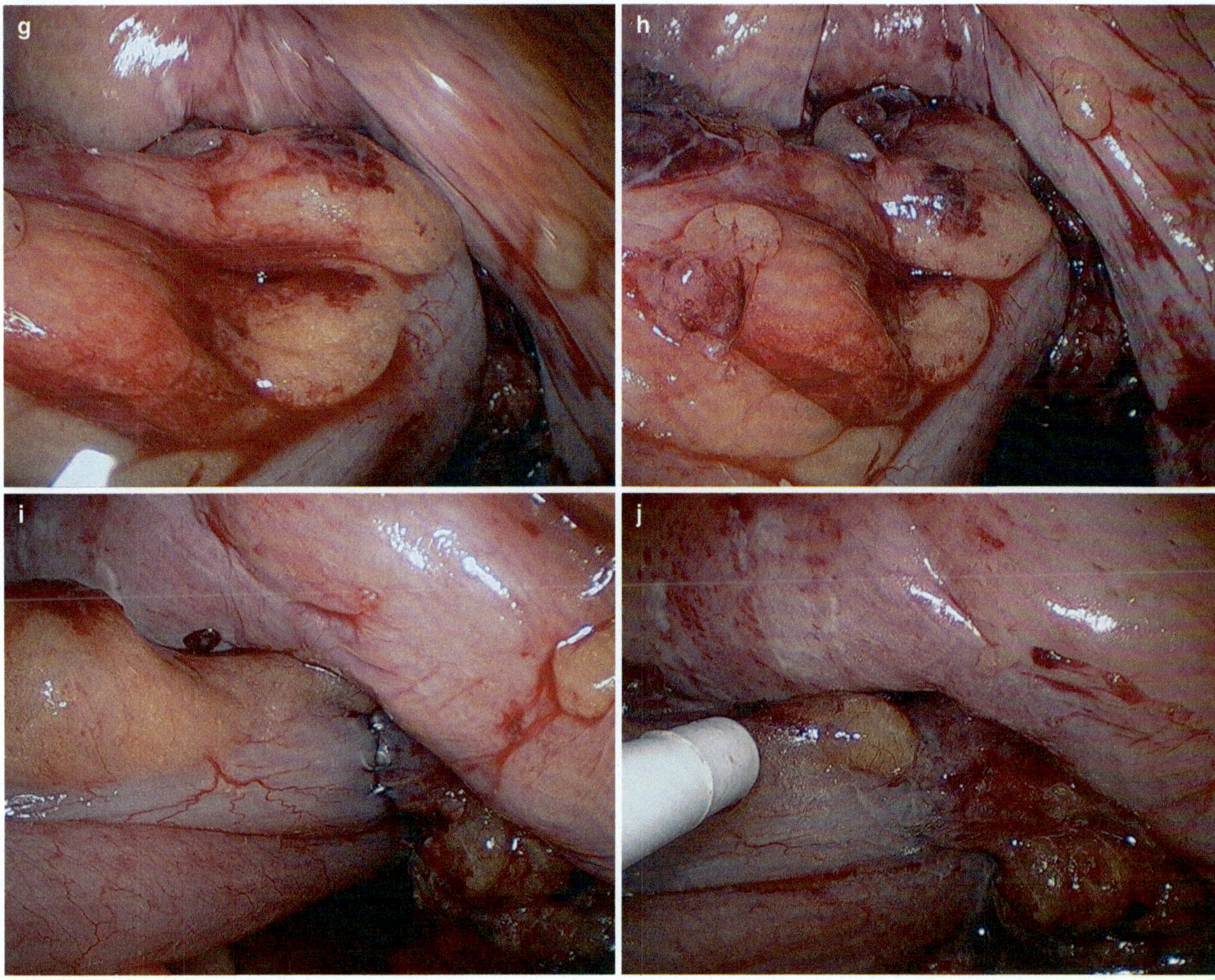

Fig. 4.29 (continued)

8. Flushing and suturing the incision.
   Routine inspection and washing were performed. After careful checking the anastomosis to exclude torsion or twist, a closed suction drain was placed near the anastomosis through the umbilical incision (Fig. 4.30).

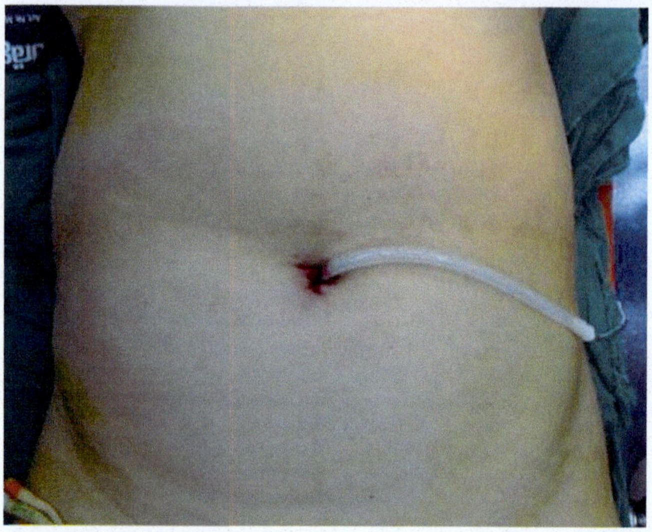

Fig. 4.30

4.4.7 Tips and Tricks

1. The patient is prepared and stabilized to a split-leg extender table.
2. The art of camera driving to provide adequate visualization is an acquired and essential skill that is particularly difficult with the rigid laparoscope. Time spent driving the scope is essential. Learning can occur in a laboratory setting.
3. It is important to be mindful of table, surgeon, and assistant positioning throughout the procedure, as all should transition as the dissection progresses.

4.5 Laparoscopic Radical Resection of Rectal Carcinoma (Dixon Technique)

4.5.1 Indications and Case Selection

Indications for laparoscopic radical resection of rectal carcinoma are identical to the indications for open surgery. Laparoscopic radical operation should be performed as early as possible if there are no contraindications. Dixon operation should be performed for the patients with rectal carcinoma, which is more than 5 cm with the inferior border of the tumor apart from dentate line.

4.5.2 Contraindications

It's identical to Sect. 4.4.2.

4.5.3 Major Instruments or Energy Sources

1. Laparoscopy System.
2. Electrocautery.
3. Harmonic scalpel.
4. Endoscopic linear and circular stapler.

4.5.4 Team Setup, Anesthesia and Position

The patient was positioned lithotomy under general anesthesia. The position of surgeon, assistants and nurses is shown in Fig. 4.31.

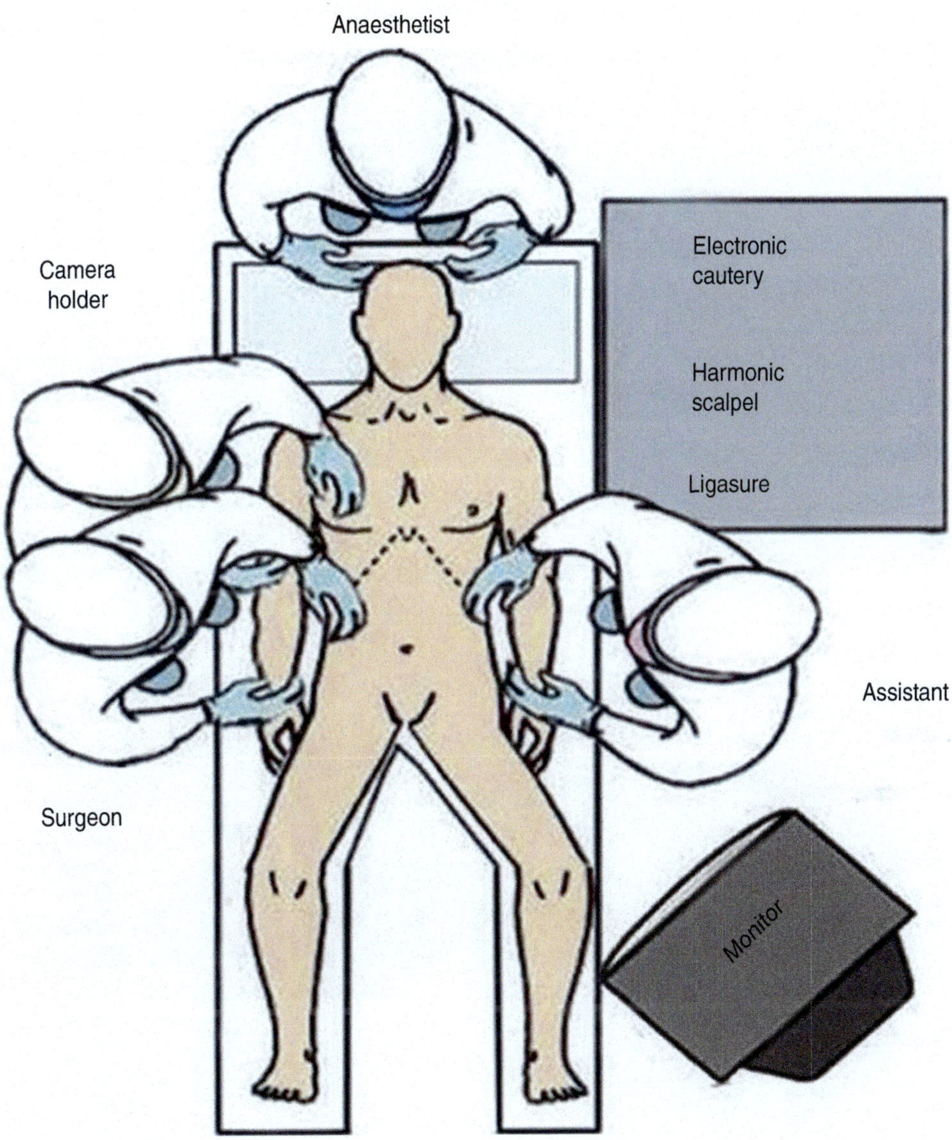

Fig. 4.31

4.5.5 Key Steps

1. Establishment of Pneumoperitoneum and Placement of Trocars.
2. Mobilization of the sigmoid colon.
3. Ligation of the inferior mesenteric vessels.
4. Mobilization of the rectum.
5. Resection of the rectum (transanal technique).
6. Colorectal anastomosis.
7. Flushing and suturing the incision.

4.5.6 Surgical Techniques

1. Establishment of Pneumoperitoneum and Placement of Trocars.
2. Mobilization of the sigmoid colon.
   The surgeon used a lateral to medial technique. The sigmoid colon was retracted medially by using an atraumatic forceps in the left hand and was mobilized from the line of Toldt to the midline by using harmonic scalpel until the peritoneal reflection was reached. Small bleeders encountered were cauterized. Mobilization of the sigmoid mesocolon was carried out inferior to the superior direction in the avascular plane between Gerota's fascia and Toldt's fascia. The medial-to-lateral dissection was continued until the left-sided colon was separated from the retroperitoneum. The left ureter and gonadal vessels were then identified and preserved (Fig. 4.32a–n).

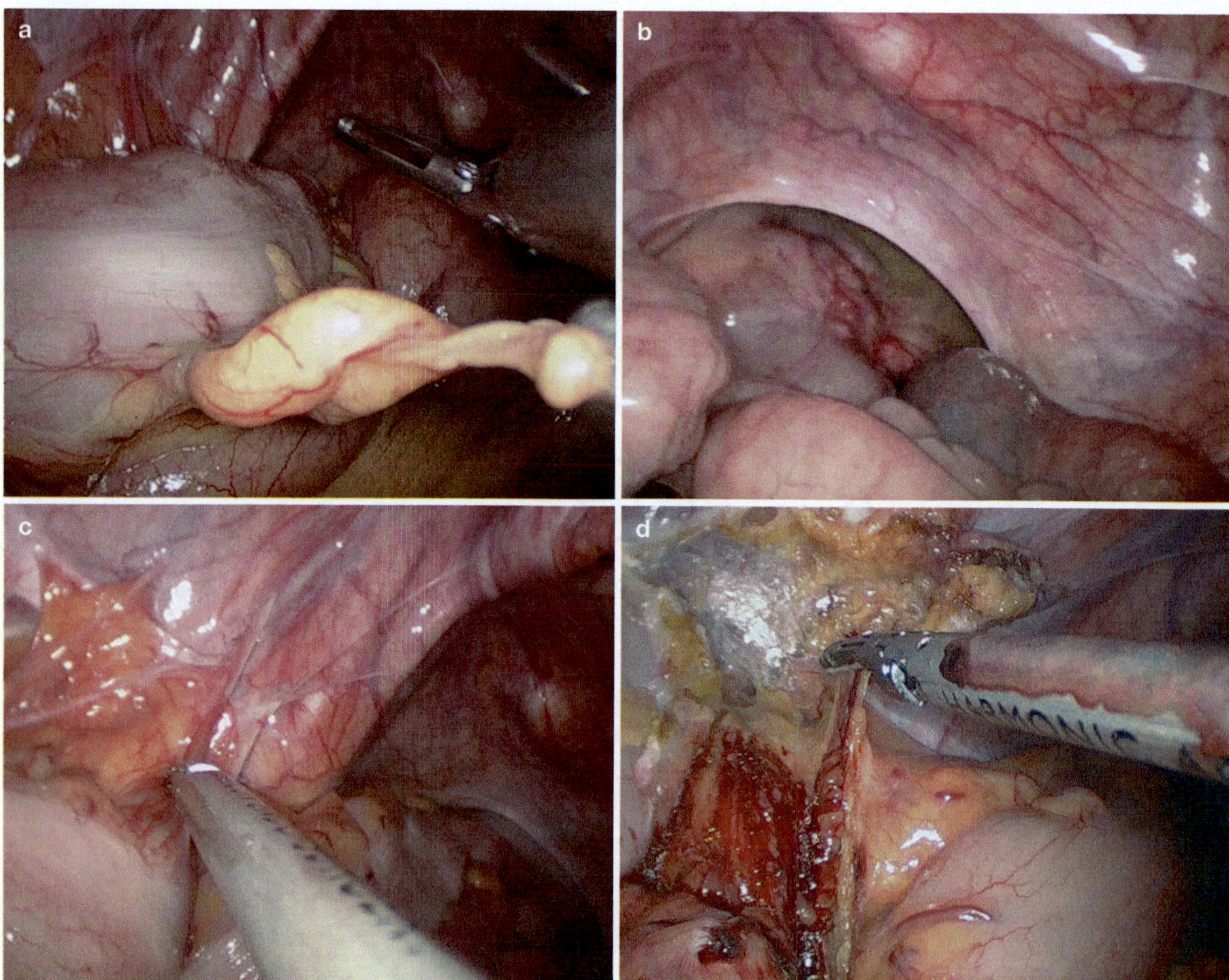

Fig. 4.32

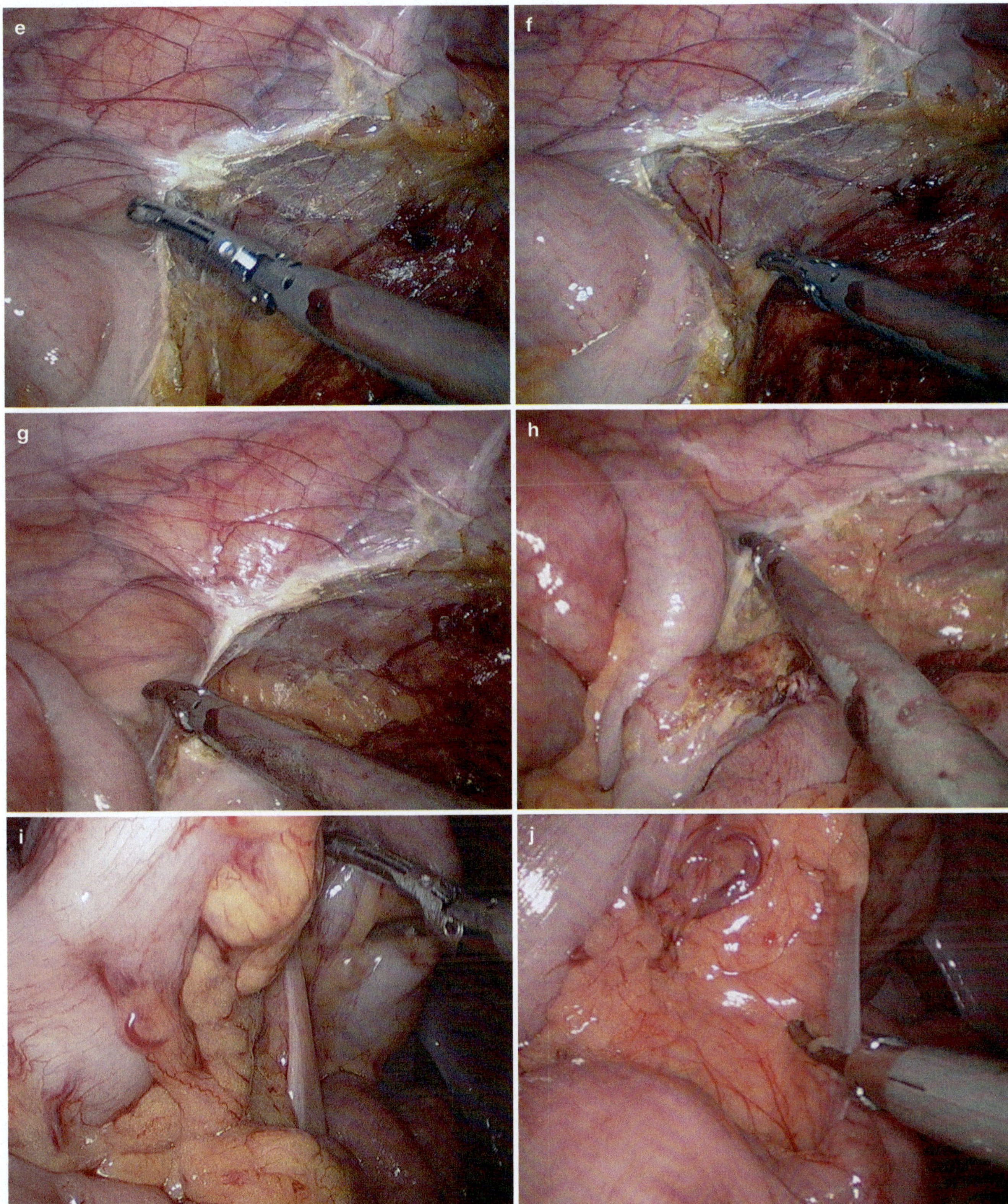

Fig. 4.32 (continued)

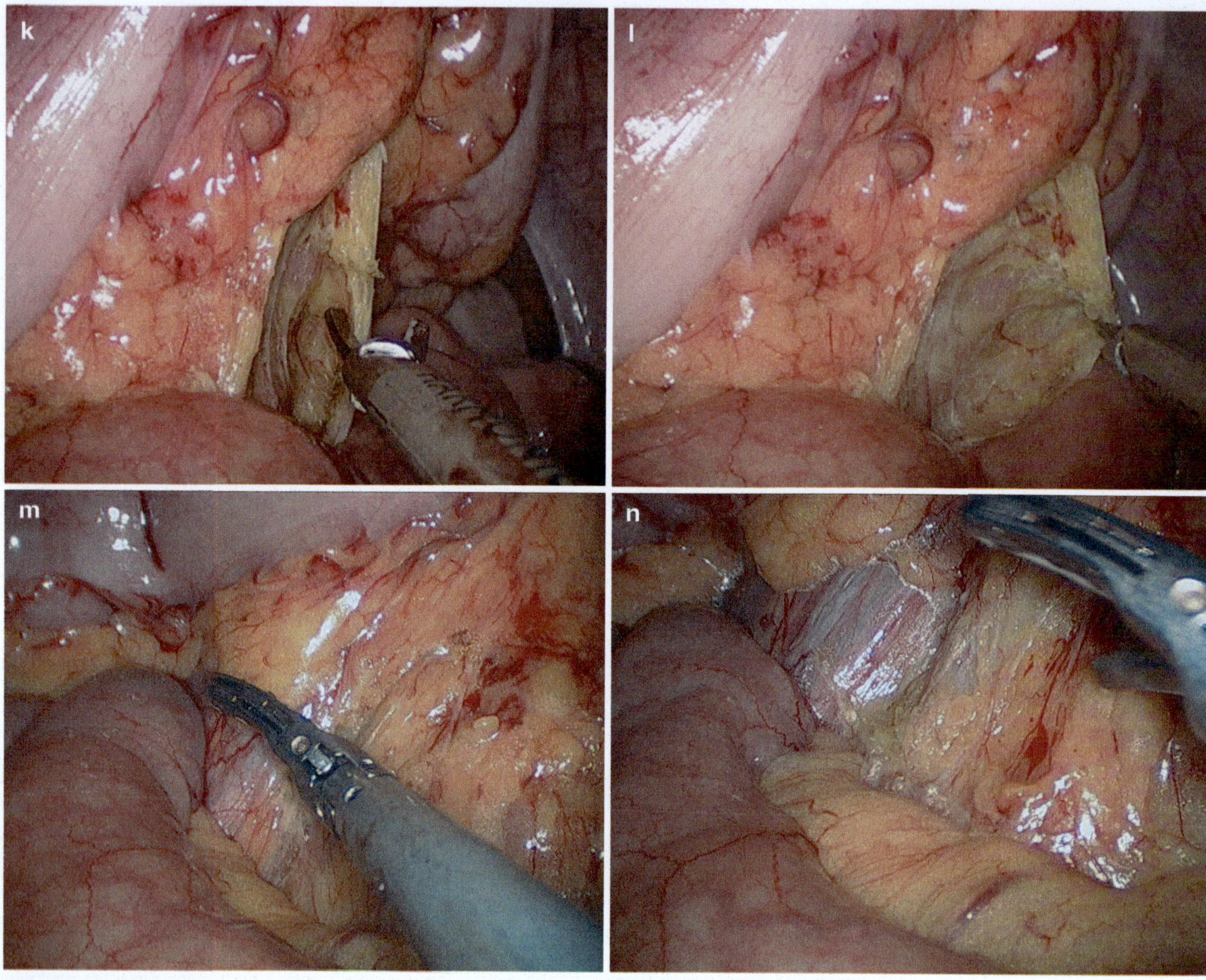

Fig. 4.32 (continued)

3. Ligation of the inferior mesenteric vessels.
   Initially, the inferior mesenteric artery (IMA) was retracted with the double fenestrated forceps, and the IMA was ligated near the origin by using clip placement or linear stapler. Thereafter, division of the inferior mesenteric vein was performed close to the Treitz ligament (Fig. 4.33a–h).

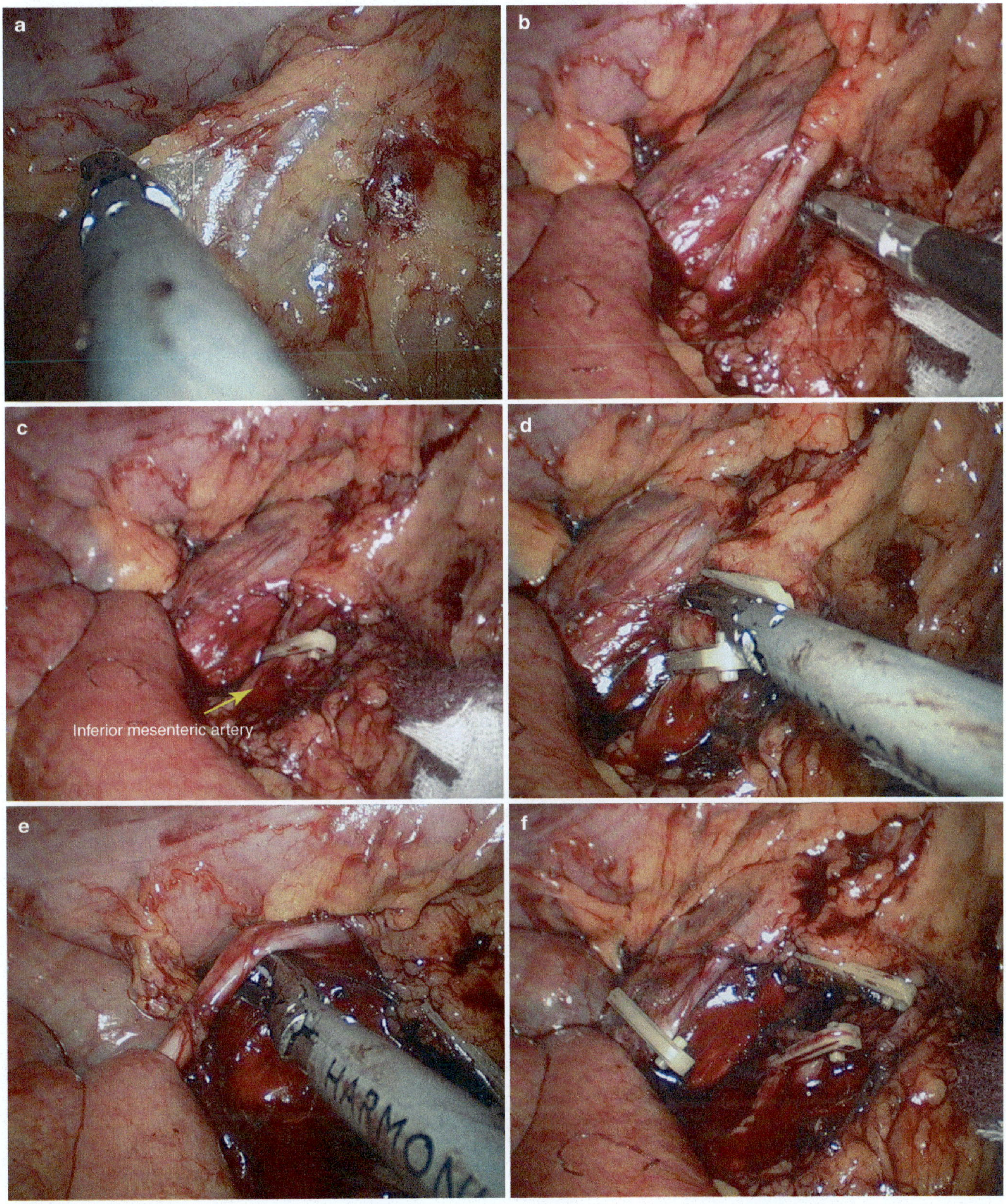

Fig. 4.33

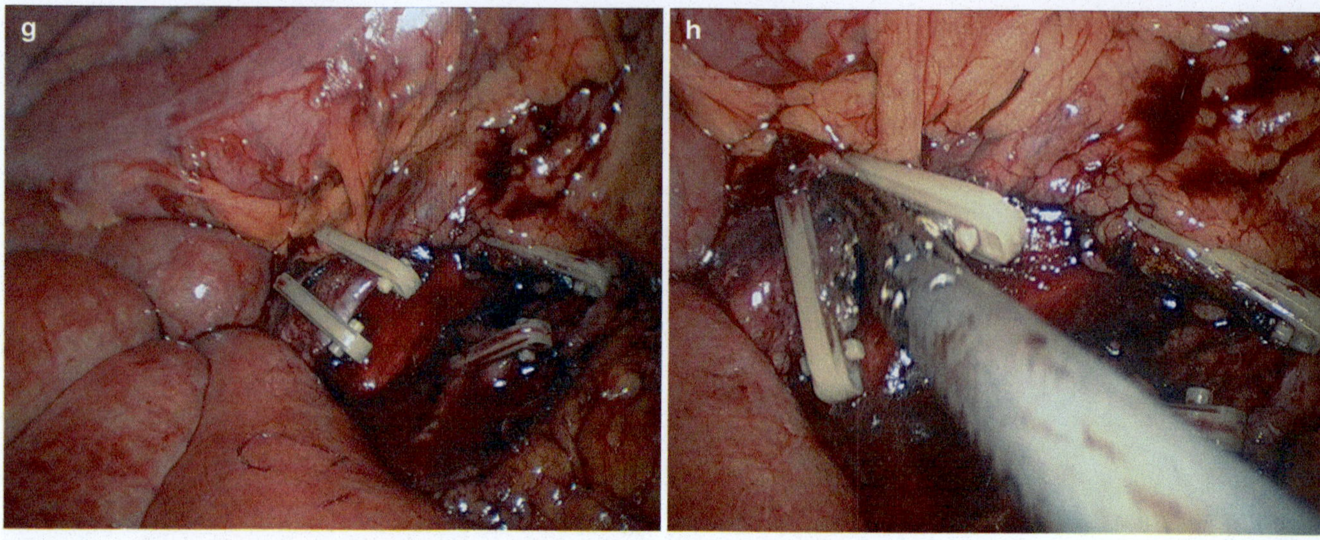

Fig. 4.33 (continued)

4. Mobilization of the rectum.
   A stay suture was introduced into the abdominal cavity through a small puncture on the lower abdominal wall. By seromuscular suture, the rectum was lifted upward to facilitate the mobilization of the posterior wall of the rectum. Rectal mobilization was initiated by dissecting the pelvic cavity along the avascular plane between the fascia propria of the rectum and the parietal fascia, and a total mesorectal excision or a partial mesorectal excision was then performed, depending on the tumor's location (Fig. 4.34a–l).

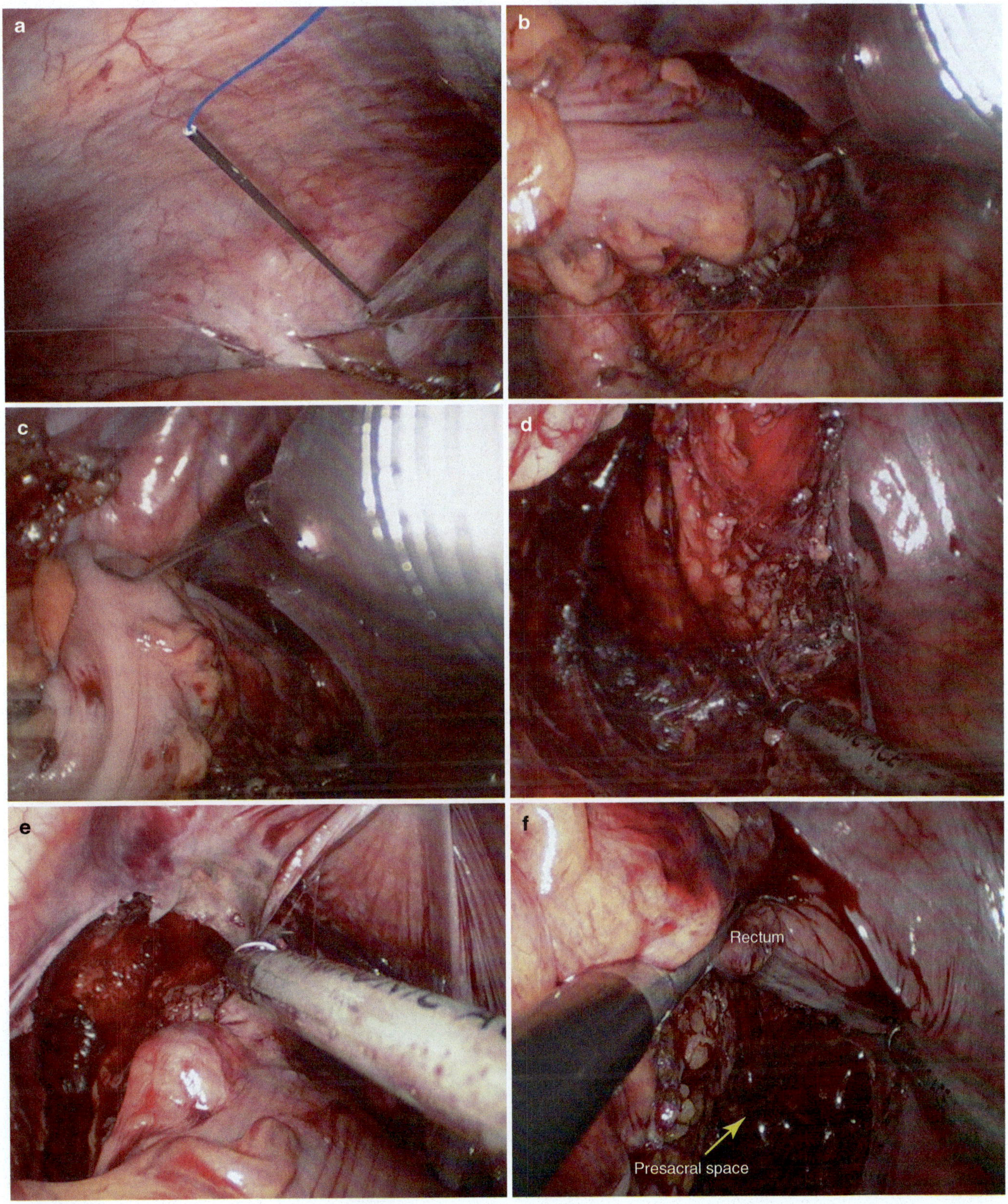

Fig. 4.34

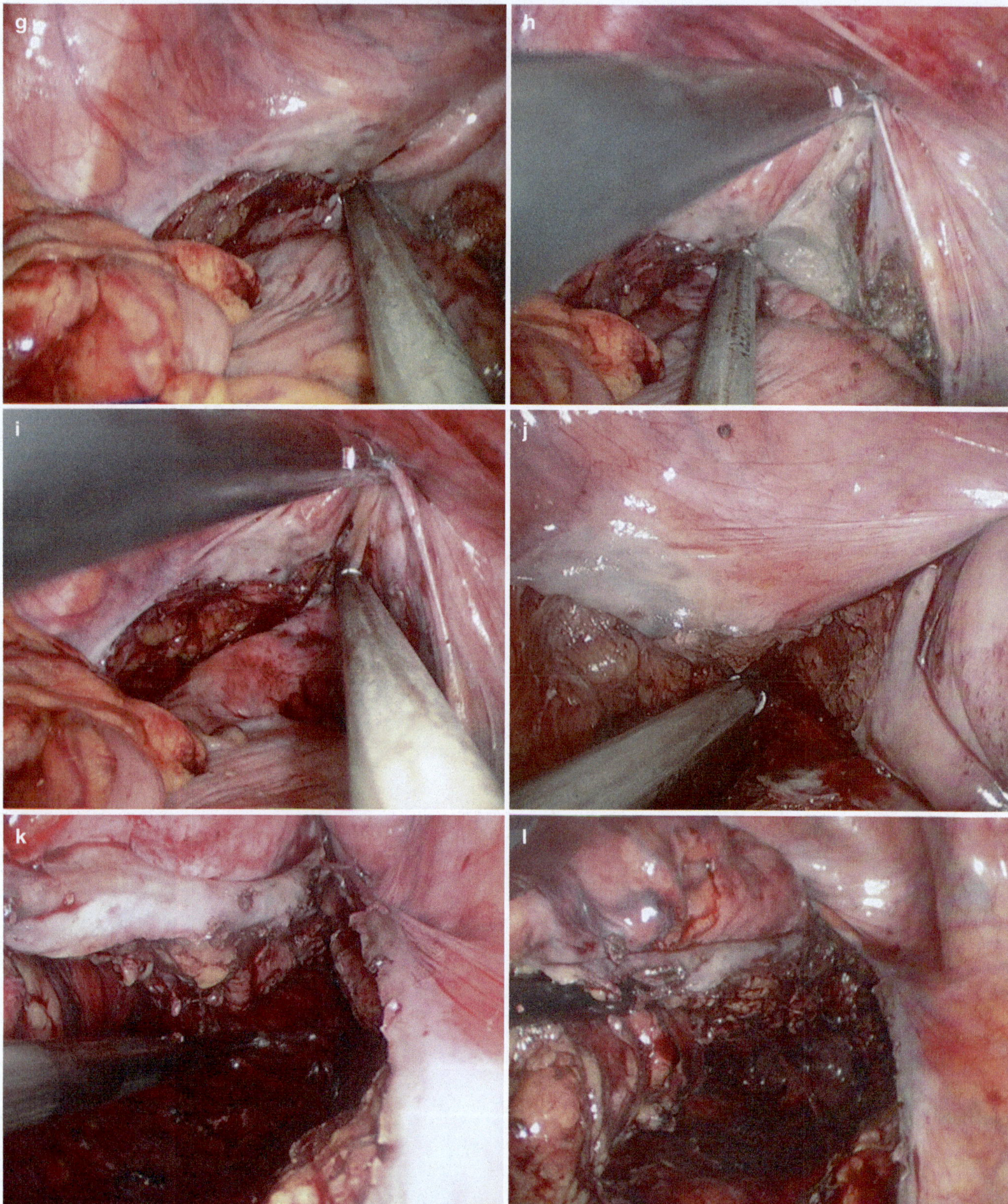

Fig. 4.34 (continued)

5. Resection of the rectum (transanal technique).
   In the case of very low rectal mass, it was difficult to transect the rectum through the umbilical incision. We used a transanal technique here. First, the sigmoid colon was transected 10 cm proximal to the mass by using flexible linear stapler. Then, an oval clamp was introduced into the rectal cavity through the anus to clip and pull out the distal rectum stump through the anus. The distal rectum was transected by using linear stapler under direct vision (Fig. 4.35a–h).

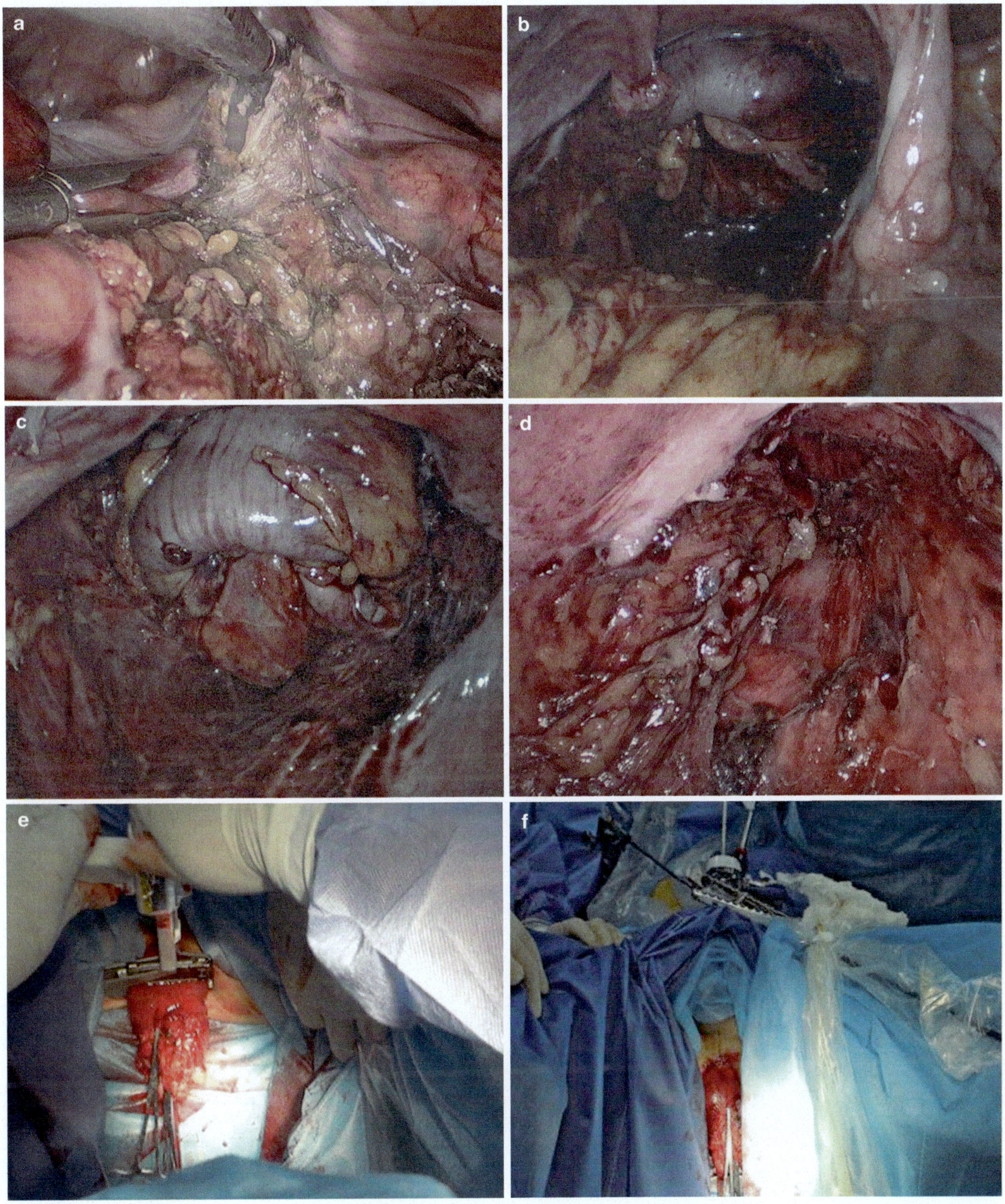

Fig. 4.35

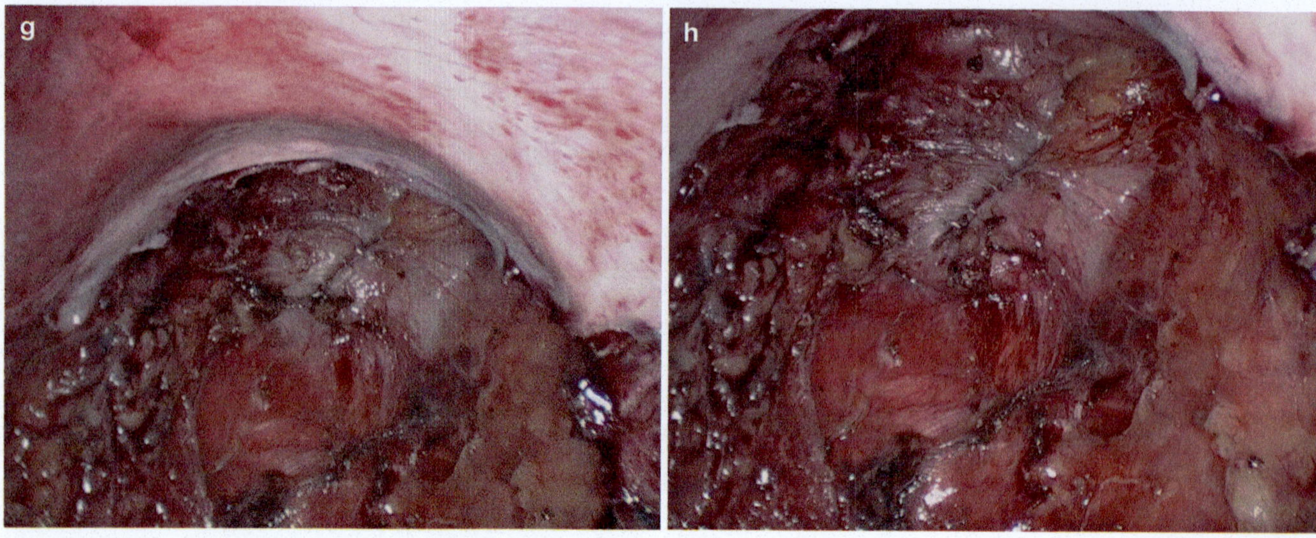

Fig. 4.35 (continued)

6. Colorectal anastomosis.

   The ports were removed and the incision was extended to 3 cm total in length to facilitate exteriorization of the specimen. The proximal sigmoid and rectum were then brought outside the abdomen. A purse-string stapler was used to divide the proximal 10 cm sigmoid colon. The anvil of the circular stapler was put into the proximal stump of the colon and embedded. Then, the stump of the colon was put back into the abdominal cavity. The handle lever of the circular stapler was implanted into the rectal lumen through the anus and punctured out through the middle point of the rectal stump where the anastomosis was to be made. The handle lever and anvil of the stapler were connected, screwed and firmly locked. After careful checking the connection part, the stapler was fired to complete the colorectal end-to-end anastomosis. Careful examination of the anastomosis was done to ensure the devoid of torsion, twist or bleeding (Fig. 4.36a–d).

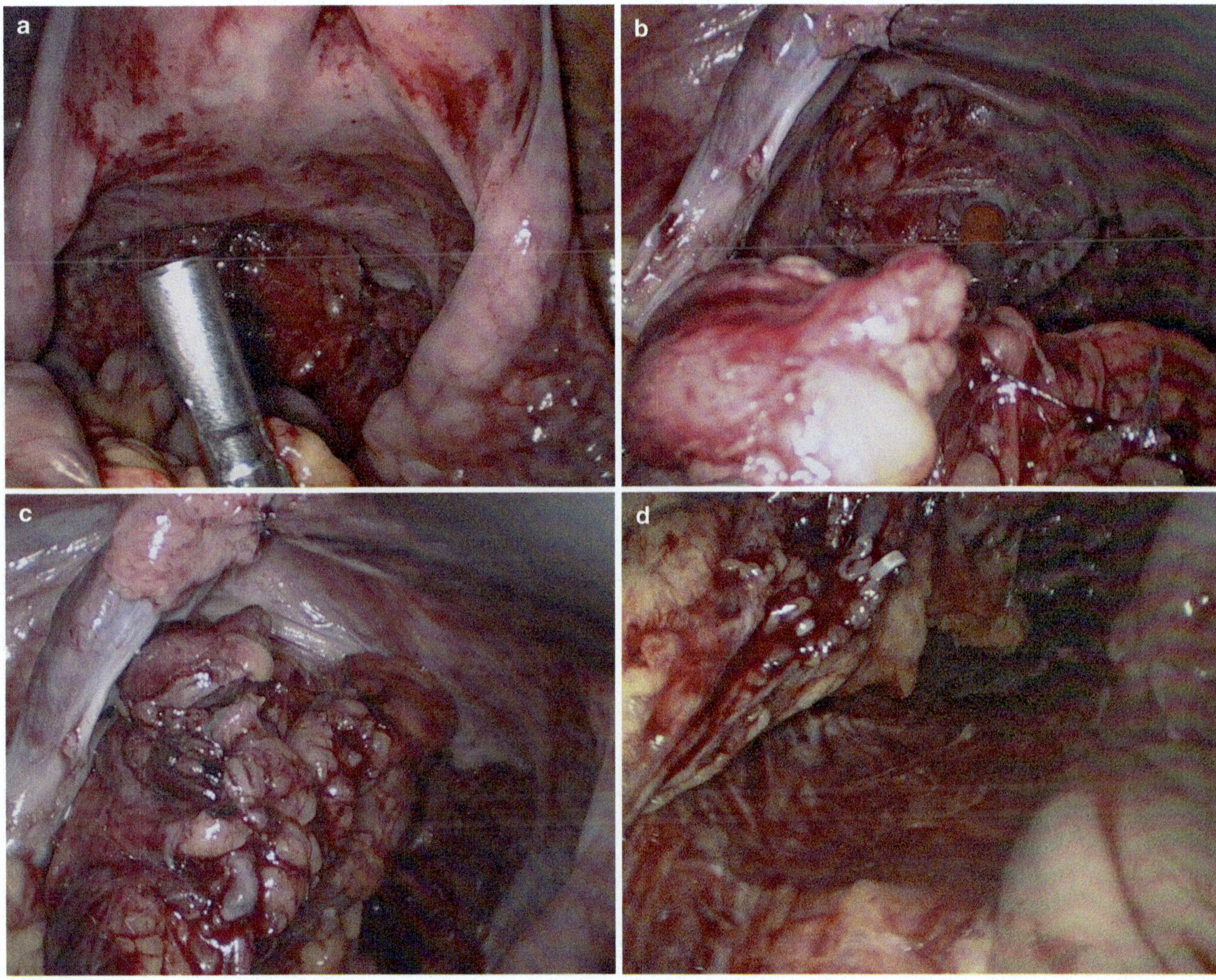

Fig. 4.36

7. Flushing and suturing the incision.
   Routine inspection and washing were performed. After careful checking the anastomosis to exclude torsion or twist, a closed suction drain was placed near the anastomosis through the umbilical incision (Fig. 4.37a, b).

4.5.7 Tips and Tricks

1. When below the peritoneal reflection, visualization can be difficult. A floppy uterus can be retracted anteriorly using a suture on a Keith needle passed under direct vision through the abdominal wall. Clips can also be used to tack a floppy ovary or fallopian tube above the broad ligament.
2. To get further separation between the vagina and the rectum, a probe can be placed into the vagina for anterior retraction or into the rectum for posterior retraction.
3. Both retraction methods can be utilized to create more operating space in the deep narrow pelvis.
4. Getting an adequate flush staple line in the low pelvis can be difficult. Dissection must be low enough to avoid injury to surrounding structures. Placing the stapler in an anterior-to-posterior fashion can make it easier to fit the rectum within the stapler jaws. The staplers are not able to articulate to 90°. By placing cephalad and posterior retraction on the anterior surface of the rectum and using 70° articulation of the stapler, a staple line that is even and flush to the levators can be created.
5. In the scenario of a long anal canal, dissecting within the levators can give additional mobilization so that when perineal pressure is applied, it is possible to get an extra 1–2 cm of rectum.
6. The stapled rectum is grasped and the colon is extracted through the wound protector. After stapling, the small bowel can be returned to the peritoneal cavity to ensure mesenteric orientation for anastomosis or stoma creation.

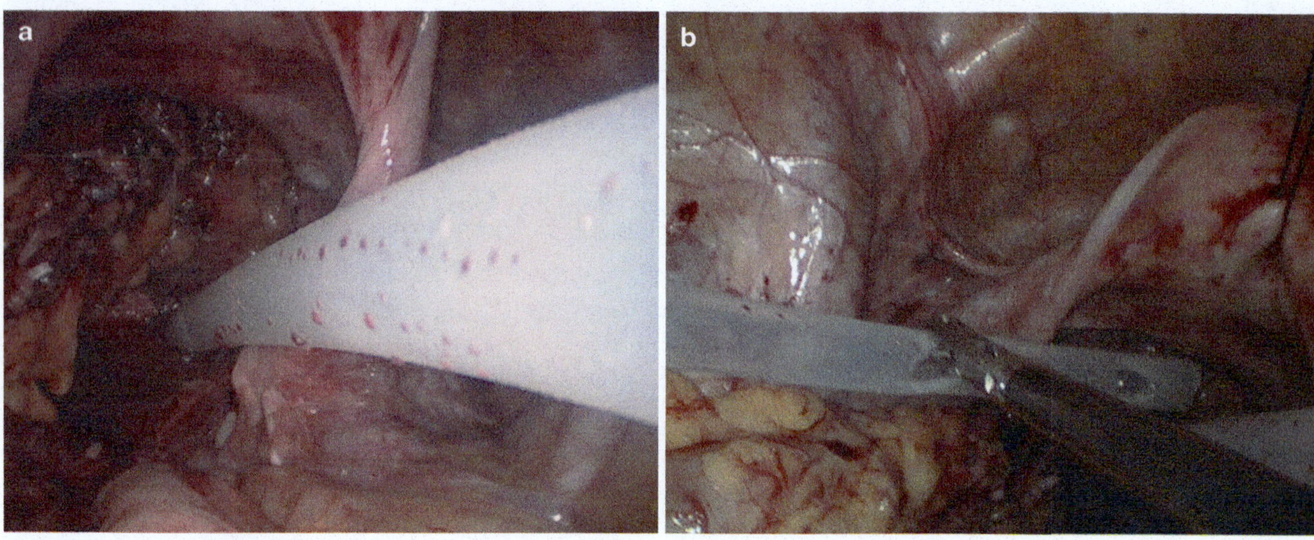

Fig. 4.37

4.6 Laparoscopic Radical Resection of Rectal Carcinoma (Miles Technique)

4.6.1 Indications and Case Selection

Miles operation should be performed for the patients with rectal carcinoma, which is less than 5 cm with the inferior border of the tumor apart from dentate line.

4.6.2 Contraindications

It's identical to Sect. 4.4.2.

4.6.3 Major Instruments or Energy Sources

1. Laparoscopy System.
2. Electrocautery.
3. Harmonic scalpel.
4. Endoscopic linear stapler.

4.6.4 Team Setup, Anesthesia and Position

The patient was positioned lithotomy under general anesthesia. The position of surgeon, assistants and nurses is shown in Fig. 4.38.

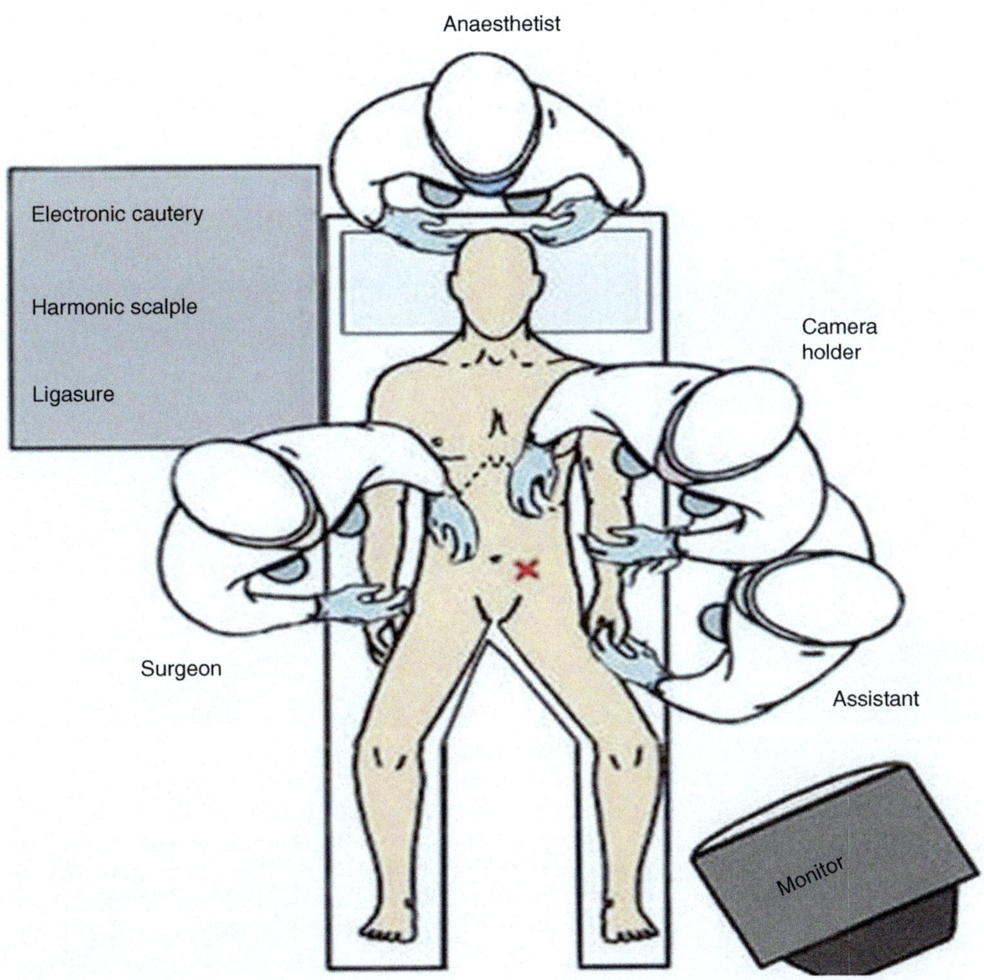

Fig. 4.38

4.6.5 Key Steps

1. Establishment of Pneumoperitoneum and Placement of Trocars.
2. Mobilization of the sigmoid colon and upper segment of the rectum.
3. Ligation of the inferior mesenteric vessels.
4. Mobilization of the rectum.
5. Transperineal resection of the rectum.
6. Establishment of artificial anus.

4.6.6 Surgical Techniques

1. Establishment of Pneumoperitoneum and Placement of Trocars.
   The single 3 cm incision was made on the left lower quadrant of the abdomen wall against the McBurney point where the stoma was to be made (Fig. 4.39).
2. Mobilization of the sigmoid colon and upper segment of the rectum.
   The surgeon used a lateral to medial technique. The sigmoid colon was retracted medially by using an atraumatic forceps in the left hand and was mobilized from the line of Toldt to the midline by using the harmonic scalpel until the peritoneal reflection was reached. Small bleeders encountered were cauterized. Mobilization of the sigmoid mesocolon was carried out inferior to the superior direction in the avascular plane between Gerota's fascia and Toldt's fascia. The medial-to-lateral dissection was continued until the left-sided colon was separated from the retroperitoneum. The left ureter and gonadal vessels were then identified and preserved (Fig. 4.39a–ab).

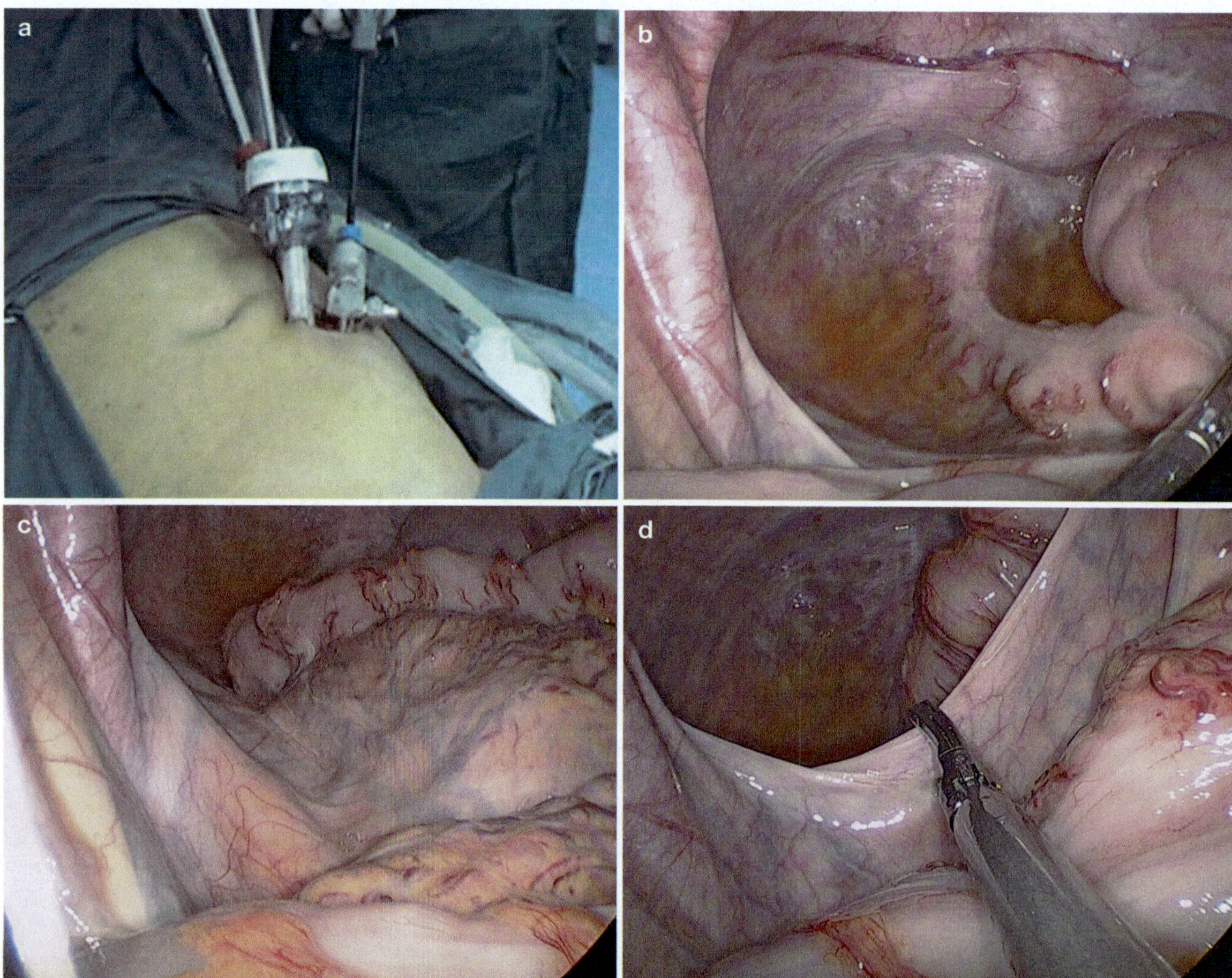

Fig. 4.39

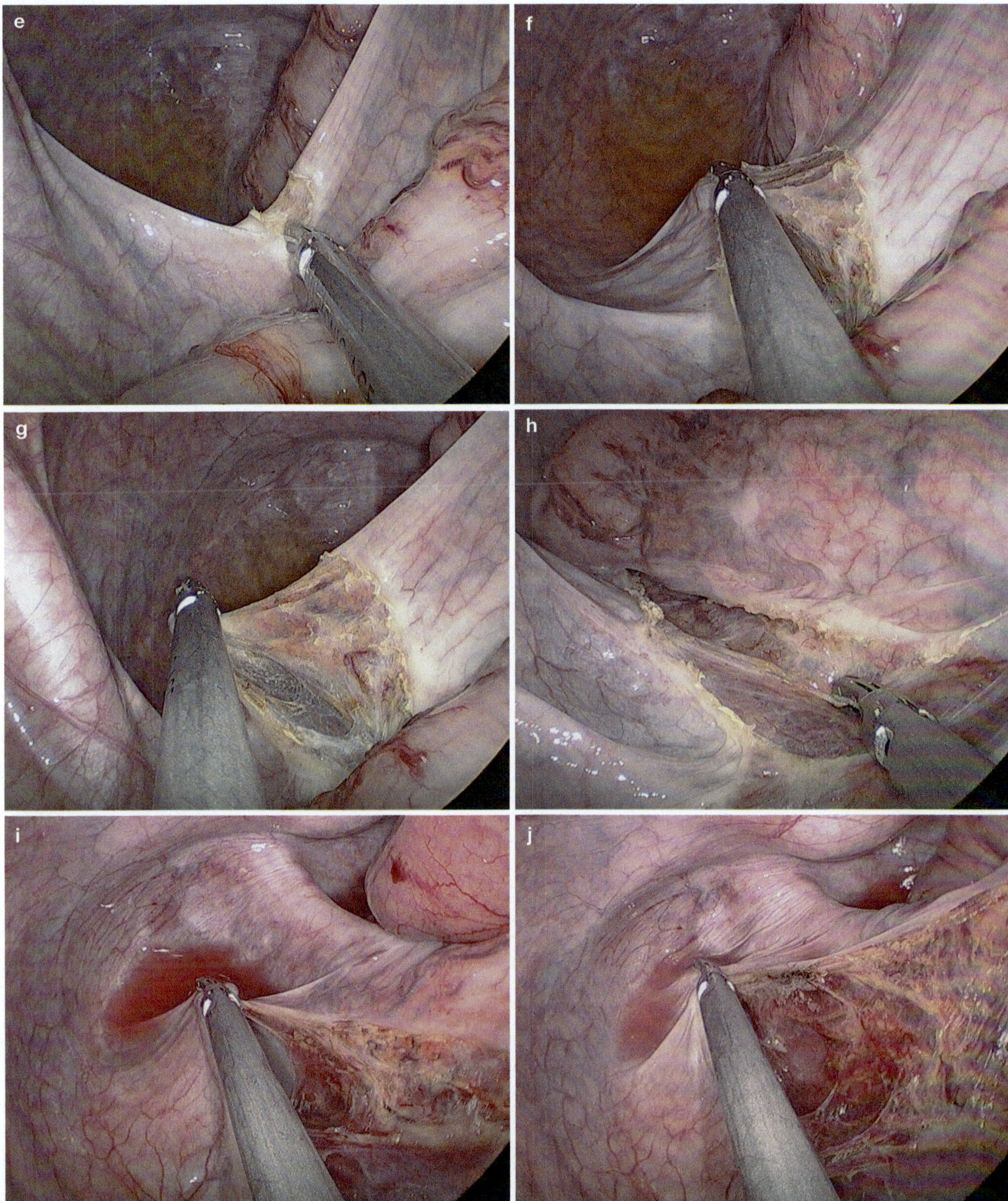

Fig. 4.39 (continued)

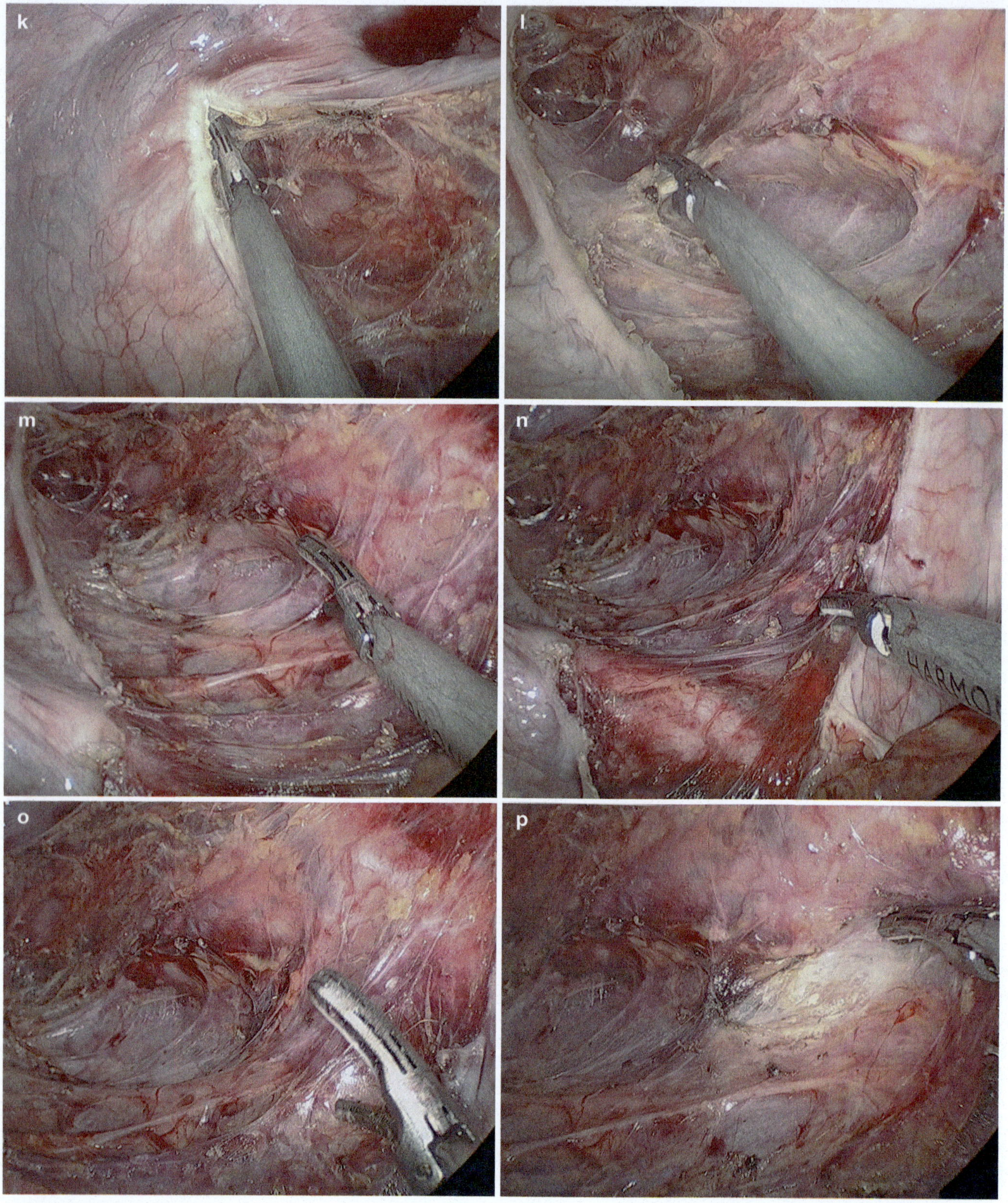

Fig. 4.39 (continued)

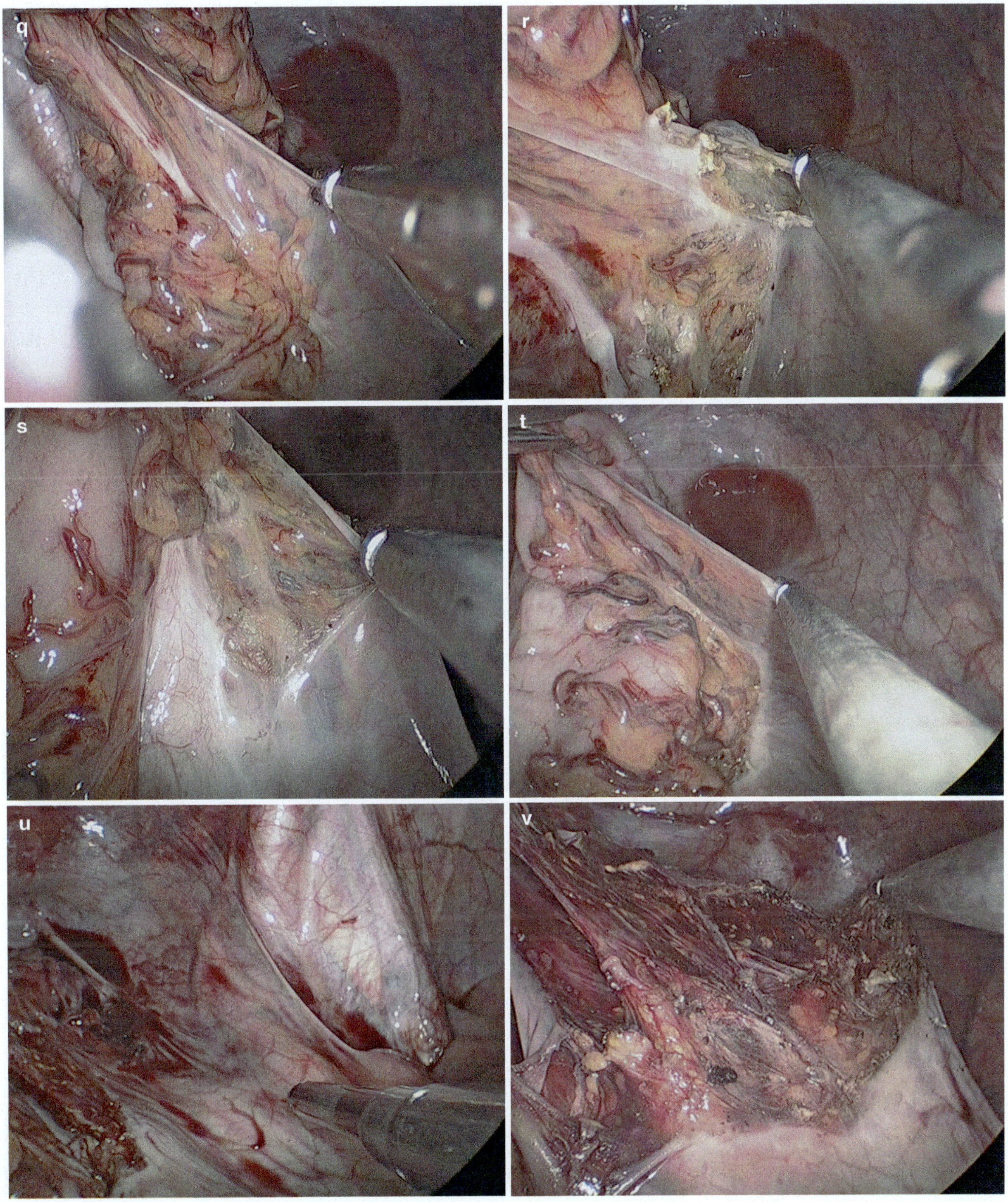

Fig. 4.39 (continued)

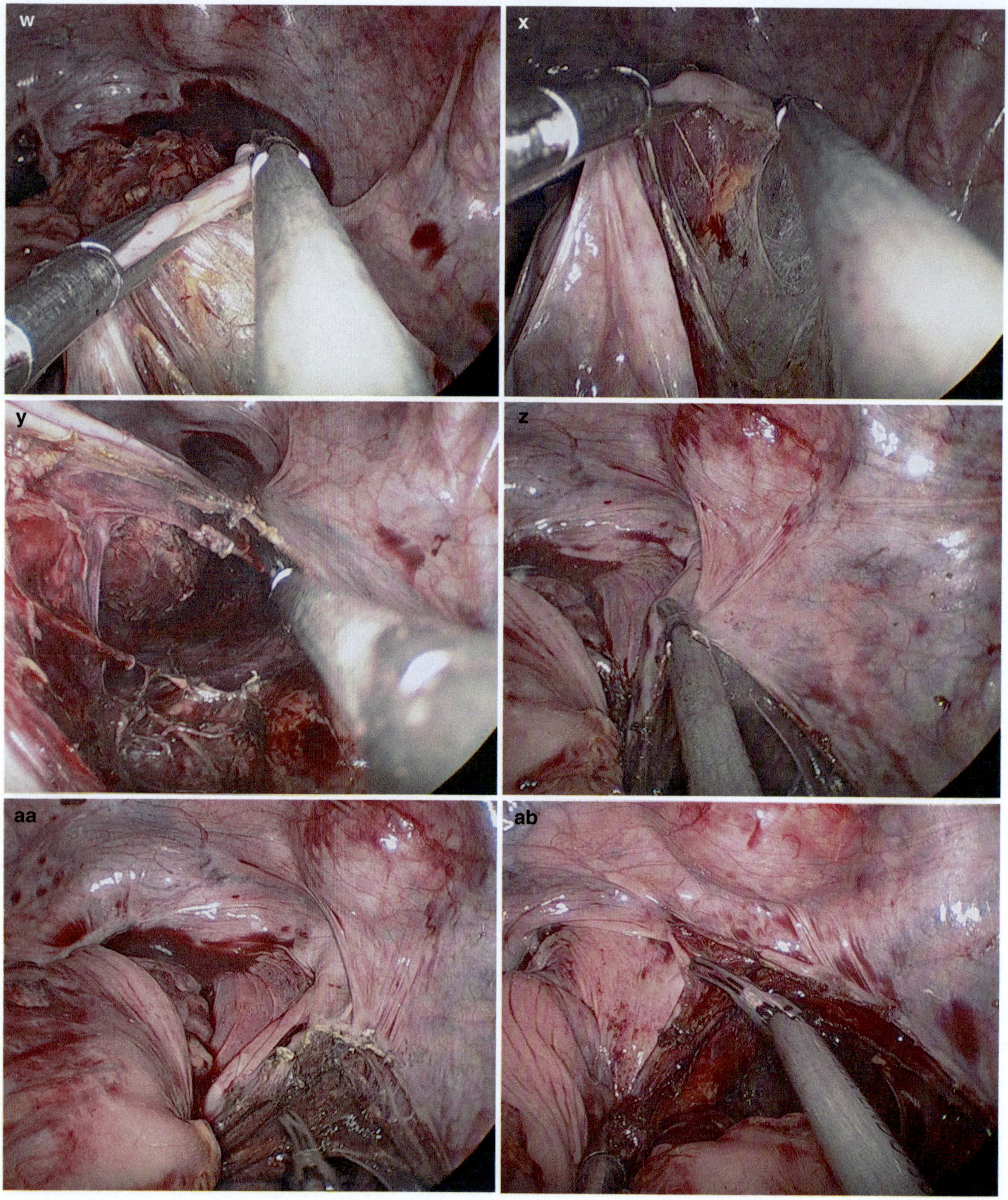

Fig. 4.39 (continued)

3. Ligation of the inferior mesenteric vessels.
   Initially, the inferior mesenteric artery (IMA) was retracted with the double fenestrated forceps, and the IMA was ligated near the origin by using clip placement or linear stapler. Thereafter, division of the inferior mesenteric vein was performed close to the Treitz ligament (Fig. 4.40a–f).

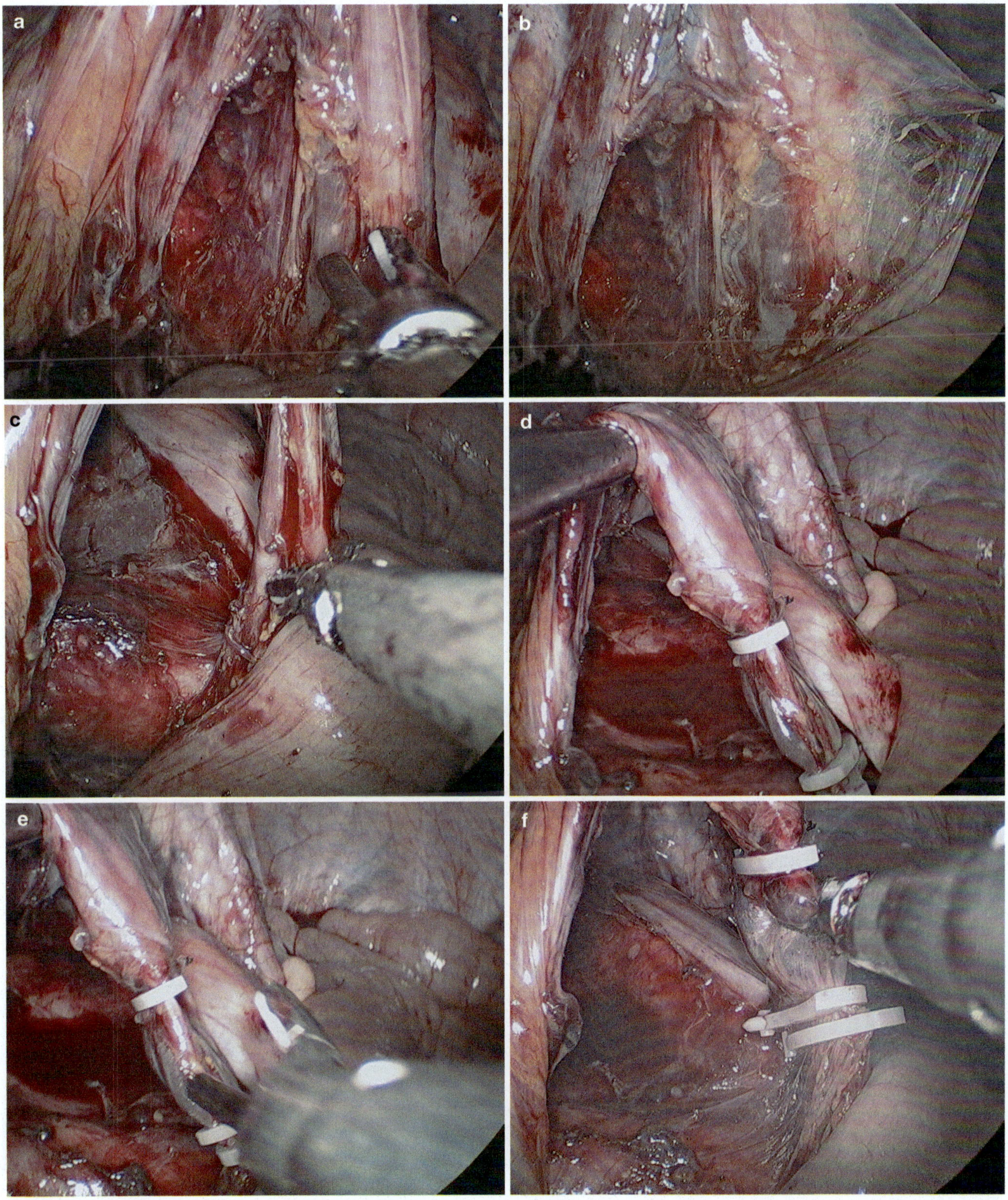

Fig. 4.40

4. Mobilization of the rectum.
Rectal mobilization was initiated by dissecting the pelvic cavity along the avascular plane between the fascia propria of the rectum and the parietal fascia, and a total mesorectal excision was then performed (Fig. 4.41a–ab).

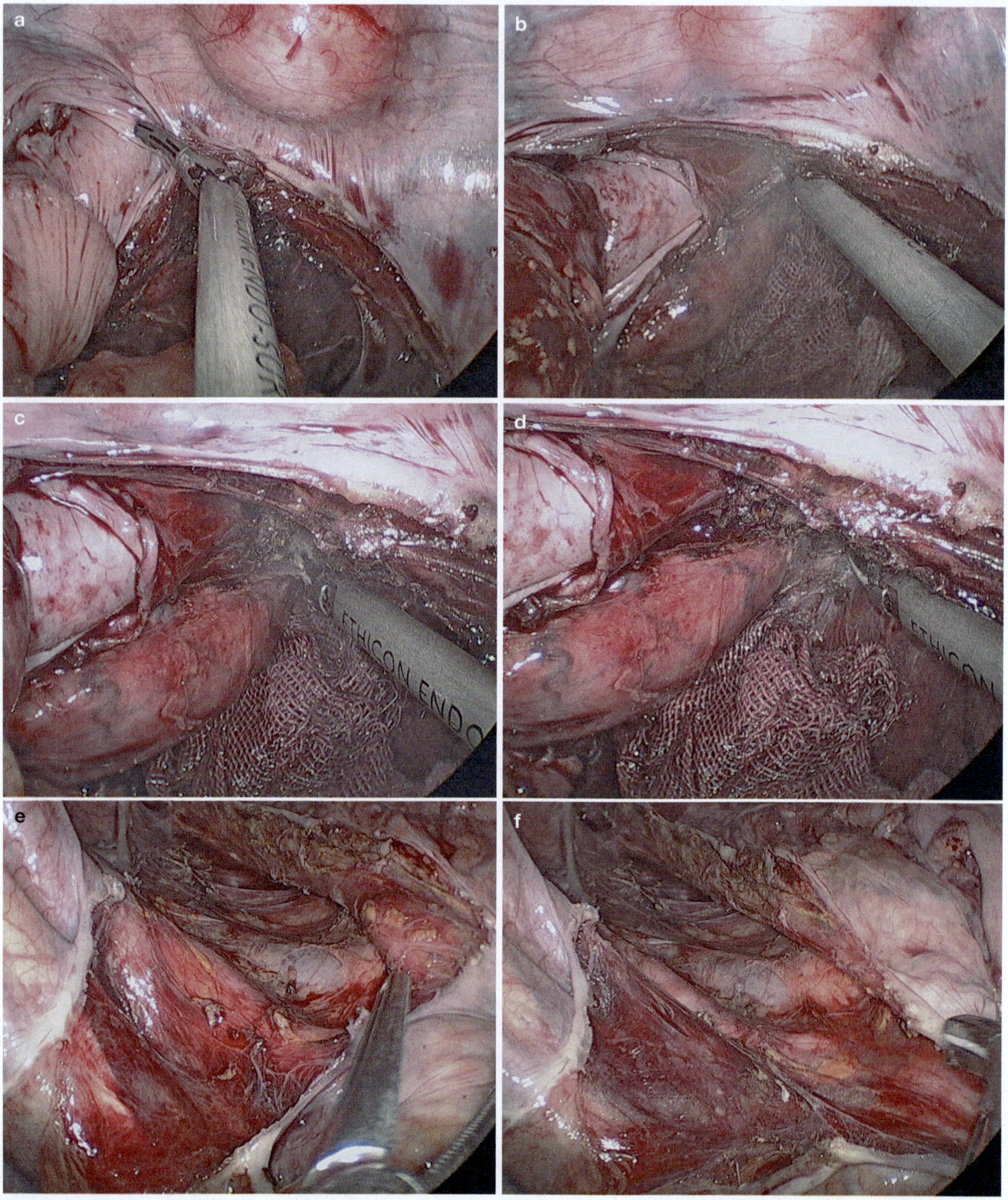

Fig. 4.41

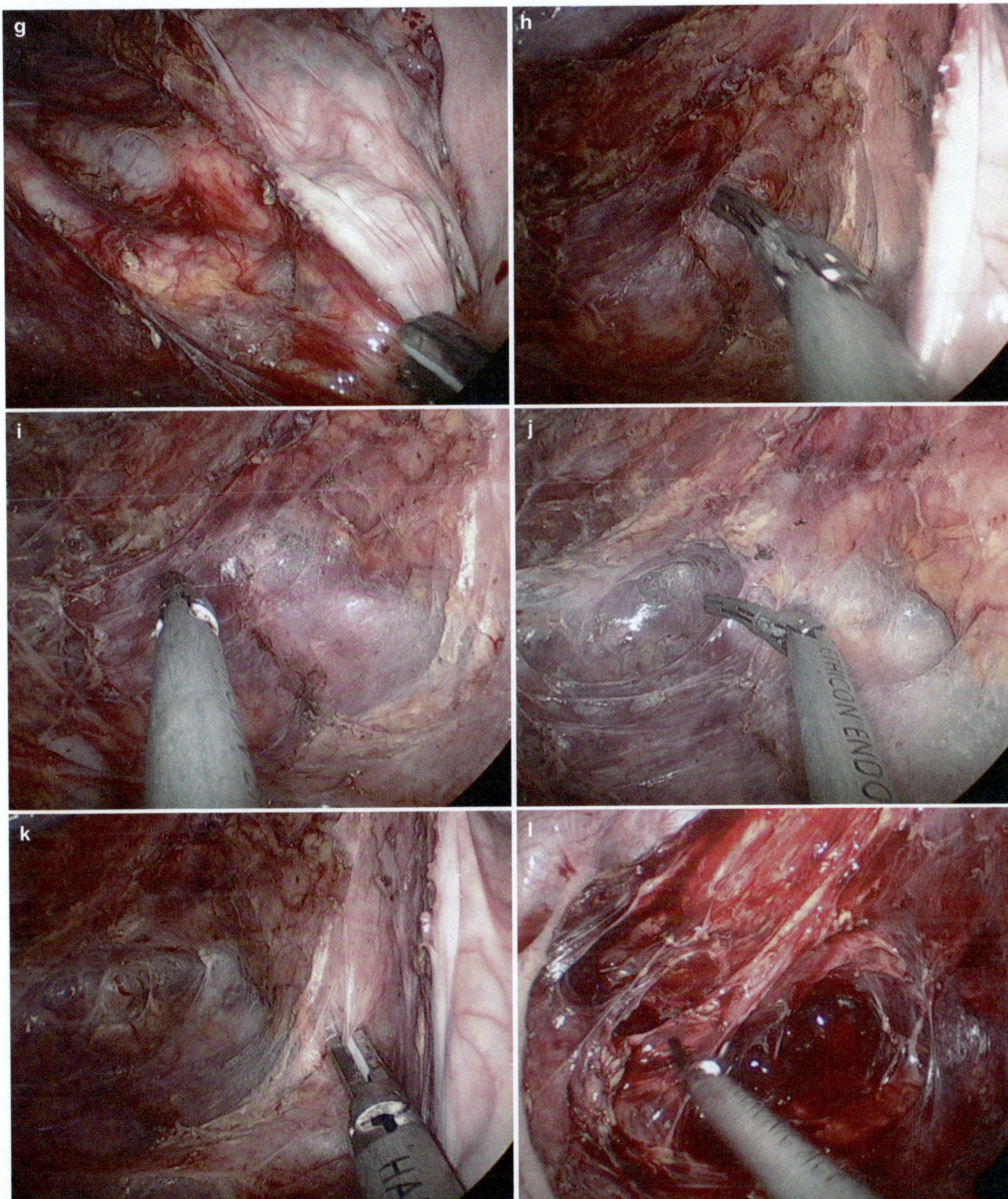

Fig. 4.41 (continued)

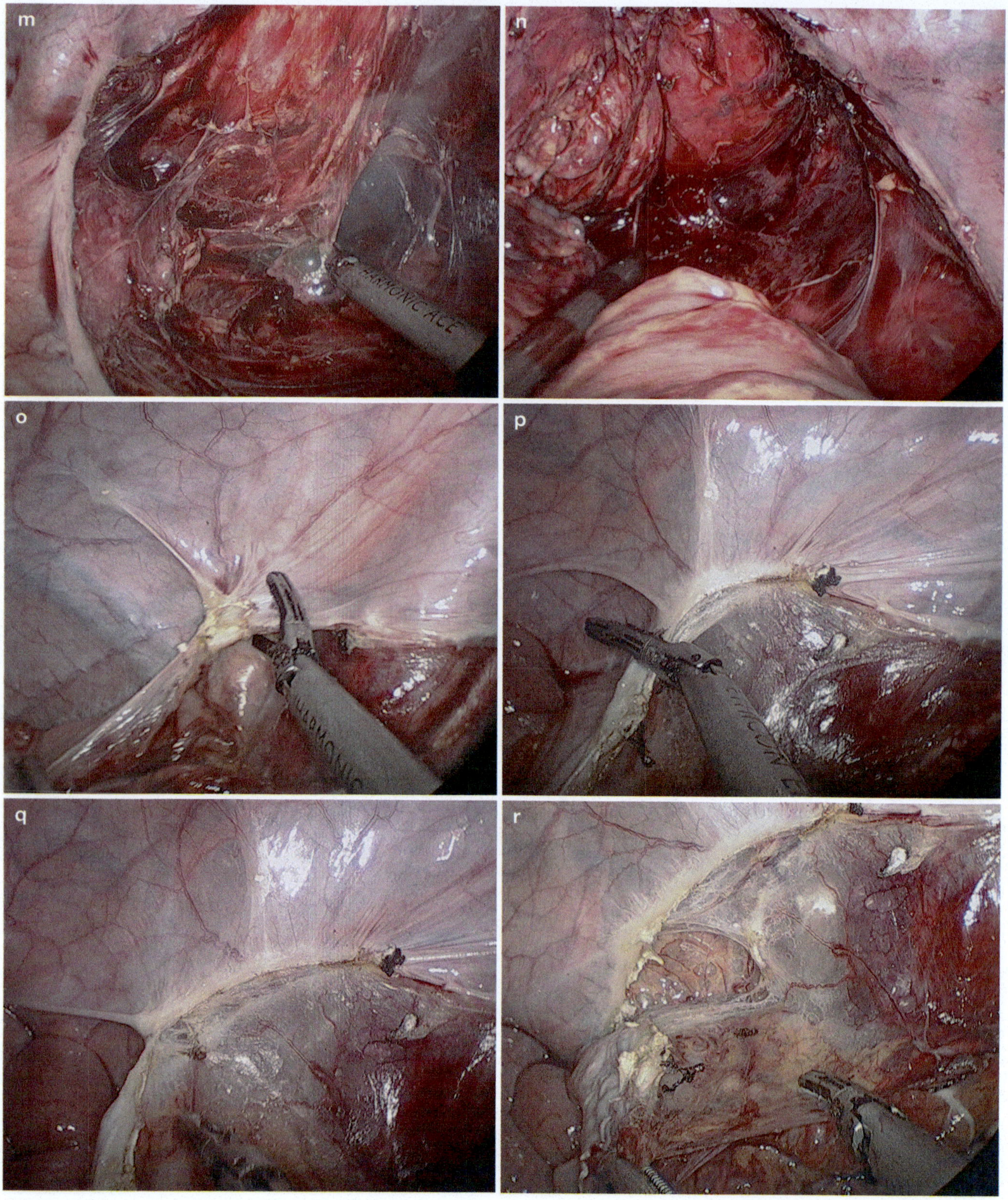

Fig. 4.41 (continued)

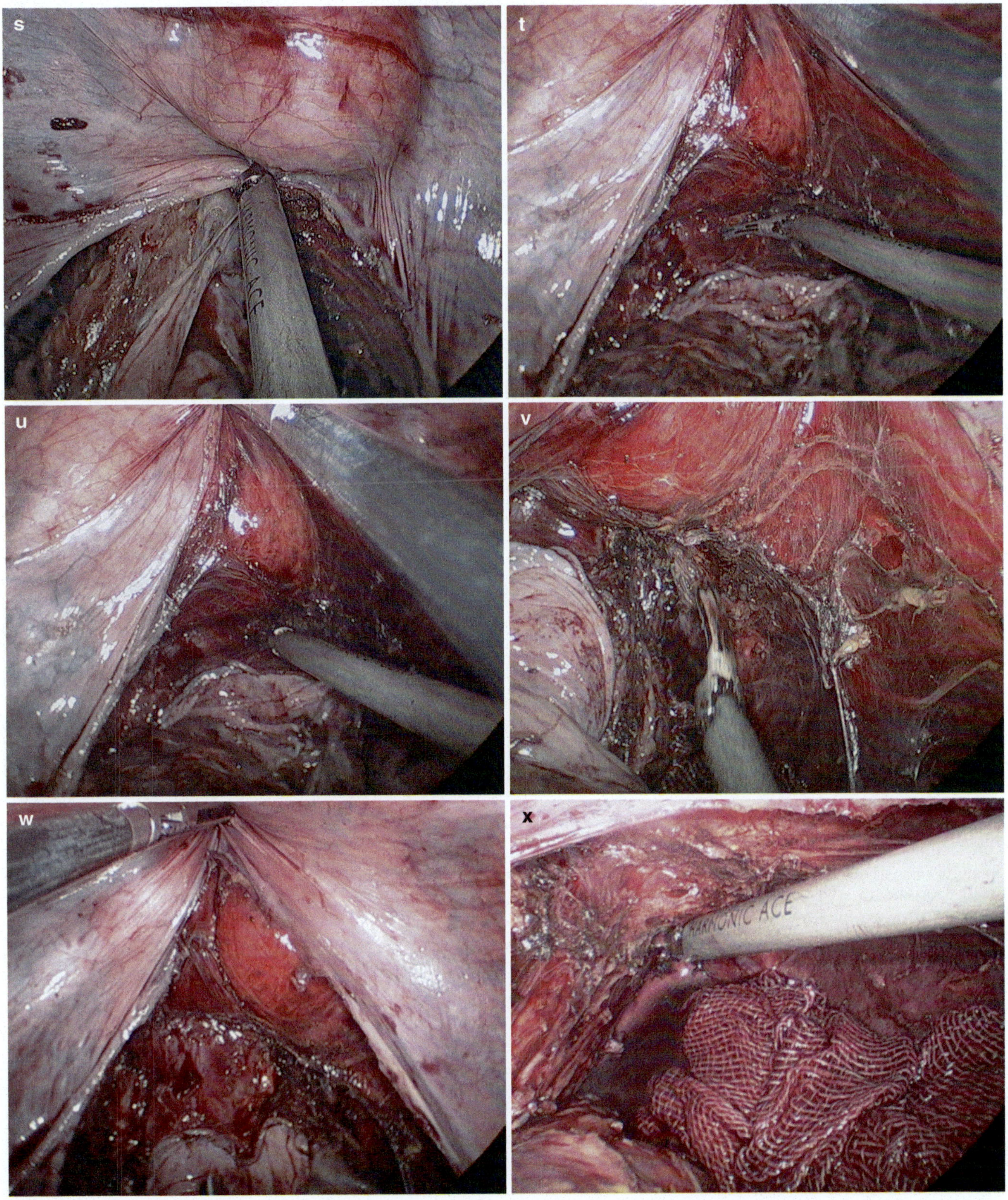

Fig. 4.41 (continued)

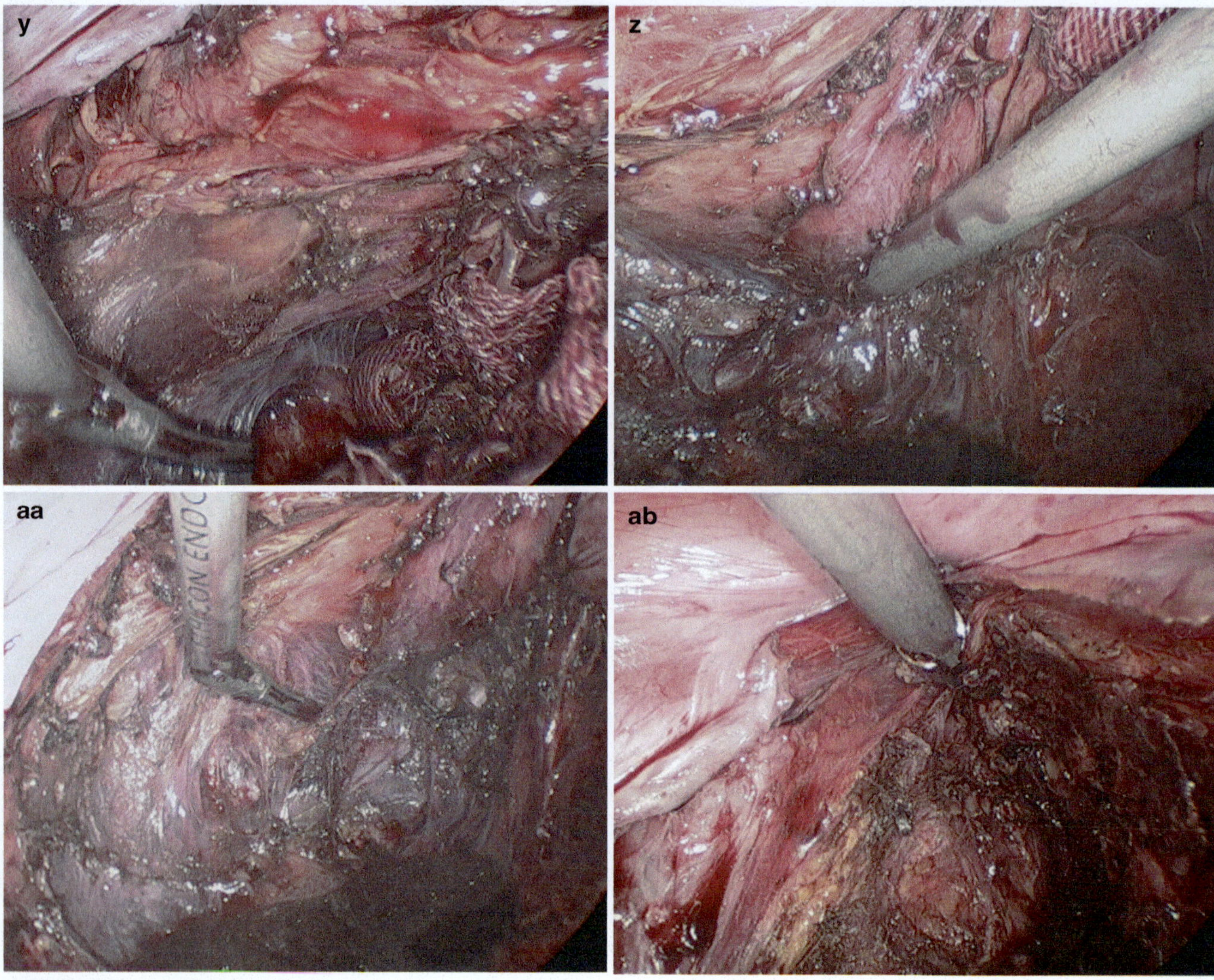

Fig. 4.41 (continued)

5. Transperineal resection of the rectum.
   After once again disinfection of the perineum, the anus was closed by interrupted suture. An oval incision was made around the anus and the lower segment of the rectum was freed layer-by-layer until it was completely fully liberated and pulled out through the anus. The sigmoid colon was transected 15 cm proximal to the mass by using linear stapler. The whole specimen was removed and the stump of the colon returned to the abdominal cavity. The perineal incision was sutured (Fig. 4.42a–h).

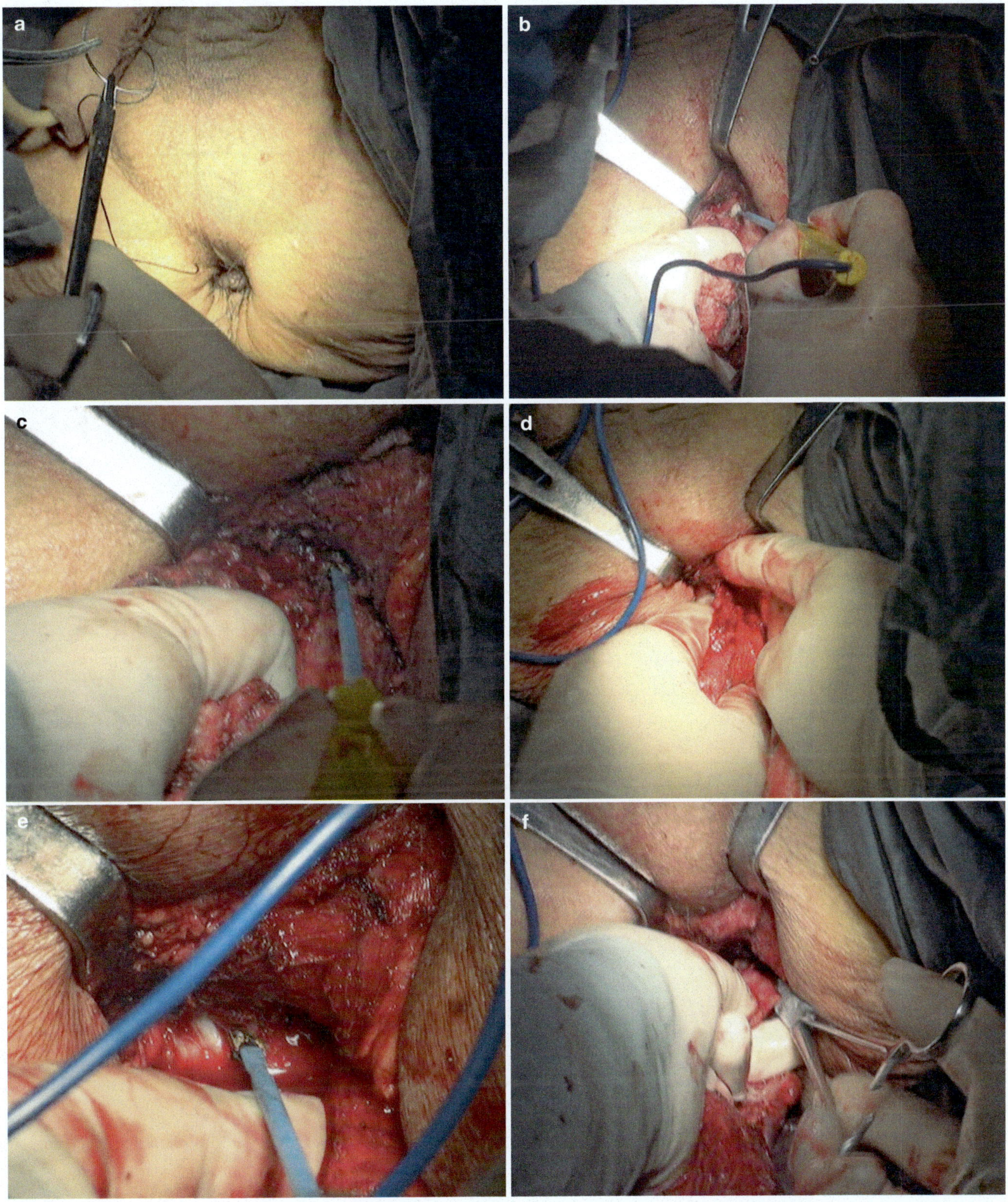

Fig. 4.42

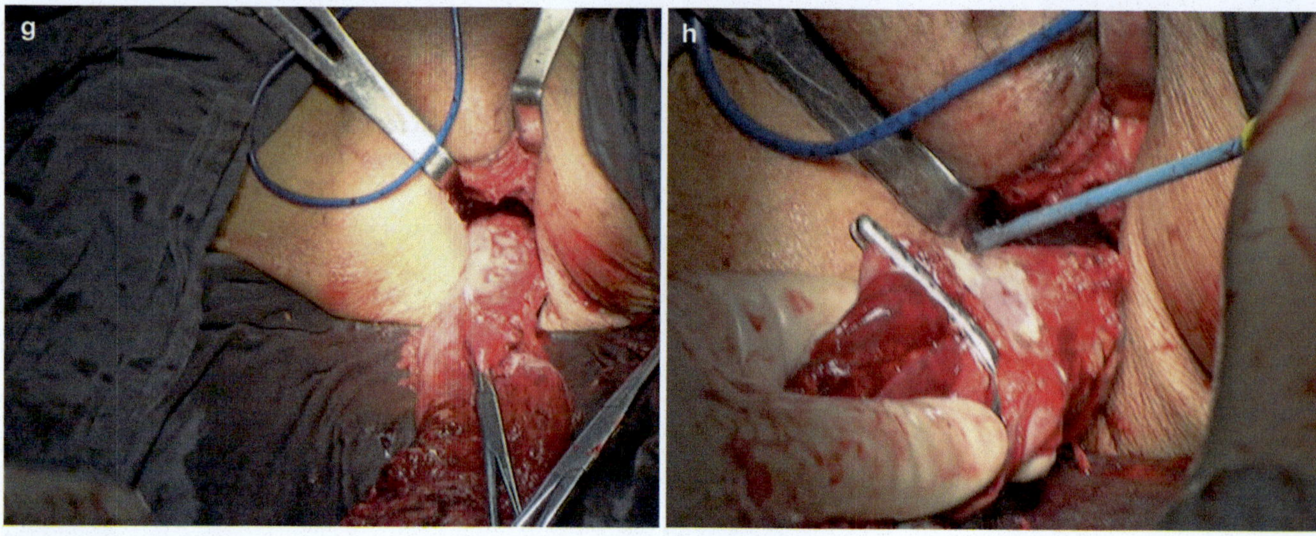

Fig. 4.42 (continued)

6. Establishment of artificial anus.
   The abdominal incision was expanded to about 3 cm and the fascial bridges among the ports were cut open. The stump of the sigmoid colon was extracted out through this single incision and an artificial anus was established (Fig. 4.43a, b).

4.6.7 Tips and Tricks

1. The right-sided dissection is difficult when operating through the stoma site as the dissection is directly below the port. Patient positioning in the maximal left-side-down position helps to maintain ergonomics while operating directly under the incision.
2. A technique for providing sufficient retraction and triangulation is using an increased table angulation and gravity to tent the mesentery over the non-dominant instrument, providing a clear view both above and below the mesentery. This technique helps to ensure safety of transection and good visualization of all structures, while not causing trauma to the bowel.
3. After sample removal, the small bowel can be returned to the peritoneal cavity to ensure mesenteric orientation for stoma creation.

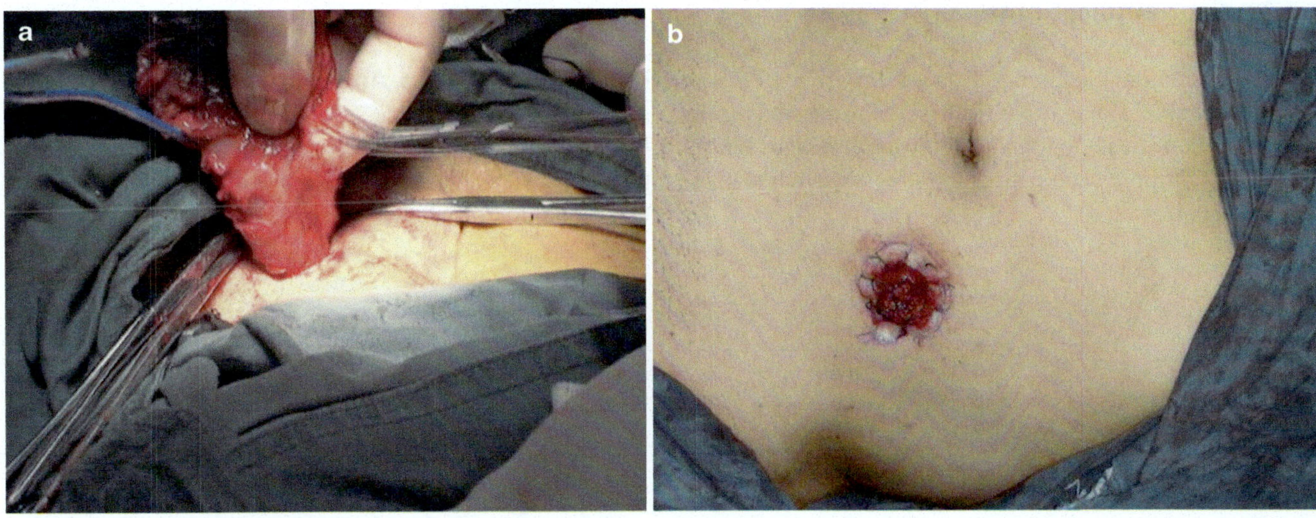

Fig. 4.43

4.7 Laparoscopic Pancolectomy

4.7.1 Indications and Case Selection

1. Patients with benign disease, including familial adenomatous polyposis coli., intractable or complicated inflammatory bowel disease, bleeding arteriovenous malformations, severe, chronic constipation, ischemic colitis or any other condition suitable for resection.
2. Patients with malignant disease, including synchronous colon carcinoma.

4.7.2 Contraindications

1. Relative contraindications: advanced disease with frozen pelvis, multiple operations with severe adhesions, very large tumors, large abdominal aortic aneurysm, advanced cirrhosis, prior gynecologic procedures, unprepared operating room.
2. Absolute contraindications: bleeding dyscrasias, severe cardiopulmonary disease, intolerance to general anesthesia, non-correctable cardiovascular disease, inadequately trained surgeon, intolerance to CO_2 and dilated bowel.

4.7.3 Major Instruments or Energy Sources

1. Laparoscopy System.
2. Electrocautery.
3. Harmonic scalpel.
4. Endoscopic linear stapler.

4.7.4 Team Setup, Anesthesia and Position

Under general anesthesia, the patient was placed in supine position with the legs apart. The position of surgeon, assistants and nurses is shown in Fig. 4.44.

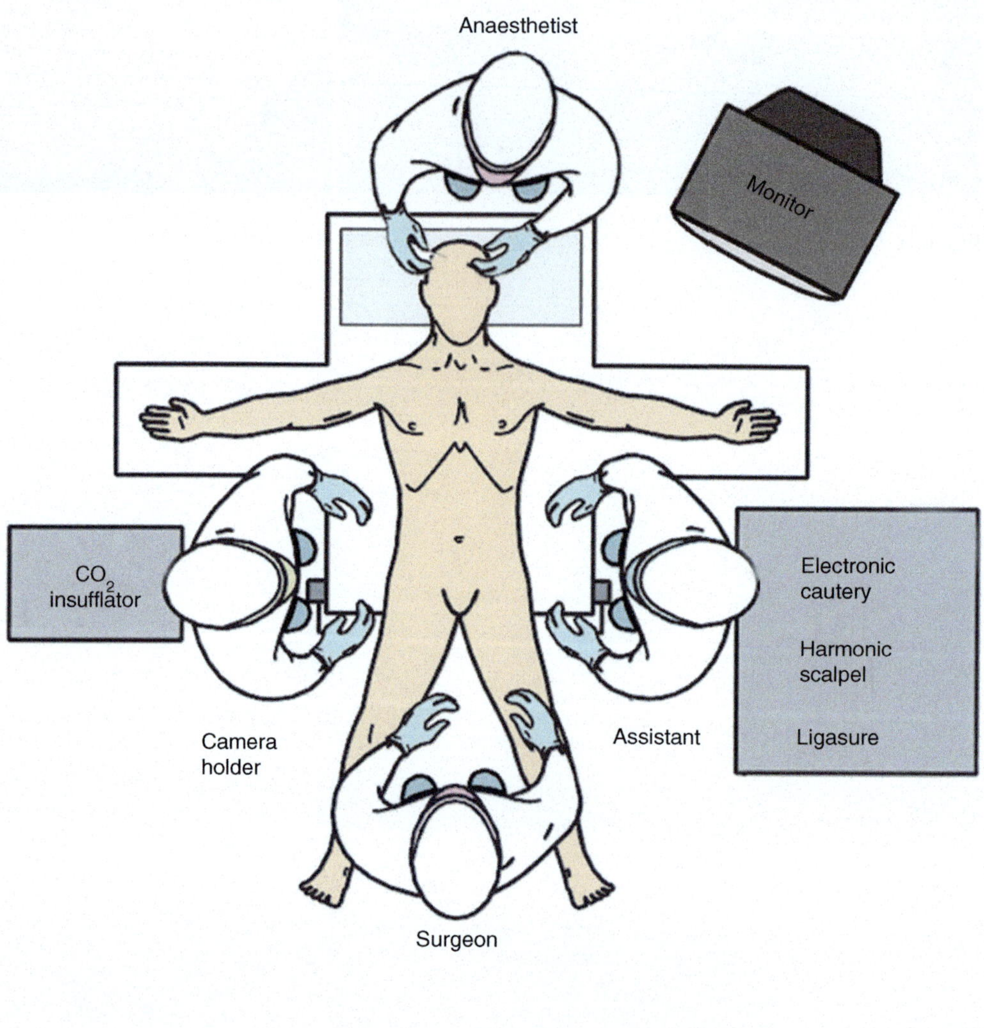

Fig. 4.44

4.7.5 Key Steps

1. Establishment of Pneumoperitoneum and Placement of Trocars.
2. Mobilization of the adhesion of the cecum.
3. Mobilization of the cecum, ascending colon and terminal ileum.
4. Mobilization of the hepatic flexure of the colon.
5. Mobilization of the transverse colon.
6. Mobilization of the splenic flexure of the colon, descending and partial sigmoid colon.
7. Transection of the sigmoid.
8. Removal of the specimen and ileosigmoid anastomosis.

4.7.6 Surgical Techniques

1. Establishment of Pneumoperitoneum and Placement of Trocars.
2. Mobilization of the adhesion of the cecum.
   The cecum was retracted medially by using an atraumatic forceps and the adhesion of the cecum was mobilized by using the harmonic scalpel (Fig. 4.45a–f).

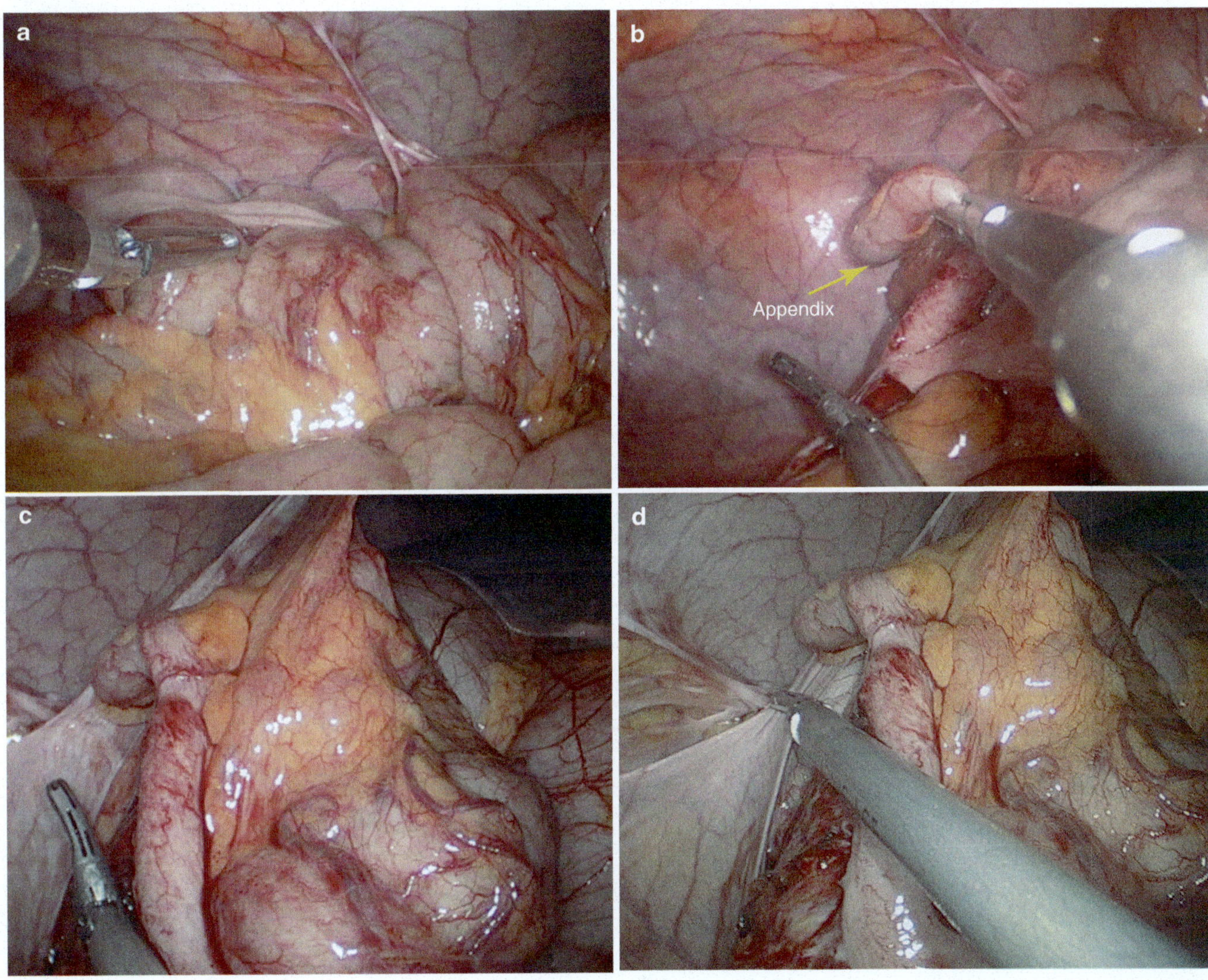

Fig. 4.45

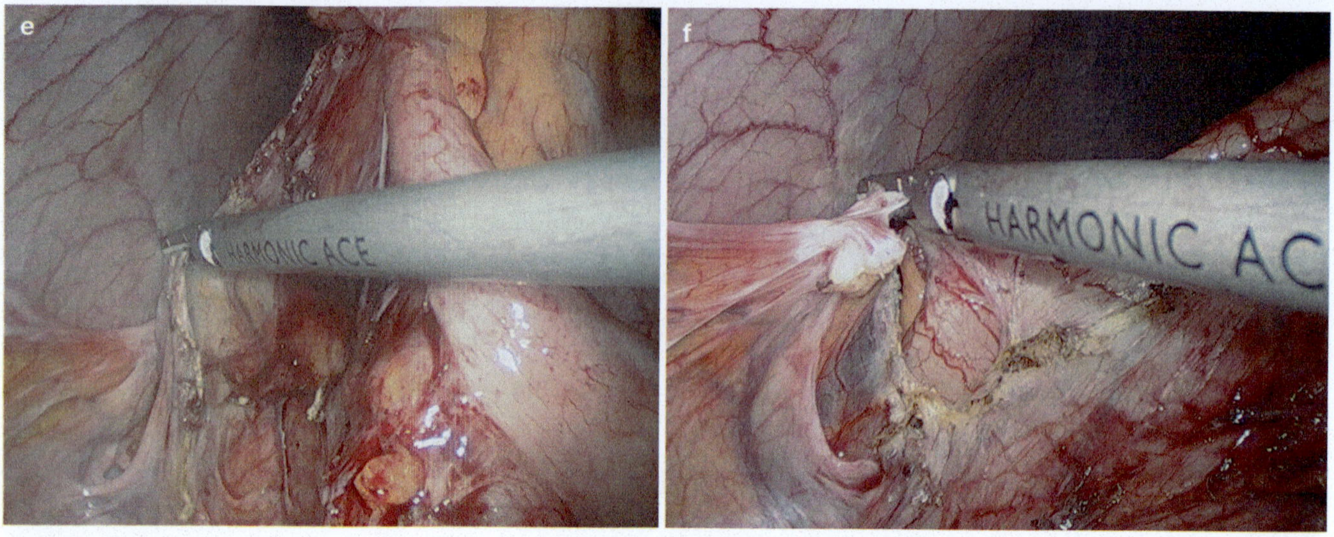

Fig. 4.45 (continued)

3. Mobilization of the cecum, ascending colon and terminal ileum.

   The surgeon used a lateral to medial technique. The ascending colon was retracted medially by using an atraumatic forceps in the left hand. The terminal ileum, cecum, and ascending colon were mobilized from the line of Toldt to the midline by using the harmonic scalpel. Small bleeders encountered were cauterized. The right ureter was identified and preserved (Fig. 4.46a–d).

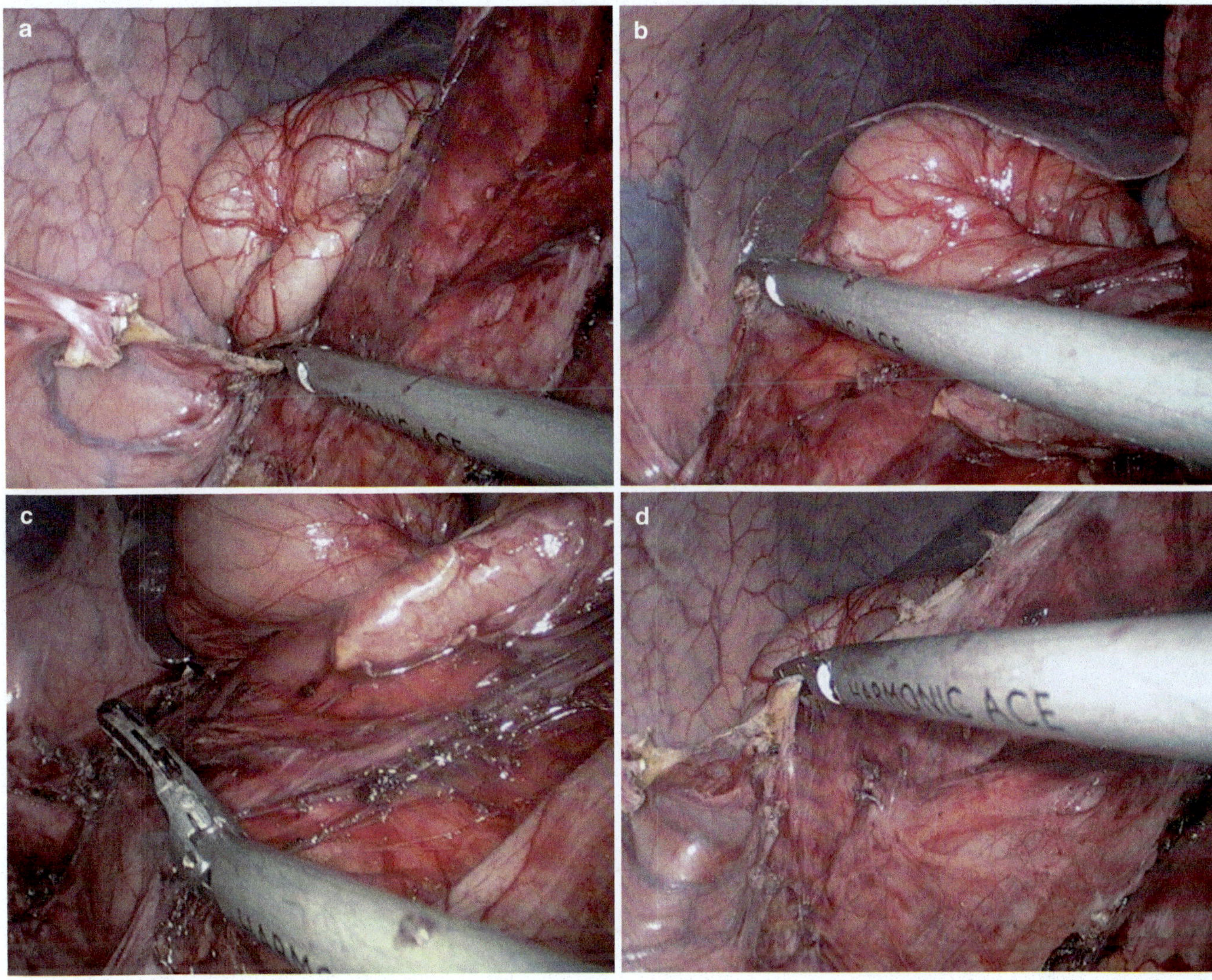

Fig. 4.46

Mobilization of the ileocolic mesentery was carried out from the inferior to superior direction in the avascular plane between Gerota's fascia and Toldt's fascia. During this procedure, the duodenum was used as a landmark for safe upward dissection. The ileocolic vessel was then isolated and separately ligated near the superior mesenteric vessel with Hemolock (Fig. 4.47a–h).

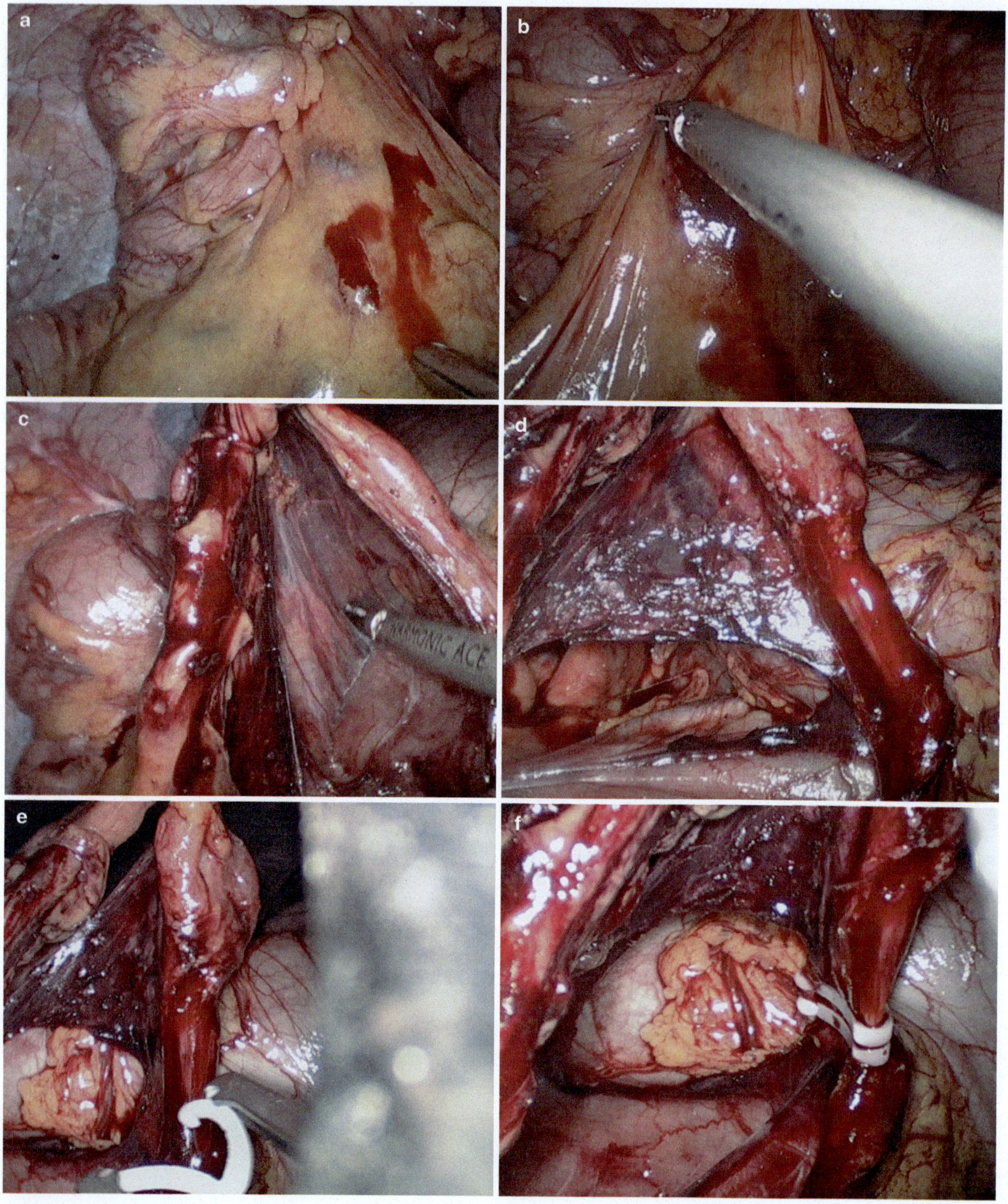

Fig. 4.47

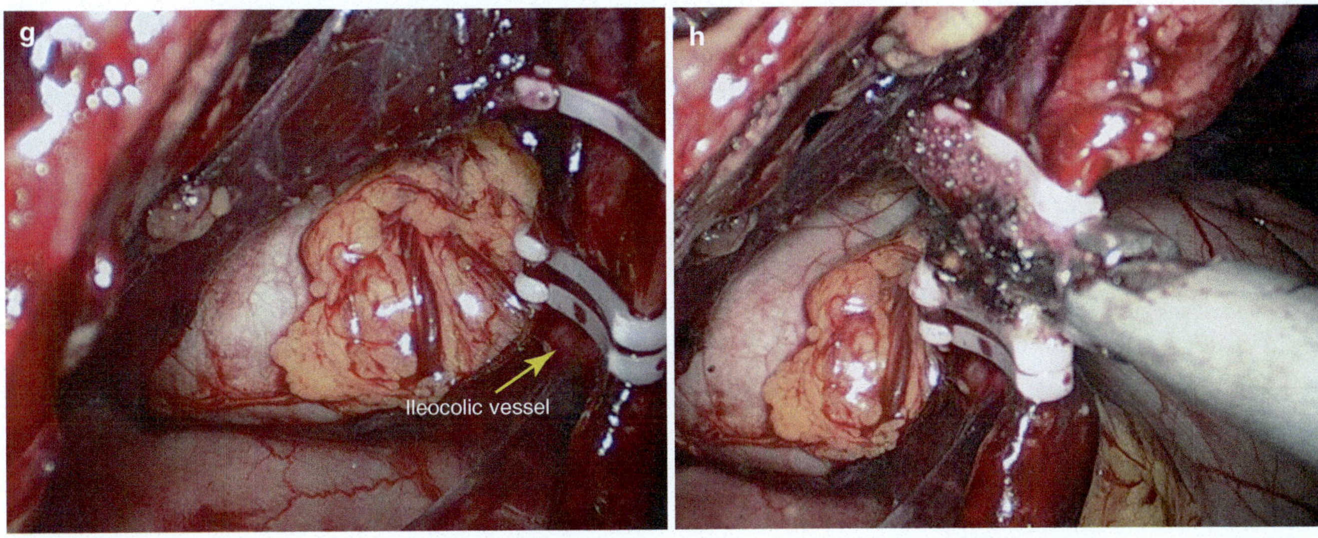

Fig. 4.47 (continued)

4. Mobilization of the hepatic flexure of the colon. Continuous mobilization upward was performed until the hepatic flexure of colon was fully freed from its attachment (Fig. 4.48a–d).

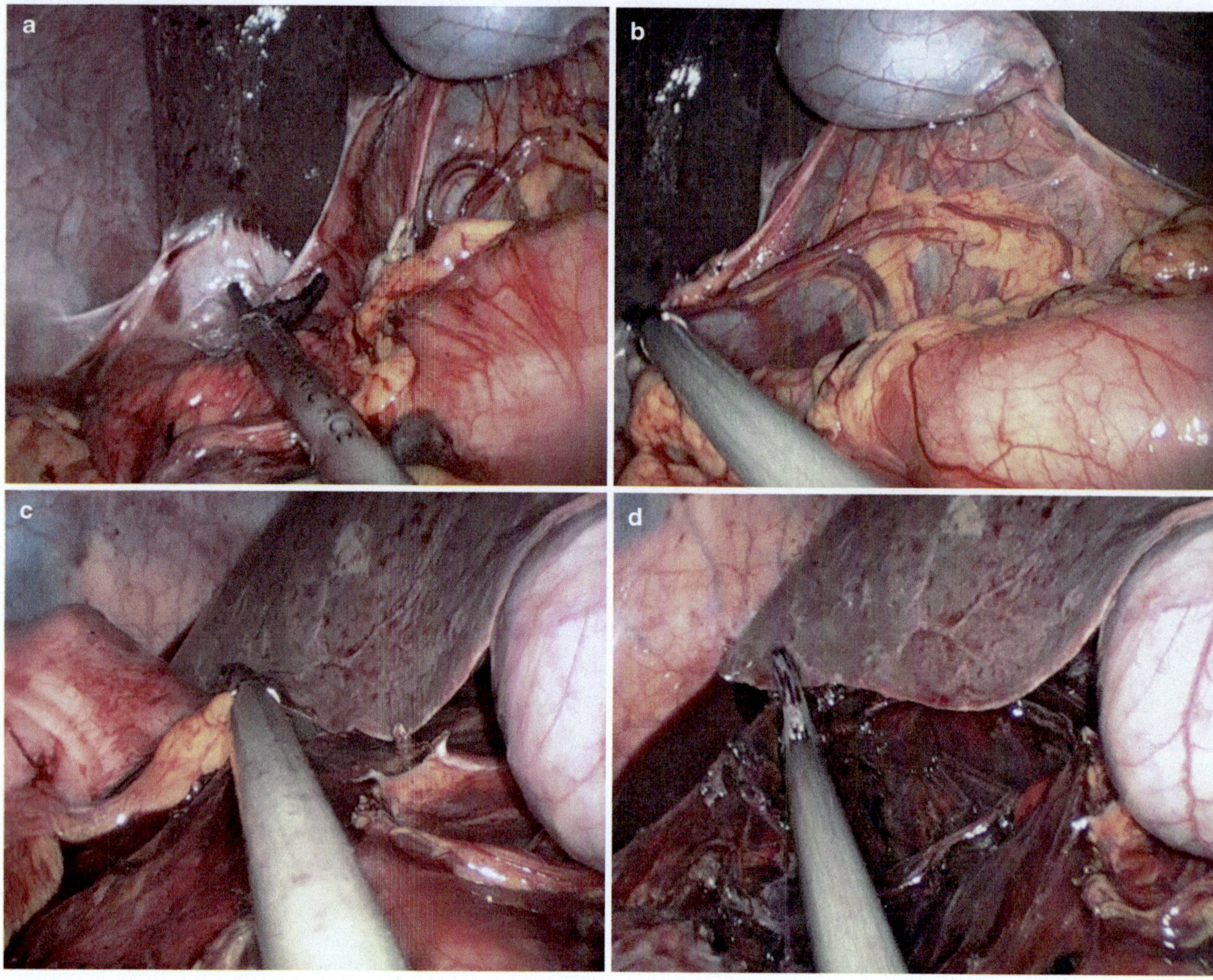

Fig. 4.48

5. Mobilization of the transverse colon.
   The hepatic flexure was retracted downward. The gastrocolic ligament was mobilized by using the harmonic scalpel. Thereafter, using a dissection along the lateral part of the middle colic vessel, the middle colic vessel was severed. The gastrocolic trunk from the superior mesenteric vein was then exposed. The duodenum was carefully protected (Fig. 4.49a–j).

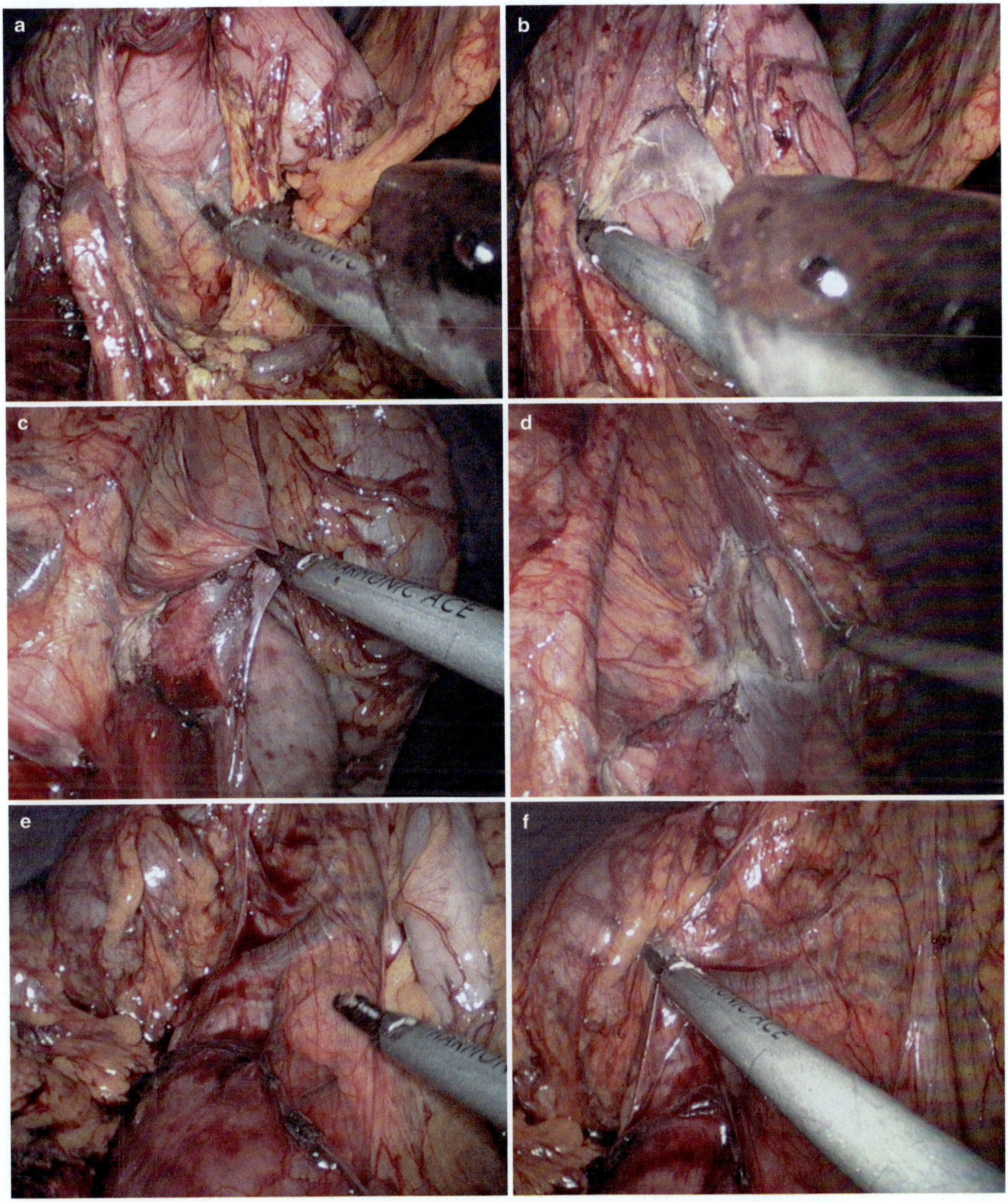

Fig. 4.49

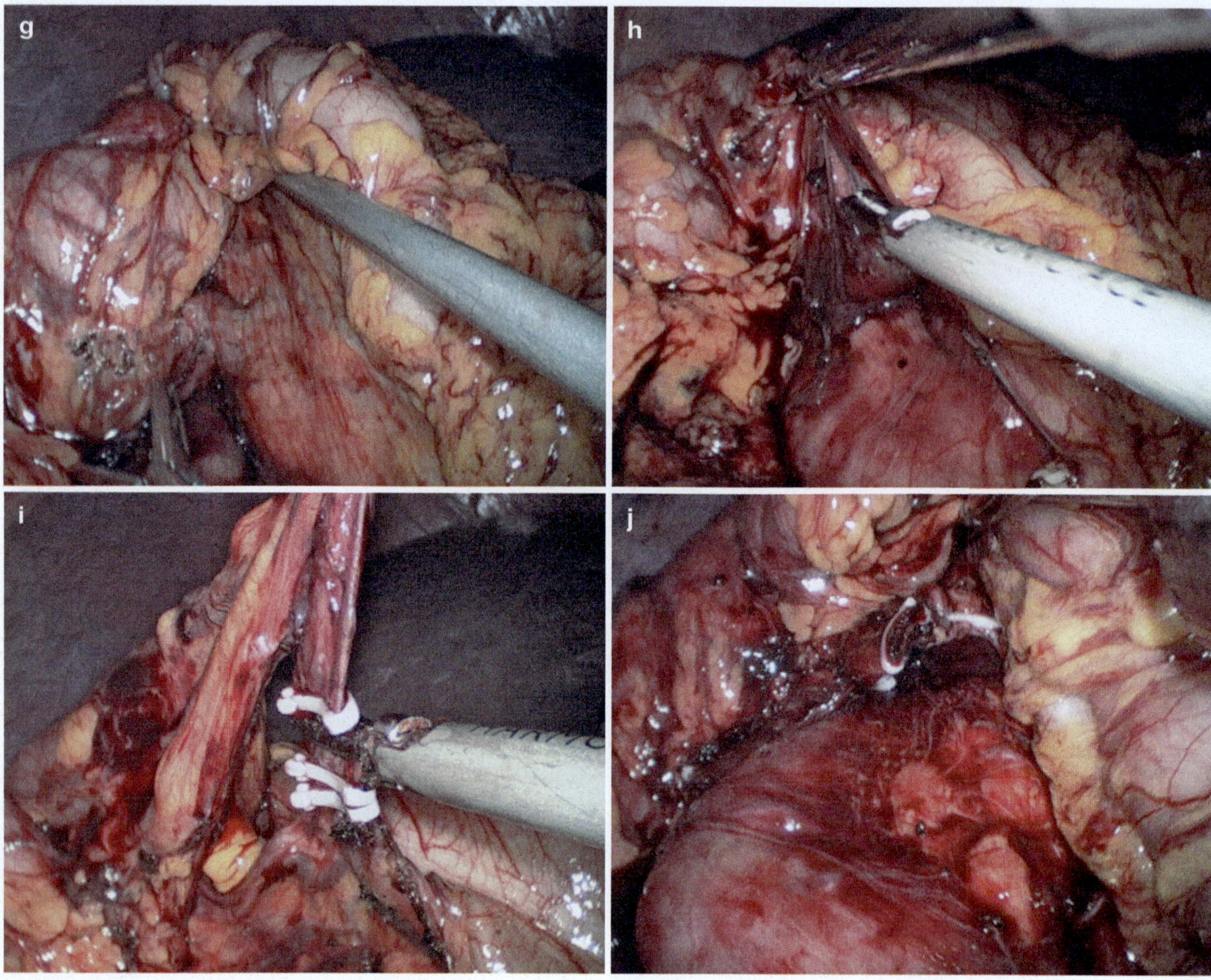

Fig. 4.49 (continued)

6. Mobilization of the splenic flexure of the colon, descending and partial sigmoid colon.
   During splenic mobilization, the double fenestrated forceps was used to retract the left-sided colon to the right side of the patients, and the splenic flexure was freed from the omentum and surrounding tissues. Continuous mobilization of the descending colon and sigmoid colon was retracted medially by using an atraumatic forceps in the left hand and was mobilized from the line of Toldt to the midline by using the harmonic scalpel. Mobilization of the descending and sigmoid mesocolon was carried out from a inferior to superior direction in the avascular plane between Gerota's fascia and Toldt's fascia. The medial-to-lateral dissection was continued until the left-sided colon was separated from the retroperitoneum. The left ureter and gonadal vessels were then identified and preserved. The inferior mesenteric artery (IMA) was retracted with the double fenestrated forceps, and the IMA was ligated near the origin by using clip placement or linear stapler. Thereafter, division of the inferior mesenteric vein was performed close to the Treitz ligament (Fig. 4.50a–d).

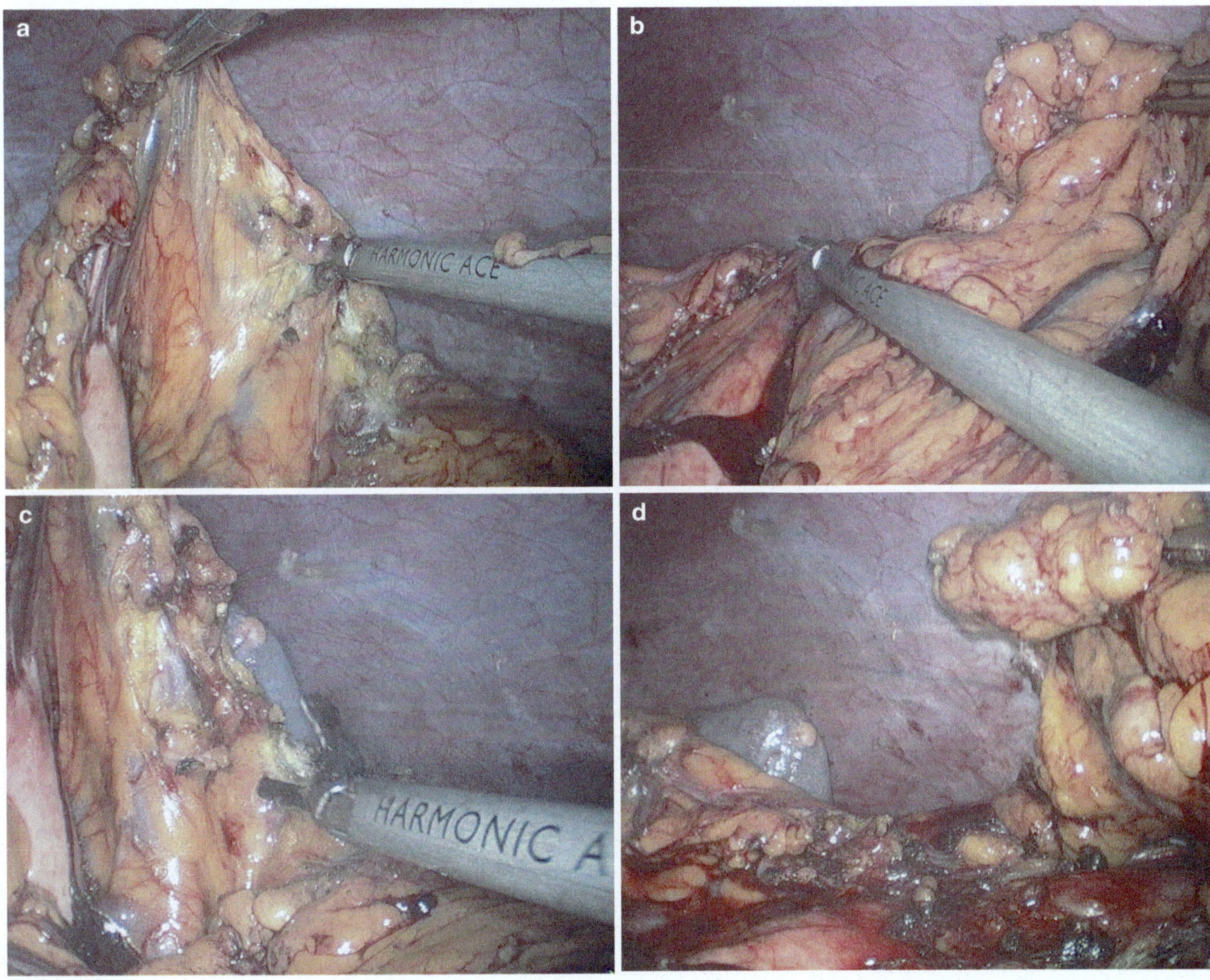

Fig. 4.50

7. Transection of the sigmoid.
   The sigmoid was transected by using flexible linear stapler (Fig. 4.51a–c).

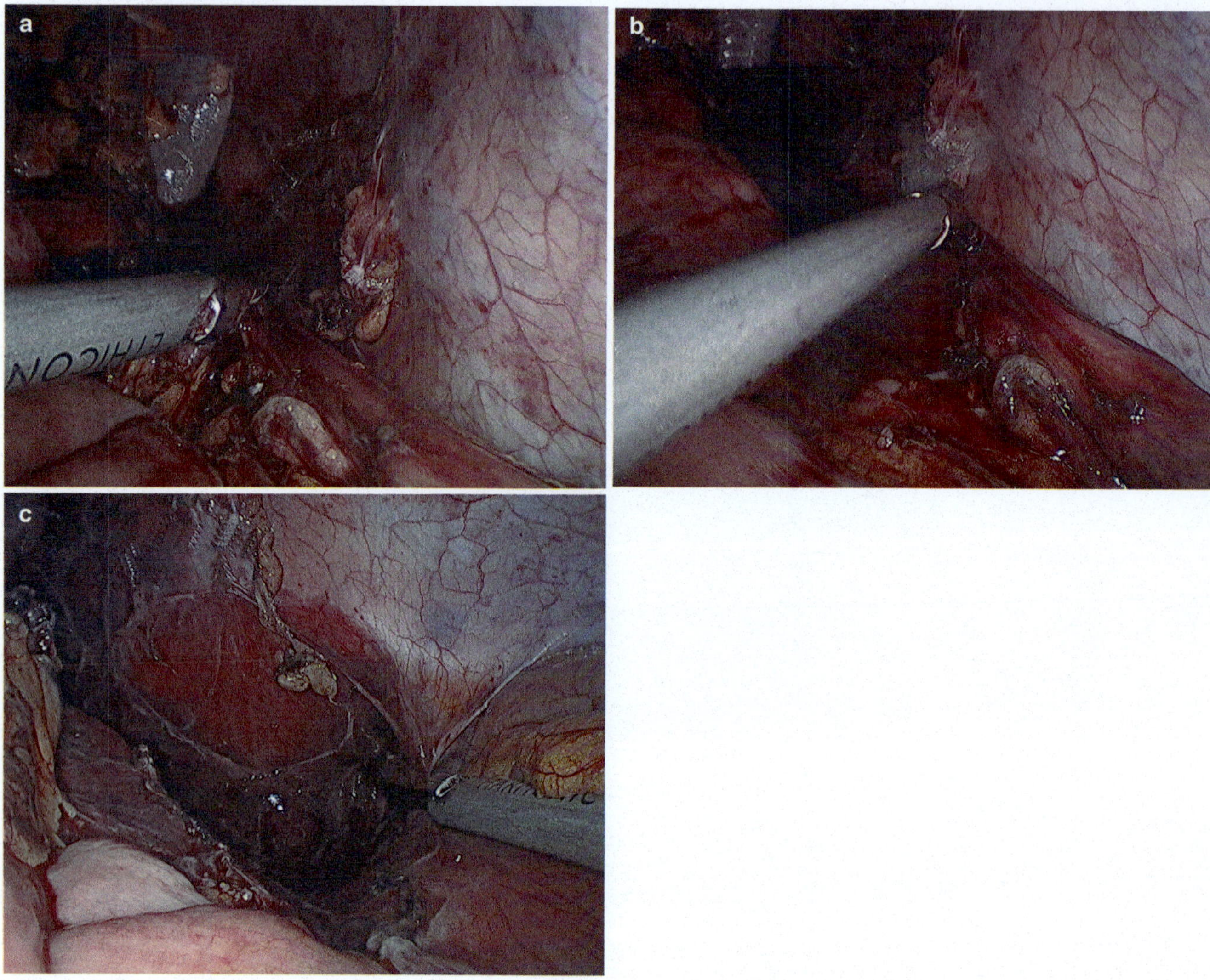

Fig. 4.51

8. Removal of the specimen and ileosigmoid anastomosis. The ports were removed and the incision was extended to 3 cm total in length to facilitate exteriorization of the specimen. The terminal ileum, cecum, ascending colon, transverse colon, descending colon and the stump of the upper sigmoid colon were then brought outside the abdomen. A purse-string stapler was used to divide the terminal 15 cm ileum. The anvil of the circular stapler was put into the proximal stump of the ileum and embedded. Then, the stump of the ileum was put back into the abdominal cavity. The handle lever of the circular stapler was implanted into the sigmoid lumen through the anus and punctured out through the middle point of the stump where the anastomosis was to be made. The handle lever and anvil of the stapler were connected, screwed and firmly locked. After careful checking the connection part, the stapler was fired to complete the colorectal end-to-end ileosigmoid anastomosis. After careful checking the anastomosis to exclude torsion or twist, a closed suction drain was placed near the anastomosis through the umbilical incision (Fig. 4.52a–f).

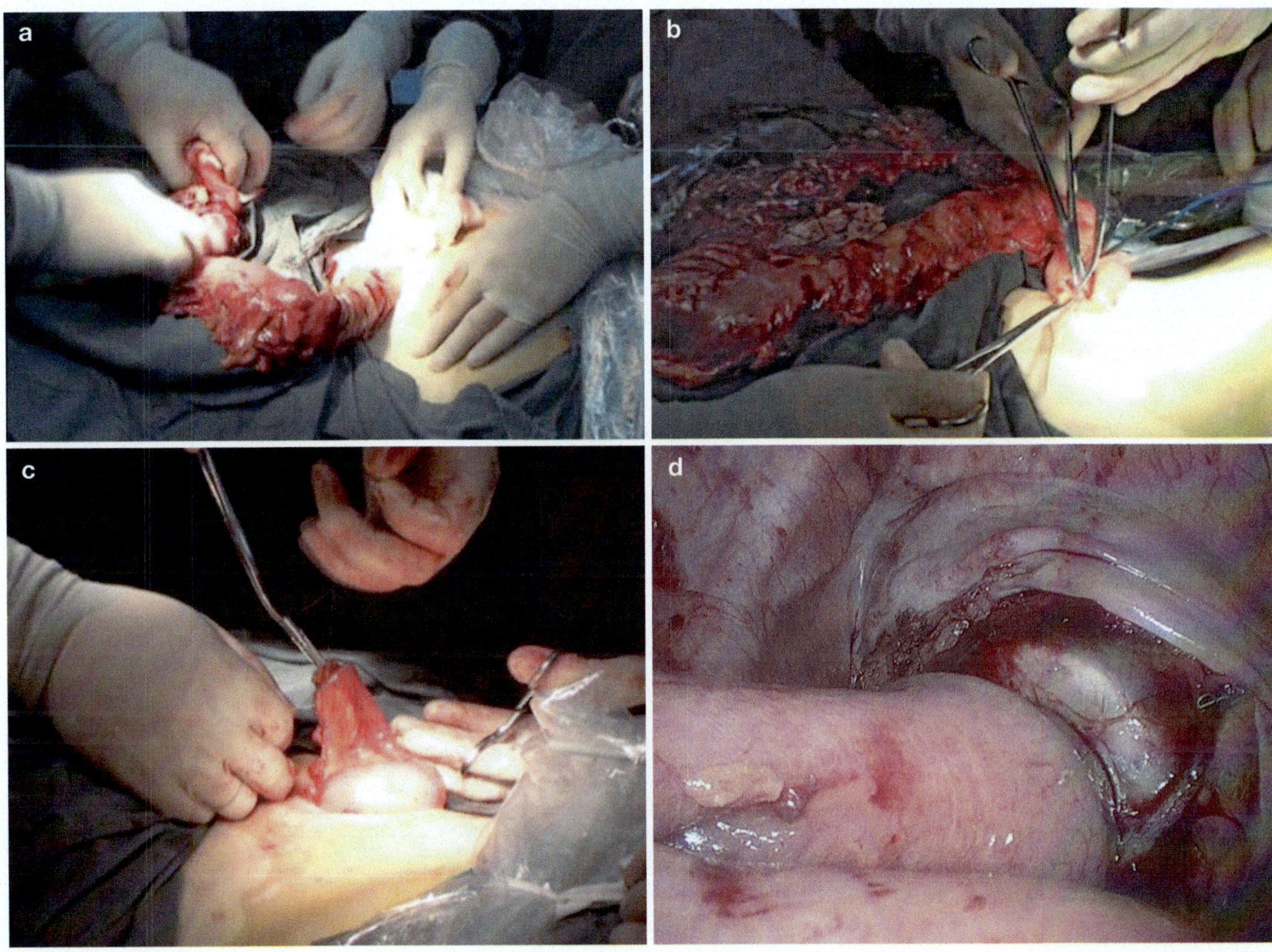

Fig. 4.52

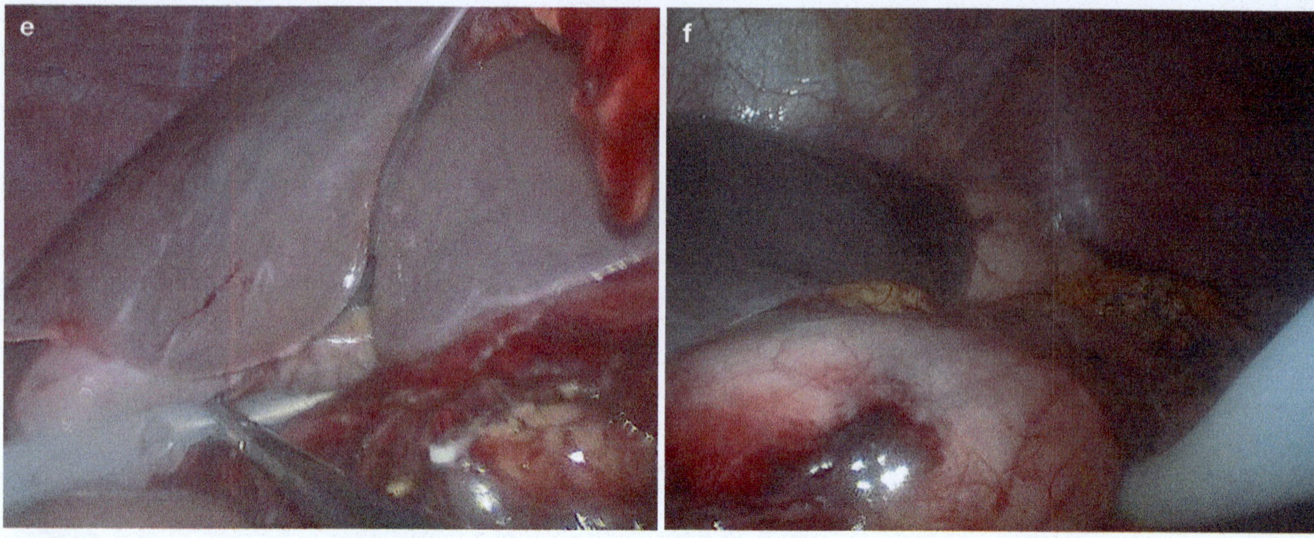

Fig. 4.52 (continued)

4.8 Laparoscopic Appendectomy

4.8.1 Indications and Case Selection

1. Patients with acute, or chronic appendicitis.
2. Patients with purulent or gangrenous appendicitis.
3. Patients with acute episode of chronic appendicitis.
4. Pregnant women with acute appendicitis who have been pregnant for less than 20 weeks.
5. However, it's more indicated for patients who are suffering from obesity or diabetes mellitus, older patients, acatalepsy, patients with much pus, or cosmetic requirements.

4.8.2 Contraindications

Appendectomy is not necessary for the patients undergoing acute appendicitis for more than 72 h, or with encapsulated mass or severe localized inflammation formed.

1. Absolute contraindications:
   (a) severe cardiorespiratory dysfunction,
   (b) inability to tolerate general anesthesia or pneumoperitoneum,
   (c) refractory coagulopathy,
2. Relative contraindications:
   (a) extensive previous surgery, or previous peritonitis leading to severe adhesion,
   (b) morbid obesity,
   (c) pregnancy (during first and third trimesters).
3. The indication for laparoscopic appendectomy in complicated or perforated appendicitis is controversial.

4.8.3 Major Instruments or Energy Sources

1. Laparoscopy System.
2. Electrocautery.
3. Harmonic scalpel.
4. Endoscopic linear stapler.

4.8.4 Team Setup, Anesthesia and Position

Under general anesthesia, the patient was placed in supine position with the arms adducted along the side. The position of surgeon, assistants and nurses is shown in Fig. 4.53.

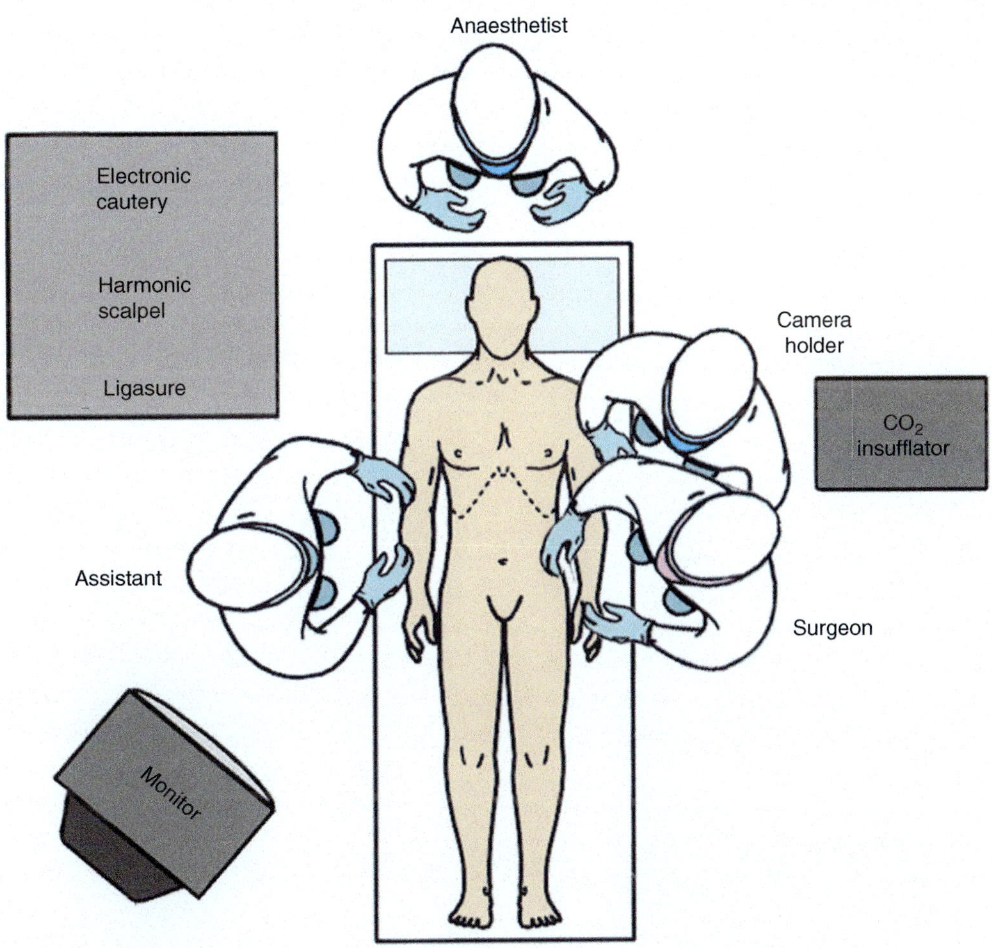

Fig. 4.53

4.8.5 Key Steps

1. Establishment of Pneumoperitoneum and Placement of Trocars.
2. Abdominal exploration and searching for the appendix.
3. Mobilization of the mesoappendix.
4. Amputation of the appendix.
5. Removal of the appendix.
6. Flushing and suturing the incision.

4.8.6 Surgical Techniques

1. Establishment of Pneumoperitoneum and Placement of Trocars.
2. Abdominal exploration and searching for the appendix. The patient was placed in Trendelenburg position with his right side elevated 30°. Using an atraumatic forceps in the left hand and a harmonic scalpel in the right hand, the appendix was located and the cecum was adequately mobilized (Fig.4.54a, b).

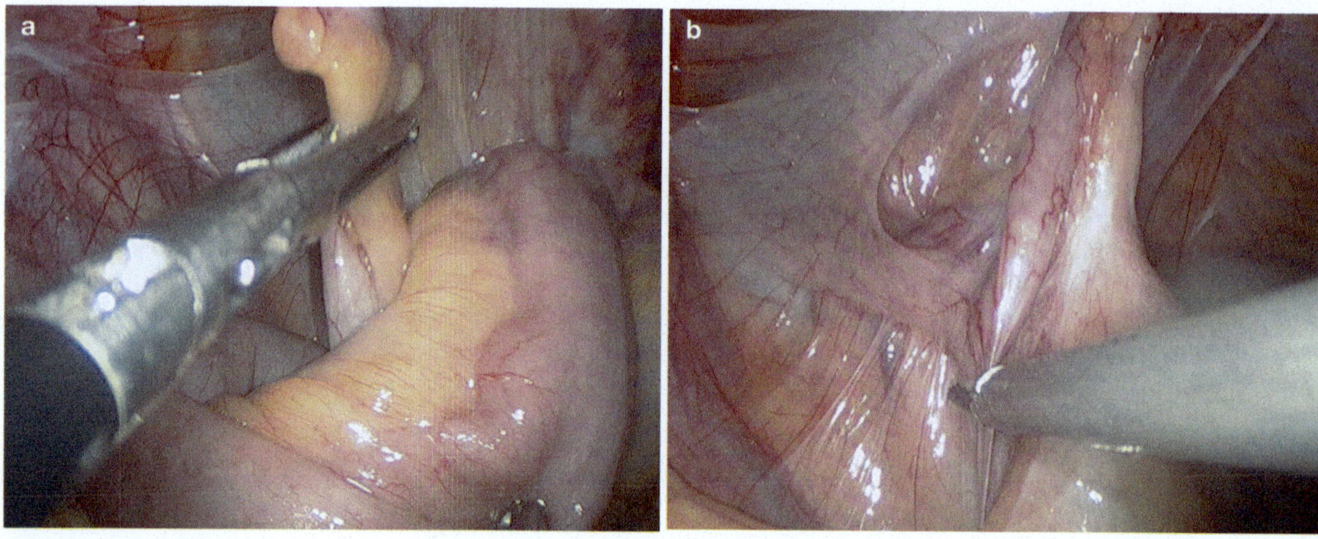

Fig. 4.54

3. Mobilization of the mesoappendix.
   The appendix tip was lifted and the mesoappendix was dissected using a harmonic scalpel to the base of the appendix. The appendiceal artery in the mesoappendix could be usually cut off directly by using the harmonic scalpel. For larger arteries, absorbable clips could be used before cutting off (Fig. 4.55a–f).

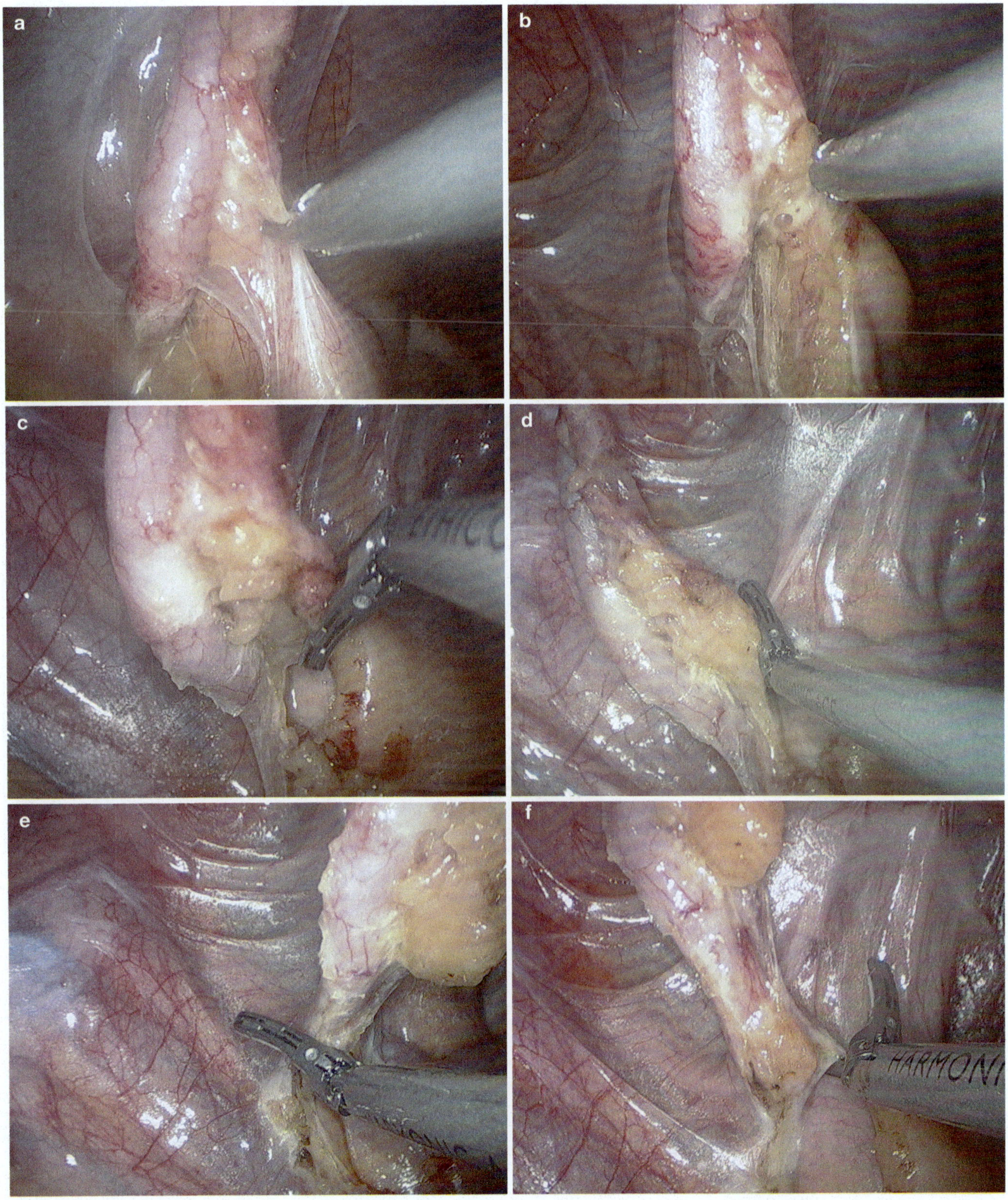

Fig. 4.55

4. Amputation of the appendix.
   In order to ligate the root of the appendix, a 10 mm hemolock forceps was needed to go through the 10 mm trocar. The 10 mm laparoscope and 5 mm harmonic scalpel were removed and a 5 mm laparoscope was inserted through the 5 mm trocar that was used for the harmonic scalpel in previous steps. The hemolock forceps was inserted through the 10 mm trocar. Thereafter, the appendix was ligated using clips (if it was less than 10 mm in diameter) or using a silk ligature if it was very large (Fig. 4.56a–d).

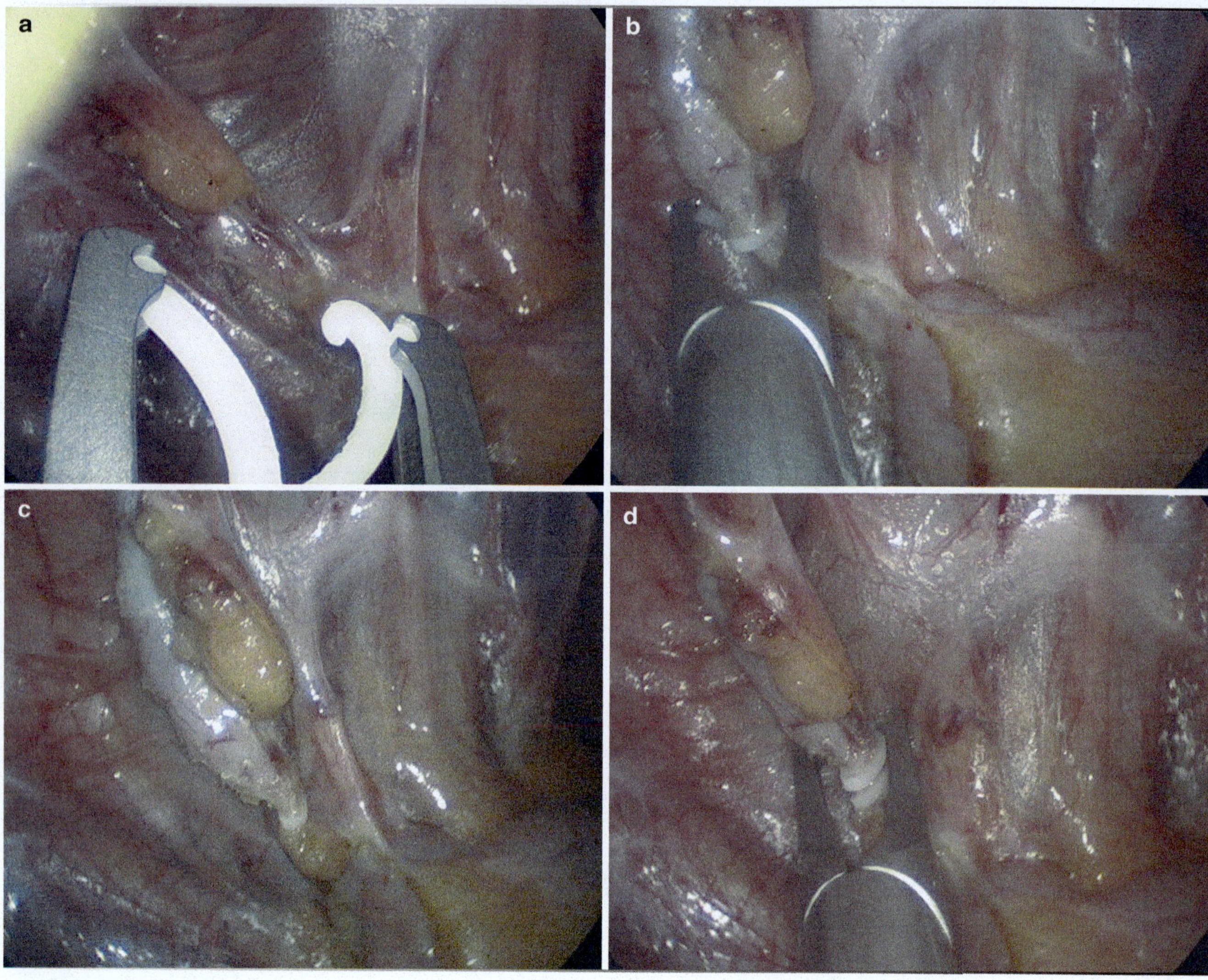

Fig. 4.56

Then, the appendix was amputated distal to the clips by using the harmonic scalpel. Checking the stump of the appendix to ensure secure clipping (Fig. 4.57a, b).

5. Removal of the appendix.
   The specimen was extracted through the 10-mm port by using a sample forceps. In case of severely polluted appendix, the sample was retrieved in a plastic bag and extracted through the 10-mm port (Fig. 4.58).

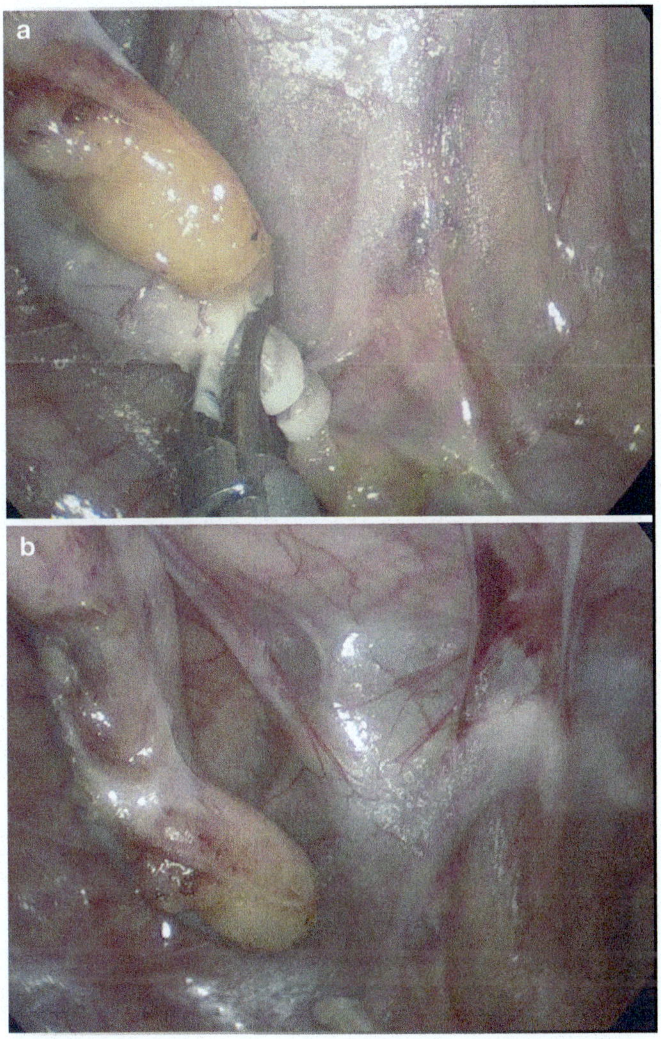

Fig. 4.57

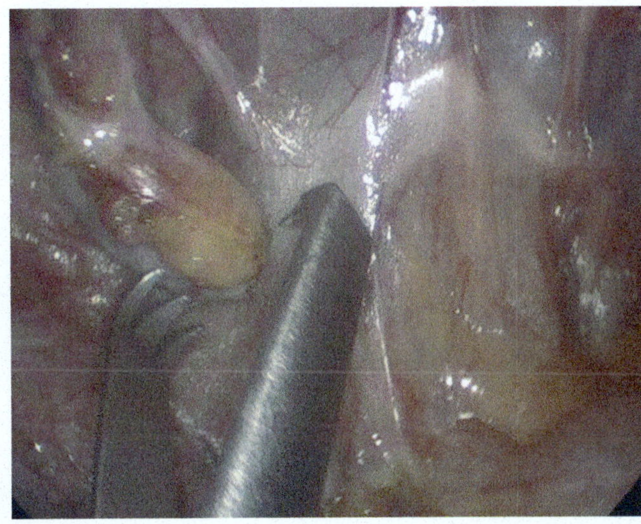

Fig. 4.58

6. Flushing and suturing the incision.
   Three trocars were reinserted and routine inspection and washing were performed before suturing the incision with absorbable stitches (Fig. 4.59a, b).

4.8.7 Tips and Tricks

1. The patient is tilted into the Trendelenburg position with their right side up.
2. The appendix should be mobilized and freed from adhesions firstly.

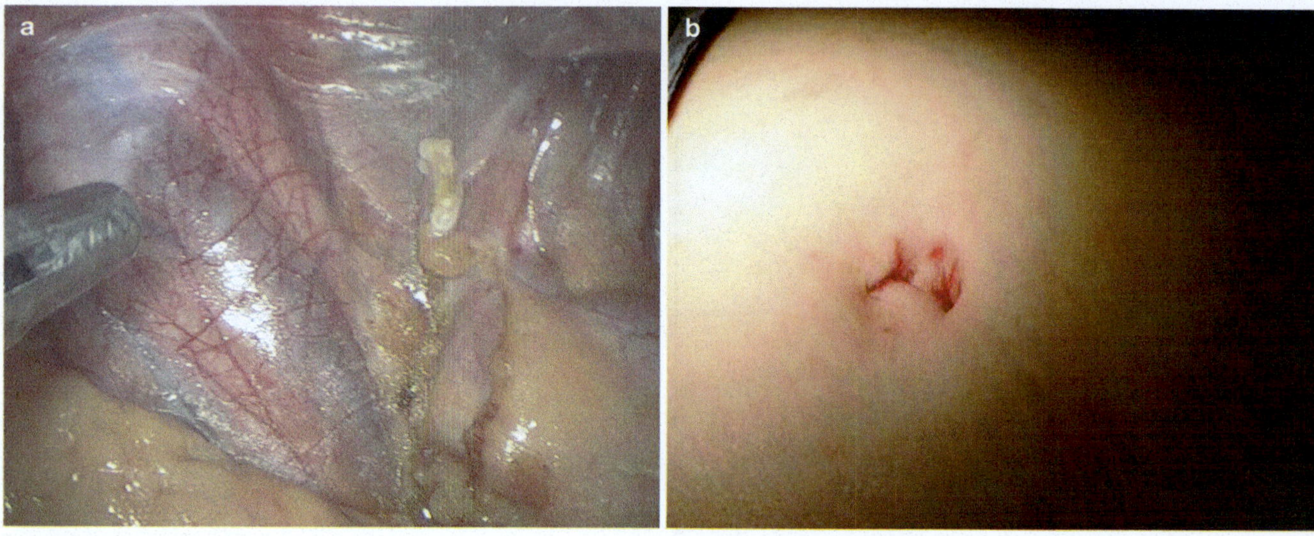

Fig. 4.59

4.9 Complications Analysis and Management

4.9.1 Haemorrhage

Haemorrhage is either primary or secondary. Primary bleeding at the time of surgery or in the immediate postoperative period is the result of poor surgical technique and failure to achieve satisfactory haemostasis.

Because of the limitation of SILS procedure, the primary reasons of haemorrhage are the lack surgical field exposure and effective retraction. Effective methods of preventing haemorrhage are an accumulation of experiences, perfect coordination between the surgeon and camera holder, and some methods that exposes the surgical field. To the definite intermediate vessels, double hemlocks clipping is still necessary. In case of haemorrhage, it is careful to avoid confusedly coagulating or blindly clipping, which can induce surrounding tissue damage. Firstly, the source of bleeding should be judged. Then, electrocoagulation, ultrasound scalpel, Ligasure or hemlock can be used to stop bleeding while sucking the surgical field. Large amount of bleeding, retraction of bleeding vessels and uncontrolled bleeding in a short time are the indications of conversion to conventional laparoscopy or open surgery.

Haemorrhage of presacral venous is the most dangerous complication of SILS rectectomy. Lacking of the assistant help, the exposure of retrorectal space is difficult in SILS rectectomy. The surgeon can't keep the dissection plane in a suitable level. The effective methods to preventing haemorrhage are good retraction and flexible cooperation of camera holder. Some assistant method such as using a suture to ligate the distal end of rectal tumor and then appropriately retracting the suture outside the abdomen can provide help to exposure the peri-rectal space. In case of haemorrhage, compression hemostasis, using hemostatic gauze or glue can be used firstly, but if the haemorrhage is hard to control, it should be converted to conventional laparoscopy or open surgery.

Haemorrhage is uncommon in SILS appendectomy. The appendicular artery can be well coagulated by ultrasound scalpel, similar to the cystic artery. But it is necessary to carefully examine whether there is active bleeding in the surgical field before the ending of SILS appendectomy.

4.9.2 Intestinal Injury

In SILS procedure, the establishment of pneumoperitoneum can form intestinal injury. But the common reasons of intestinal injury are: (1) The bowel is injured by excessively clamping. Especially when the surgeon retracts hard on the bowel to exposure the surgical field, and the retracted bowel, which can't be observed, is within the laparoscopic visual field. (2) Due to the lacking of necessary assistance, the bowels that are not related to operation accumulate close to the surrounding of energy devices. (3) In vitro, anastomosis via narrow umbilical incision can form crashing injury by strenuous retraction of bowel. So the surgeon should keep appropriate strength in operation to avoid rough handling. Changing the body position can keep the bowels which are not related to operation far from the energy devices. The umbilical incision can be enlarged appropriately. When the bowel is retraced outside the abdomen, the dissected mesentery should be dragged outside firstly and then the bowels.

4.9.3 Urinary Injury

The ureter injury is the most common injured urinary organ in SILS colorectal surgery. The injury of ureter is similar to conventional laparoscopy by blindly ligation of large tissue in case of unclear anatomical level. So, dissecting the bowel under direct vision plays an important role in preventing ureter injury. In rectal surgery, the most common injured parts of ureter are left lumber segment and bilateral pelvic segments. In SILS surgery, "cross hands" can induce greater interferences between operational instruments and laparoscope, which is against the exposure of left area of rectum when dissecting the left side of rectum. At this moment, extra attention should be paid to the anatomical level and if it's necessary, the ureter should be exposed and protected. Dissecting from the inside to the outside in the procedure of dissociating rectum and sigmoid colon is more favorable to distinguish the anatomical level of ureter. In case of injury, the ureter should be repaired in time.

Membranous and bulbous parts of urethra are the possible injured parts in SILS rectal surgery. Assistant retraction in SILS can help to expose the anatomical level and prevent the injury of urethra.

4.9.4 Complications of Anastomotic Stoma

In our SILS colorectal surgery, the enteroenterostomy or embedding the head stake of stapler is in vitro via the umbilical incision. This can reduce the anastomotic difficulties of SILS colorectal surgery and the time of operation. So the anastomotic leakage and stenosis in SILS are uncommon. However, due to the smaller umbilical incision, it can't provide a complete vision of the mesenteric direction preparing for anastomosis, so the anastomotic direction may be wrong under this condition. At the end of the procedure, the whole anastomotic bowel should be carefully examined under laparoscopy and an exact correct anastomotic direction should be confirmed. Choosing a right type of stapler can prevent the anastomotic stenosis.

4.9.5 Internal Hernia

Internal hernia is uncommon in conventional laparoscopy or open surgery, but it is possible in SILS colorectal surgery. The intraoperative suture in SILS is difficult, so closing dissected mesentery is always ignored. This is the primary reason of internal hernia formation. So, if the mesenteric gap is large in SILS right hemicolectomy and transverse colectomy, closing the mesenteric gap is recommended.

References

1. Jacobs M, Verdeja JC, Goldstein HS. Minimally invasive colon resection (laparoscopic colectomy). Surg Laparosc Endosc. 1991;1:144–50.
2. Martel G, Crawford A, Barkun JS, Barkun JS, Boushey RP, Ramsay CR, Fergusson DA. Expert opinion on laparoscopic surgery for colorectal cancer parallels evidence from a cumulative meta-analysis of randomized controlled trials. PLoS One. 2012;7:e35292.
3. Huang MJ, Liang JL, Wang H, Huang MJ, Liang JL, Wang H, Kang L, Deng YH, Wang JP. Laparoscopic-assisted versus open surgery for rectal cancer: a meta-analysis of randomized controlled trials on oncologic adequacy of resection and long-term oncologic outcomes. Int J Colorectal Dis. 2011;26:415–21.
4. Ma Y, Yang Z, Qin H, Wang Y. A meta-analysis of laparoscopy compared with open colorectal resection for colorectal cancer. Med Oncol. 2011;28:925–33.
5. Lourenco T, Murray A, Grant A, McKinley A, Krukowski Z, Vale L. Laparoscopic surgery for colorectal cancer: safe and effective? – A systematic review. Surg Endosc. 2008;22:1146–60.
6. Siddiqui MR, Sajid MS, Qureshi S, Cheek E, Baig MK. Elective laparoscopic sigmoid resection for diverticular disease has fewer complications than conventional surgery: a meta-analysis. Am J Surg. 2010;200:144–61.
7. Cirocchi R, Farinella E, Trastulli S, Sciannameo F, Audisio RA. Elective sigmoid colectomy for diverticular disease. Laparoscopic vs open surgery: a systematic review. Colorectal Dis. 2012;14:671–83.
8. Lu CC, Lin SE, Chung KC, Rau KM. Comparison of clinical outcome of single-incision laparoscopic surgery using a simplified access system with conventional laparoscopic surgery for malignant colorectal disease. Colorectal Dis. 2012;14:e171–6.
9. Chen WT, Chang SC, Chiang HC, Lo WY, Jeng LB, Wu C, Ke TW. Single-incision laparoscopic versus conventional laparoscopic right hemicolectomy: a comparison of short-term surgical results. Surg Endosc. 2011;25:1887–92.
10. Kim SJ, Ryu GO, Choi BJ, Kim JG, Lee KJ, Lee SC, Oh ST. The short-term outcomes of conventional and single-port laparoscopic surgery for colorectal cancer. Ann Surg. 2011;254:933–40.
11. Lai C, Edwards T, Clements D, Coleman M. Single port laparoscopic right colonic resection using a 'vessel-first' approach. Colorectal Dis. 2012;14:1138–44.
12. Papaconstantinou HT, Thomas JS. Single-incision laparoscopic colectomy for cancer: assessment of oncologic resection and short-term outcomes in a case-matched comparison with standard laparoscopy. Surgery. 2011;150:820–7.
13. Fujii S, Watanabe K, Ota M, Watanabe J, Ichikawa Y, Yamagishi S, Tatsumi K, Suwa H, Kunisaki C, Taguri M, Morita S, Endo I. Single-incision laparoscopic surgery using colon-lifting technique for colorectal cancer: a matched case–control comparison with standard multiport laparoscopic surgery in terms of short-term results and access instrument cost. Surg Endosc. 2012;26:1403–11.
14. Poon JT, Cheung CW, Fan JK, Lo OS, Law WL. Single-incision versus conventional laparoscopic colectomy for colonic neoplasm: a randomized, controlled trial. Surg Endosc. 2012;26:2729–34.
15. Ramos-Valadez DI, Ragupathi M, Nieto J, Patel CB, Miller S, Pickron TB, Haas EM. Single-incision versus conventional laparoscopic sigmoid colectomy: a case-matched series. Surg Endosc. 2012;26:96–102.
16. Rijcken E, Mennigen R, Argyris I, Senninger N, Bruewer M. Single-incision laparoscopic surgery for ileocolic resection in Crohn's disease. Dis Colon Rectum. 2012;55:140–6.
17. Huscher CG, Mingoli A, Sgarzini G, Mereu A, Binda B, Brachini G, Trombetta S. Standard laparoscopic versus single-incision laparoscopic colectomy for cancer: early results of a randomized prospective study. Am J Surg. 2012;204:115–20.
18. Lee SW, Milsom JW, Nash GM. Single-incision versus multiport laparoscopic right and hand-assisted left colectomy: a case-matched comparison. Dis Colon Rectum. 2011;54:1355–61.
19. Waters JA, Guzman MJ, Fajardo AD, Selzer DJ, Wiebke EA, Robb BW, George VV. Single-port laparoscopic right hemicolectomy: a safe alternative to conventional laparoscopy. Dis Colon Rectum. 2010;53:1467–72.
20. Champagne BJ, Lee EC, Leblanc F, Stein SL, Delaney CP. Single-incision vs straight laparoscopic segmental colectomy: a case-controlled study. Dis Colon Rectum. 2011;54:183–6.
21. Champagne BJ, Papaconstantinou HT, Parmar SS, Nagle DA, Young-Fadok TM, Lee EC, Delaney CP. Single-incision versus standard multiport laparoscopic colectomy: a multicenter, case-controlled comparison. Ann Surg. 2012;255:66–9.
22. Adair J, Gromski MA, Lim RB, Nagle D. Single-incision laparoscopic right colectomy: experience with 17 consecutive cases and comparison with multiport laparoscopic right colectomy. Dis Colon Rectum. 2010;53:1549–54.
23. Gaujoux S, Maggiori L, Bretagnol F, Ferron M, Panis Y. Safety, feasibility, and short-term outcomes of single port access colorectal surgery: a single institutional case-matched study. J Gastrointest Surg. 2012;16:629–34.
24. Kanakala V, Borowski DW, Agarwal AK, Tabaqchali MA, Garg DK, Gill TS. Comparative study of safety and outcomes of single-port access versus conventional laparoscopic colorectal surgery. Tech Coloproctol. 2012;16:423–8.
25. McNally ME, Todd Moore B, Brown KM. Single-incision laparoscopic colectomy for malignant disease. Surg Endosc. 2011;25:3559–65.
26. Wolthuis AM, Penninckx F, Fieuws S, D'Hoore A. Outcomes for case-matched single-port colectomy are comparable with conventional laparoscopic colectomy. Colorectal Dis. 2012;14:634–41.
27. Papaconstantinou HT, Sharp N, Thomas JS. Single-incision laparoscopic right colectomy: a case-matched comparison with standard laparoscopic and hand-assisted laparoscopic techniques. J Am Coll Surg. 2011;213:72–80; discussion 80–2.
28. Chambers WM, Bicsak M, Lamparelli M, Dixon AR. Single-incision laparoscopic surgery (SILS) in complex colorectal surgery: a technique offering potential and not just cosmesis. Colorectal Dis. 2011;13:393–8.
29. Zhou YM, Wu LP, Zhao YF, Xu DH, Li B. Single-incision versus conventional laparoscopy for colorectal disease: a meta-analysis. Dig Dis Sci. 2012;57:2103–12.

Hepatobiliary Surgery

5

Abstract

Carl Langenbuch first reported the procedure of cholecystectomy in 1882. He used an open approach then which remained unchanged for more than 100 years (Bittner, Langenbecks Arch Surg 389:157–163, 2004). In 1987, Philippe Mouret performed the first video-assisted laparoscopic cholecystectomy (LC) in Lyon, France (Kaiser and Corman, Surg Oncol Clin N Am 10:483–492, 2001). LC was a significant advancement, removing many of the objections that patients had to go under open cholecystectomy. It is now considered world-wide as the "golden standard" because of its unquestionable advantages in terms of smaller incision, reduced postoperative pain, shorter hospital stay, and faster return to normal activities when compared to the traditional open approach (Soper et al., Arch Surg 127:917–921, 1992; Schirmer et al., Ann Surg 213:665–676, 1991; Johansson et al., Br J Surg 92:44–49, 2005). Laparoendoscopic single-site cholecystectomy (SILSC), which emerged as a form of natural orifice surgery, was first described in 1995 (Navarra et al., Br J Surg 84:695, 1997). Hypothetically, the benefits of laparoendoscopic single-site surgery (SILS) would include those of the conventional multiport laparoscopic procedures in association with improved cosmetic results and patient satisfaction as the operation is performed through just one incision.

The application of SILSC is in its infancy, but gaining significant momentum. Experience with single incision laparoscopic technique, is growing rapidly. With advancements in laparoscopic techniques and the development of new instruments, more complex operations are being approached laparoscopically, including resection of malignant intestinal tumors (Lai et al., Arch Surg 144:143–147, 2009; Adani et al., Surgery 145:452, 2009; Sarpel et al., Ann Surg Oncol 16:1572–1577, 2009; Choh and Madura, Surg Clin North Am 89:53–77, 2009). Laparoscopic biliary-enteric anastomosis has been reported for benign biliary tract disease (O'Rourke et al., Am J Surg 187:621–624, 2004; Chokshi et al., J Laparoendosc Adv Surg Tech A 19:87–91, 2009). All of these have made it possible to perform laparoscopic bile duct exploration, bile duct reconstruction, biliary bypass, and resection of congenital choledochal cyst and high cholangiocarcinomas, all through a single incision. Besides that, some complex hepatic procedures such as liver resection has been reported using the SILS technique (Binenbaum et al., Arch Surg 144:734–738, 2009; Hodgett et al., J Gastrointest Surg 13:188–192, 2009; Hong et al., J Laparoendosc Adv Surg Tech A 19:75–78, 2009; Fagotti et al., Fertil Steril 92:1168.e13–1168.e16, 2009; Fader and Escobar, Gynecol Oncol 114:157–161, 2009).

S. Wu et al. (eds.), *Atlas of Single-Incision Laparoscopic Operations in General Surgery*,
DOI 10.1007/978-94-007-6955-7_5, © Springer Science+Business Media Dordrecht 2013

Evidence to support routine use of single incision laparoscopic hepatobiliary surgery is still lacking, but this approach can be considered an alternative and may be applied in a selected group of patients. Despite the rapid uptake of SILS techniques, it has become increasingly clear that there still remain issues that need to be addressed; among which, safety is of utmost importance. SILS hepatobiliary surgery requires a unique technical skill set, with ergonomic and technical demands that are different from conventional laparoscopic skills, exhibiting a learning curve even for expert laparoscopic surgeons. Only through a fully implemented system of proficiency-based progression can competent laparoscopic surgeons be ensured to further advance the technique. It is the intention of this section to detail our current techniques for SILS hepatobiliary surgery.

Keywords
Cholecystectomy • Calot's triangle • Common bile duct exploration • Choledochoscope • J tube • Cholecystojejunostomy • Ligament of Treitz • Jejunojejunostomy • Cholangiojejunostomy • Hepatoduodenal ligament • Roux-en-Y conduit • Choledochalcystectomy • Hepaticojejunostomy • Interposition of the Ileum • Liver Cyst Fenestration • Partial Hepatectomy

5.1 Laparoscopic Cholecystectomy

5.1.1 Indications and Case Selection

1. Patients generally have documented cholelithiasis and symptoms attributable to a diseased gallbladder, including cholecystolithiasis, polypoid lesions of gallbladder, chronic cholecystitis, acute cholecystitis with symptomatic relief after treatment, etc.
2. Prophylactic laparoscopic cholecystectomy for asymptomatic cholelithiasis may be justified for certain patients, such as patients complicated with diabetic mellitus, cardiorespiratory dysfunction in stable phase, Sickle cell disease, total parenteral nutrition, chronic immunosuppression, no immediate access to health care facilities (e.g., missionaries, military personnel, Peace Corps workers, relief workers), incidental cholecystectomy for patients undergoing laparoscopic procedure for other indications.
3. Other indications for laparoscopic cholecystectomy include acalculous cholecystitis (e.g., biliary dyskinesia), gallstone pancreatitis, gallbladder polyps greater than 1 cm in diameter and porcelain gallbladder.

5.1.2 Contraindications

1. Absolute contraindications to performing laparoscopic cholecystectomy include the inability to tolerate general anesthesia or pneumoperitoneum, suspicion of carcinoma, refractory coagulopathy.
2. Relative contraindications to performing laparoscopic cholecystectomy include advanced acute cholecystitis, Mirizzi syndrome, previous upper abdominal surgery, cholangitis, diffuse peritonitis, Cirrhosis or portal hypertension, chronic obstructive pulmonary disease, cholecystenteric fistula, morbid obesity, pregnancy (during first and third trimesters).

5.1.3 Major Instruments or Energy Sources

1. Laparoscopy System.
2. Holding forceps.
3. Harmonic scalpel.

5.1.4 Team Setup, Anesthesia and Position

Under general anesthesia, the patient was placed in supine position with the arms adducted along the side. The position of surgeon, assistants and nurses is shown in Fig. 5.1.

Fig. 5.1

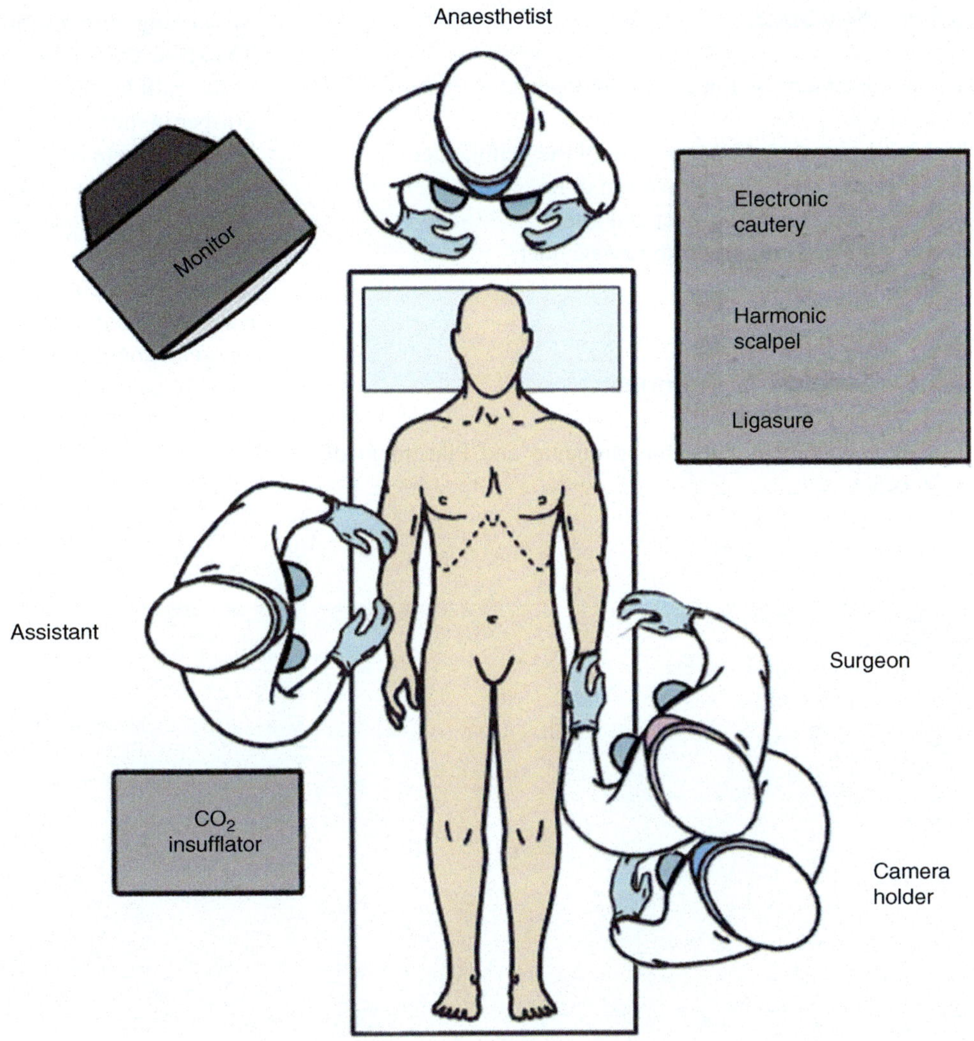
Anaesthetist
Monitor
Electronic cautery
Harmonic scalpel
Ligasure
Assistant
Surgeon
CO2 insufflator
Camera holder

5.1.5 Key Steps

1. Establishment of Pneumoperitoneum and Placement of Trocars.
2. Mobilizing the inferior margin of the gallbladder.
3. Mobilizing the superior margin of the gallbladder.
4. Mobilizing the cystic duct and artery.
5. Ligating and cutting off the cystic duct.
6. Taking out gallbladder.

5.1.6 Surgical Techniques

1. Establishment of Pneumoperitoneum and Placement of Trocars.
2. Mobilizing the inferior margin of the gallbladder.
   To expose the inferior margin of the gallbladder, the body of the gallbladder was lifted superiorly and medially by a grasper in the surgeon's left hand. The serosal layer of the inferior margin of the gallbladder was cut open by a harmonic scalpel in the surgeon's right hand along the borderline between the gallbladder and the liver. A loose connective tissue layer could be found and dissected between the hepatic plate and the gallbladder. Mobilization was performed as much as possible towards the superior margin through the loose connective tissue layer behind the gallbladder from the neck to the fundus (Fig. 5.2a–i).

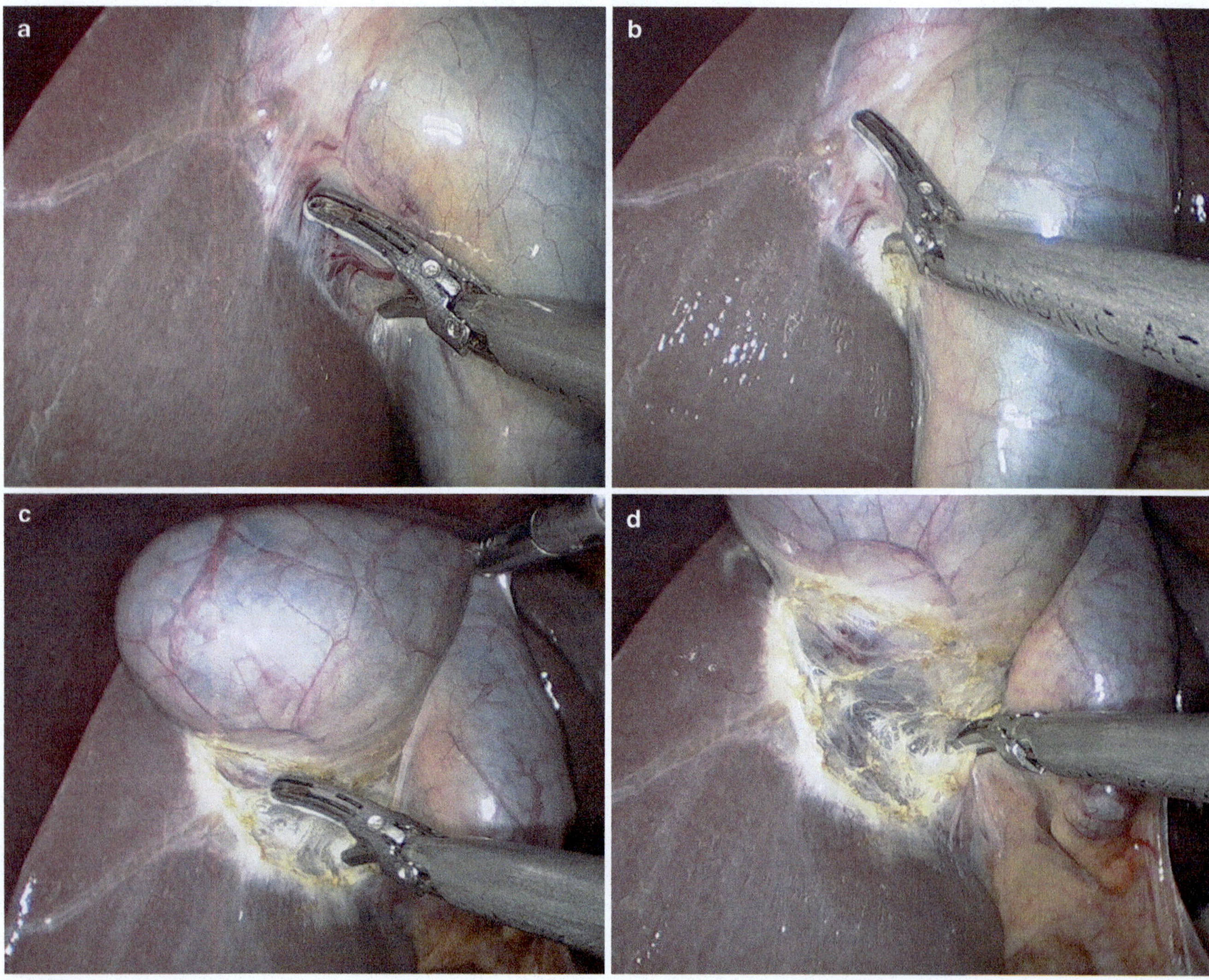

Fig. 5.2

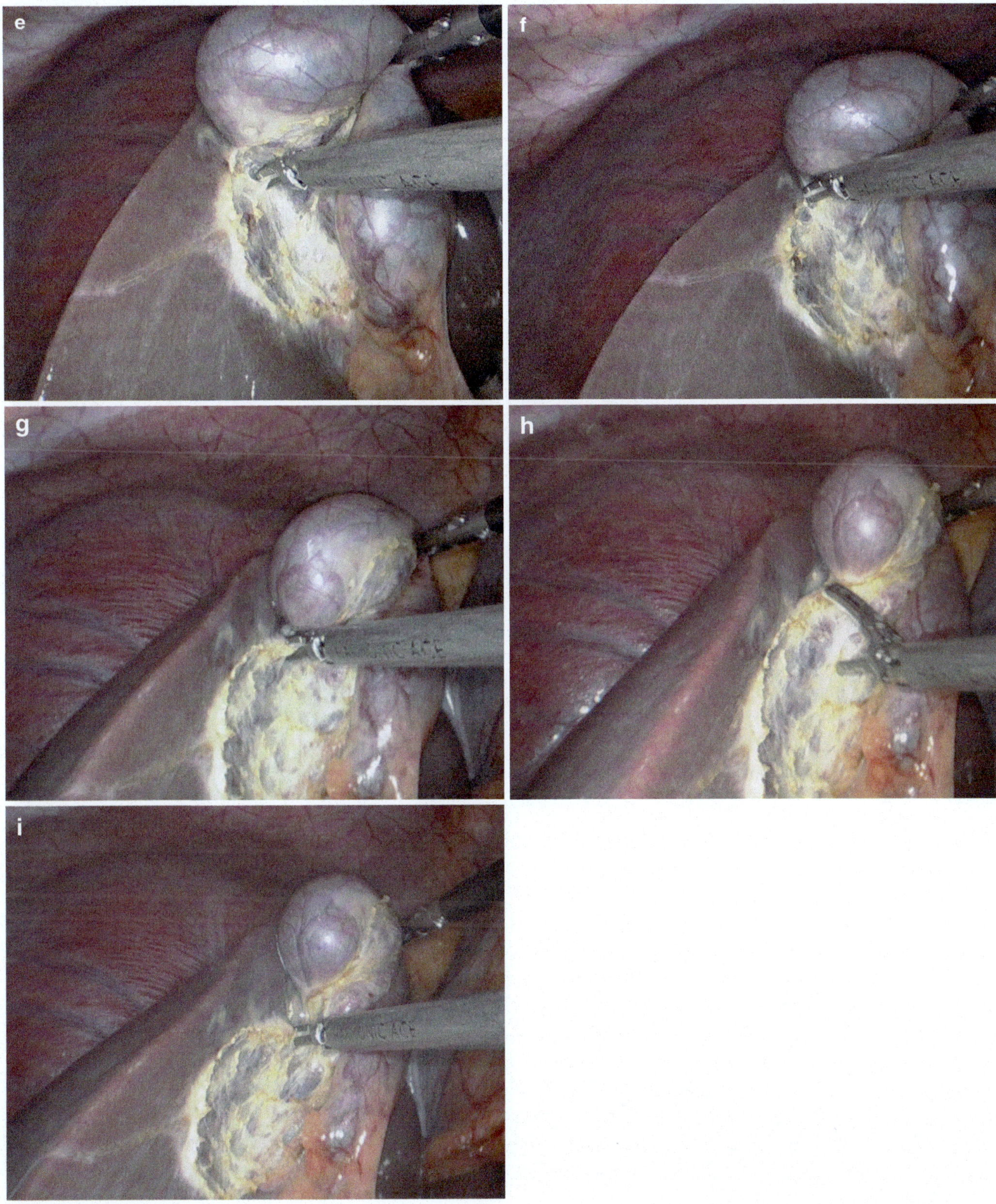

Fig. 5.2 (continued)

3. Mobilizing the superior margin of the gallbladder.
   To expose the superior margin of the gallbladder, the margin of liver was pushed back by the grasper in the left hand and the fundus of the gallbladder was released drooping freely. The serosal layer of the superior margin of the gallbladder was cut open by the harmonic scalpel in the right hand from the fundus to the neck until reaching the boundary of Calot's triangle. The mobilization was performed also through the loose connective tissue layer between the hepatic plate and gallbladder until meeting the space previously dissected in the previous step (Fig. 5.3a, b).

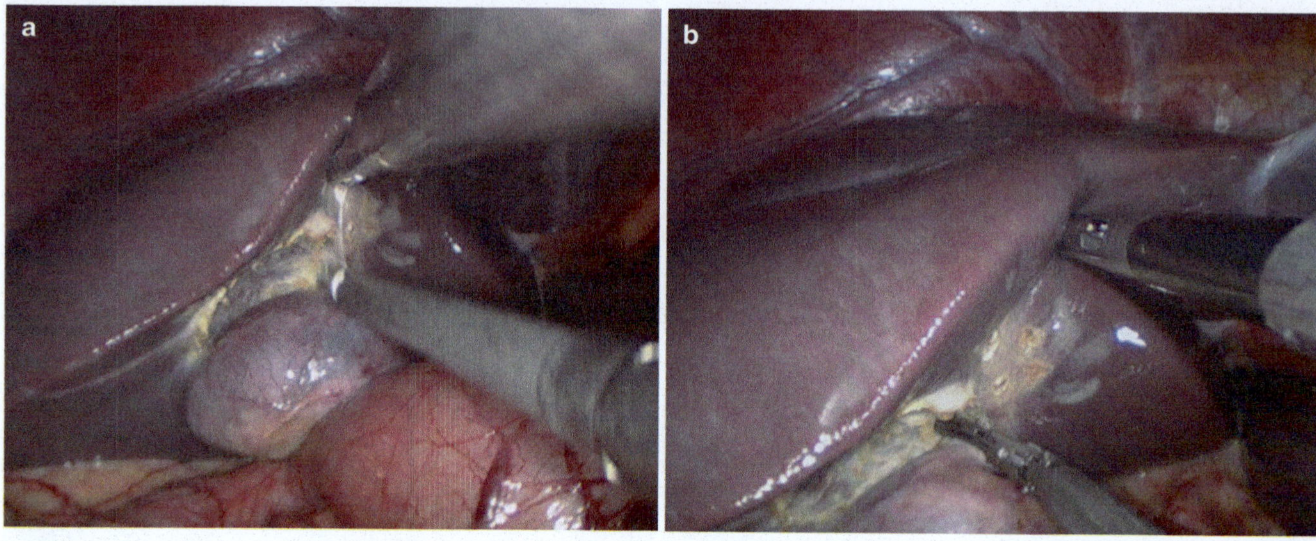

Fig. 5.3

4. Mobilizing the cystic duct and artery.

   After previous mobilization, the body of gallbladder was freed completely from liver. To expose the cystic duct, the body of gallbladder was vertically pulled upward by grasper in the left hand. And the lateral region of cystic duct was dissected by the harmonic scalpel. Then, the gallbladder was pulled laterally and downward to expose the medial region of cystic duct. In this region, cystic artery could be found and dissected by the harmonic scalpel. In this step, much attention must be paid to avoid bile duct injury. When the gallbladder was pulled upward, the cystic duct and bile duct were in a shape of inverted "T". The hepatic duct may be pulled up sometimes. In this situation, the bile duct is prone to be injured. The lateral region and medial region may need to be dissected alternately according to specific circumstance and the arrangement of the three instruments should shift accordingly (Fig. 5.4a–n).

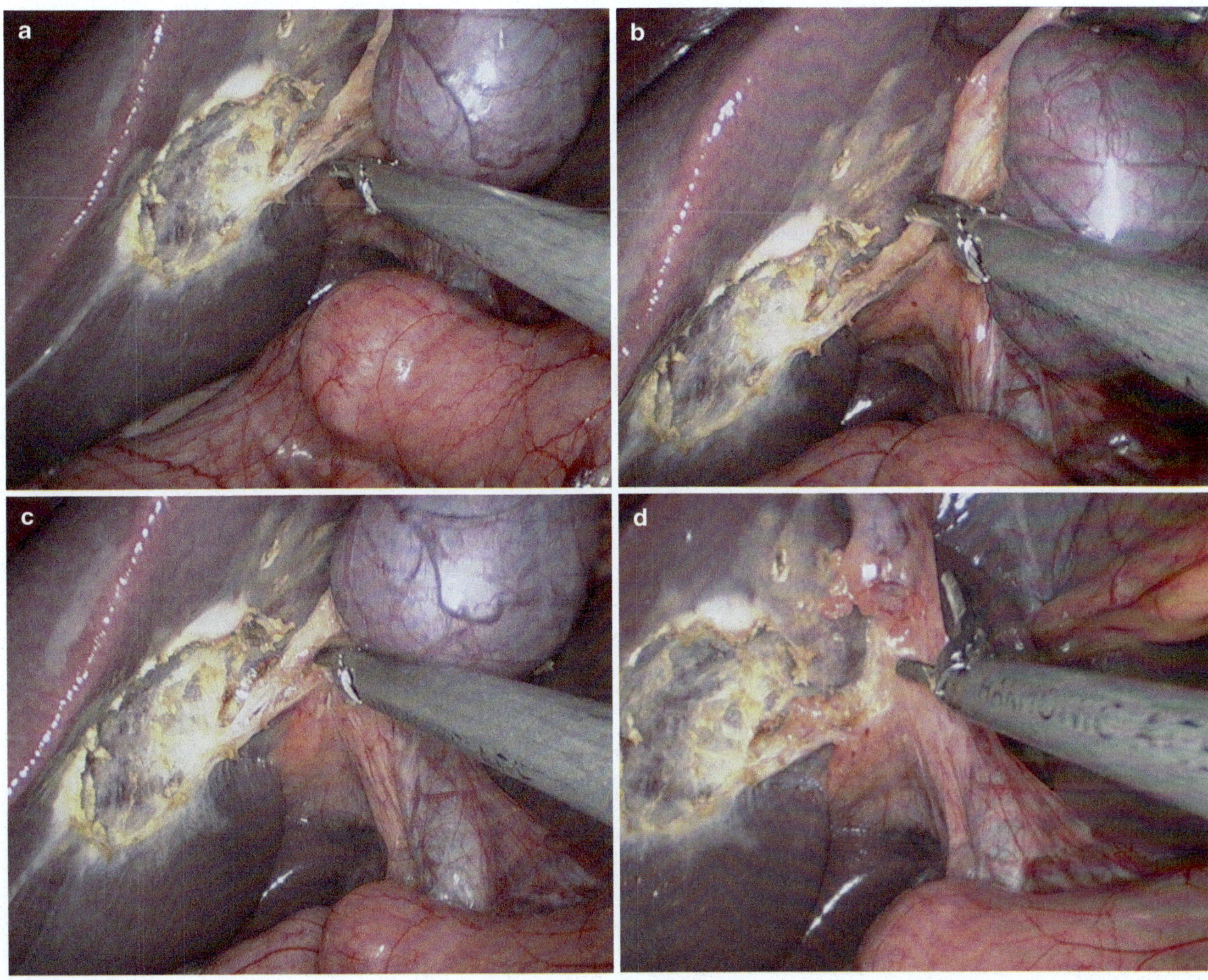

Fig. 5.4

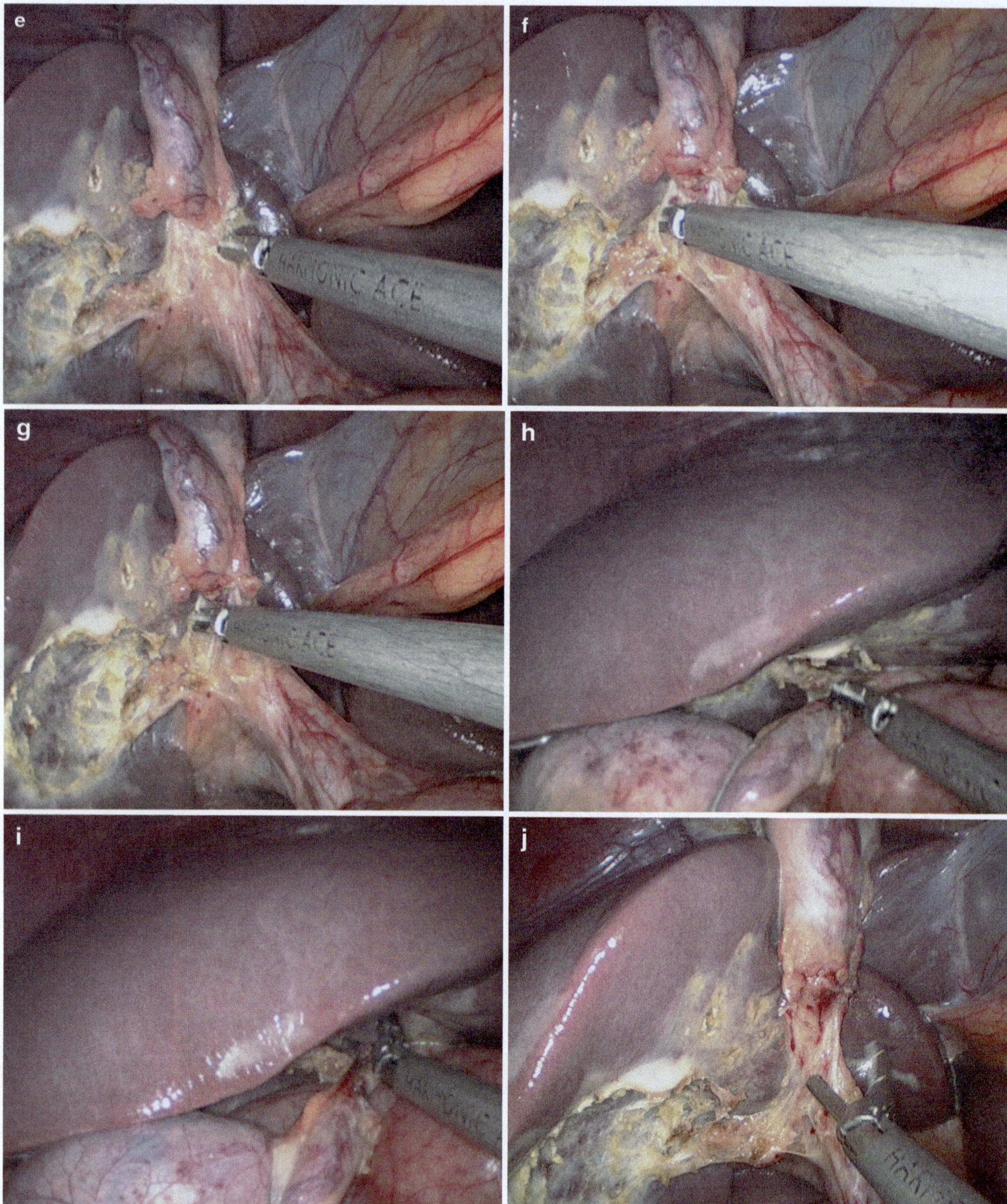

Fig. 5.4 (continued)

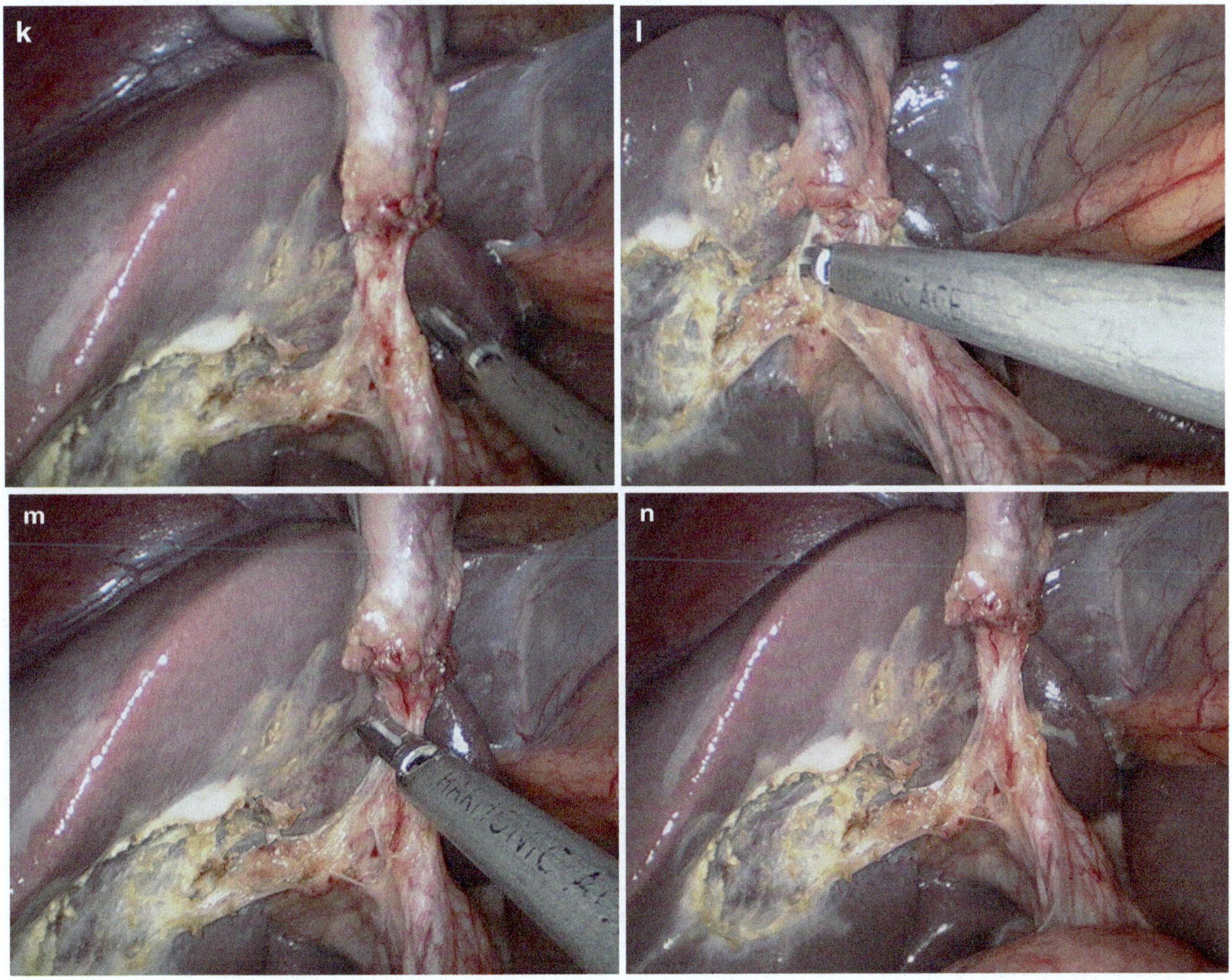

Fig. 5.4 (continued)

5. Ligating and cutting off the cystic duct.
   In order to ligate the cystic duct, a 10 mm hemolock forceps was needed to go through the 10 mm trocar. The 10 mm laparoscope and 5 mm harmonic scalpel were removed and a 5 mm laparoscope was inserted through the 5 mm trocar that was used for the harmonic scalpel in previous steps. The hemolock forceps was inserted through the 10 mm trocar. The gallbladder was pulled upward by the grasper in the left hand to expose the cystic duct. The cystic duct was double ligated by two hemolock clips. When the hemolock forceps was replaced by a harmonic scalpel to cut off the cystic duct through the 10 mm trocar, the scalpel went alone the same track as the hemolock forceps (Fig. 5.5a–f).

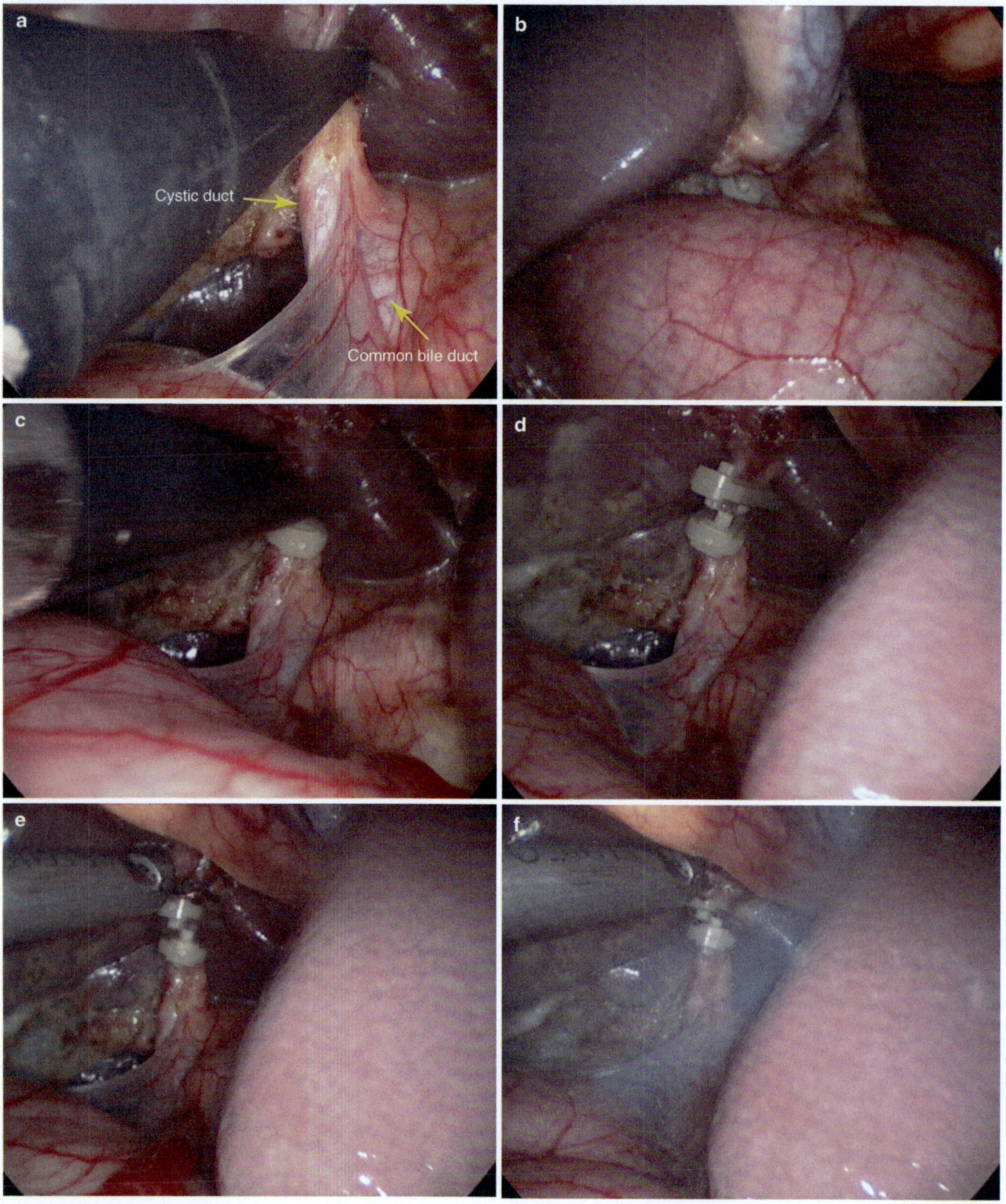

Fig. 5.5

6. Taking out gallbladder.
   A 10 mm specimen forceps was inserted through the 10 mm trocar to grasp the end of the cystic duct. Under the monitoring of 5 mm laparoscope from above, the gallbladder was pulled towards the incision. The 10 mm trocar was removed and the opening end of cystic duct was pulled out of the incision. Bile and stones were cleared under direct vision and then the gallbladder was taken out easily. Three trocars were reinserted and routine inspection and washing were performed before suturing the incision with absorbable stitches (Fig. 5.6a, b).

5.1.7 Tips and Tricks

1. The patient is placed in the reversed Trendelenberg position with right side elevated like the conventional laparoscopic cholecystectomy. The operating surgeon and the assistant stands on the left side.
2. The grasper introduced through the right trocar is used to retract the gallbladder up and to the left. The dissection of the gallbladder from the liver bed using harmonic scalpel should start from the right edge of the gallbladder.
3. The cystic duct and the artery are isolated. The segment five of the liver is seen in the window created, with the cystic duct seen as the only structure entering the gallbladder (critical view). The cystic duct is left intact as it serves as an additional point of fixation.

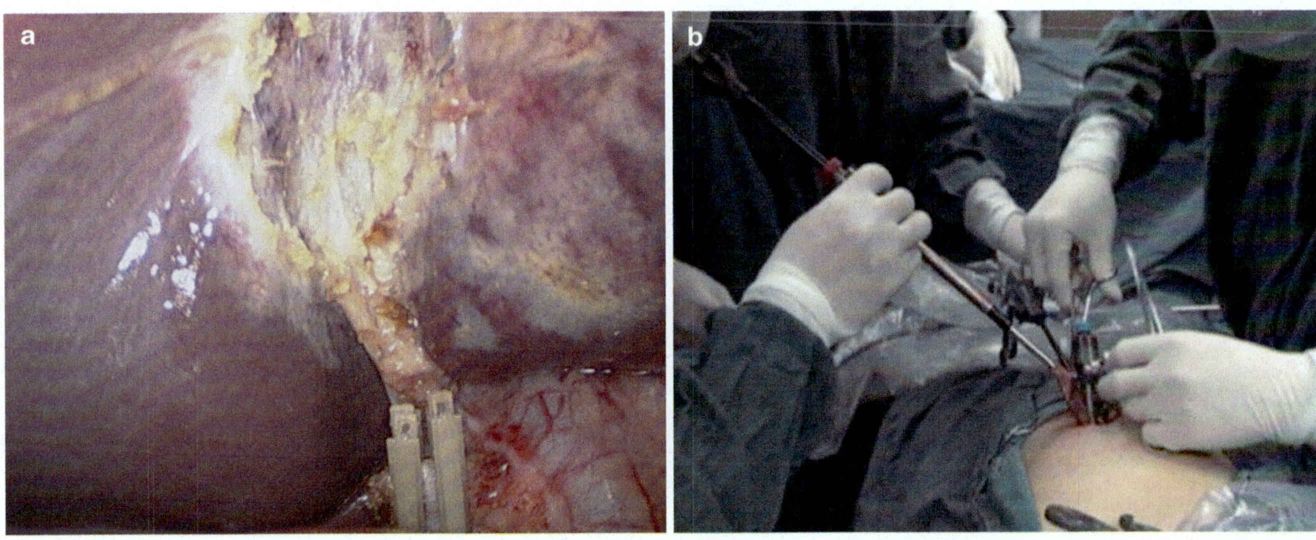

Fig. 5.6

5.2 Laparoscopic Common Bile Duct Exploration

5.2.1 Indications and Case Selection

1. Patients with primary, or secondary extrahepatic bile duct stones complicated with cholecystolithiasis, which should be: (1) Large stones (>10 mm). (2) Multiple stones. (3) Stone location proximal to the cystic duct/common bile duct junction. (4) Narrow/tortuous cystic duct, etc. And it should be with dilated common bile duct (6–10 mm).
2. Failed laparoscopic transcystic exploration or preoperative endoscopic stone extraction.
3. Biliary ascariasis.

5.2.2 Contraindications

1. Inability to tolerate general anesthesia or pneumoperitoneum.
2. Suspicion of carcinoma.
3. Refractory coagulopathy.
4. Residual, or regenerated stone after biliary surgery.
5. Severe adhesion around the bile ducts.
6. Stenosis of bile duct.
7. Intrahepatic bile duct stone, and hepatectomy is considered.

5.2.3 Major Instruments or Energy Sources

1. Laparoscopy System.
2. Holding forceps.
3. Harmonic scalpel.
4. Cholangioscope.

5.2.4 Team Setup, Anesthesia and Position

It is the same as Sect. 5.1.4.

5.2.5 Key Steps

1. Dissection of gallbladder.
2. Incision of common bile duct and removal of the stones.
3. Choledocoscopy exploration and removal of the stones.
4. Placement of J tube.
5. Closure of the common bile duct.
6. Resection of gallbladder.

5.2.6 Surgical Techniques

1. Dissection of gallbladder.
   Dissection of gallbladder was performed as described in the cholecystectomy section, with the cyst duct clipped but uncut.
2. Incision of common bile duct and removal of the stones.
   The gallbladder was maintained in position, which helped to expose the common bile duct (CBD). After CBD and its diameter were clearly identified, a longitudinal incision of 1–1.5 cm was then made over the anterior wall. Once the duct was opened, nearby stones were grasped and removed directly with grasper or Semm's spoon forceps (Fig. 5.7a–f).

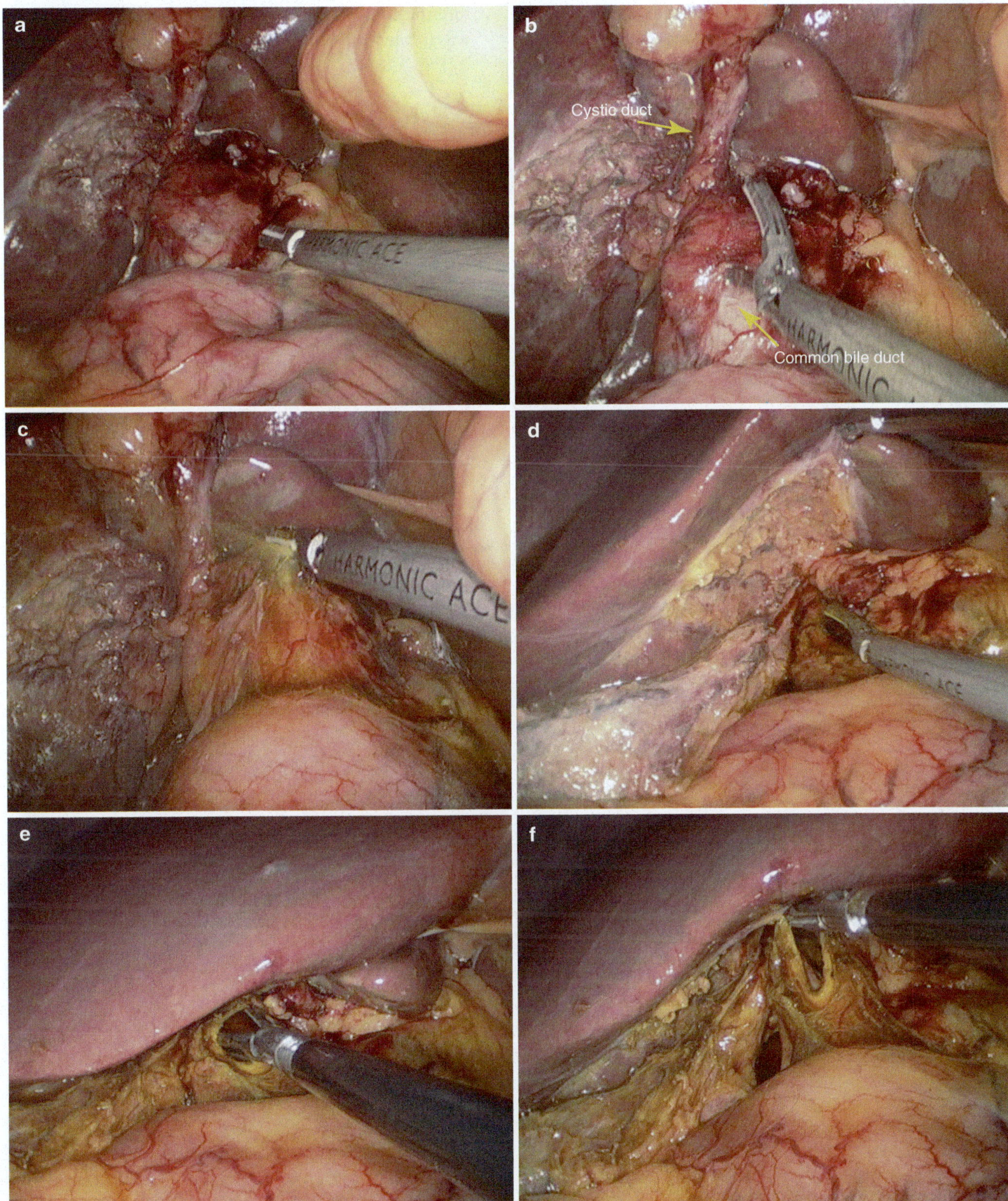

Fig. 5.7

3. Choledocoscopy exploration and removal of the stones. A flexible choledochoscope was then passed through the 5-mm port to perform visually guided extraction of any other residual stones. The superior biliary tract and the inferior biliary tract were explored in turn. When a stone was located, a Dormia retrieval basket was used to extract it (Fig. 5.8a–d).

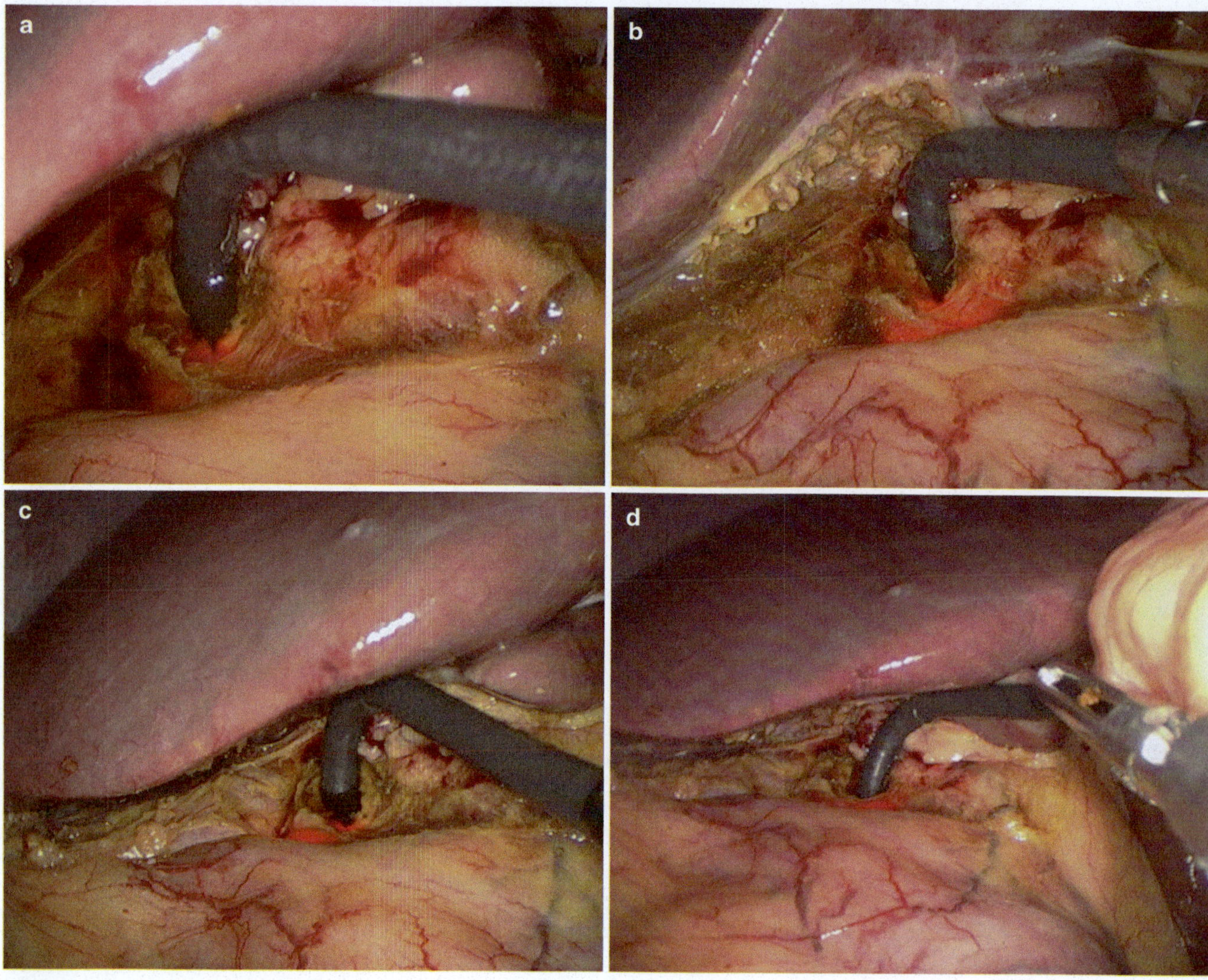

Fig. 5.8

4. Placement of J tube.

   Once clearance of CBD stones was confirmed and no presence of edema or inflammation was observed, a guidewire was passed through the instrument channel of the choledochoscope and advanced through the ampulla of Vater into the duodenum, after which the scope was removed, leaving the guidewire in place. A J-tube was then threaded along the guidewire into the CBD, through the ampulla of Vater, and into the duodenum. With one end of the J-tube in the lumen of the duodenum, the guidewire was removed and the J-tube was retained in the CBD. A completion check choledochoscopy was performed to ensure exact positioning of the J-tube before primary choledochorrhaphy (Fig. 5.9a–f).

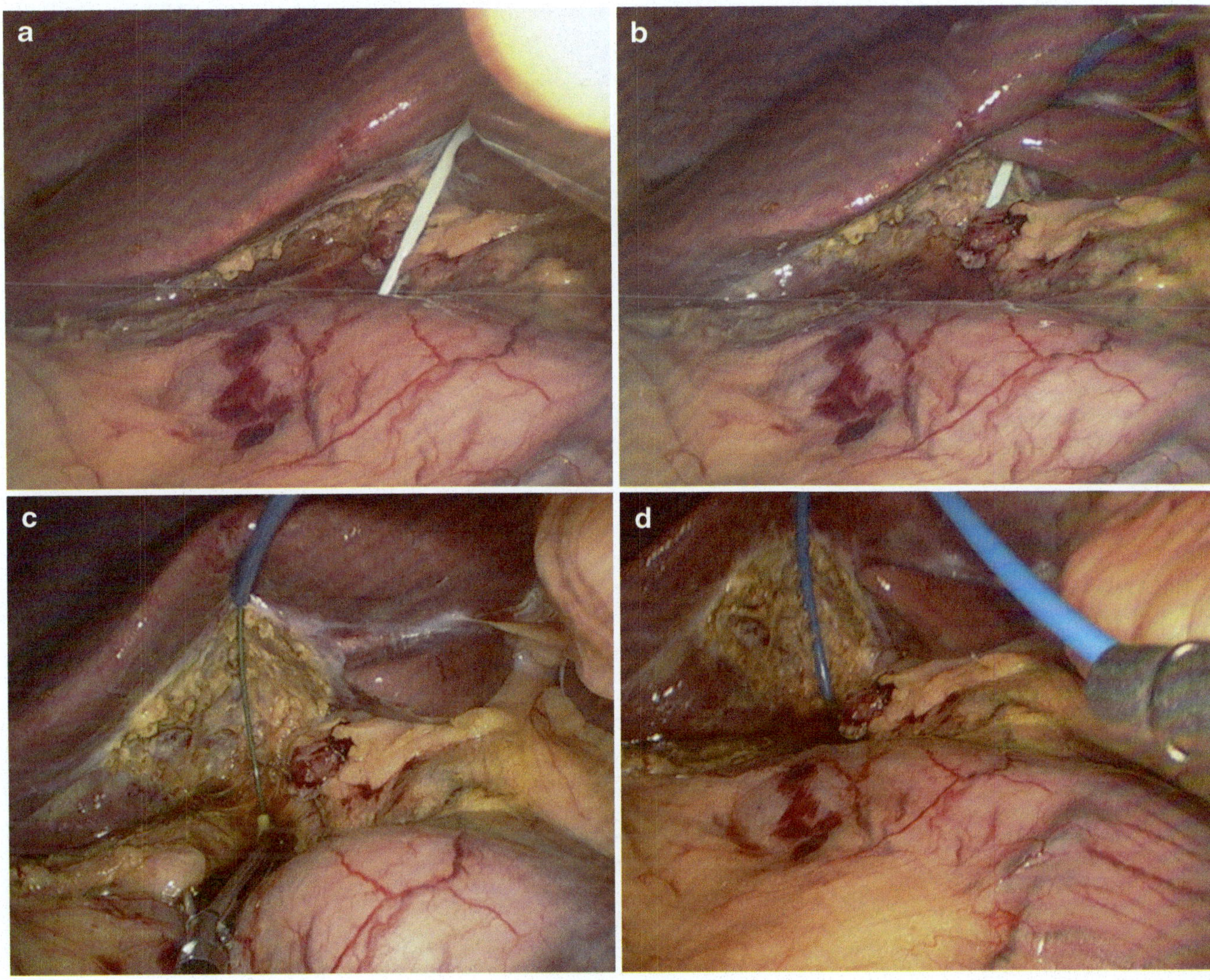

Fig. 5.9

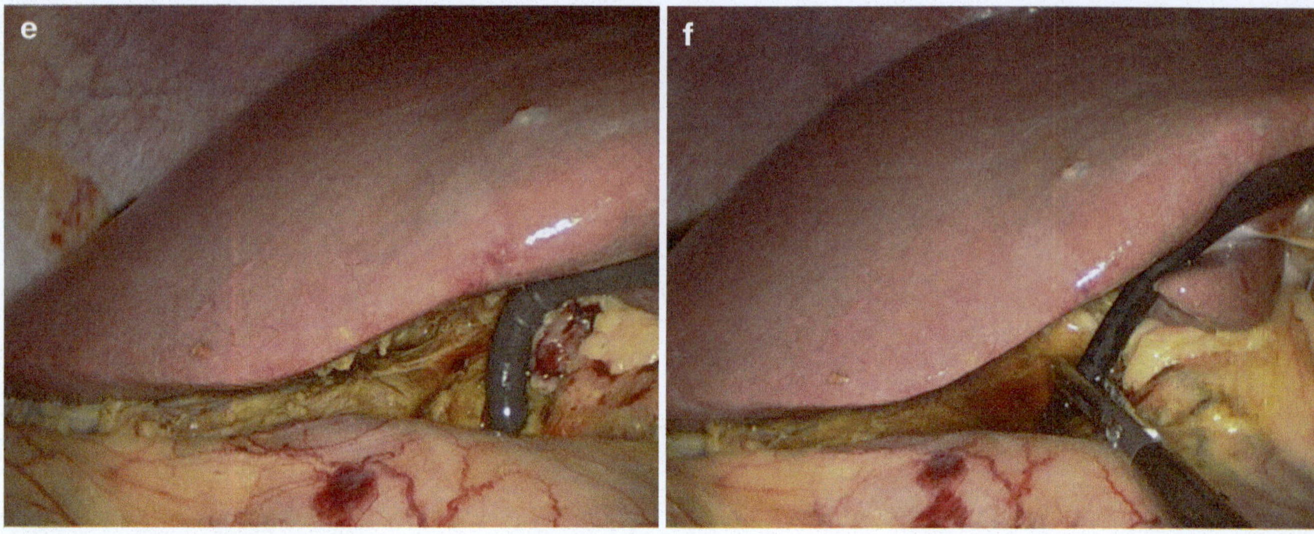

Fig. 5.9 (continued)

5. Closure of the common bile duct.
   Primary closure of the choledochotomy was performed longitudinally using absorbable 3/0 Vicryl suture(s). If the diameter of CBD was less than 1.5 cm, interrupted suture would work (Fig. 5.10a–f).

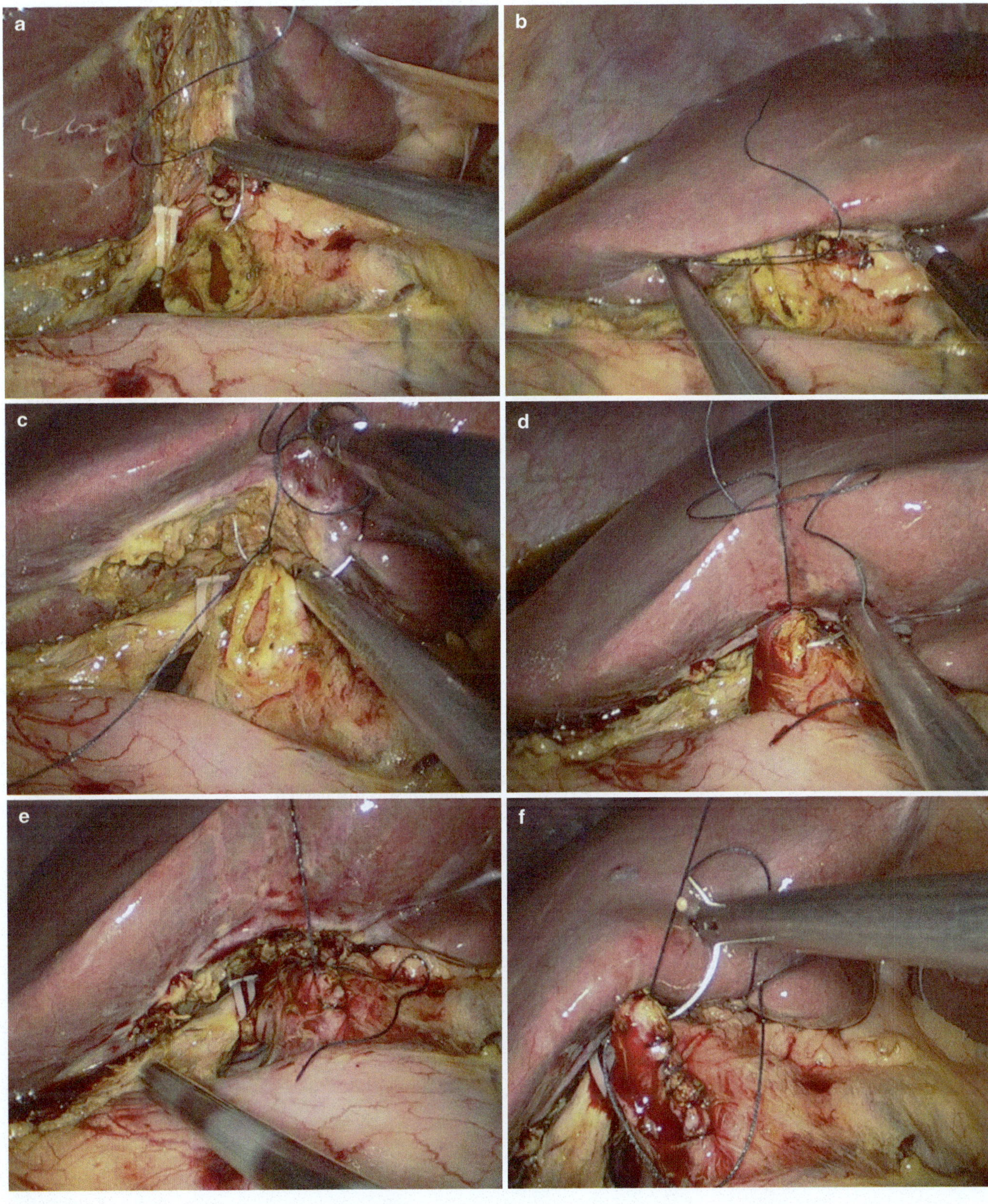

Fig. 5.10

6. Resection of gallbladder.
   Removal of gallbladder was performed as described in the cholecystectomy section. A drain was pulled in through the incision and placed in the foramen of Winslow (Fig. 5.11).

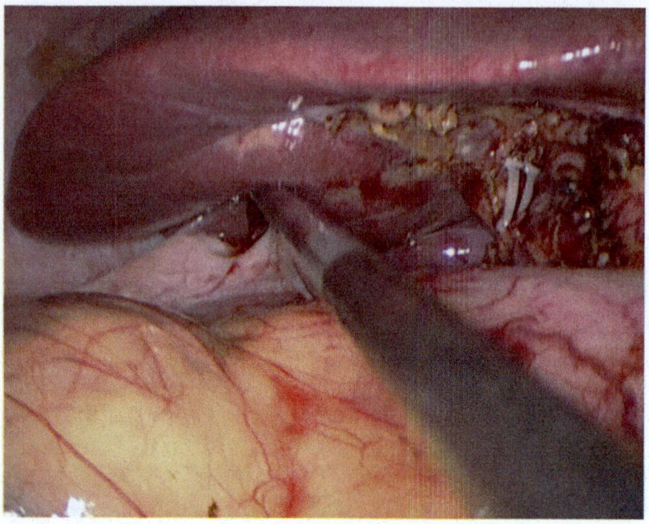

Fig. 5.11

5.2.7 Tips and Tricks

1. The ENBD, ERBD or J-type tube was introduced into the common bile duct preoperatively or intraoperatively for T-tube-free laparoscopic choledocholithtomy.
2. ENBD and ERBD drainage: A 7Fr ENBD tube (Cook, Winston-Salem, NC, USA) or an 8.5Fr 5-cm ERBD tube (Cook, Winston-Salem, NC, USA) was placed preoperatively in the CBD of patient without sphincterotomy. The ERBD tubes were commonly removed by endoscopy on postoperative week 2. Cholangiography was scheduled to confirm the absence of residual stones in the biliary tract before the ENBD tubes were removed.
3. Pigtail J-tube drainage: The use of the pigtail J-tube is ideal for patients with large single or multiple stones primarily in the CBD. Once clearance of CBD stones is confirmed, a pigtail J-tube can be employed as an internal drainage/stent for biliary tree decompression in the presence of distal ductal edema or spasm. A guidewire was passed through the instrument channel of the choledochoscope and advanced through the ampulla of Vater into the duodenum, after which the scope was removed, leaving the guidewire in place. A pigtail J-tube (HuaMei, Zhangjiagang, Jiangsu, China) was then threaded along the guidewire into the CBD, through the ampulla of Vater, and into the duodenum. With one end of the J-tube in the lumen of the duodenum, the guidewire was removed and the J-tube was retained in the CBD. This was facilitated by the coils on both ends of the J-tube, which provided a self-retaining mechanism. A completion check choledochoscopy was performed to ensure exact positioning of the J-tube before primary choledochorrhaphy with interrupted or continuous 3/0 absorbable Vicryl suture(s). The position of the pigtail J-tube was further confirmed with fluoroscopy before the J-tube was removed and the patient was discharged.
4. No biliary drainage: We performed primary choledochorrhaphy with interrupted 3/0 absorbable Vicryl suture leaving no biliary drainage for the patients who had absence of distal ductal edema or spasm during the completion check choledochoscopy.

5.3 Laparoscopic Cholecystojejunostomy

5.3.1 Indications and Case Selection

1. Obstruction in the inferior segment of common bile duct, e.g. radical resection is improper for carcinoma of head of pancreas in later period.
2. Staging operation for carcinoma of head of pancreas.
3. Malignant obstruction in the inferior segment of common bile duct, in which document dilated cystic duct is identified.

5.3.2 Contraindications

1. Patients with obstruction in cystic duct due to malignant change in later period.
2. Patients with low insertion of cystic duct into the common hepatic duct, which is easily obstructed by tumor.
3. Patients with cholangiocarcinoma in the middle or superior segment.
4. Patients with gallbladder stone or common bile duct stone.

5.3.3 Major Instruments or Energy Sources

1. Laparoscopy System.
2. Holding forceps.
3. Harmonic scalpel.
4. Endoscopic linear stapler.

5.3.4 Team Setup, Anesthesia and Position

Under general anesthesia, the patient was placed in supine position with the legs apart. The position of surgeon, assistants and nurses is shown in Fig. 5.12.

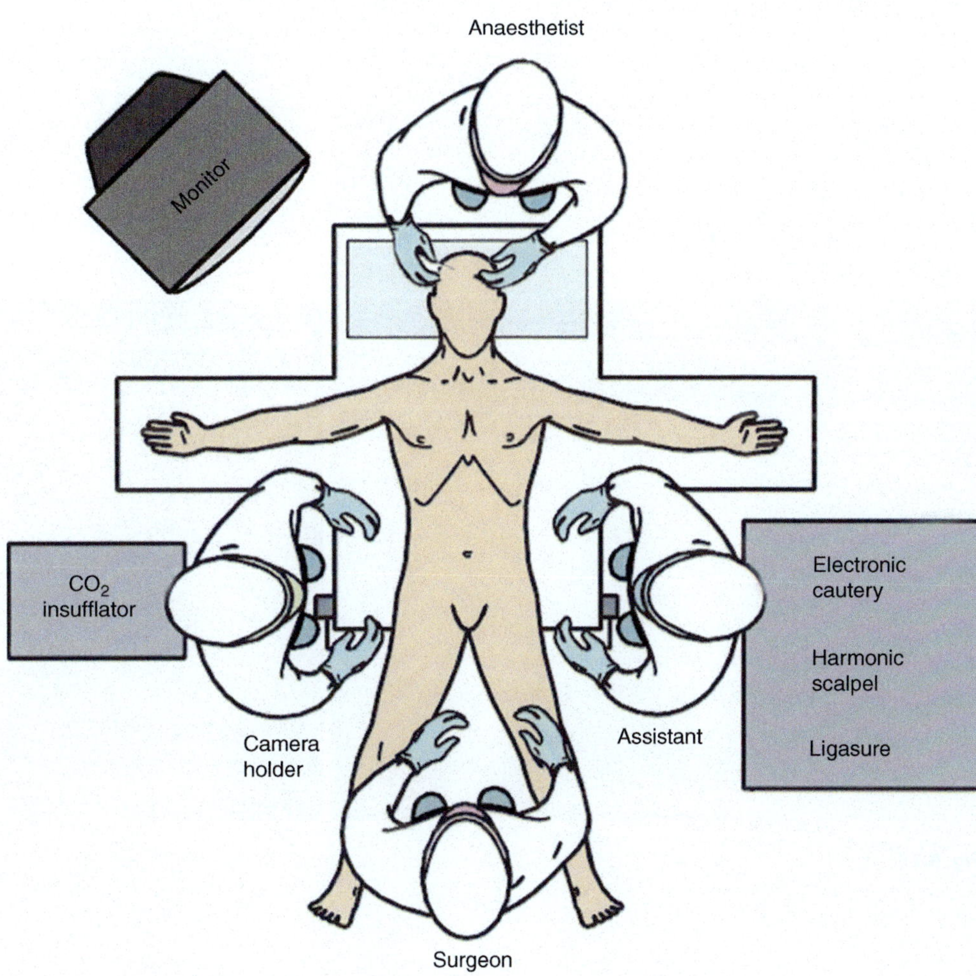

Fig. 5.12

5.3.5 Key Steps

1. Exploration of the lesion.
2. Dissection of upper jejunum.
3. Anastomosis of gallbladder and jejunum.
4. Side-to-side jejunojejunostomy.
5. Irrigation and drainage.

5.3.6 Surgical Techniques

1. Exploration of the lesion.
   The procedure began with a general exploration of the abdomen, particularly to confirm the radiological patent hepatocystic junction.
2. Dissection of upper jejunum.
   First, an upper jejunal loop (the first loop) was identified by a descending (ligament of Treitz) exploration of the small intestine. A suitable loop (45–50 cm) distally to the ligament of Trietz that could easily and comfortably reach the sub-hepatic space was passed in an anterior colic manner without tension and approximated to the gallbladder (Fig. 5.13a–h).

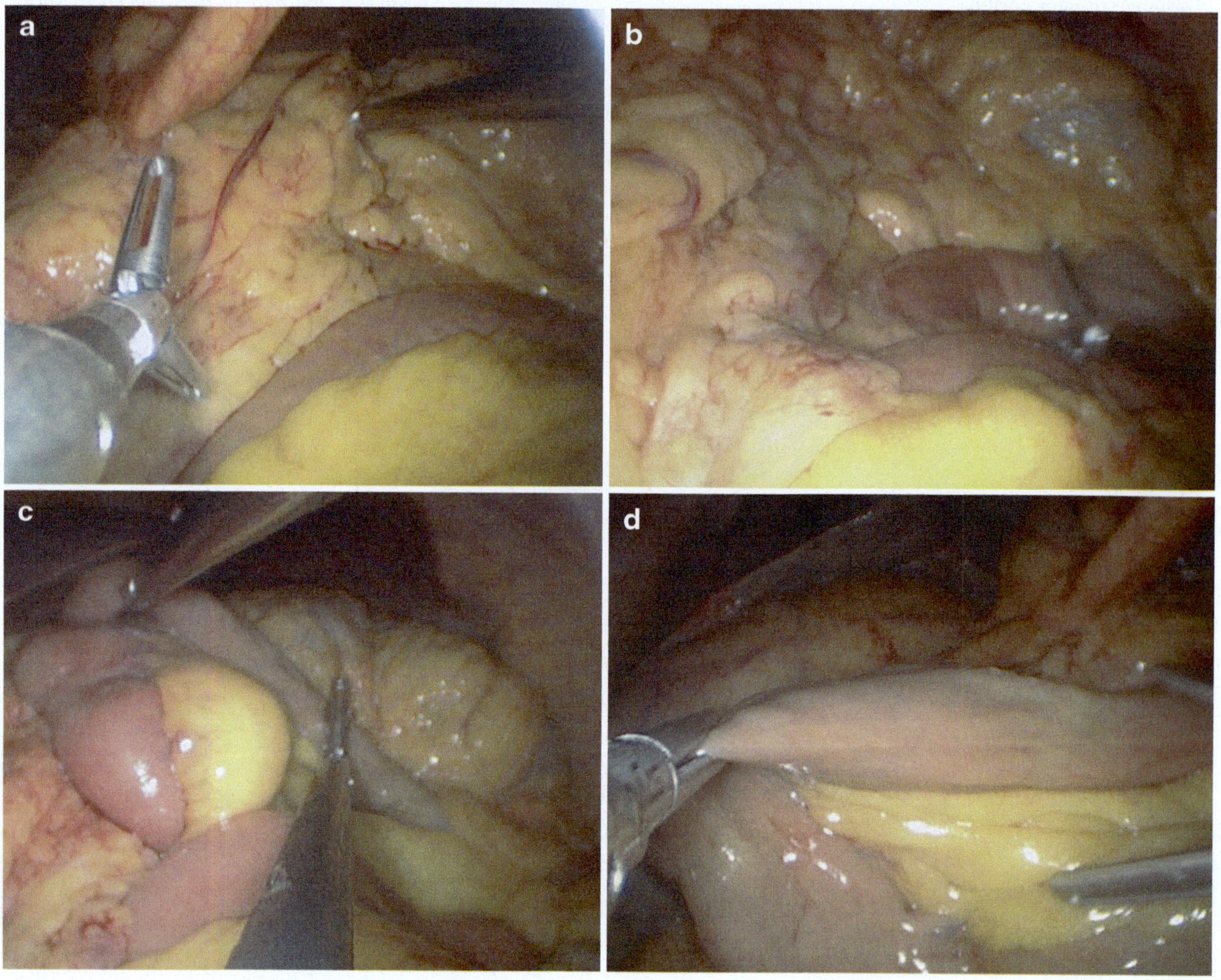

Fig. 5.13

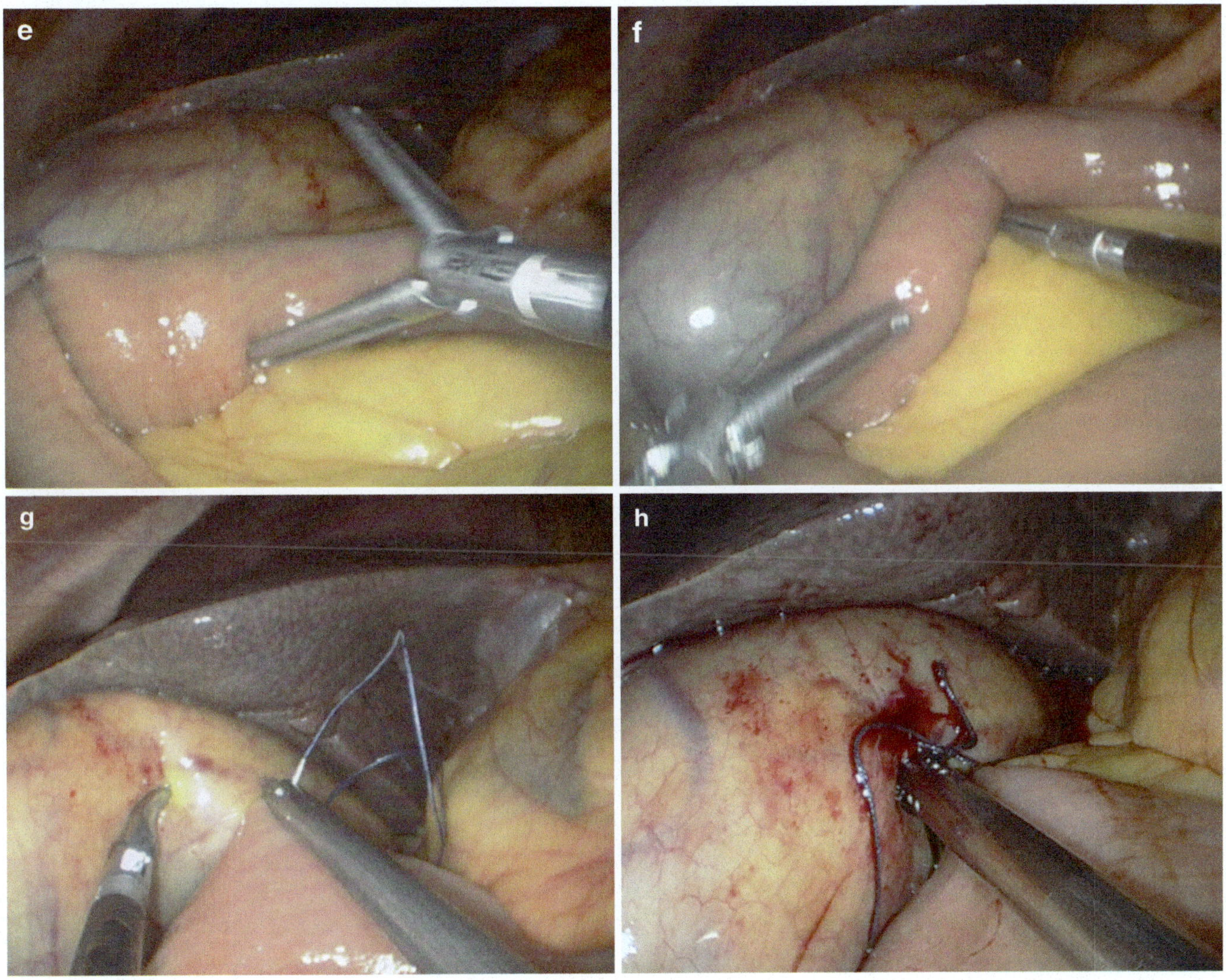

Fig. 5.13 (continued)

3. Anastomosis of gallbladder and jejunum.
   A small incision was made in the body of the gallbladder, and the bile evacuated (Fig. 5.14a, b).

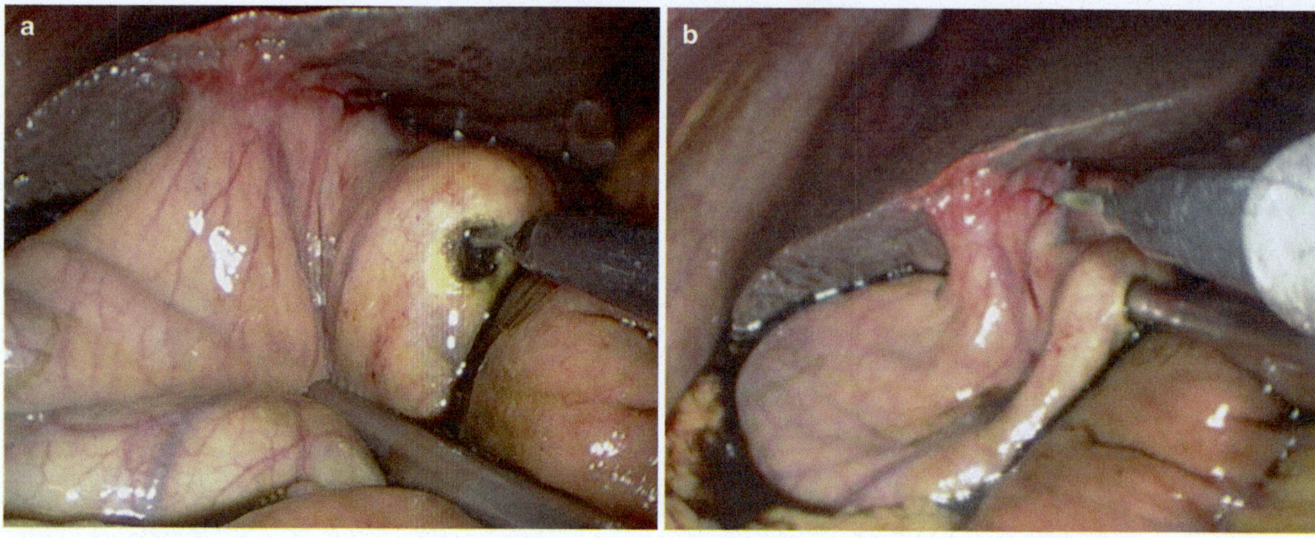

Fig. 5.14

A similar incision was made on the predesigned antimesenteric part of the approximated jejunum. The jaws of the Endo-GIA stapler was introduced through these two incisions and pushed to its full length, closed, and fired (Fig. 5.15a–d).

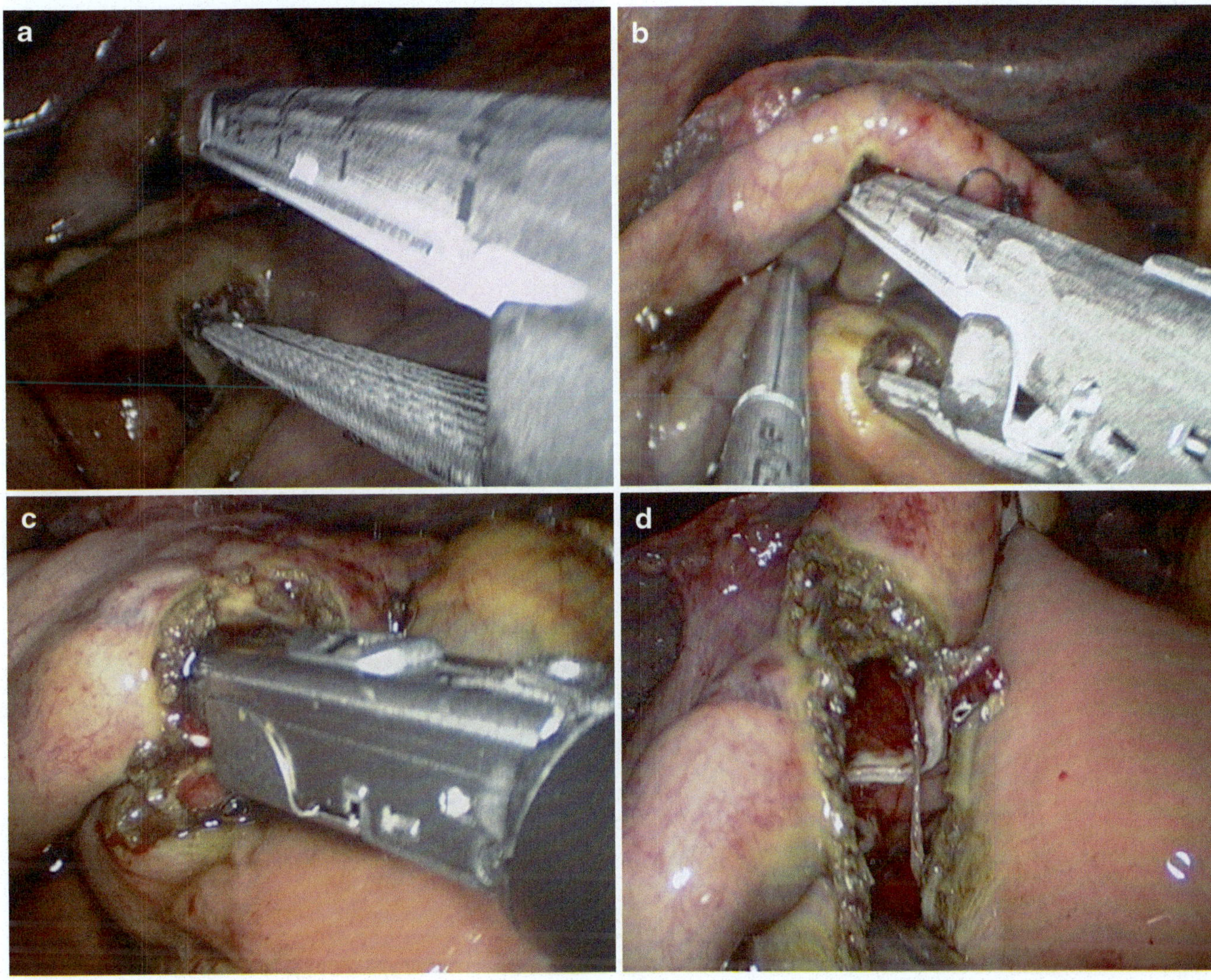

Fig. 5.15

The two entry sites were combined as one. They were closed by using 3/0 absorbable Vicryl sutures (Fig. 5.16a–f).

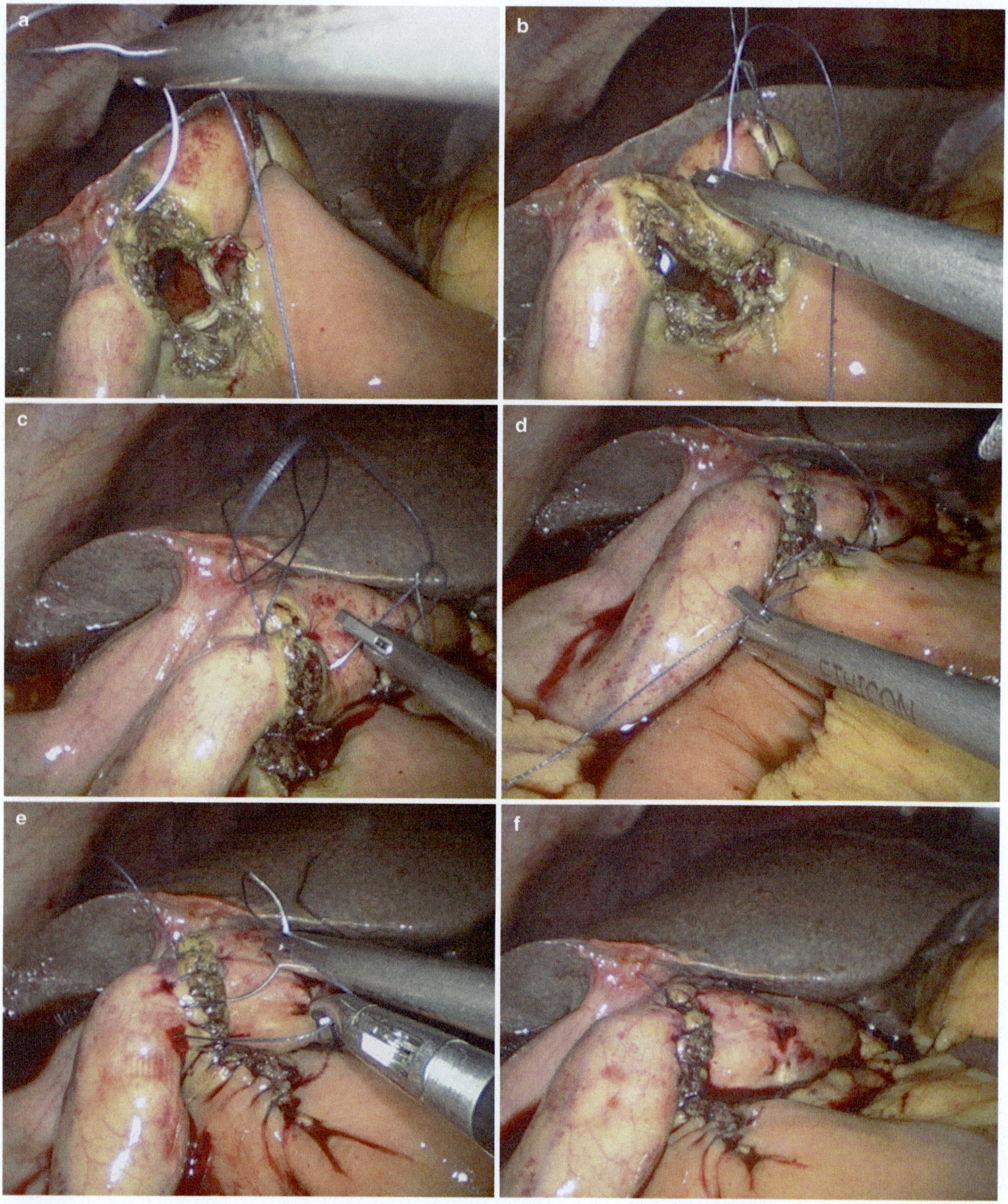

Fig. 5.16

4. Side-to-side jejunojejunostomy.
   The patient was then placed in the position with a 15° tile to the right. The anti-mesenteric part of the first and second (45–50 cm distally to the anastomosis) loops of jejunum were pulled together for enteroenterostomy (Fig. 5.17a, b).

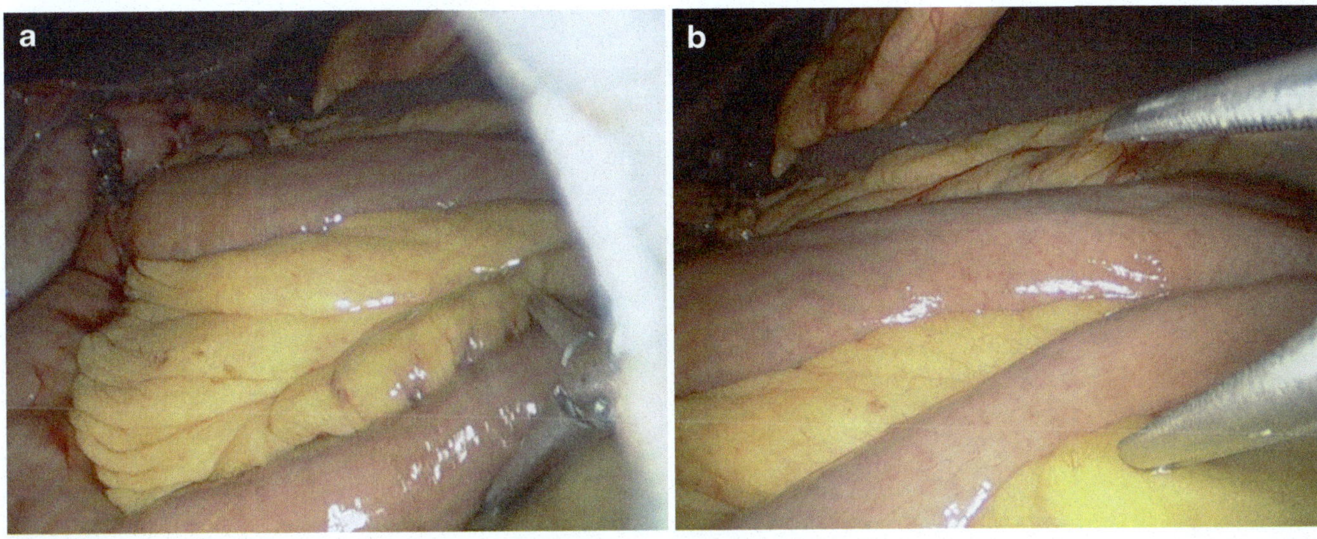

Fig. 5.17

A 0.5 cm incision was separately made on both anti-mesenteric part of the jejunum (Fig. 5.18a, b).

The jaws of the Endo-GIA stapler was introduced through these two incisions and pushed to its full length, closed, and fired. Making sure there was no mesenteric volvulus (Fig. 5.19a–d).

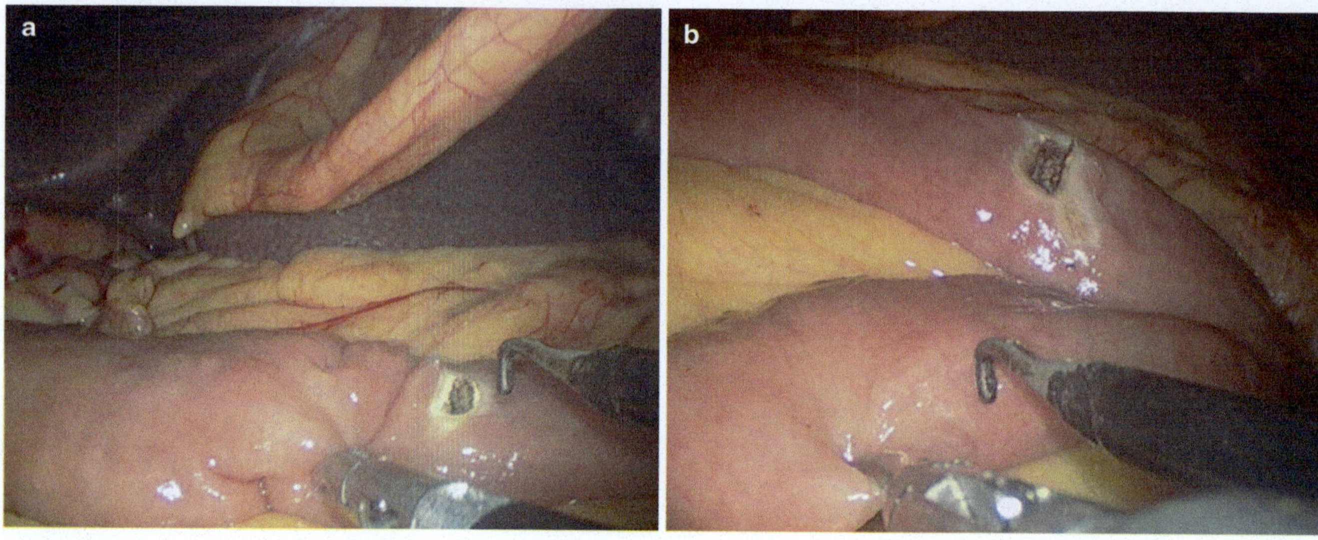

Fig. 5.18

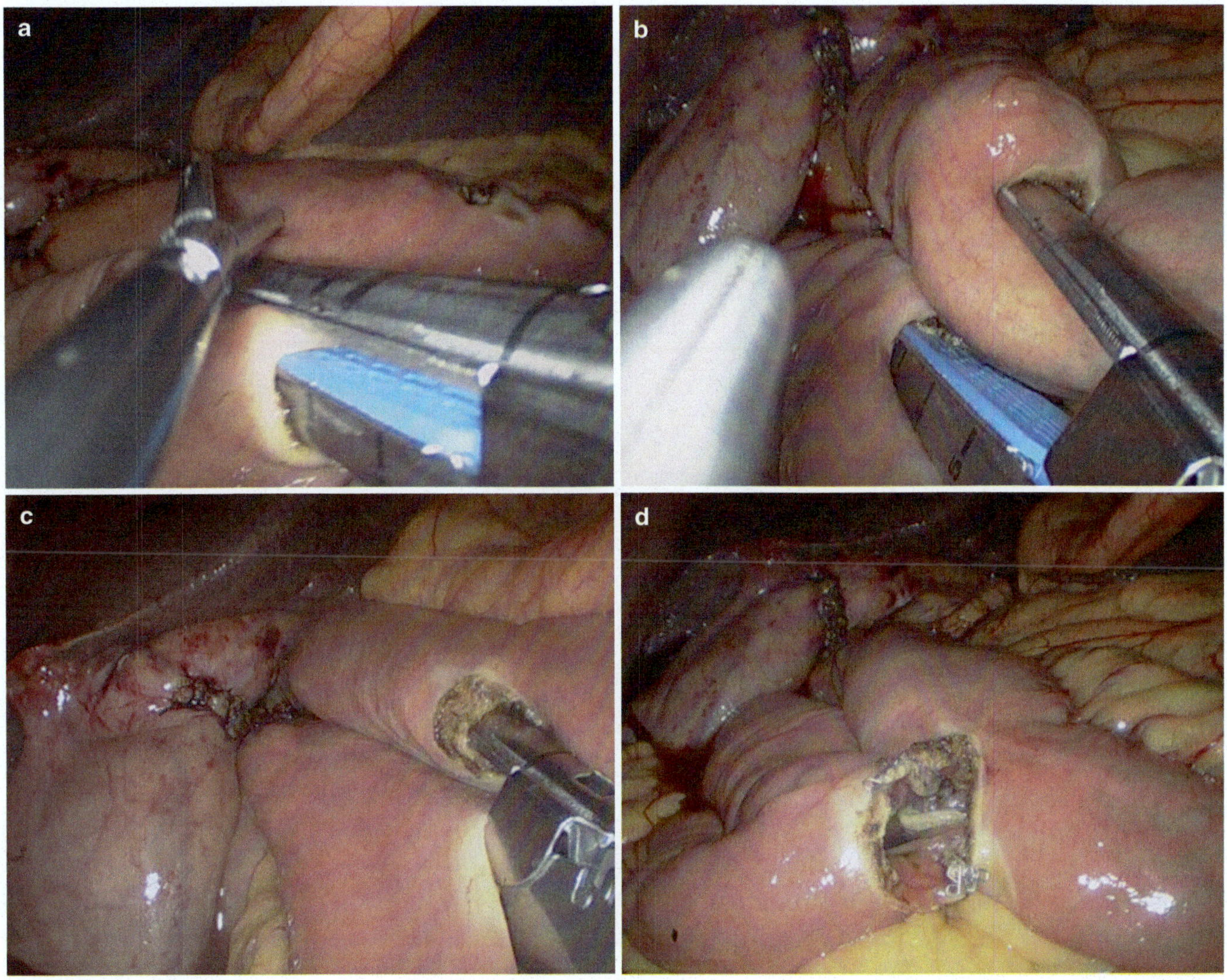

Fig. 5.19

The common opening left behind after the removal of the stapler was closed by 3/0 absorbable Vicryl sutures (Fig. 5.20a–h).

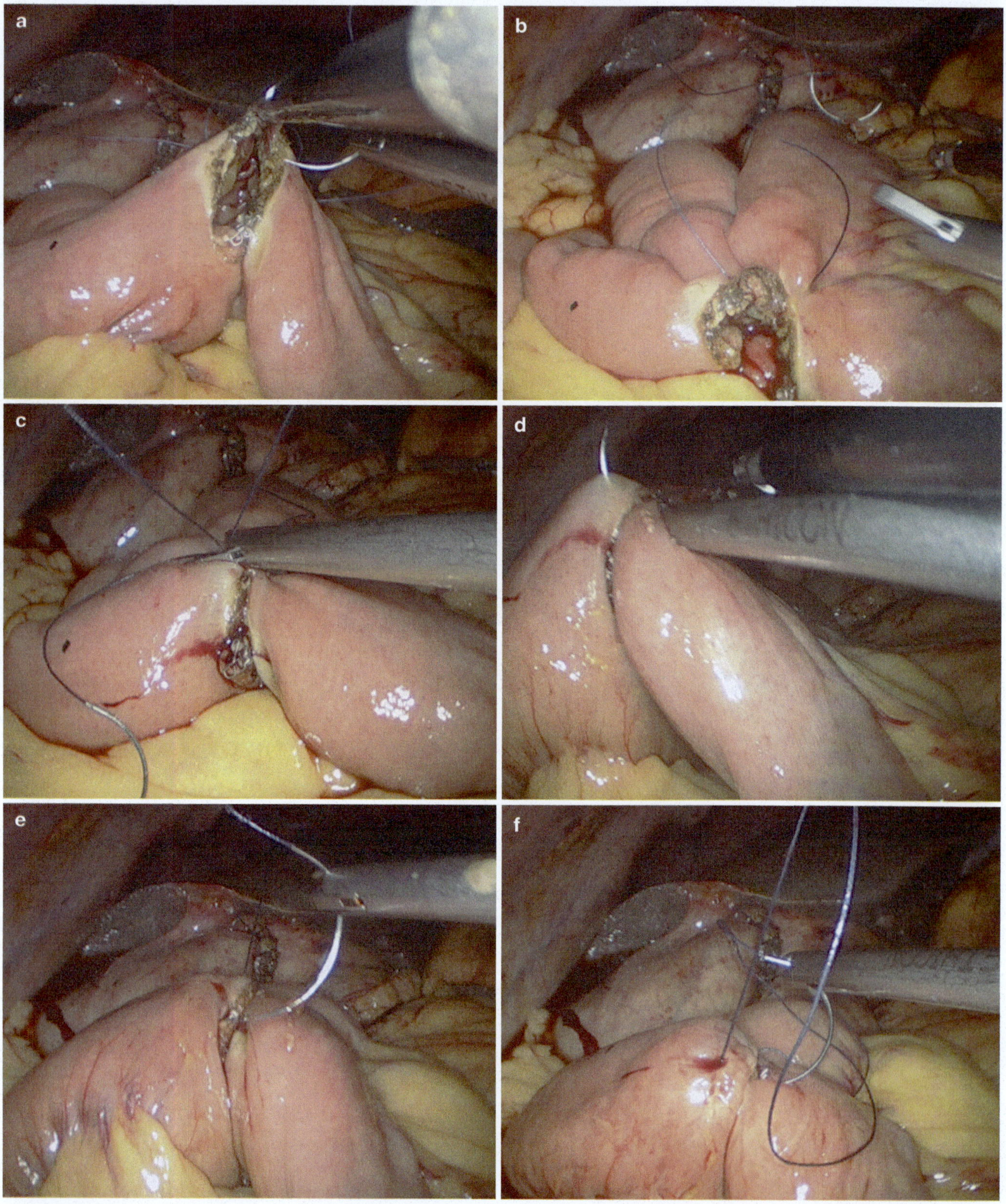

Fig. 5.20

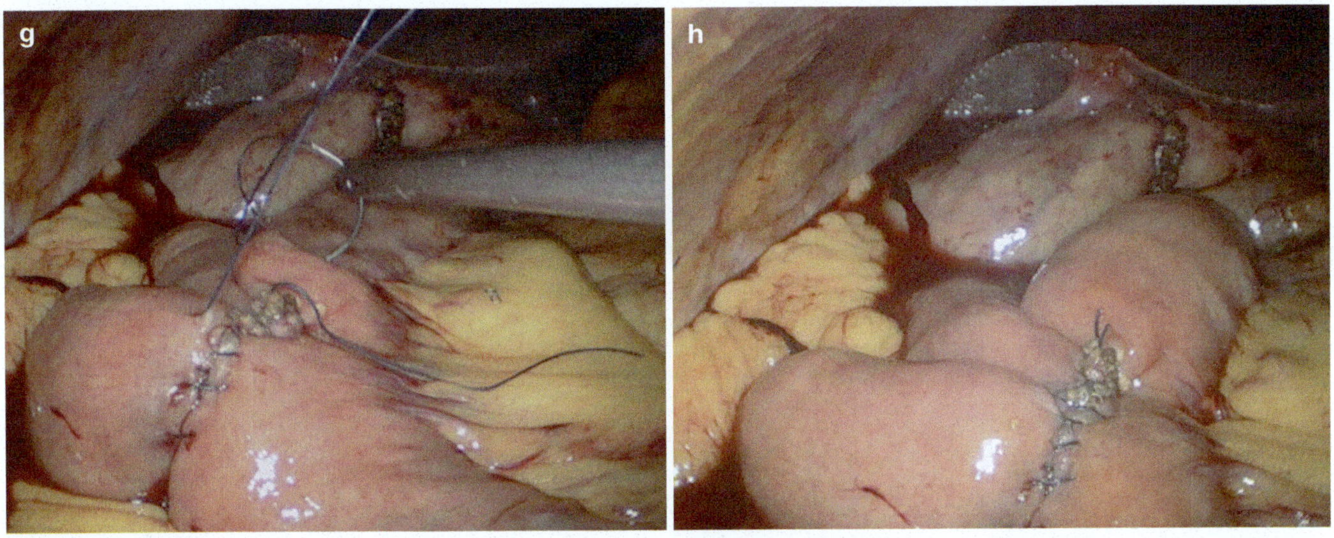

Fig. 5.20 (continued)

5. Irrigation and drainage.
   After adequate flushing of the surgical field, a drain was placed behind the anastomosis of cholecystojejunostomy through the umbilicus (Fig. 5.21a–d).

5.3.7 Tips and Tricks

1. The patency of the hepatocystic junction, and the junction of the cystic duct with the common hepatic duct was more than 1 cm away from the proximal extent of the tumors should be confirmed.
2. Two percutaneous transfascial retraction sutures (3/0 Prolene. Ethicon, US) could be placed at the right and left costal margins to achieve adequate exposure not only to facilitate anastomosis but also throughout the whole procedure. One suture was placed at one end of the anastomotic line between the fundus of the gallbladder and intestine, and the other was at one end of the anastomotic line between the two segments of intestine

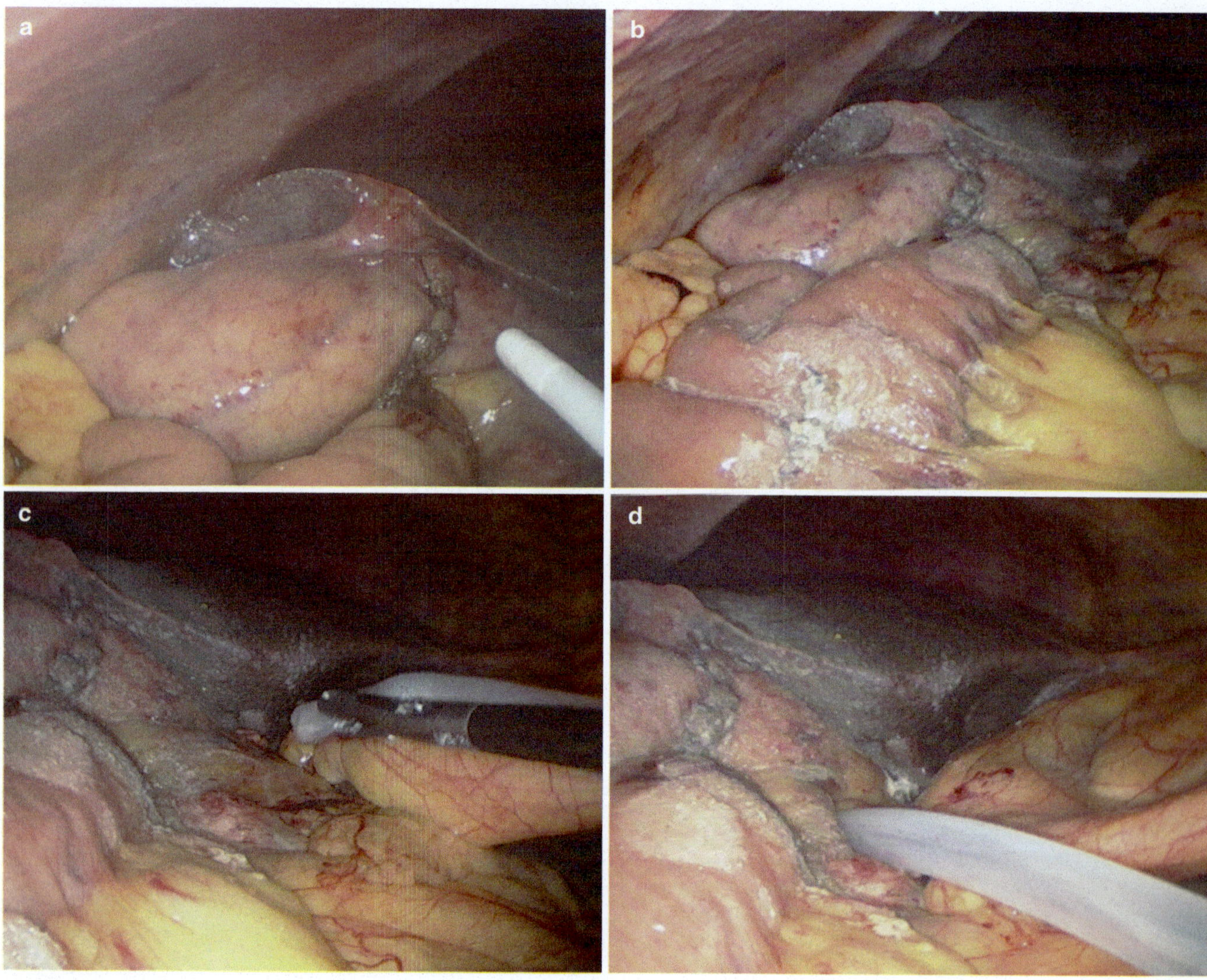

Fig. 5.21

5.4 Laparoscopic Cholangiojejunostomy

5.4.1 Indications and Case Selection

1. Benign stenosis of extrahepatic bile duct.
2. Striction in the terminal of common bile duct.
3. Paraduodenal papilla diverticulum, such causing recurrent pancreatitis and cholangitis.
4. Congenital anomalies of biliary system, e.g. reconstruction of biliary tract after cyst resection for congenital cystic dilatation of common bile duct.
5. Biliary alimentary anastomotic stoma striction.
6. Carcinoma of gallbladder or head of pancreas, which is difficult to resect.
7. Carcinoma of the middle segment of bile duct.

5.4.2 Contraindications

Patients with intrahepatic bile duct striction or stone should be the contraindicated to perform laparoscopic cholangiojejunostomy.

5.4.3 Major Instruments or Energy Sources

1. Laparoscopy System.
2. Holding forceps.
3. Harmonic scalpel.
4. Endoscopic linear stapler.

5.4.4 Team Setup, Anesthesia and Position

Under general anesthesia, the patient was placed in supine position with the legs apart. The position of surgeon, assistants and nurses is shown in Fig. 5.22.

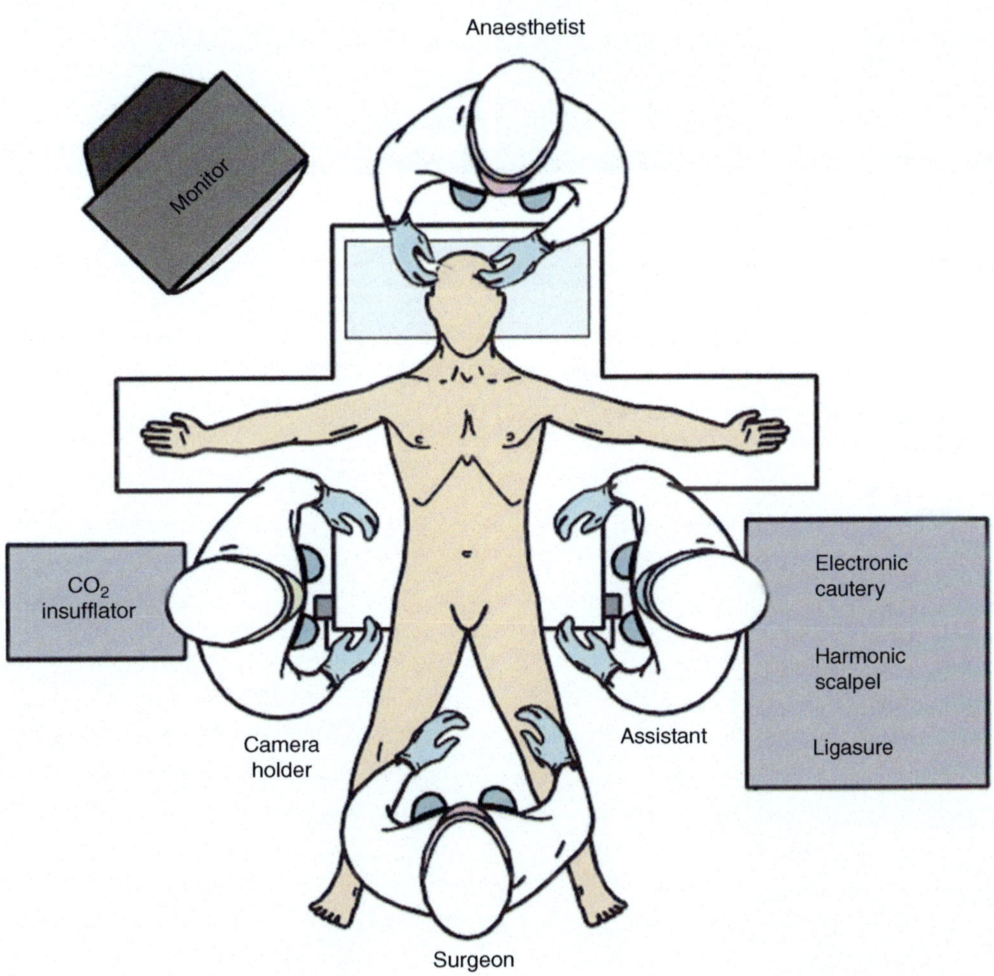

Fig. 5.22

5.4.5 Key Steps

1. Dissection of gallbladder.
2. Skeletonization of hepatoduodenal ligament.
3. Transection of common bile duct.
4. Transection of common hepatic duct.
5. Dissection of jejunum.
6. Cholangiojejunostomy.
7. Jejunojejunostomy.
8. Specimen retraction.
9. Irrigation and drainage.

5.4.6 Surgical Techniques

1. Dissection of gallbladder.
   The gallbladder was removed from the liver bed without transecting the cystic duct (Fig. 5.23a, b).

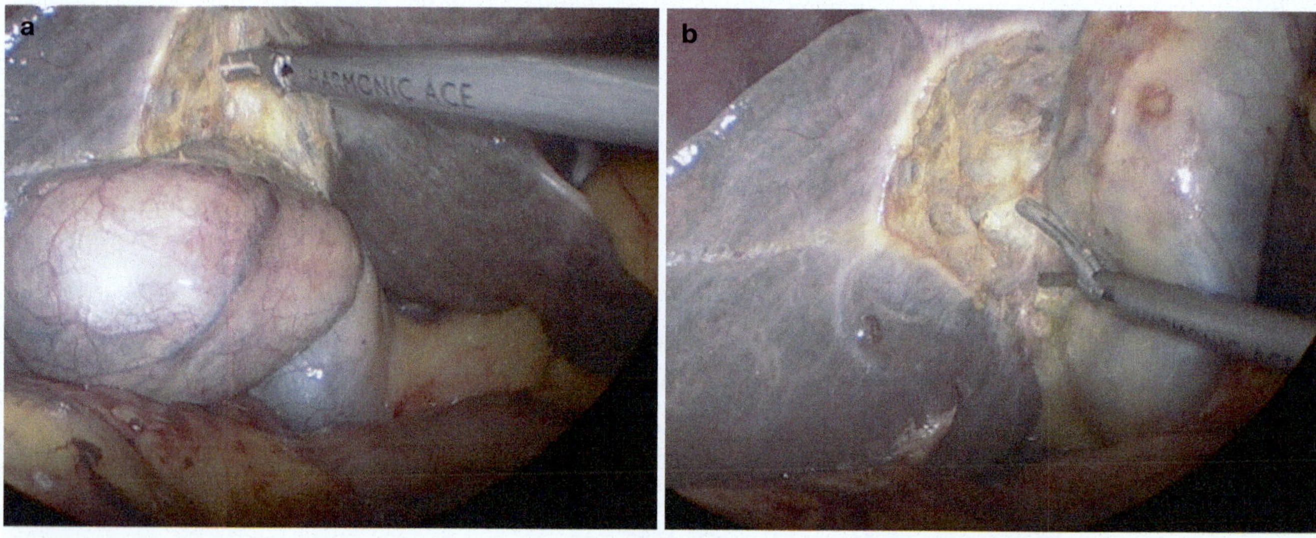

Fig. 5.23

2. Skeletonization of hepatoduodenal ligament.
   A percutaneous transfascial retraction suture was placed below the xiphoid process to achieve adequate exposure. Lymph nodes and connective tissues lateral and posterior to the bile duct were mobilized using the 5-mm harmonic scalpel, leading to complete skeletonization of the proper hepatic artery, portal vein and common bile duct (CBD) (Fig. 5.24a–r).

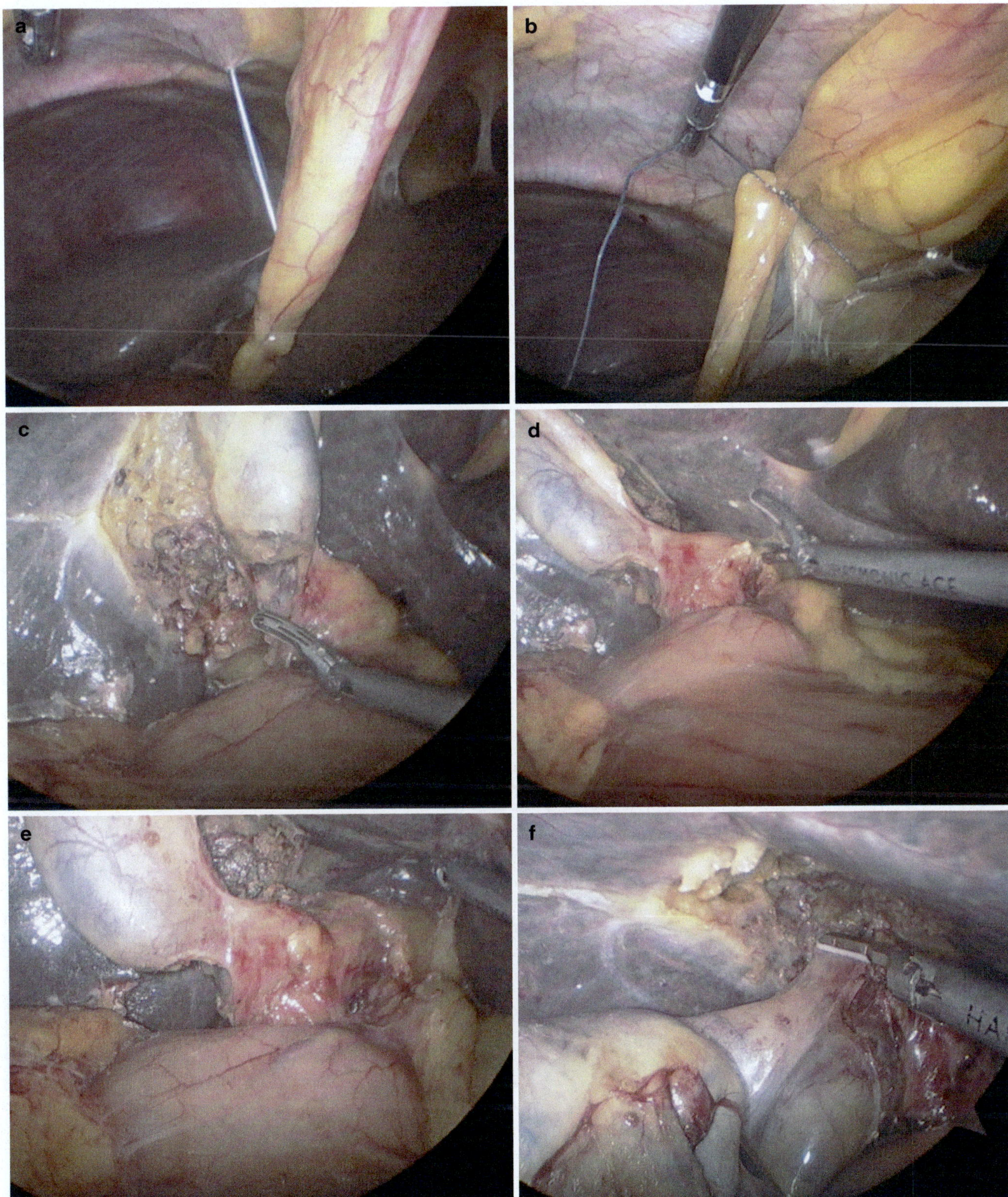

Fig. 5.24

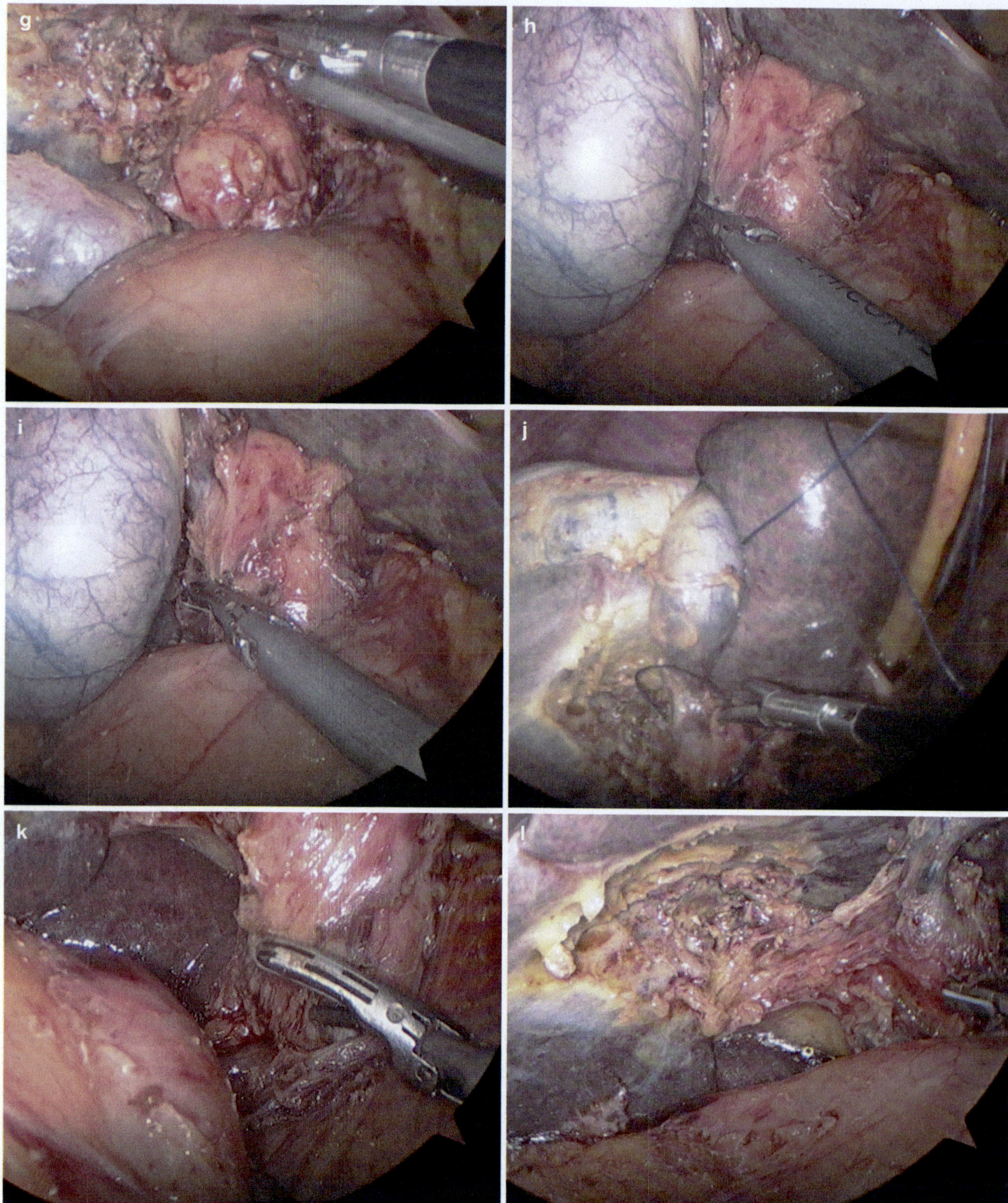

Fig. 5.24 (continued)

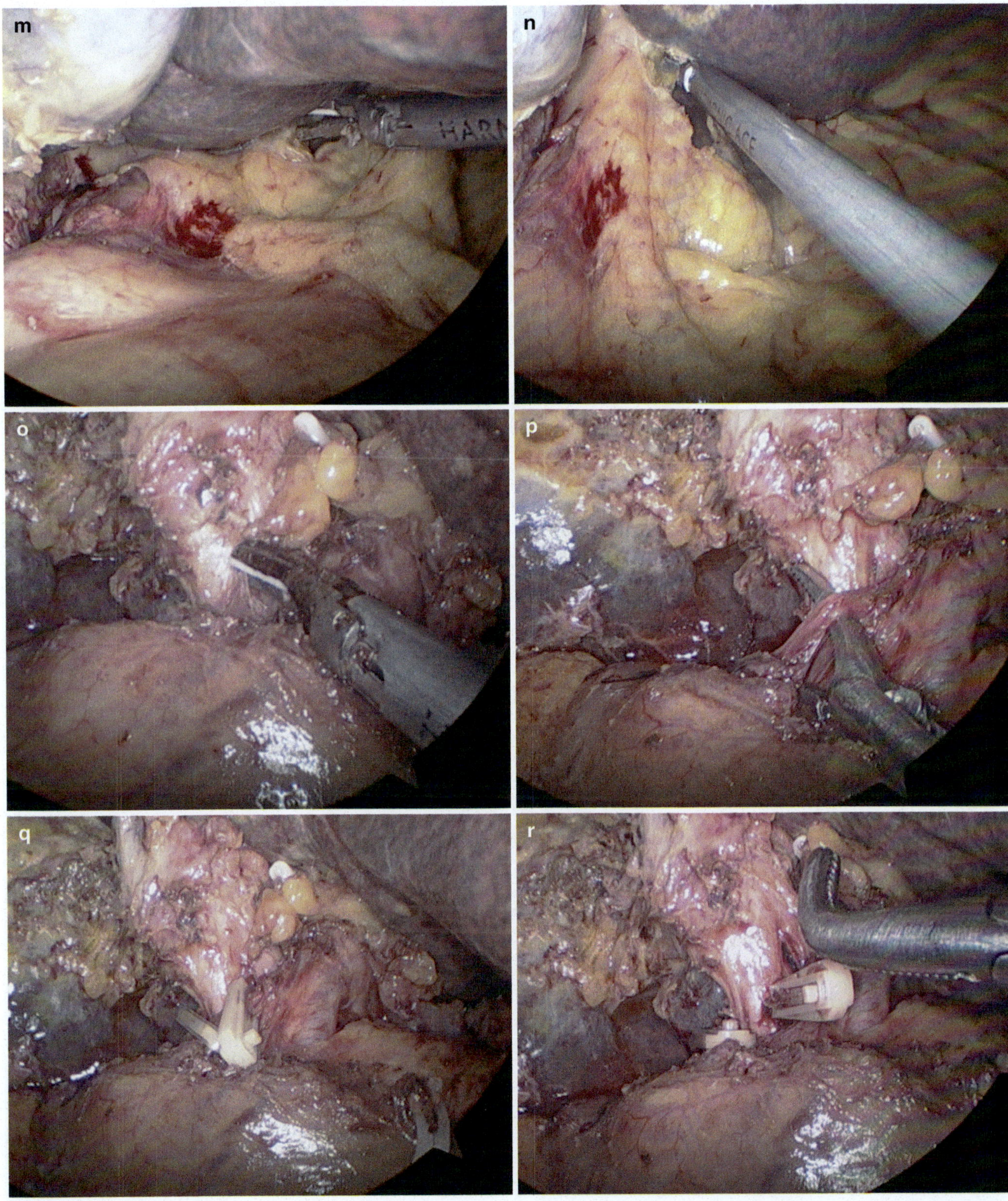

Fig. 5.24 (continued)

3. Transection of common bile duct.
   The CBD was transected at the superior edge of duodenum (2 cm distally to the inferior margin of tumor) (Fig. 5.25a–h).

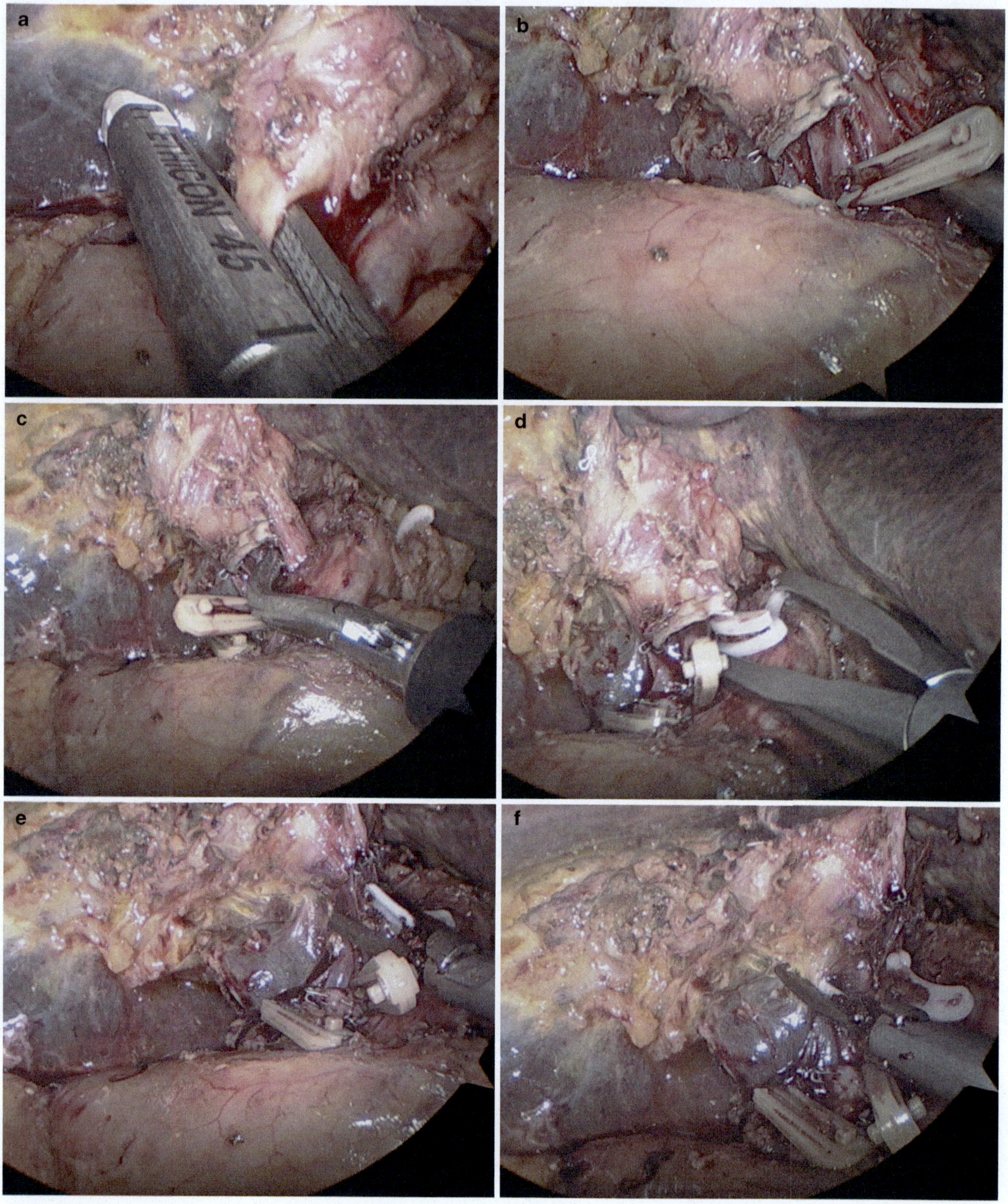

Fig. 5.25

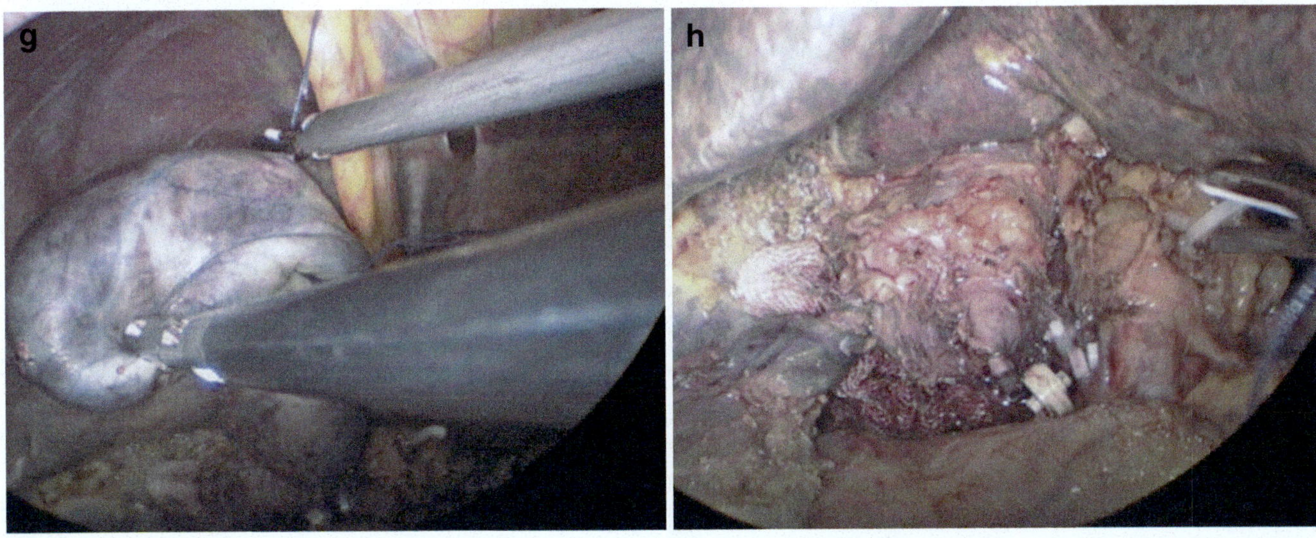

Fig. 5.25 (continued)

4. Transection of common hepatic duct.
   Dissection was next extended further in the cephalad direction, and the common hepatic duct or extrahepatic right and left bile ducts were divided at least 2 cm away from the superior margin of the tumor. The surgical specimen was removed and included the distal common hepatic duct, the common bile duct with the attached gallbladder, and the regional node-bearing tissue (Fig. 5.26a–i).

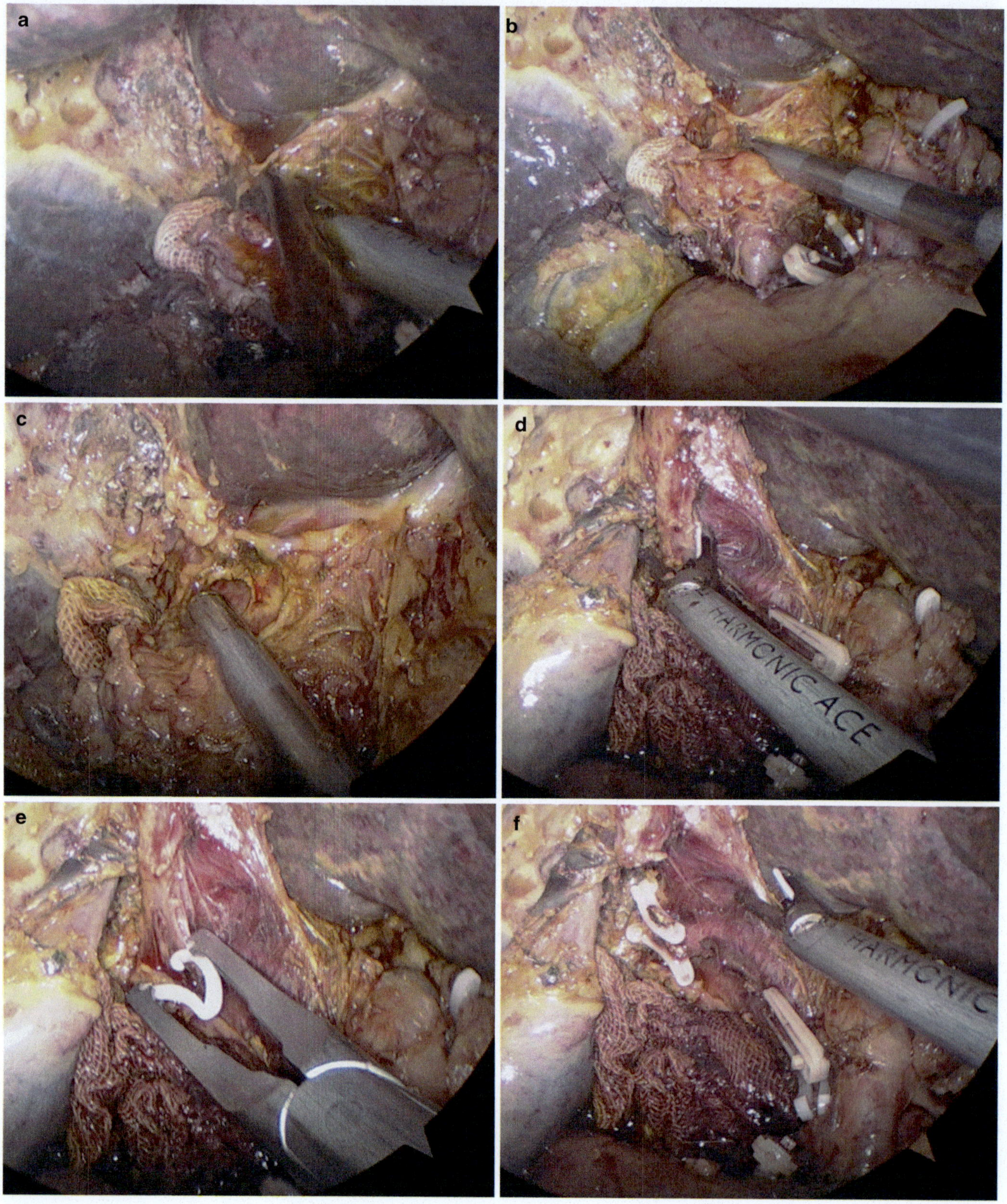

Fig. 5.26

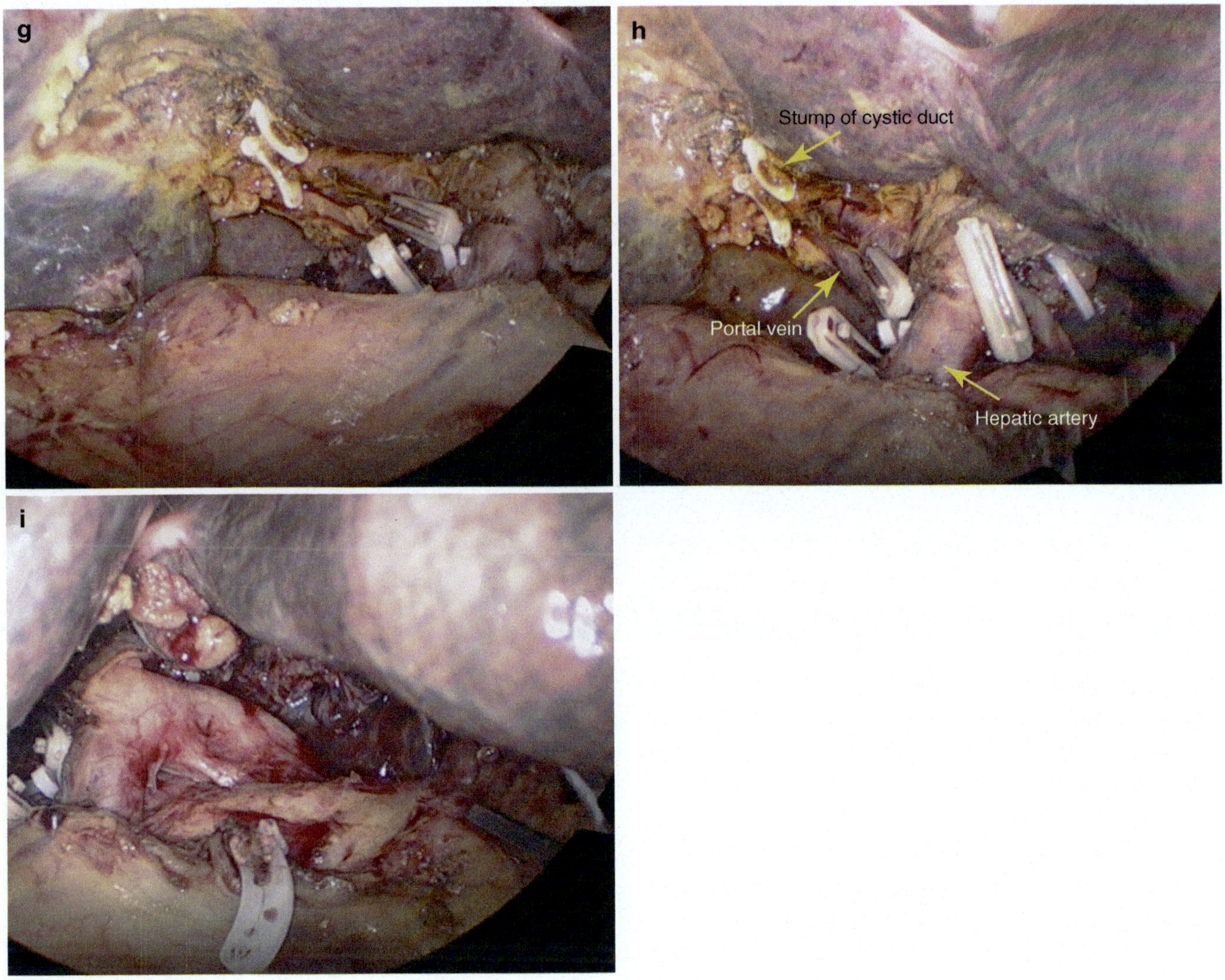

Fig. 5.26 (continued)

5. Dissection of jejunum.
   The first jejunal loop 10–15 cm distally to the ligament of Treitz that comfortably reached the sub-hepatic space was used to create a Roux-en-Y conduit. It was divided using the GIA stapler (Fig. 5.27a–e).

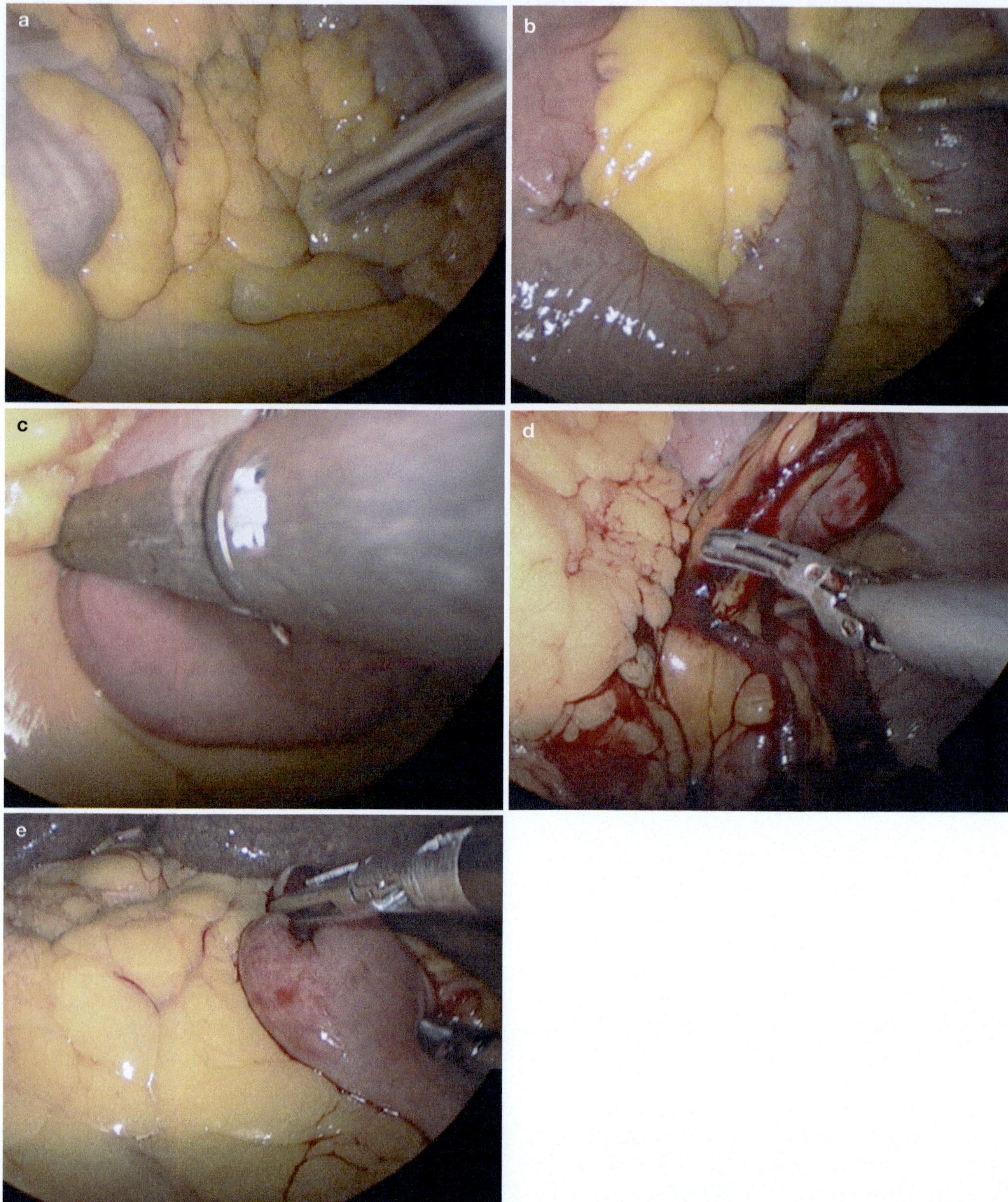

Fig. 5.27

6. Cholangiojejunostomy.
   The distal part of the jejunal loop was brought through a window in the transverse mesocolon toward the severed common duct. The end-to-side choledochojejunal anastomosis was constructed on the anti-mesenteric part of the loop (5 cm to the end) by 3/0 absorbable Vicryl suture (Fig. 5.28a–n).

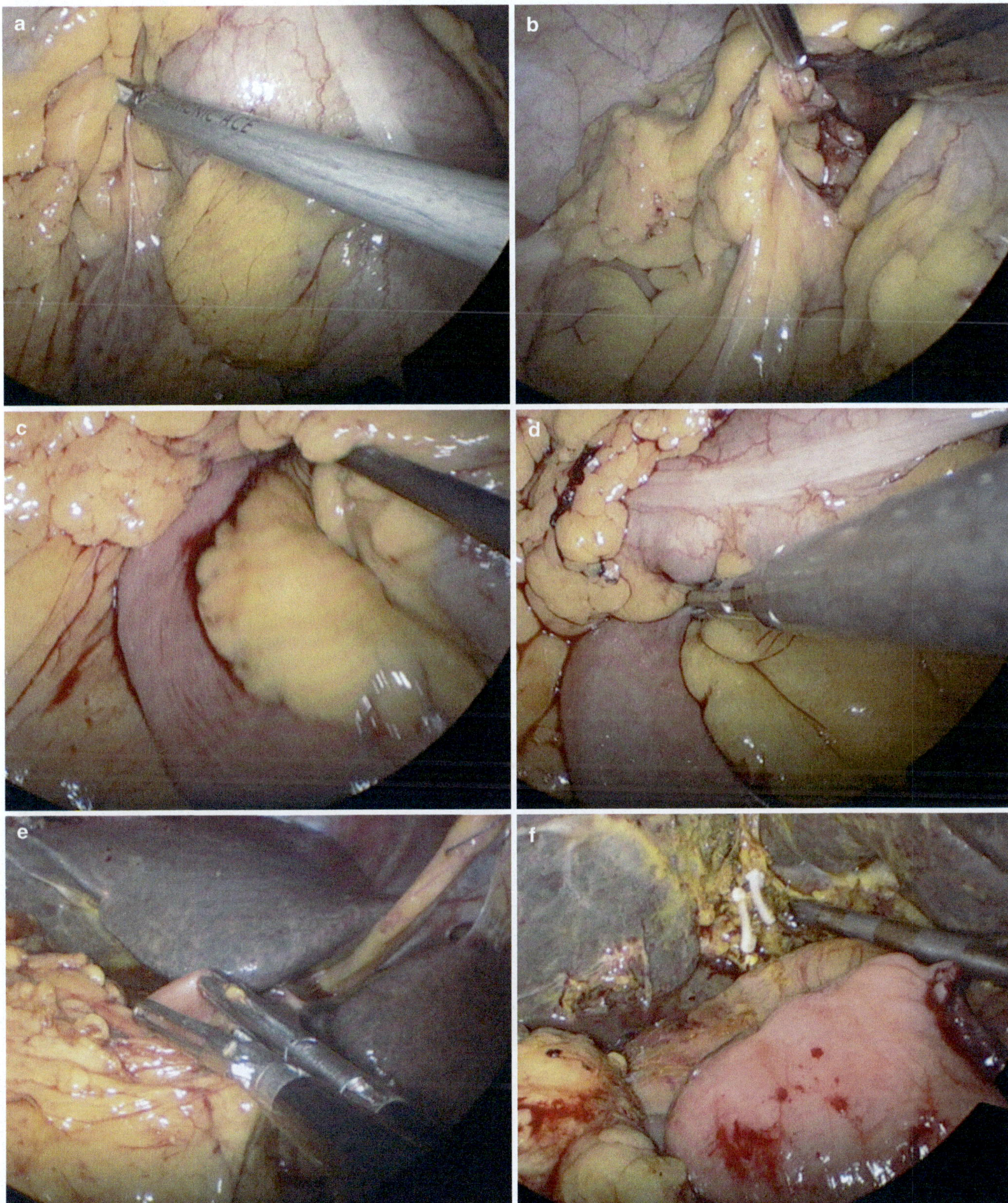

Fig. 5.28

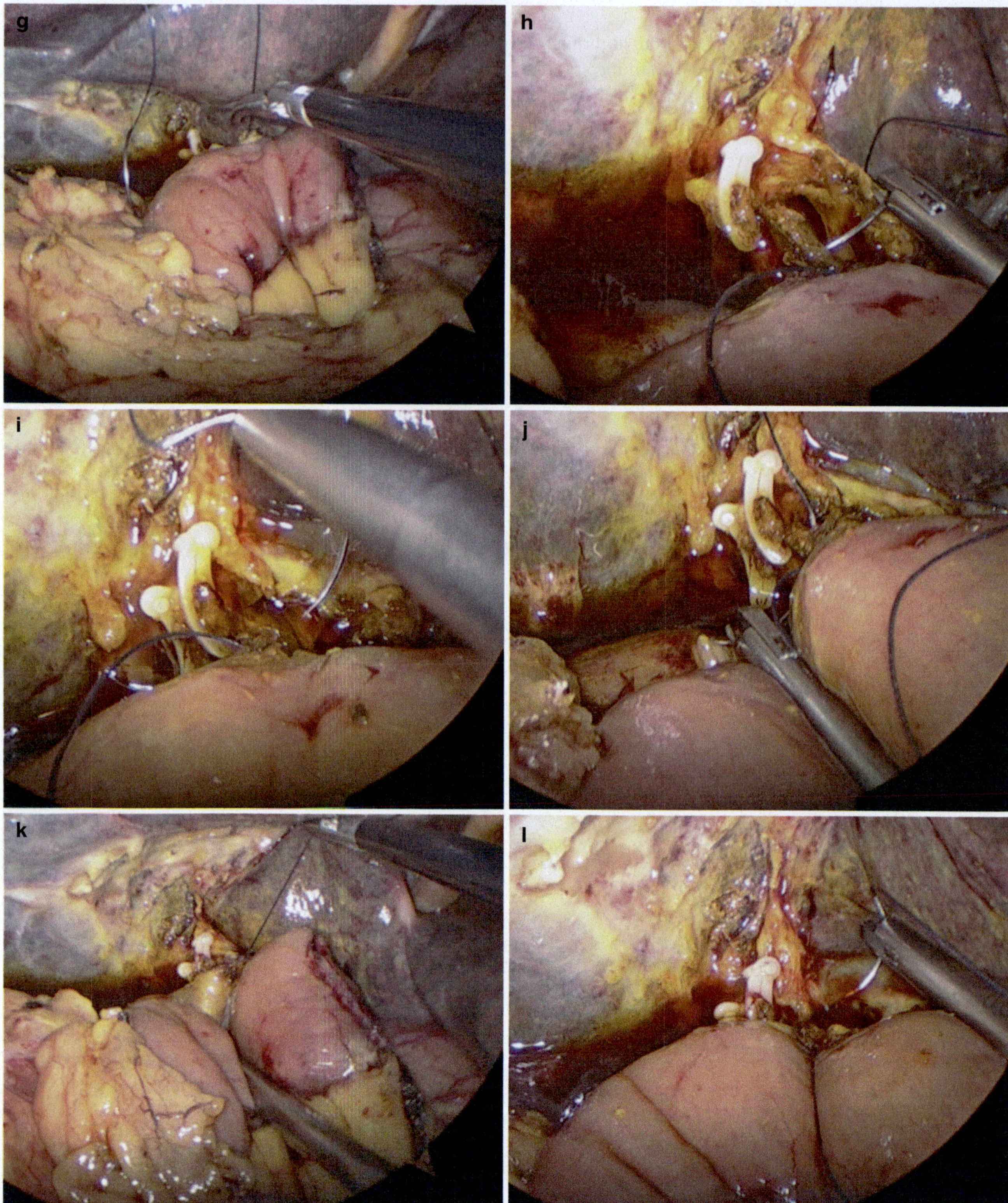

Fig. 5.28 (continued)

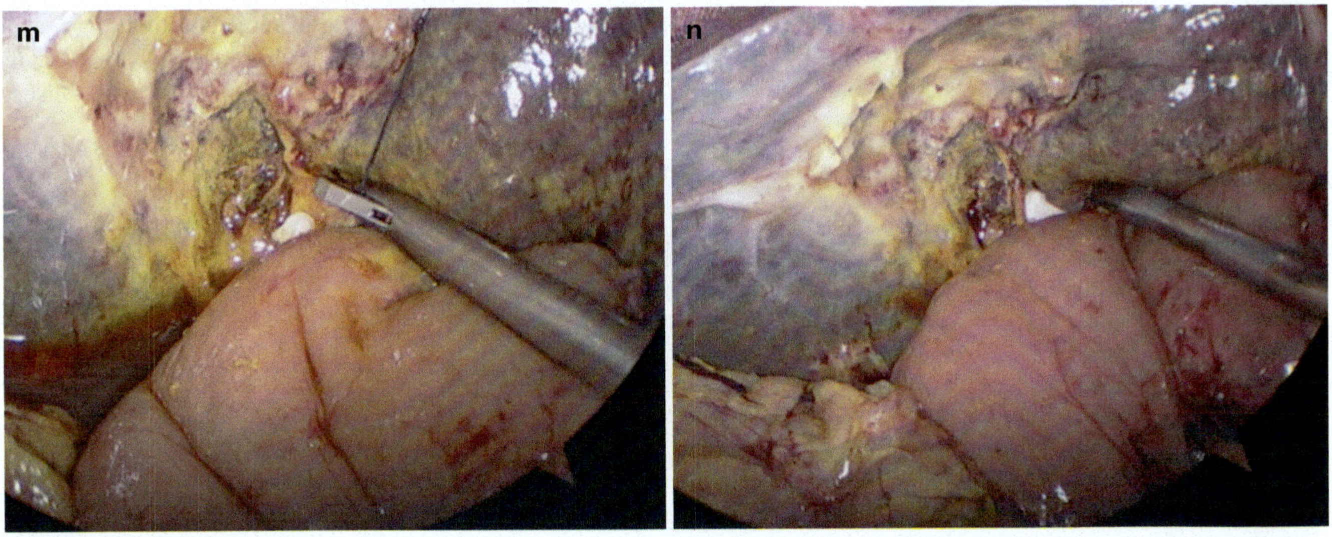

Fig. 5.28 (continued)

7. Jejunojejunostomy.
   The proximal afferent loop was sutured in a side-to-side/end-to-side manner to the ascending limb of jejunum (45 cm distal to the choledochojejunal anastomosis) extracorporeally. Once the jejunojejunostomy was completed, the intestine was sent into the abdominal cavity and pneumoperitoneum was then reestablished (Fig. 5.29a–c).

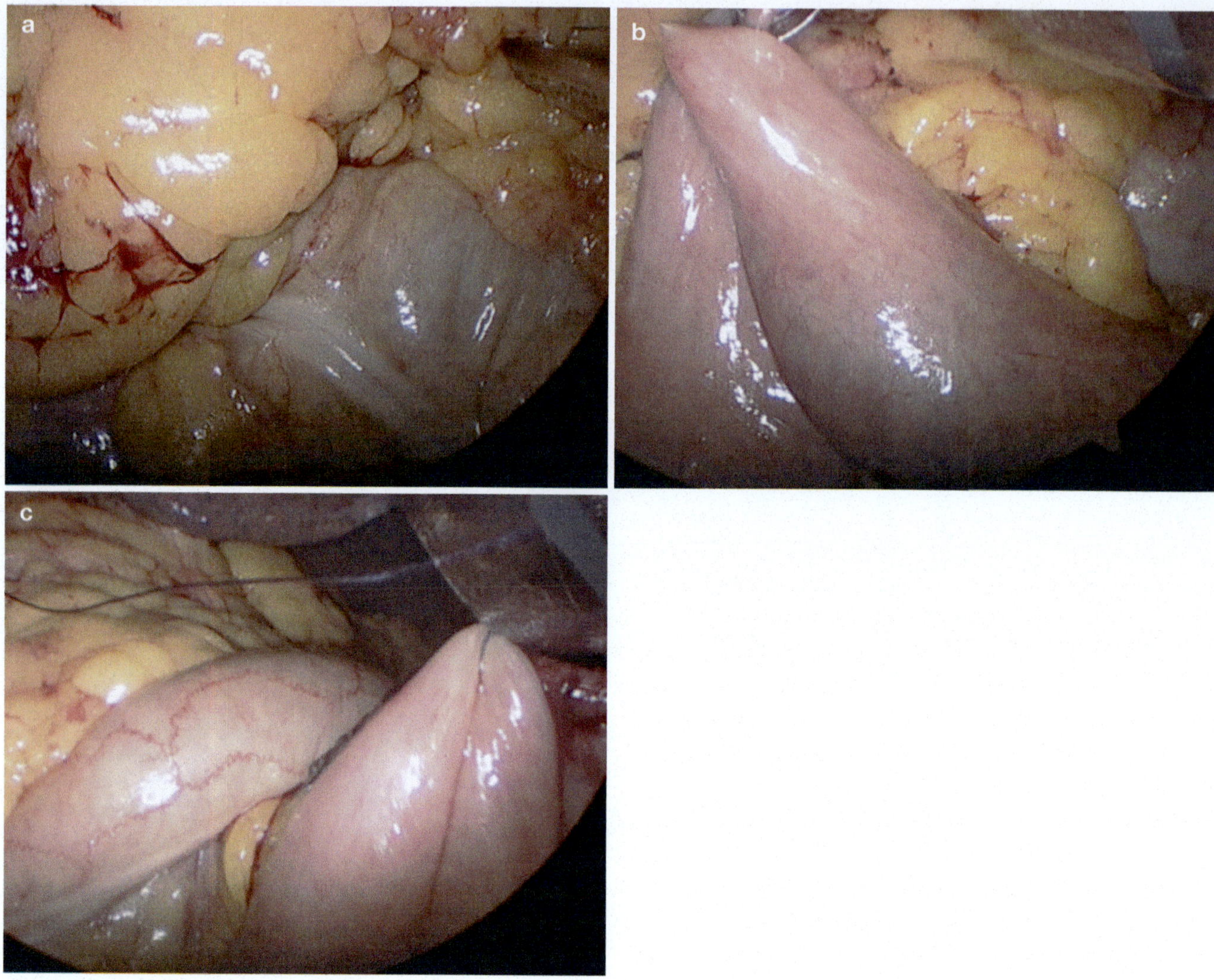

Fig. 5.29

8. Specimen retraction.
   The specimen bag was retracted through the umbilical incision (Fig. 5.30a, b).

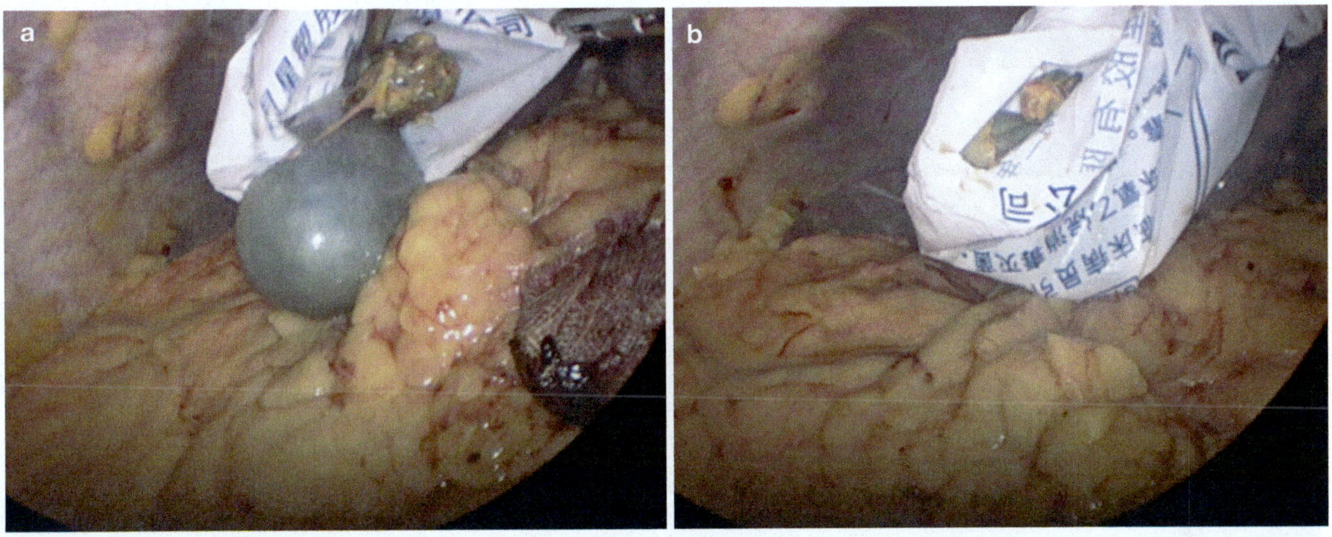

Fig. 5.30

9. Irrigation and drainage.
   After adequate flushing the surgical field, a sub-hepatic drain was placed close to the choledochojejunal anastomosis through the umbilicus (Fig. 5.31a–d).

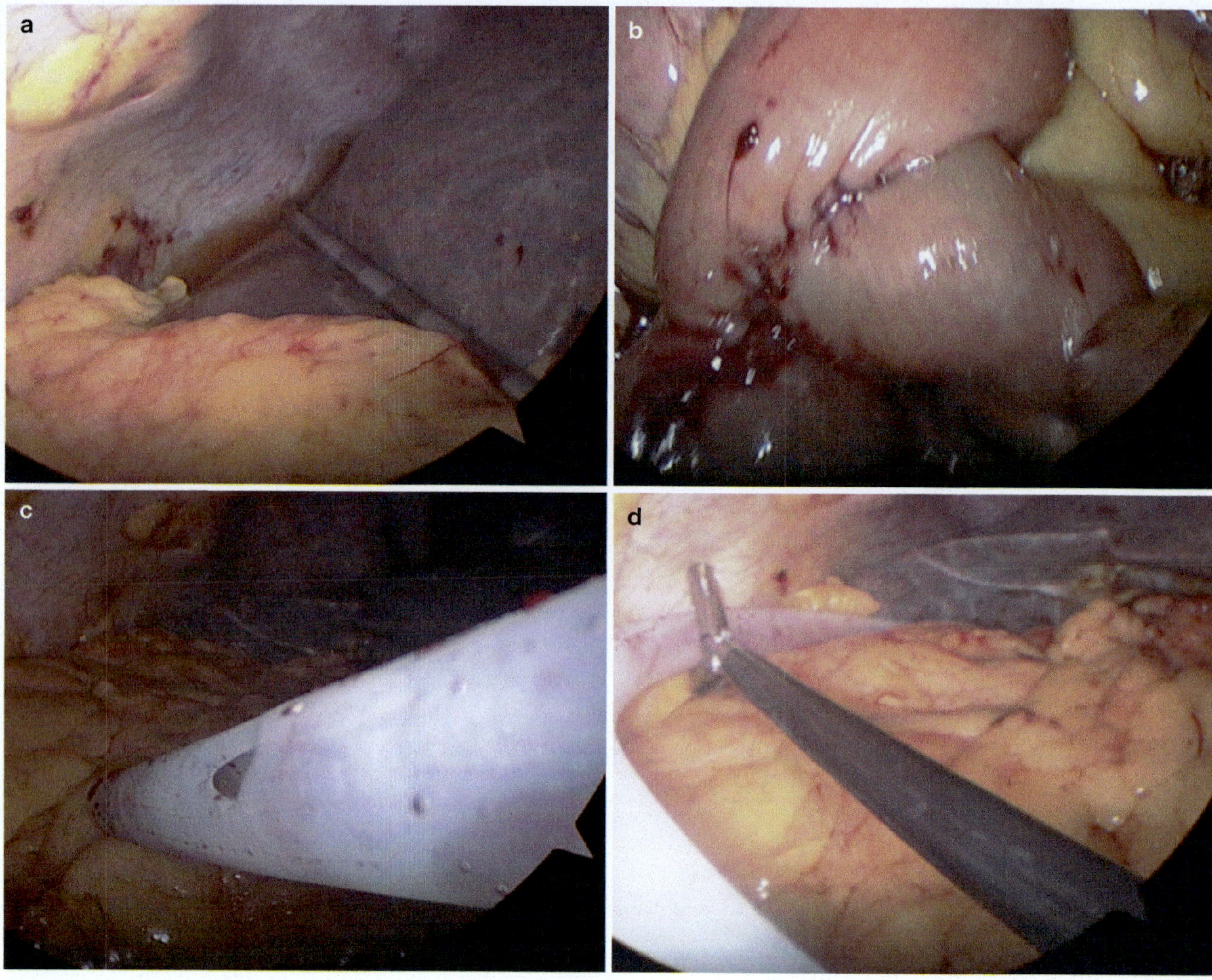

Fig. 5.31

5.5 Laparoscopic Choledochalcystectomy with Jejunal Roux-en-Y Reconstruction

5.5.1 Indications and Case Selection

1. Type I and II choledochalcyst.
2. Relapse of symptoms or complications after cyst internal drainage.
3. Highly suspicious of malignant change of cyst.

5.5.2 Contraindications

1. Any contraindications to open liver resection.
2. Patients who cannot tolerate pneumoperitoneum or general anesthesia.
3. Type III, IV and V choledochalcyst.

5.5.3 Major Instruments or Energy Sources

1. Laparoscopy System.
2. Holding forceps.
3. Harmonic scalpel.
4. Endoscopic linear stapler.

5.5.4 Team Setup, Anesthesia and Position

Under general anesthesia, the patient was placed in supine position with the legs apart. The position of surgeon, assistants and nurses is shown in Fig. 5.32.

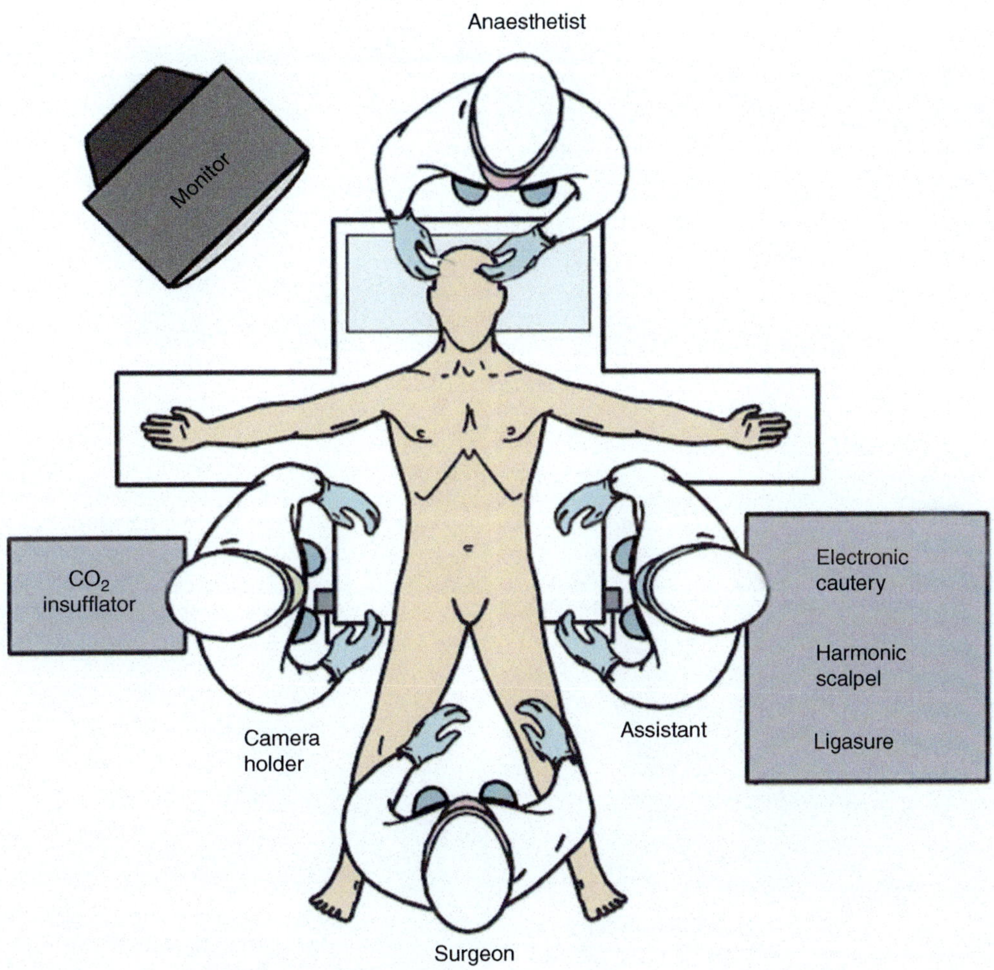

Fig. 5.32

5.5.5 Key Steps

1. Dissection of gallbladder.
2. Dissection of cyst.
3. Hepaticojejunostomy and jejunojejunostomy.

5.5.6 Surgical Techniques

1. Dissection of gallbladder.
   Dissection of gallbladder was performed as described in the cholecystectomy section (Fig. 5.33a–j).

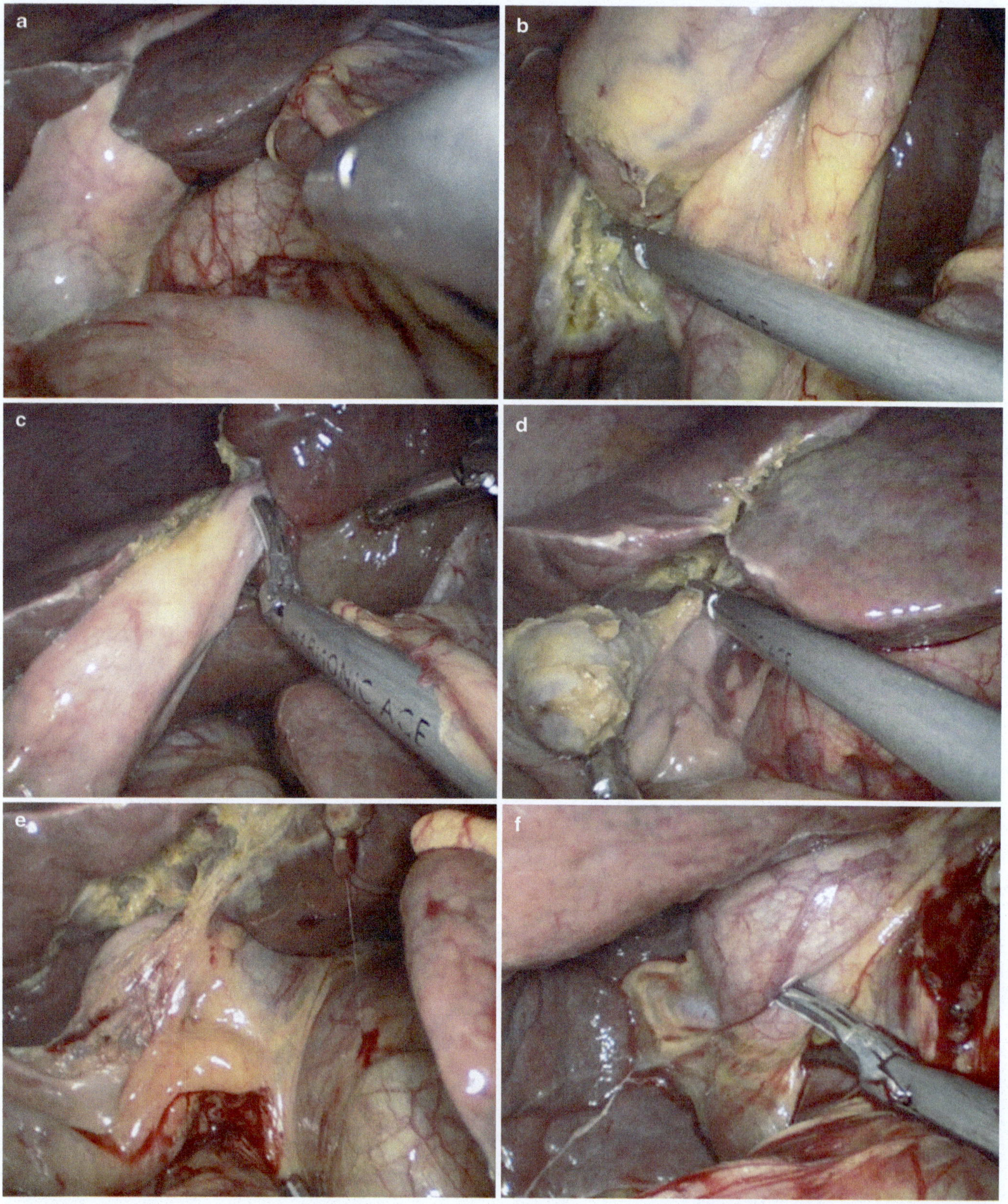

Fig. 5.33

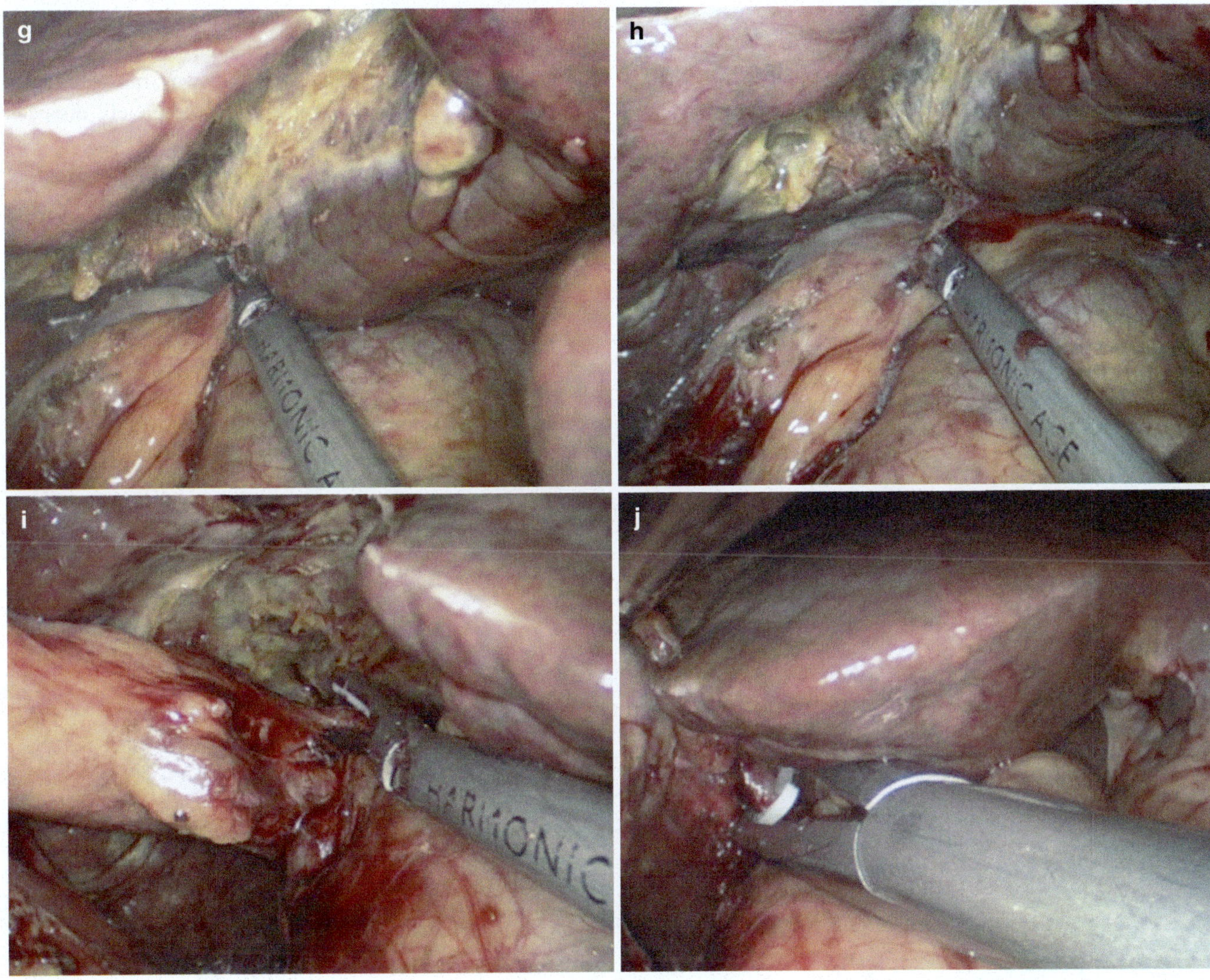

Fig. 5.33 (continued)

2. Dissection of cyst.
   Placement of stay suture below the xiphoid process was performed as described in the fourth section of this chapter. CBD was verified by a puncture in its anterior surface. After confirmation, the hepatic common bile (HCB) was transected, and then the distal portion of HCB was pulled downward. The dissection was extended along the cyst. After confirming the transitional area of choledochal cyst at the head of the pancreas, the CBD was transected distal to the cyst, and the cyst was then completely dissected (Fig. 5.34a–q).

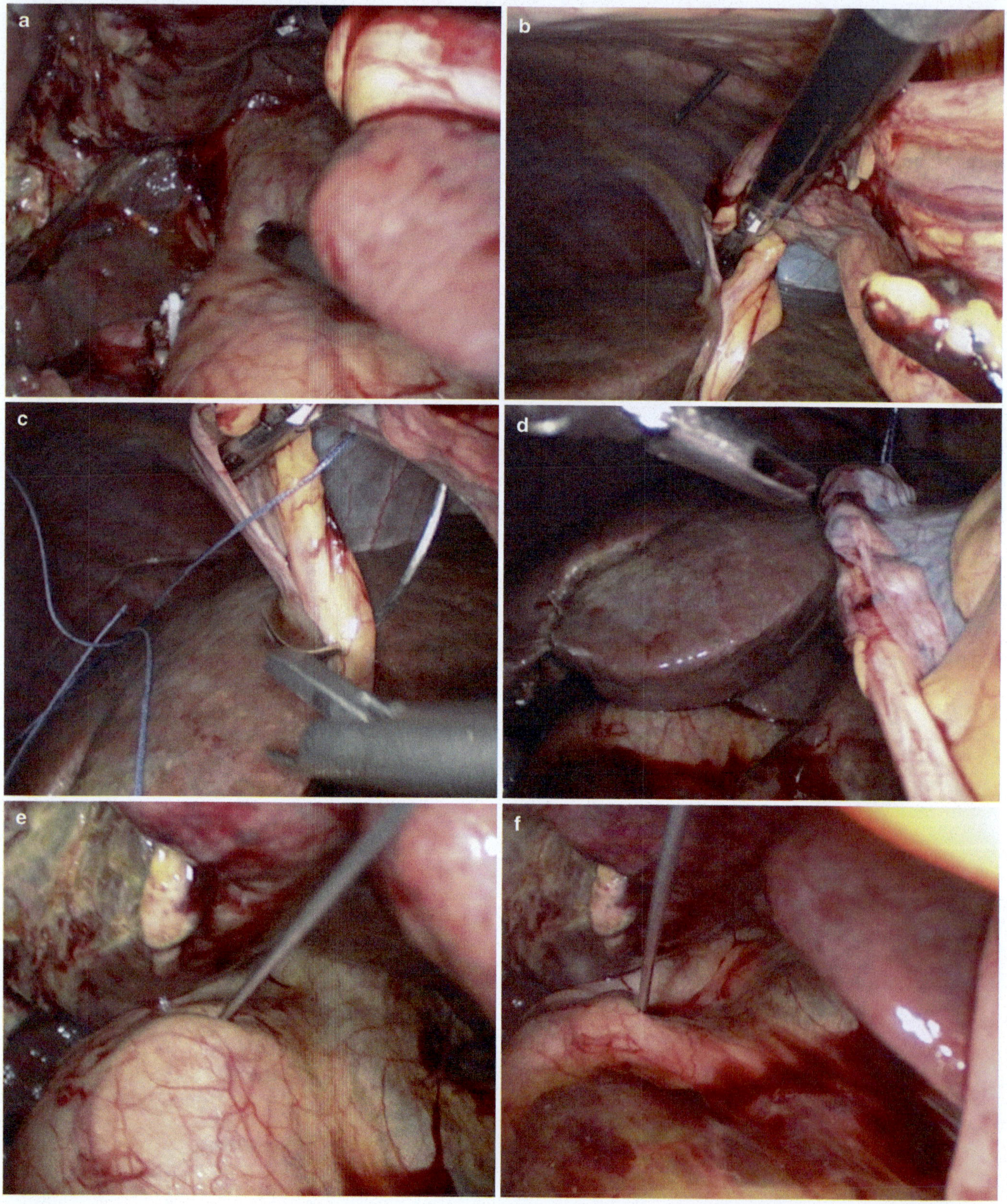

Fig. 5.34

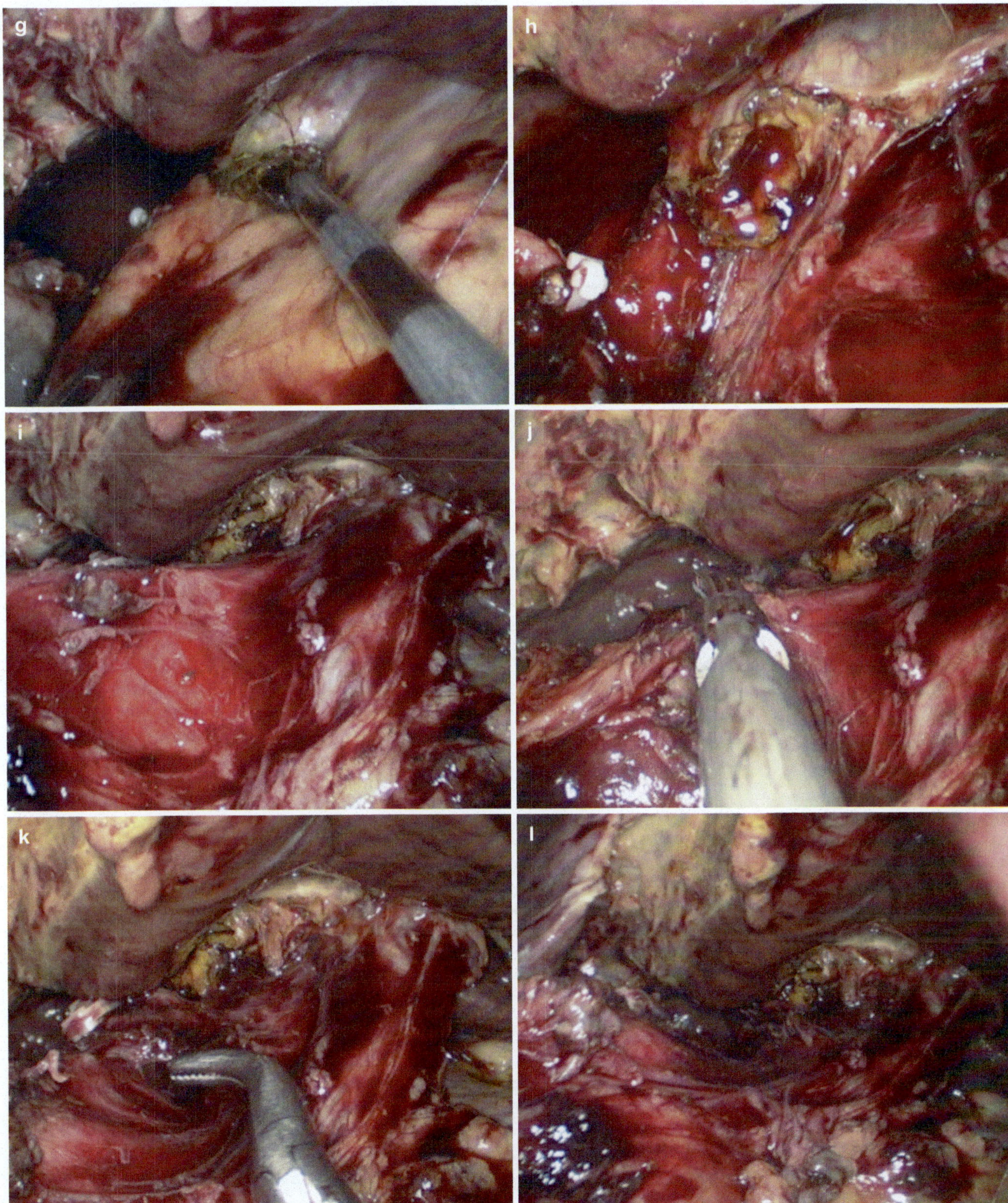

Fig. 5.34 (continued)

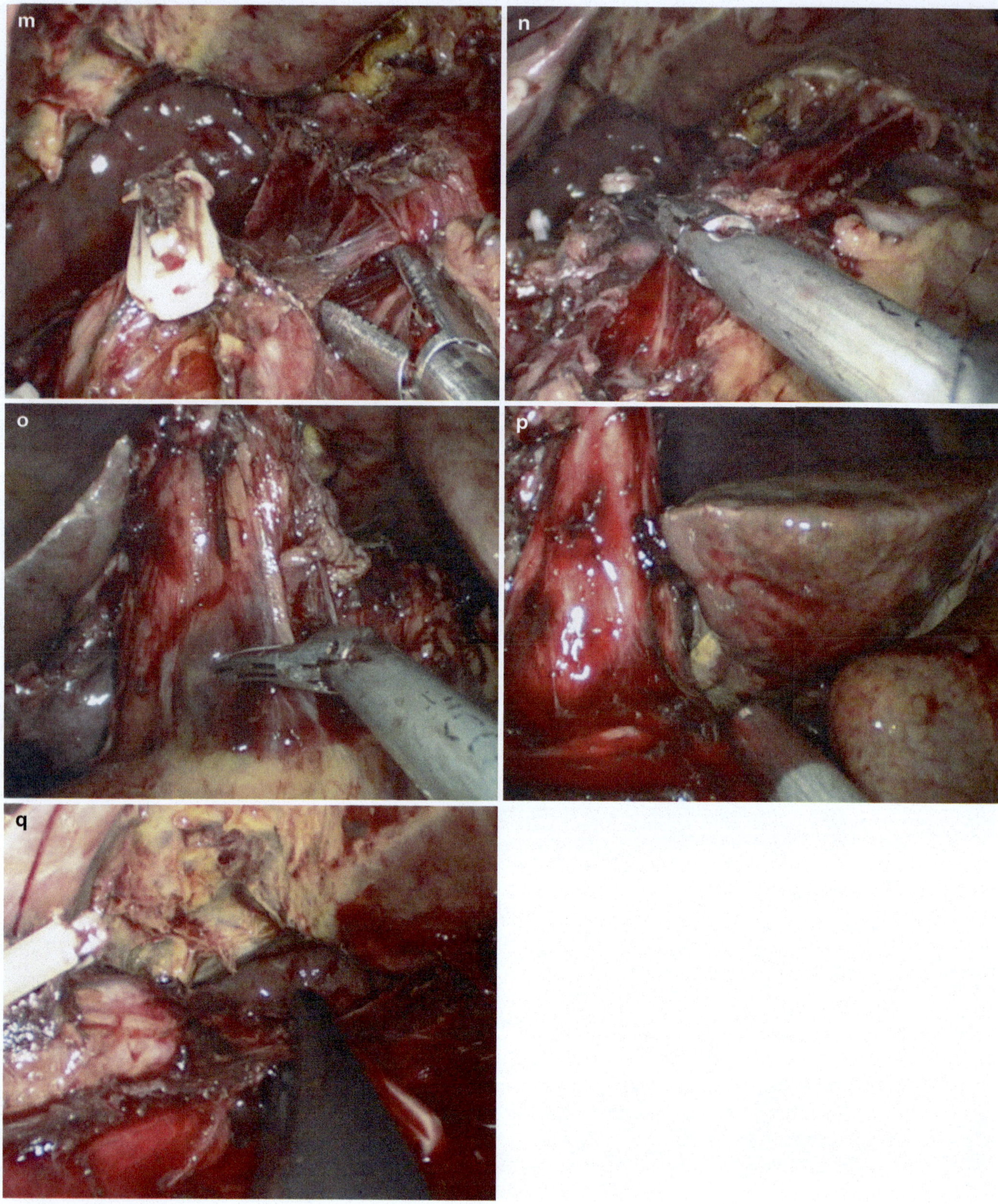

Fig. 5.34 (continued)

3. Hepaticojejunostomy and jejunojejunostomy.
   Hepaticojejunostomy and jejunojejunostomy (Roux-en-Y reconstruction) was performed as described in the fourth section of this chapter (Fig. 5.35a–h).

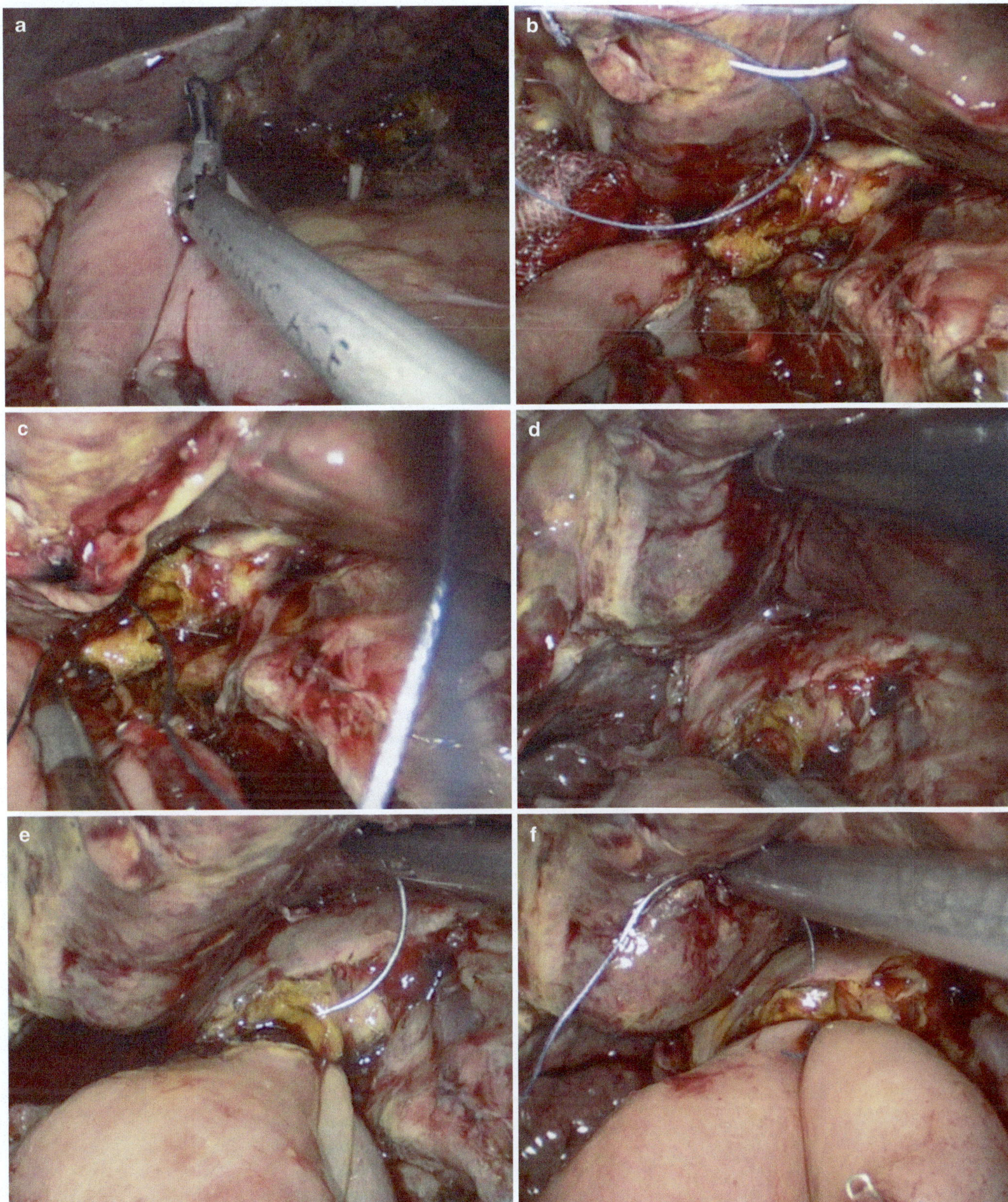

Fig. 5.35

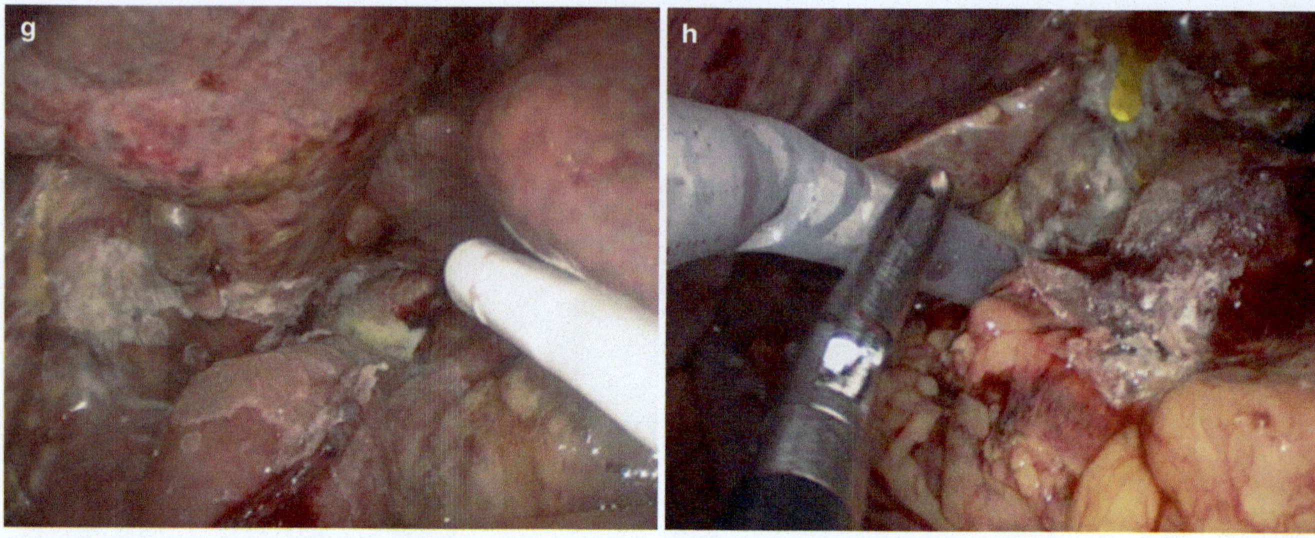

Fig. 5.35 (continued)

5.6 Laparoscopic Cholecystojejunostomy with Interposition of the Ileum

5.6.1 Indications and Case Selection

1. Obstruction in the inferior segment of common bile duct, e.g. radical resection is improper for carcinoma of head of pancreas in later period.
2. Staging operation for carcinoma of head of pancreas.
3. Malignant obstruction in the inferior segment of common bile duct, in which document dilated cystic duct is identified.

5.6.2 Contraindications

1. Patients with obstruction in cystic duct due to malignant change in later period.
2. Patients with low insertion of cystic duct into the common hepatic duct, which is easily obstructed by tumor.
3. Patients with cholangiocarcinoma in the middle or superior segment.
4. Patients with gallbladder stone or common bile duct stone.

5.6.3 Major Instruments or Energy Sources

1. Laparoscopy System.
2. Holding forceps.
3. Harmonic scalpel.
4. Endoscopic linear stapler.

5.6.4 Team Setup, Anesthesia and Position

It is the same as Sect. 5.5.4.

5.6.5 Key Steps

1. Exploration of lesion.
2. Dissection of terminal ileum.
3. Creation of an ileal segment with its mesentery pedicle.
4. Anastomosis between gallbladder and ileal segment.
5. Jejuno-ileostomy.

5.6.6 Surgical Techniques

1. Exploration of lesion.
   Exploration was performed as described in section three (Fig. 5.36).

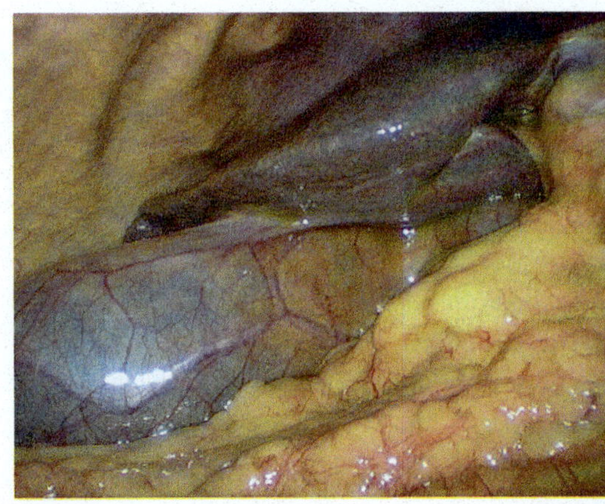

Fig. 5.36

2. Dissection of terminal ileum.
   A segment of ileum was divided between 15 and 60 cm from the ileocecal junction (Fig. 5.37a–d).

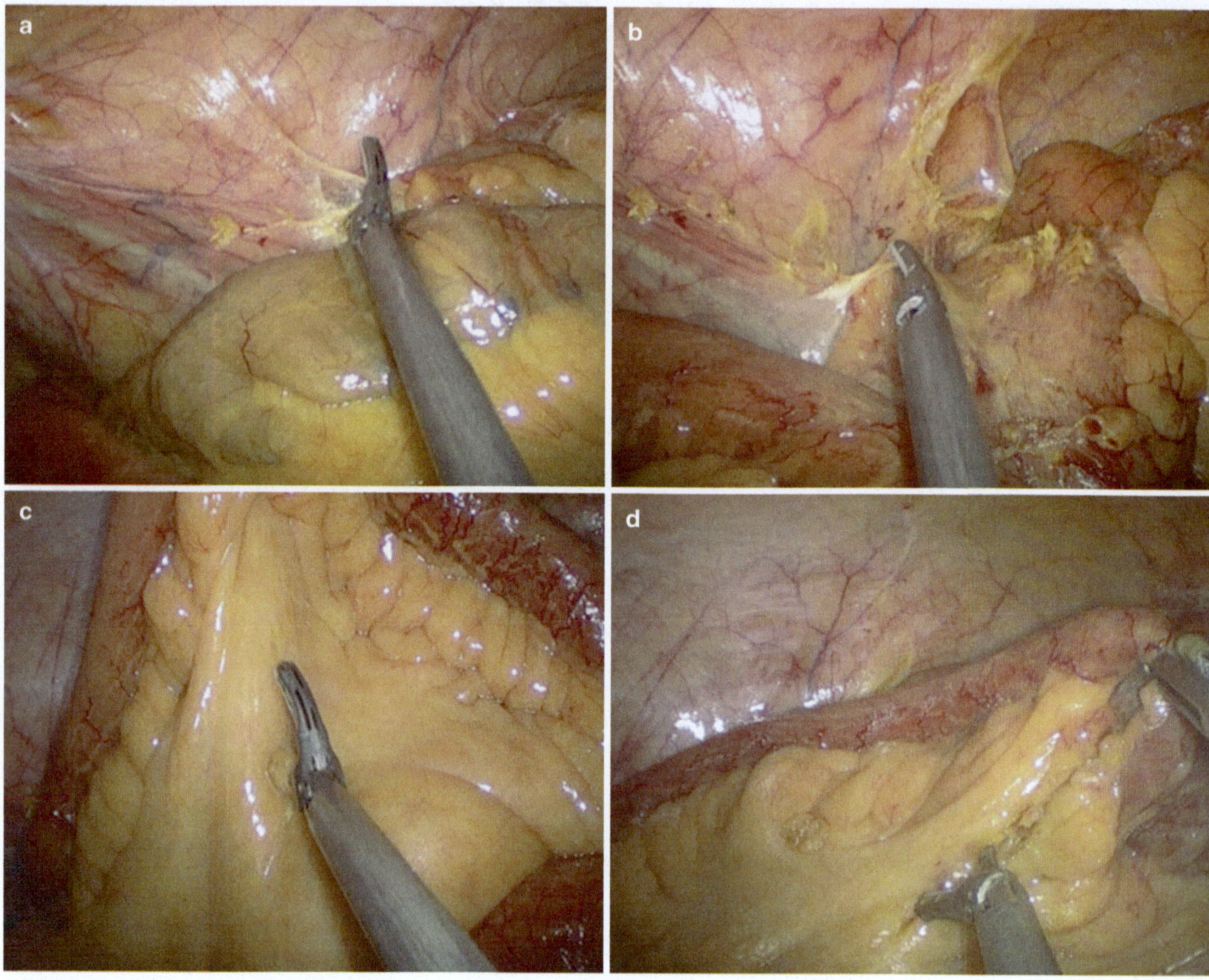

Fig. 5.37

3. Creation of an ileal segment with its mesentery pedicle. A distal ileal segment of 45 cm was transected along with its mesentery pedicle by using Endo-GIA (Fig. 5.38a–n).

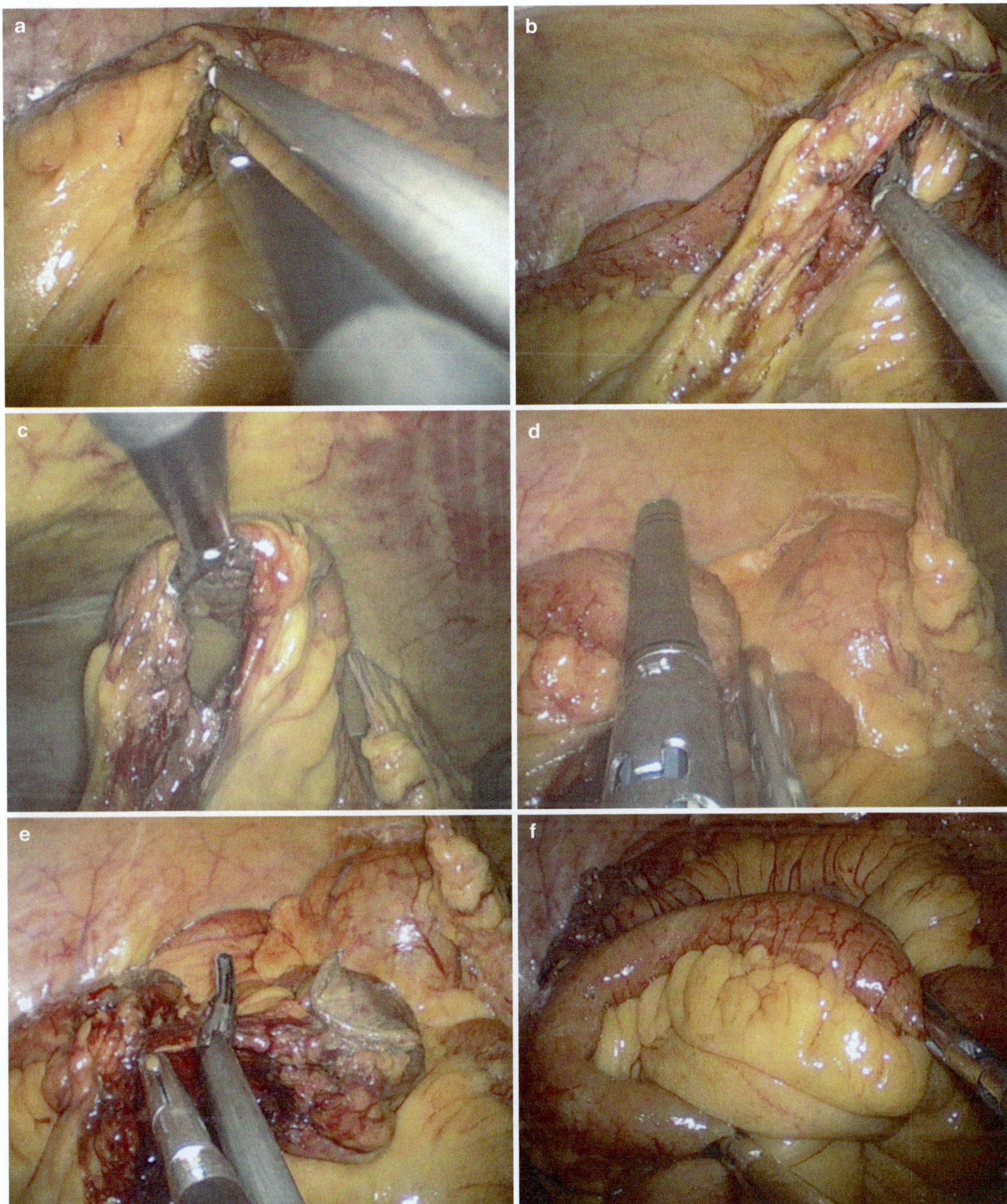

Fig. 5.38

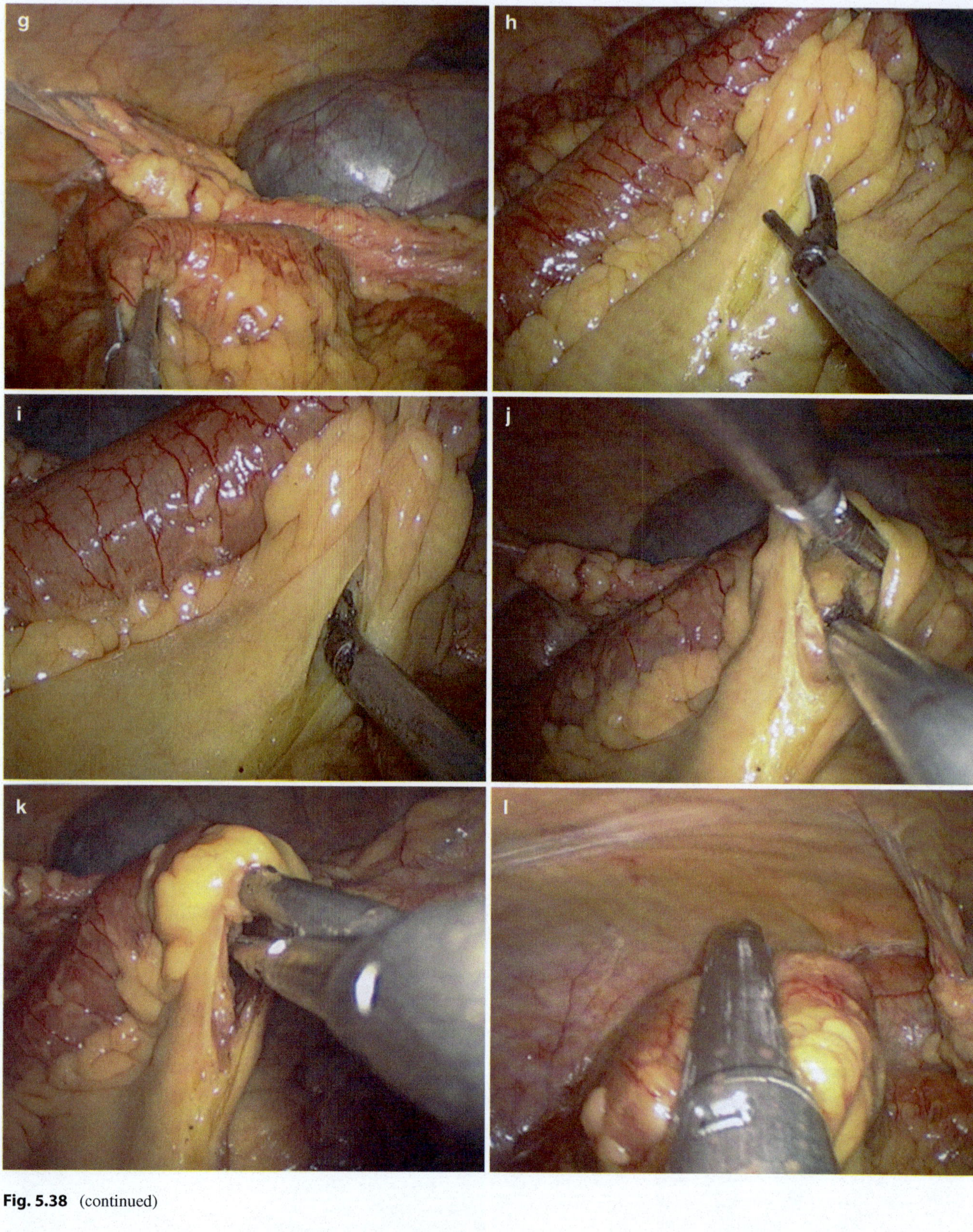

Fig. 5.38 (continued)

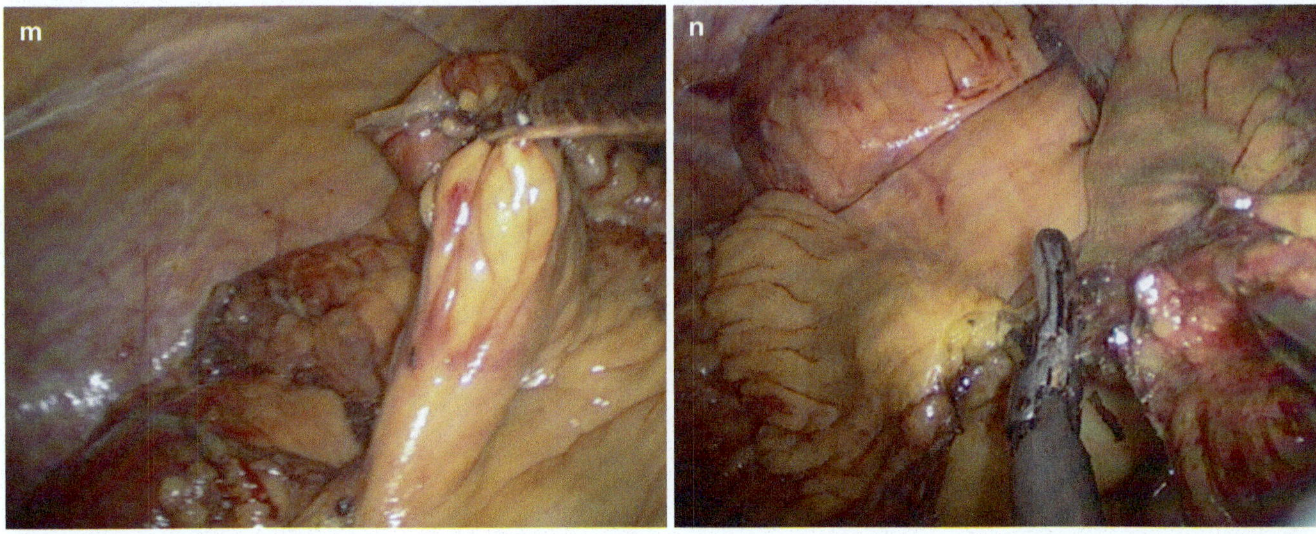

Fig. 5.38 (continued)

4. Anastomosis between gallbladder and ileal segment.
   The ileal segment was pulled upward and side-to-side anastomosis between the gallbladder and proximal ileal segment was performed as described in the cholecystojejunostomy section (Fig. 5.39a–u).

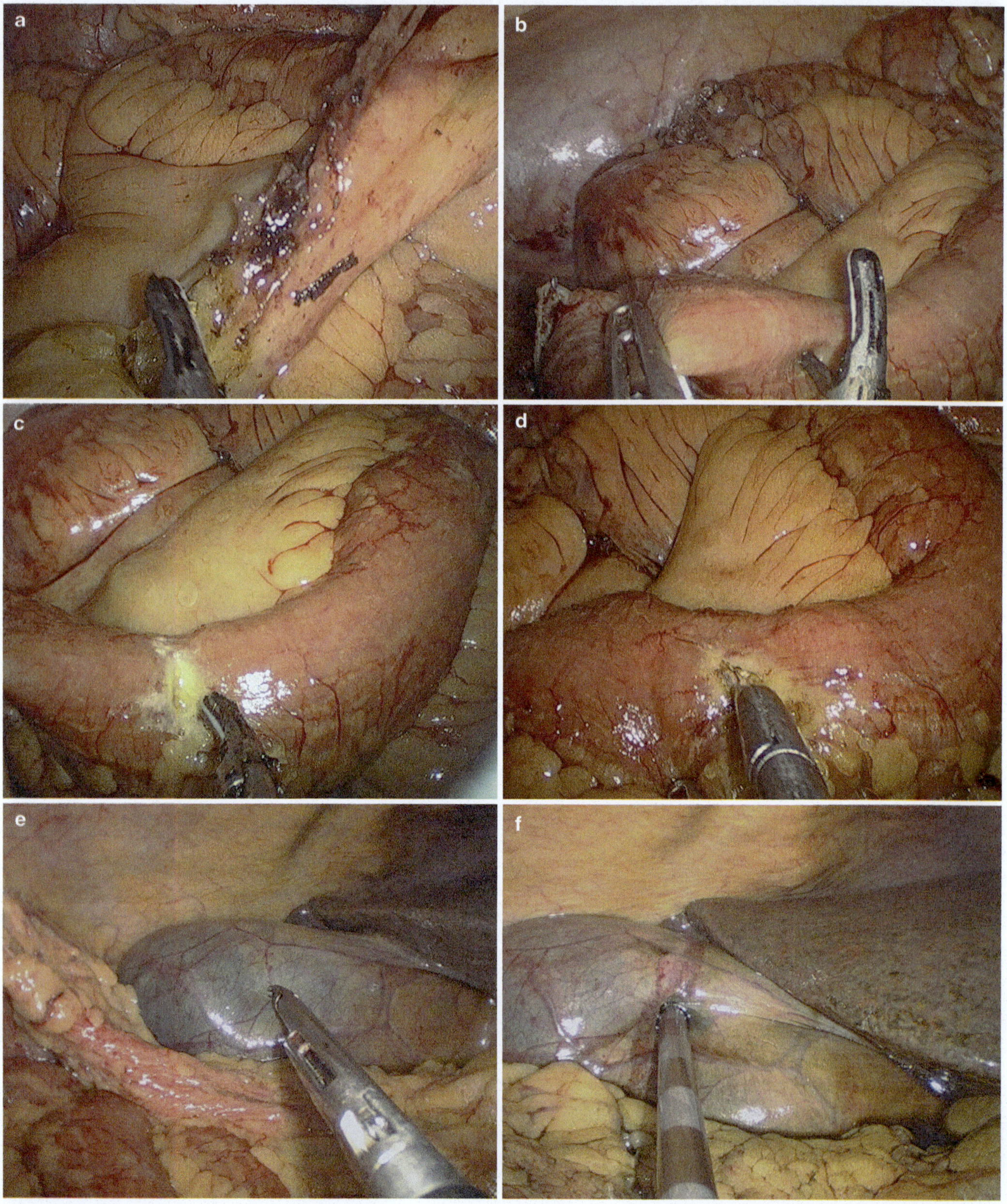

Fig. 5.39

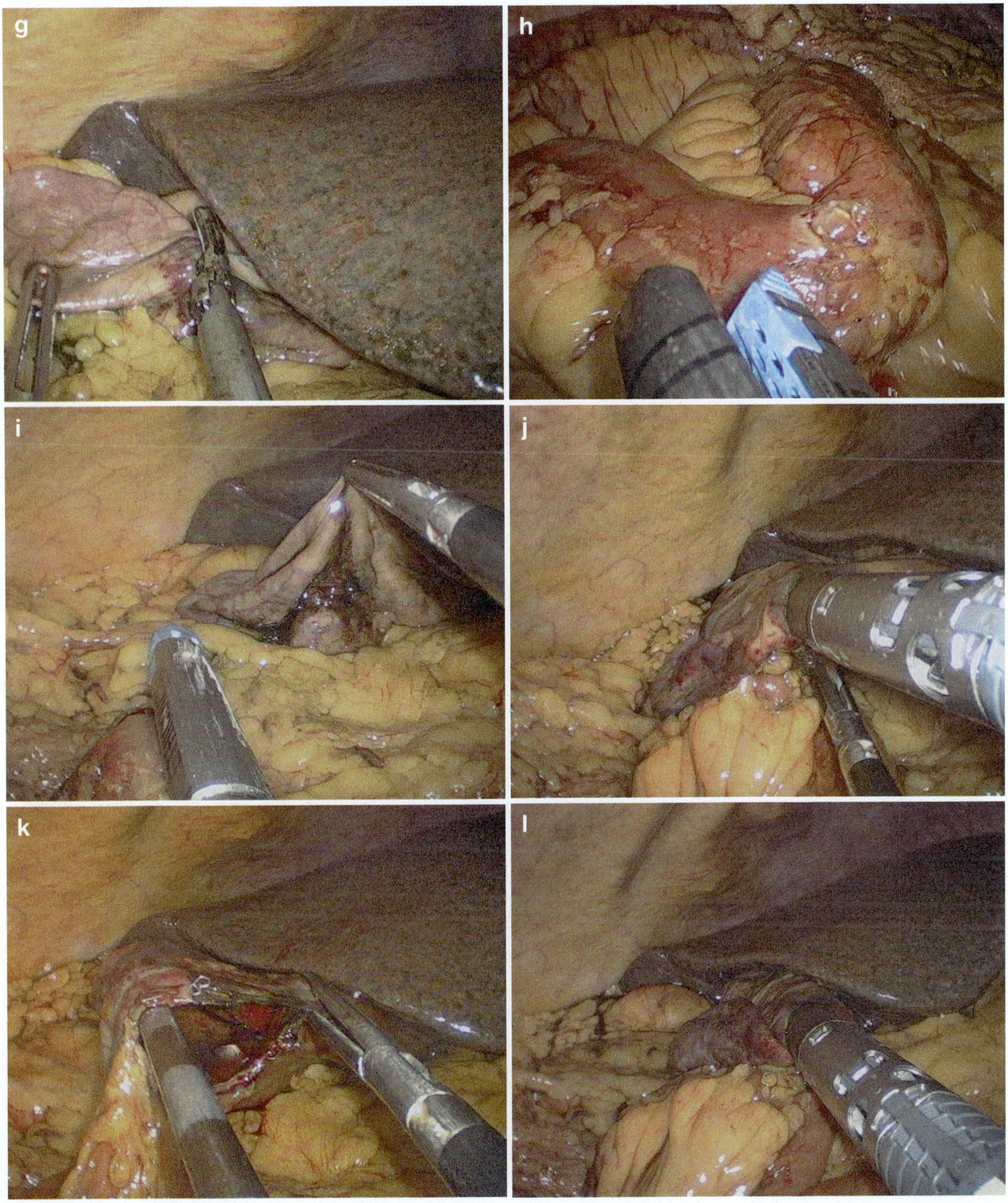

Fig. 5.39 (continued)

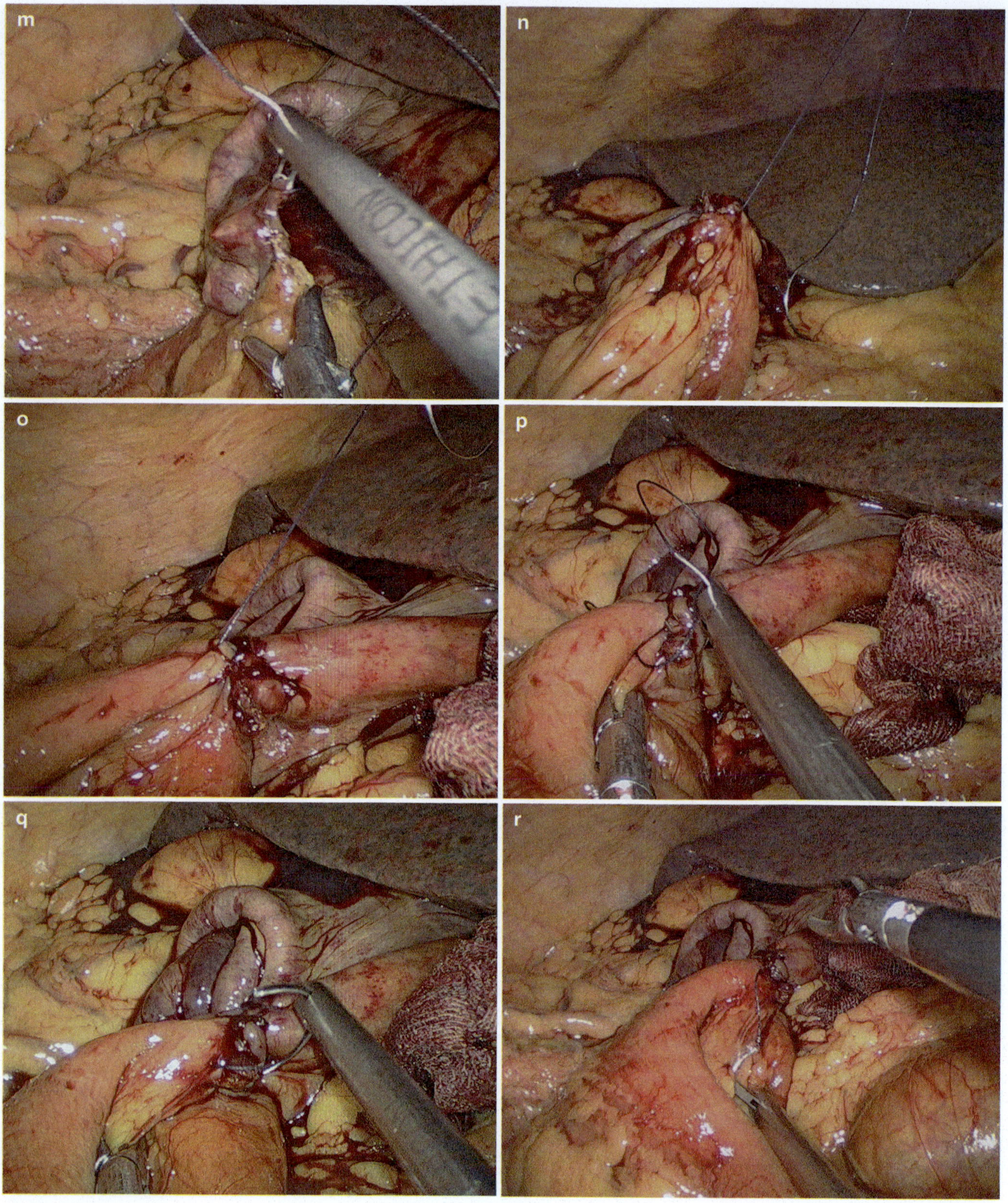

Fig. 5.39 (continued)

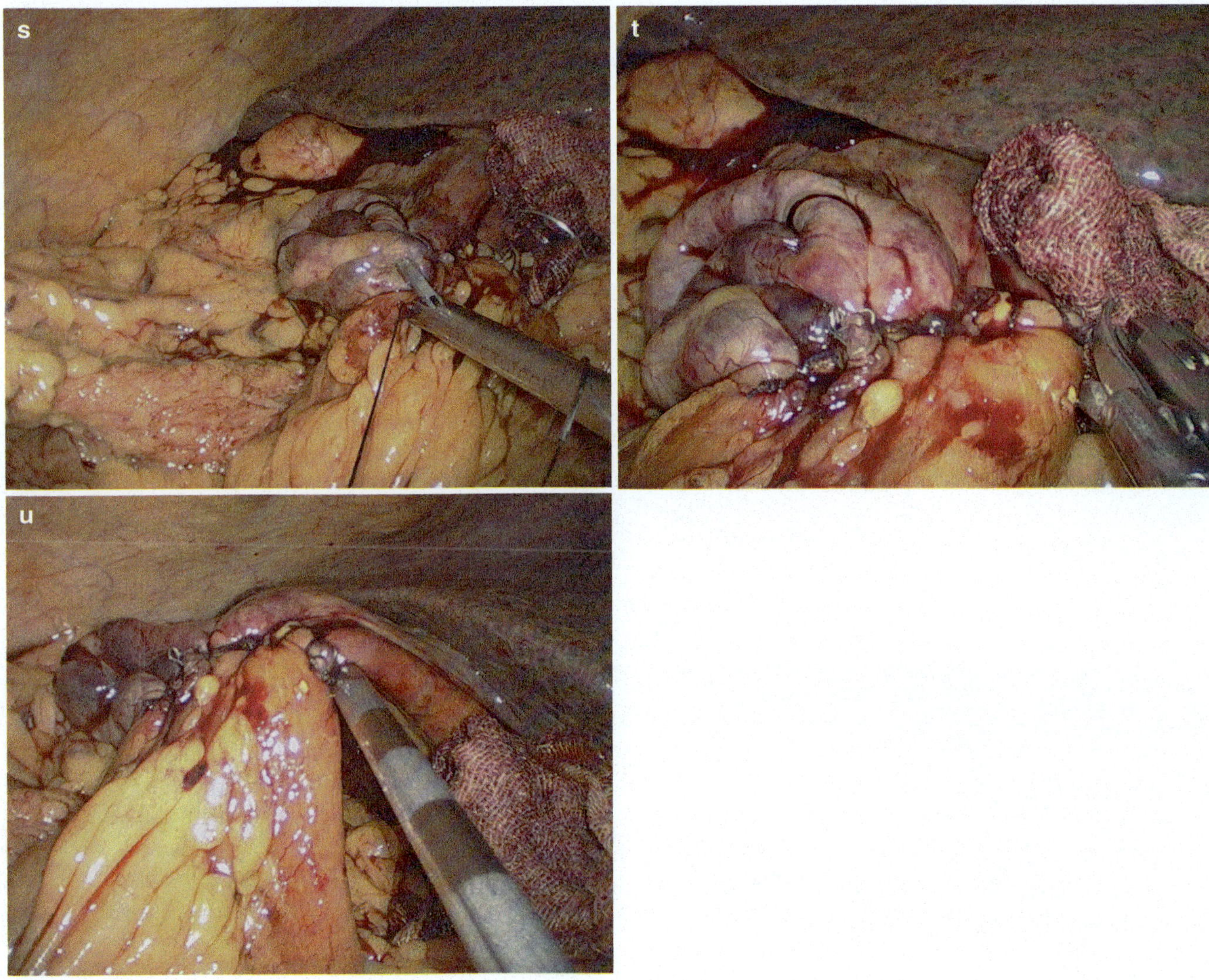

Fig. 5.39 (continued)

5. Jejuno-ileostomy.
The distal end of transected ileal segment was interposed and anastomosed to the upper jejunal loop (15 cm from the ligament of Treitz) in a side-to-side way as described in the cholecystojejunostomy section. Continuity of small bowel was restored extracorporally by end-to-end ileo-ileal anastomosis (Fig. 5.40a–f).

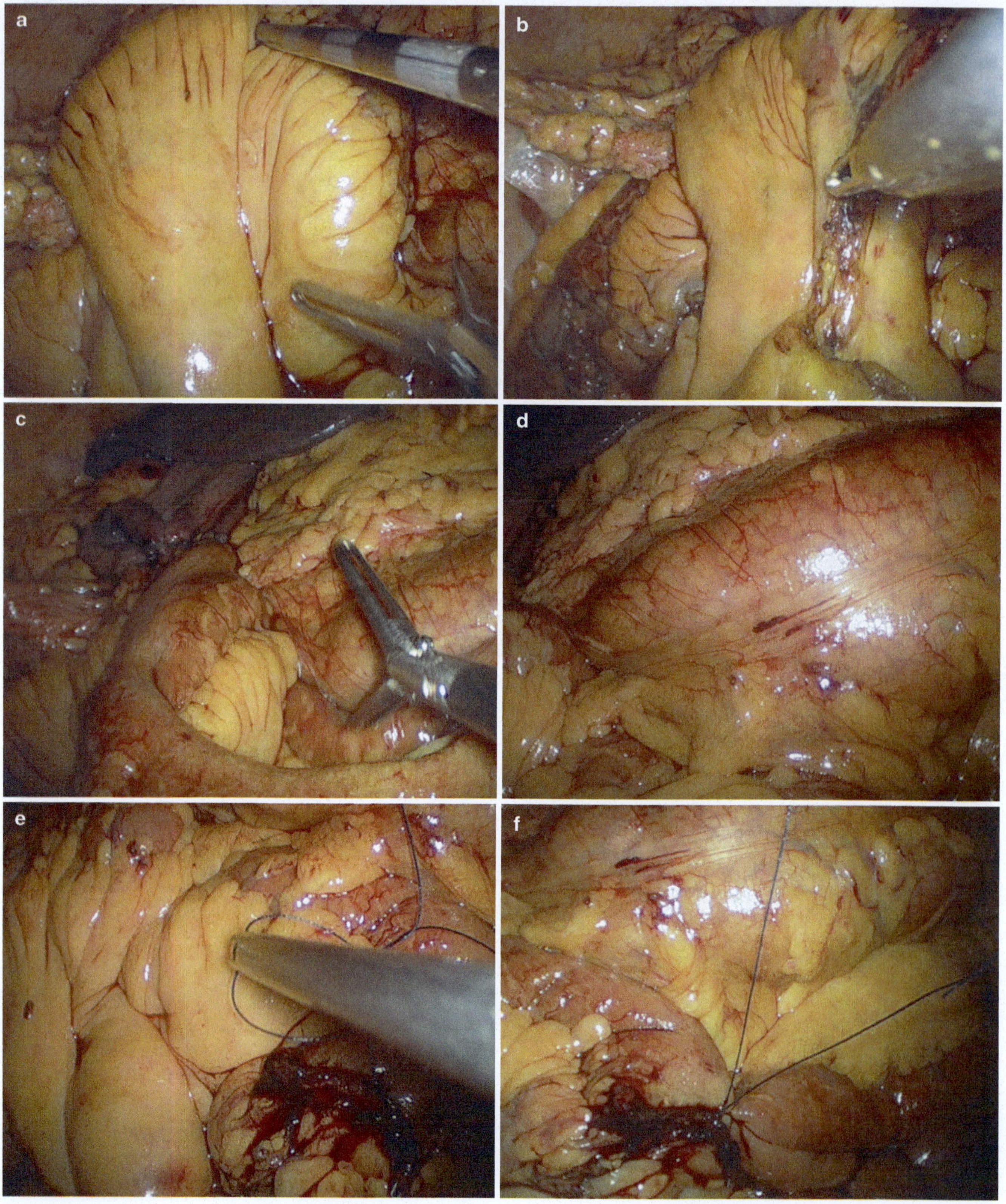

Fig. 5.40

5.7 Laparoscopic Liver Cyst Fenestration

5.7.1 Indications and Case Selection

1. Patients with symptomatic single cyst with the diameter larger than 5 cm, which is located in the liver superficially.
2. Patients with a limited number of large and superficial cysts that can be individually treated as single cysts to establish a large communication between the cyst and the peritoneal cavity.
3. Patients with cysts treated by alcohol and other non-operative procedures ineffectively.

5.7.2 Contraindications

1. Inability to tolerate general anesthesia or pneumoperitoneum.
2. Refractory coagulopathy
3. Cysts located deep in the liver, which are difficult to manage operatively.
4. There are communications between the cysts and intrahepatic ducts.
5. Cysts complicated with hemorrhage and infection.

5.7.3 Major Instruments or Energy Sources

1. Laparoscopy System.
2. Holding forceps.
3. Harmonic scalpel.

5.7.4 Team Setup, Anesthesia and Position

Under general anesthesia, the patient was placed in supine position with the arms adducted along the side. The position of surgeon, assistants and nurses is shown in Fig. 5.41.

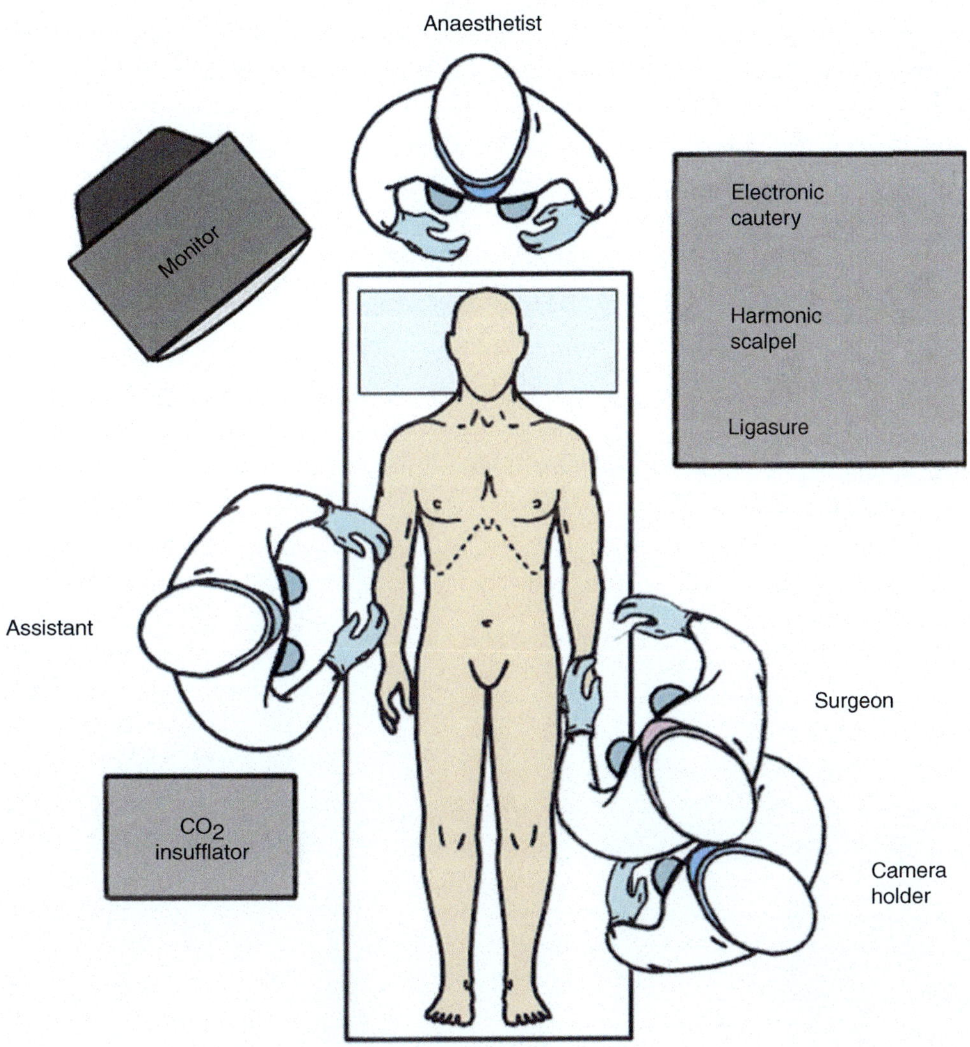

Fig. 5.41

5.7.5 Key Steps

1. Exploration of lesion and identification and aspiration of the cyst.
2. Fenestration of the cyst.
3. Irrigation and check of the abdominal cavity.
4. Drainage and closure of the incision.

5.7.6 Surgical Techniques

1. Exploration of lesion and identification and aspiration of the cyst.
   After a brief exploration of the abdomen, the main cyst was punctured. Aspiration was performed to make a definite judgment about the cyst liquid (Fig. 5.42a, b).

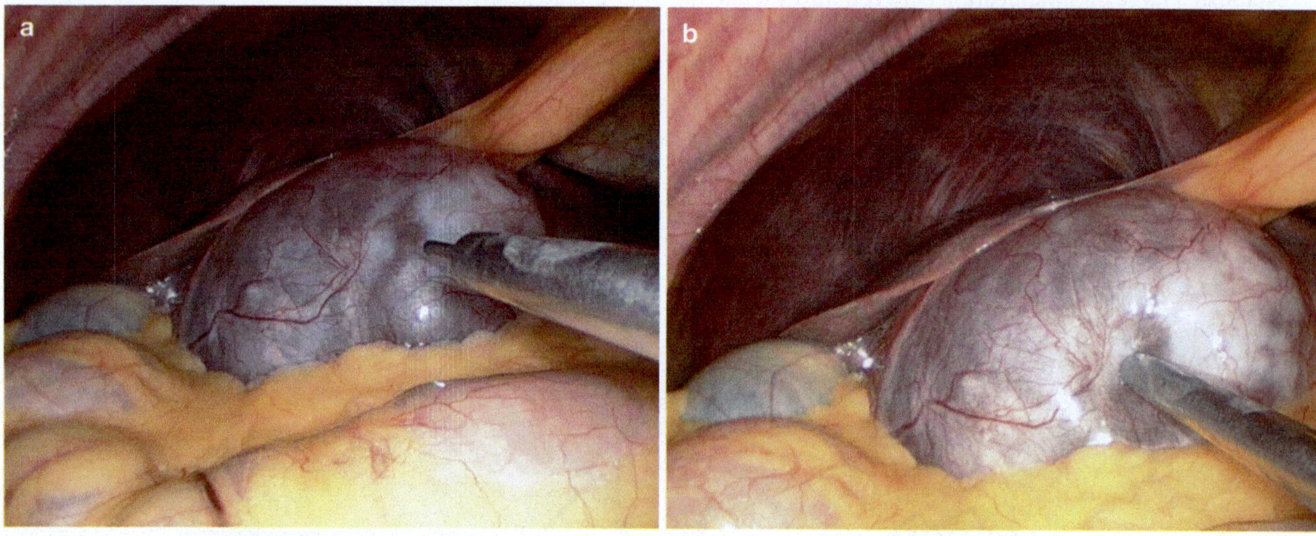

Fig. 5.42

2. Fenestration of the cyst.
   A suction drain was placed close to the opening and the main part of the liquid was suctioned out of the abdomen. The decompressed cyst was entered and resected with and ultrasonic dissector (Fig. 5.43a–h).

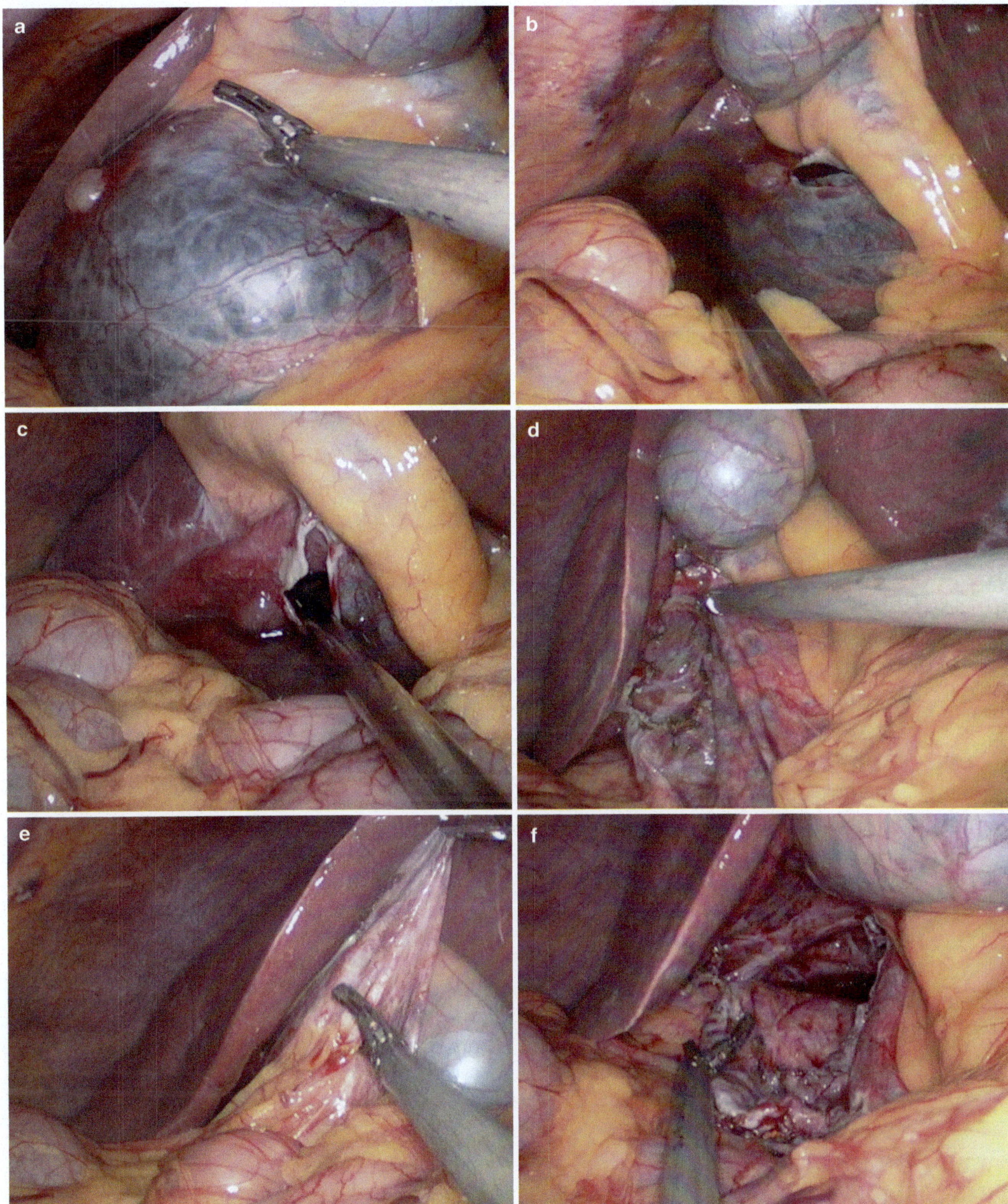

Fig. 5.43

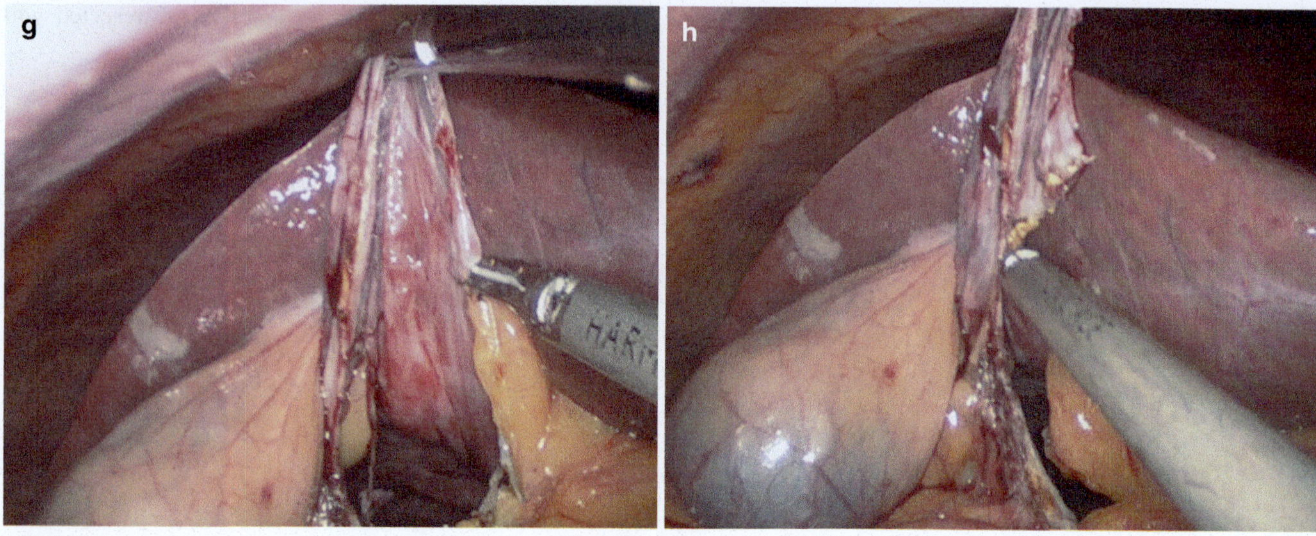

Fig. 5.43 (continued)

3. Irrigation and check of the abdominal cavity.
   A careful control of the internal part of the cyst must be performed in case of bile leakage or hemorrhage. After adequate flushing the surgical field, a drain could be placed if necessary (Fig. 5.44a, b).

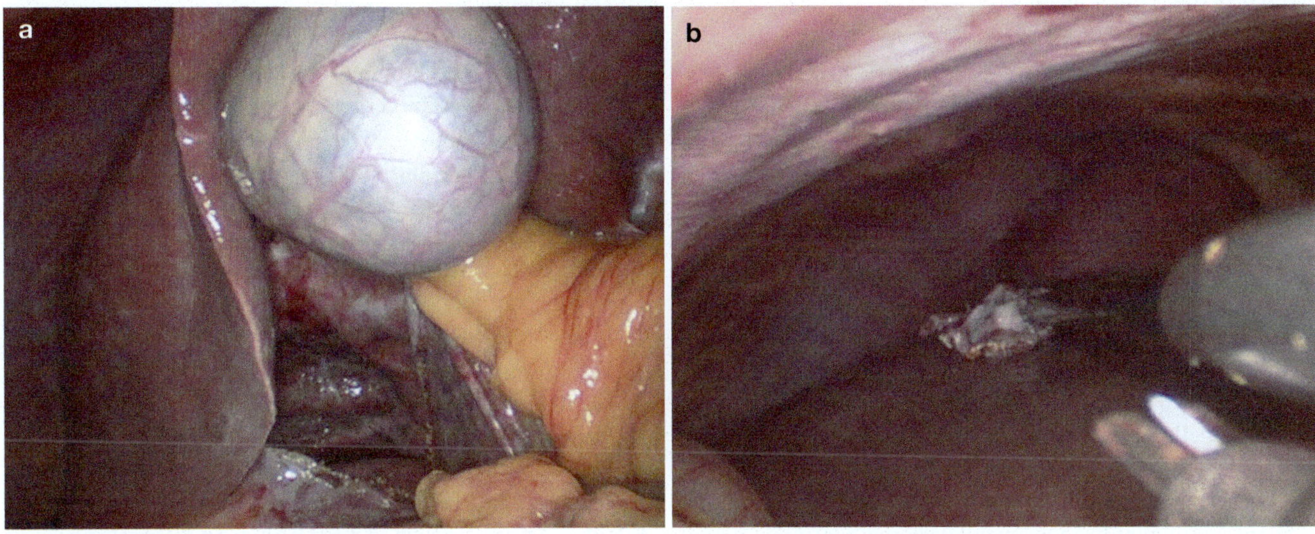

Fig. 5.44

5.7.7 Tips and Tricks

Using the harmonic scalpel (harmonic ACE 5 mm, Ethicon Endo-Surgery, Somerville), a liver cyst fenestration was carried out in the typical manner.

5.8 Laparoscopic Partial Hepatectomy

5.8.1 Indications and Case Selection

1. Benign liver lesions.
2. Symptomatic hemangioma.
3. Symptomatic focal nodular hyperplasia.
4. Adenoma.
5. Symptomatic giant hepatic cyst.
6. Malignant liver lesions.
7. Hepatocellular carcinoma.
8. Colorectal carcinoma metastasis.
9. Others, including liver donor hepatectomy for liver transplant, malignant lesions, or indeterminate lesions (cannot rule out cancer).

5.8.2 Contraindications

1. Any contraindications to open liver resection.
2. Patients who cannot tolerate pneumoperitoneum or general anesthesia.
3. Dense adhesions that cannot be lysed laparoscopically.
4. Lesions too close to major vasculature.
5. Lesions too large to be safely manipulated laparoscopically.
6. Resection that requires extensive portal lymphadenectomy.

5.8.3 Major Instruments or Energy Sources

1. Laparoscopy System.
2. Holding forceps.
3. Harmonic scalpel.
4. Endoscopic Linear Stapler.

5.8.4 Team Setup, Anesthesia and Position

Under general anesthesia, the patient was placed in supine position with the arms adducted along the side. The position of surgeon, assistants and nurses is shown in Fig. 5.45.

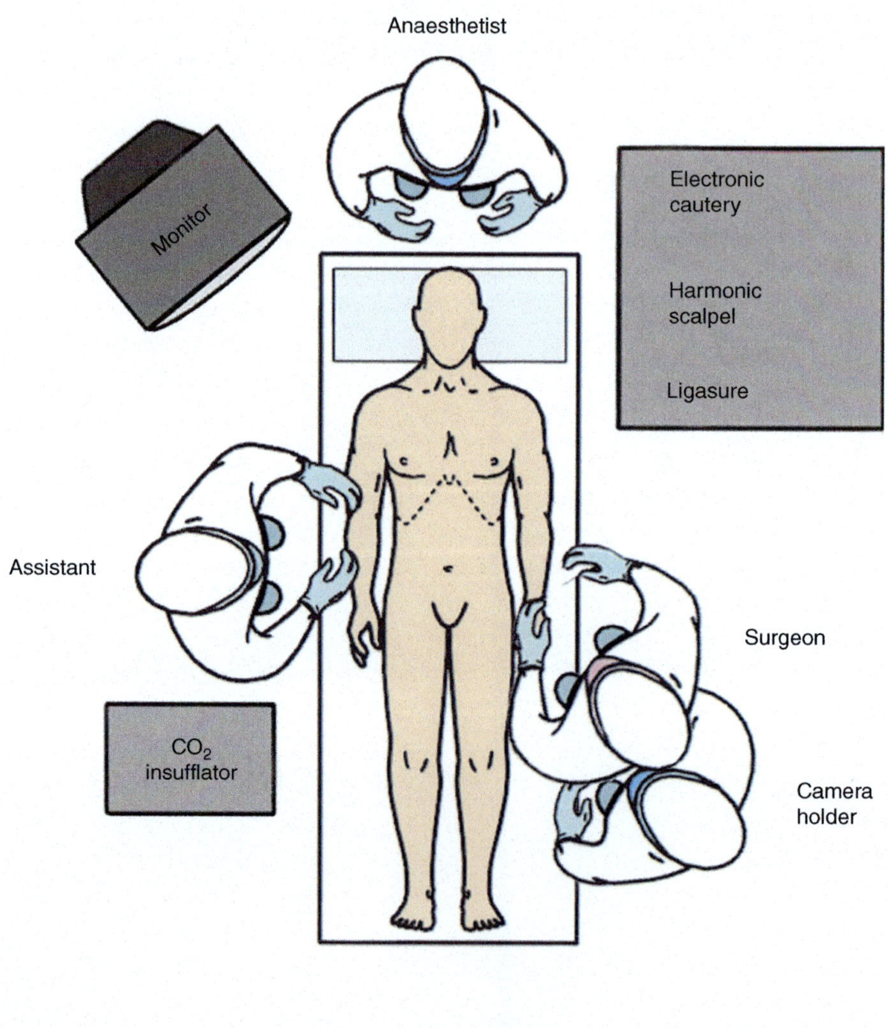

Fig. 5.45

5.8.5 Key Steps

1. Exploration of abdominal cavity and identification of the lesion.
2. Dissection of hepatic ligament.
3. Resection of liver tissue.
4. Retrieval of the specimen.
5. Irrigation and drainage.

5.8.6 Surgical Techniques

1. Exploration of abdominal cavity and identification of the lesion.
   The mass involving the left hepatic lobe was identified and exploration of the peritoneal cavity was performed to rule out the possibility of an extrahepatic cause (Fig. 5.46a–d).

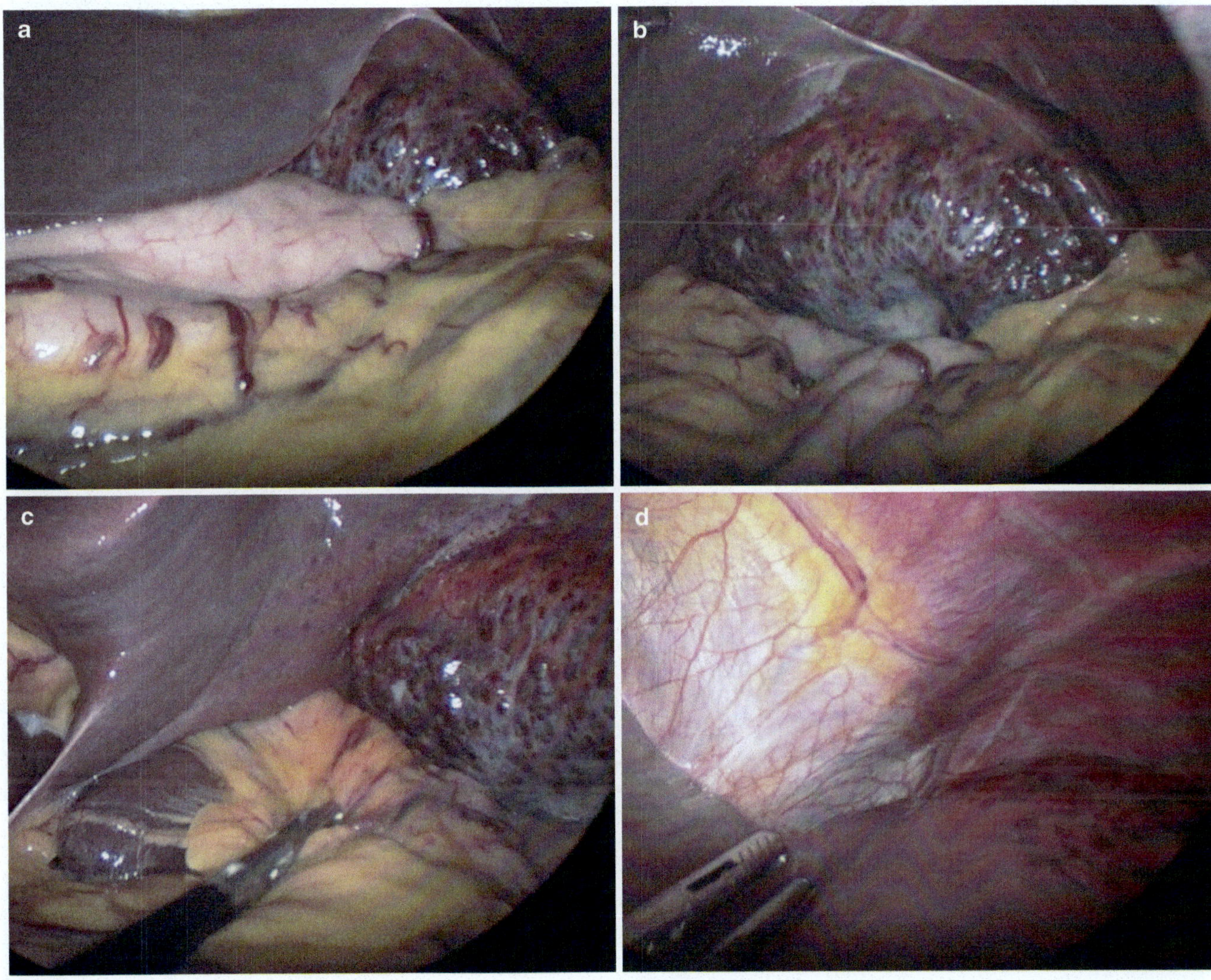

Fig. 5.46

2. Dissection of hepatic ligament.
   The patient was positioned in a reverse Trendelenburg position. The left triangular ligament was divided by means of ultrasonic scalpel in order to expose the left lobe (Fig. 5.47a–f).

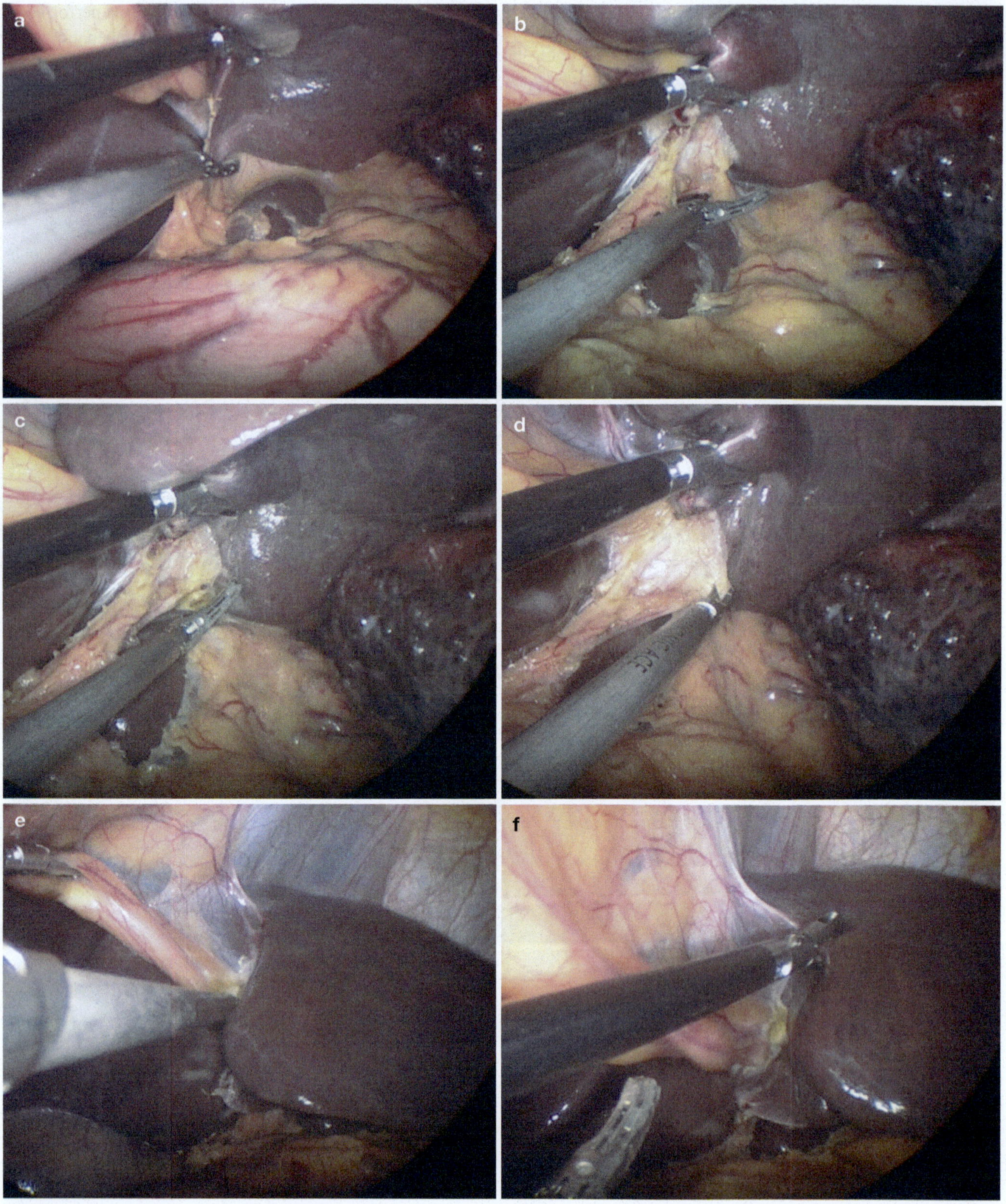

Fig. 5.47

3. Resection of liver tissue.
   The liver parenchymal transection line was marked with cautery hook. Liver transection was performed using ultrasonic scalpel (Fig. 5.48a–f).

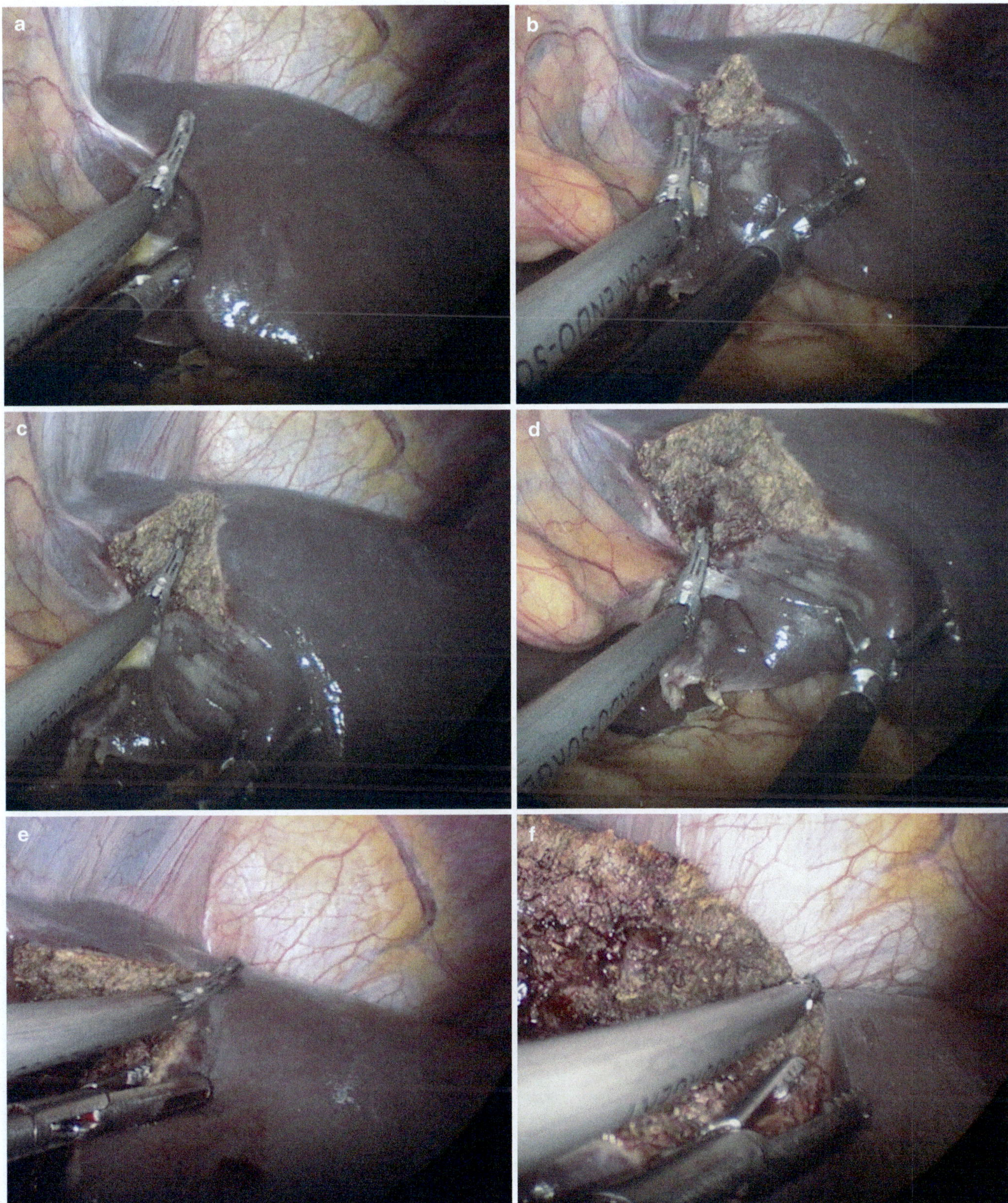

Fig. 5.48

Hemostasis and liver division surface coagulation were completed with Ligasure device. Some vascular and bile duct structures could be ligated and transected by Endo-GIA (Fig. 5.49a–k).

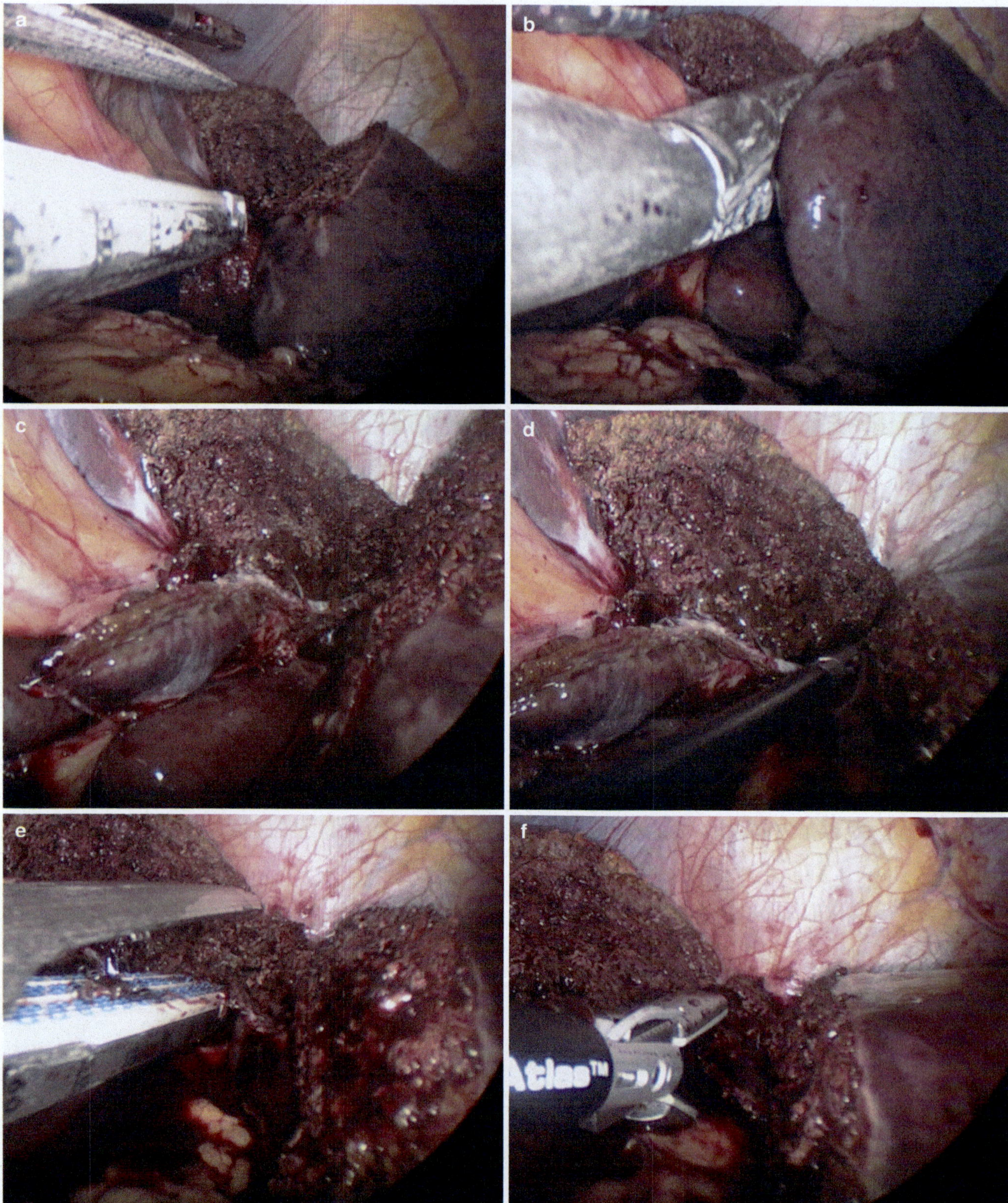

Fig. 5.49

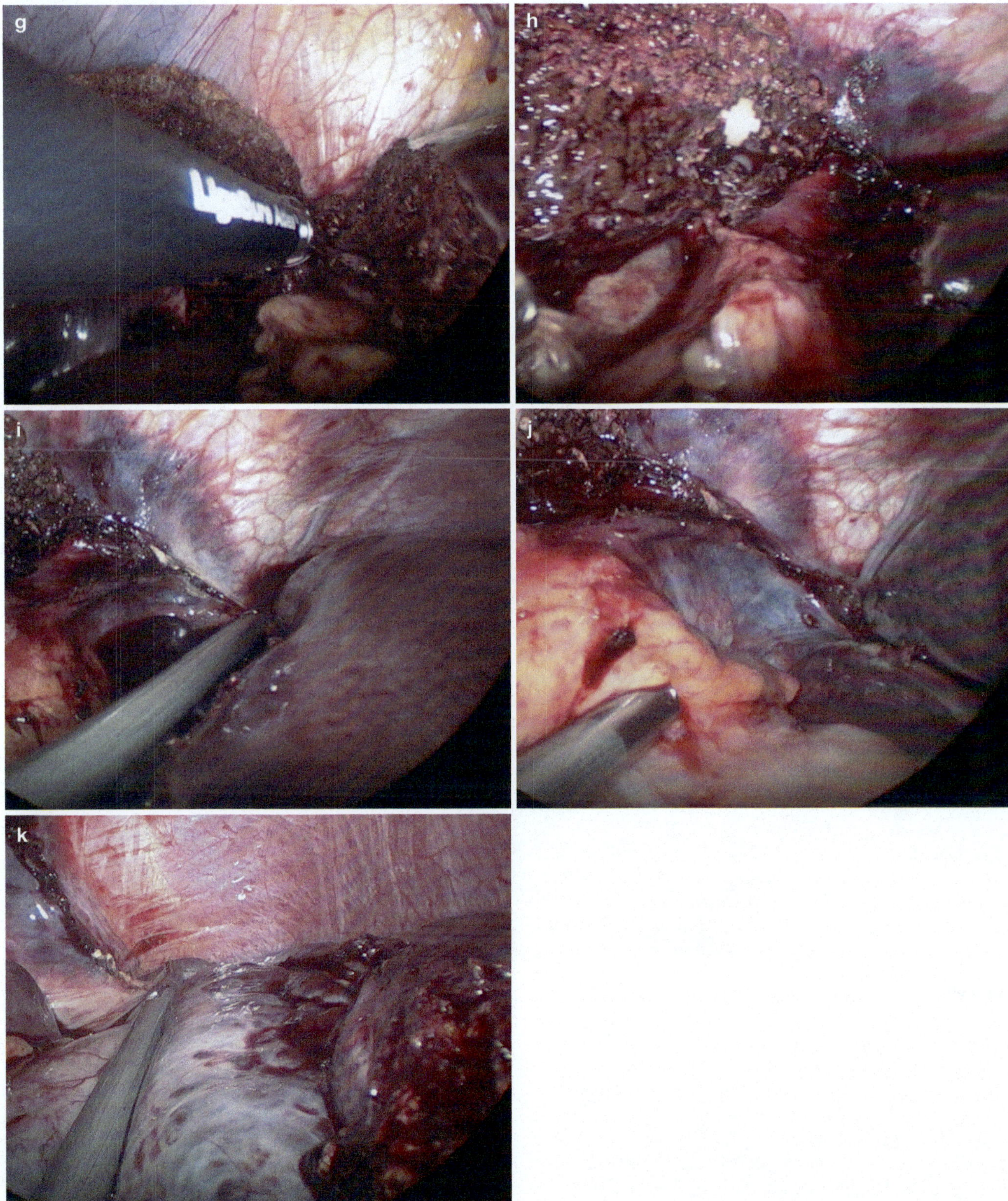

Fig. 5.49 (continued)

4. Retrieval of the specimen.
   The resected left hepatic lobe was then put in a plastic bag and completely removed through the umbilical incision (Fig. 5.50a–c).

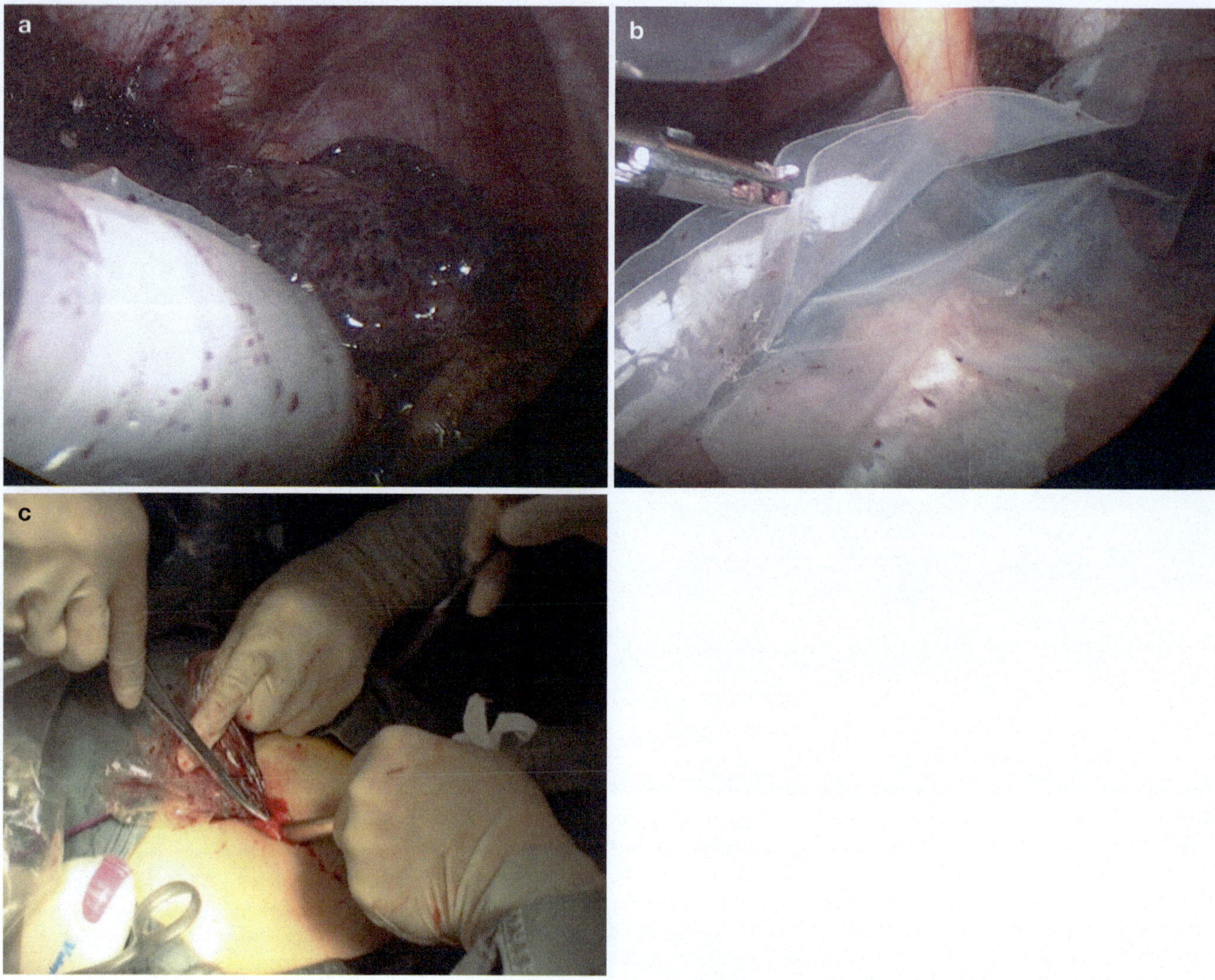

Fig. 5.50

5. Irrigation and drainage.
   After final inspection for the site of bleeding and bile leakage, aided by saline irrigation, the drainage tubes were placed in the foramen of Winslow and near the stump of liver separately (Fig. 5.51a, b).

5.8.7 Tips and Tricks

1. For left lateral segmentectomies, the liver was mobilized from the falciform ligament and left triangular ligament using the Harmonic Scalpel (Ethicon Endo-Surgery, Inc.)
2. Intraoperative ultrasound could be performed using a laparoscopic ultrasound probe. The site of the tumor was confirmed, and the transection plane with appropriate margins was marked using diathermy.

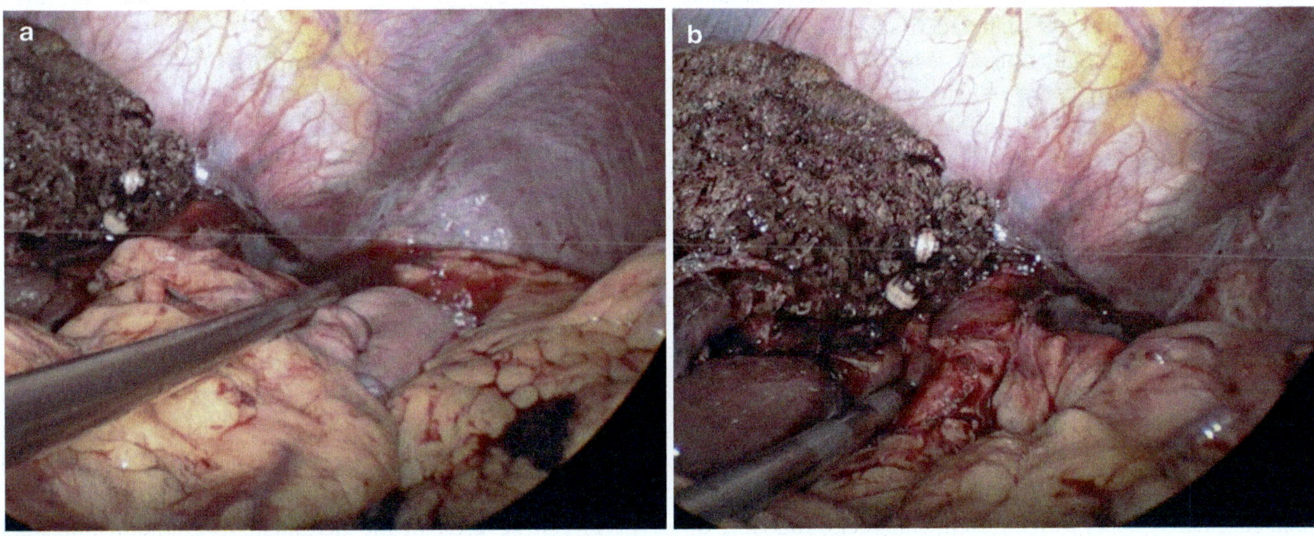

Fig. 5.51

5.9 Complications Analysis and Management

5.9.1 Haemorrhage

The most common reason of haemorrhage in laparoscopic cholecystectomy is sever inflammation in the cystic triangle, which tends to form obscure anatomical structure and injure the cystic artery. But such cases aren't suitable for SILS. In SILS cholecystectomy, cystic artery can be excellently coagulated by ultrasound scalpel. It is notable that the ultrasound scalpel working time and clamped tissue thickness determine the effect of coagulation. Intraoperative haemorrhage can also be induced by liver parenchyma injury accompanied with deeper wound surface of gallbladder bed. Electrocantery and haemostatic gauze can stop bleeding easily.

In SILS biliary surgery, massive bleeding can be induced by the injury of hepatic artery or portal vein. In SILS surgery, the lack of triangle relationship and limitation of motion may injure the vessels in the hepatoduodenal ligament during the dissection of the extrahepatic bile ducts. In case of massive haemorrhage around the common bile duct in SILS biliary surgery, local compression hemostasis by gauze and converting to open surgery should be decided as soon as possible.

The application of SILS in liver diseases is limited. So, the occurrence of massive bleeding is not high. For intrahepatic vascular systems with different diameters, choosing the proper cutting and coagulating instruments is absolutely essential. The chose of ultrasound scalpel, LigaSure, linear stapler or Hemolock is decided by the diameters of Gllisson's sheath. After the lobe or tumor had been completely removed, a bipolar electrocauterizer or argon beam coagulator was used for hemostasis of the liver wound.

5.9.2 Biliary Injury and Bile Leakage

In SILS cholecystectomy and biliary exploration, vague anatomical relationship caused by local inflammation can induce laceration of extrahepatic bile duct, cutting and burning of bile duct, partly or completely clamped bile duct and even transaction. In this case, conversion to open surgery is always necessary. So, how to identify correct anatomical structure and choosing proper cases for SILS is the basis of avoiding biliary injury. More attention should be paid to the direction and strength of gallbladder retraction in SILS procedure. Excessive gallbladder retraction can cause jerking and angulating the common bile duct. In this case, gallbladder dissection may injury the sidewall of common hepatic duct and the clamping of cystic duct may cause a partial or complete clamping of the common bile duct. Bile leakage in SILS liver resection is always caused by dissecting the intrahepatic bile duct with unsuitable instruments. For larger bile ducts, clamping with Hemolock is recommended. Careful examination of bile leakage from liver wound and a proper placement of drainage are important methods to prevent postoperative bile leakage. Clamping and local suture can be used to deal with intraoperative bile leakage. For postoperative bile leakage, if the patient doesn't have abdominal pain, fever and peritonitis symptoms, the drainage is adequate and conservative treatment will be considered.

5.9.3 Secondary Common Bile Duct Stone

Except for missing common bile duct stone before the operation, most postoperative common bile duct stones in SILS cholecystectomy are dropped from gallbladder. No matter what kind of dissecting sequence is used in SILS cholecystectomy, the gallbladder will be inevitable moved before the cystic duct was being clamped. So the possibility of gallbladder stone dropping into the common bile duct is existent. If the gallbladder stones is multiple, and the volume of stone is smaller (less than 3 mm), or the patients have the history of biliary pancreatitis, informed consent on the possibility of secondary common bile duct stones should be given before the operation. Endoscopic sphincterotomy (EST) can be used in the treatment of common bile duct stones.

5.9.4 Bile Duct Residual Stones

In SILS biliary exploration, the choledochoscope and basket enter the abdomen through the umbilical incision. In the surgical field, the choledochoscope and basket are parallel to the common bile duct. Though it is easier to observe and retract the intrahepatic bile duct stones, the stones in the distal end are difficult and often missed easily. Intraoperatively combined with duodenoscope or ERCP can identify the existence of residual stones in common bile duct while confirming whether the distal end of the C tube is in the duodenum.

5.9.5 Bile Duct Stenosis

Excess tissue of bile duct side wall can induce postoperative bile duct stenosis, especially in the case when the common bile duct diameter is less than 1 cm. Do not involved too much of bile duct side wall in the suture. SILS is not suitable in cases when the diameter of common bile duct is less than 5 mm.

References

1. Bittner R. The standard of laparoscopic cholecystectomy. Langenbecks Arch Surg. 2004;389:157–63.
2. Kaiser AM, Corman ML. History of laparoscopy. Surg Oncol Clin N Am. 2001;10:483–92.
3. Soper NJ, Stockmann PT, Dunnegan DL, Ashley SW. Laparoscopic cholecystectomy. The new 'gold standard'? Arch Surg. 1992;127:917–21.
4. Schirmer BD, Edge SB, Dix J, Hyser MJ, Hanks JB, Jones RS. Laparoscopic cholecystectomy. Treatment of choice for symptomatic cholelithiasis. Ann Surg. 1991;213:665–76. discussion 677.
5. Johansson M, Thune A, Nelvin L, Stiernstam M, Westman B, Lundell L. Randomized clinical trial of open versus laparoscopic cholecystectomy in the treatment of acute cholecystitis. Br J Surg. 2005;92:44–9.
6. Navarra G, Pozza E, Occhionorelli S, Carcoforo P, Donini I. One-wound laparoscopic cholecystectomy. Br J Surg. 1997;84:695.
7. Lai EC, Tang CN, Ha JP, Li MK. Laparoscopic liver resection for hepatocellular carcinoma. Ten-year experience in a single center. Arch Surg. 2009;144:143–7.
8. Adani GL, Aprile G, Baccarani U, Risaliti A, De Anna D, Lorenzin D, et al. Benefit of laparoscopy for rectal resection in patients operated simultaneously for synchronous liver metastases: preliminary experience. Surgery. 2009;145:452.
9. Sarpel U, Hefti MM, Wisnievsky JP, Roayaie S, Schwartz ME, Labow DM. Outcome for patients treated with laparoscopic versus open resection of hepatocellular carcinoma: case-matched analysis. Ann Surg Oncol. 2009;16:1572–7.
10. Choh MS, Madura 2nd JA. The role of minimally invasive treatments in surgical oncology. Surg Clin North Am. 2009;89:53–77.
11. O'Rourke RW, Lee NN, Cheng J, Swanstrom LL, Hansen PD. Laparoscopic biliary reconstruction. Am J Surg. 2004;187:621–4.
12. Chokshi NK, Guner YS, Aranda A, Shin CE, Ford HR, Nguyen NX. Laparoscopic choledochal cyst excision: lessons learned in our experience. J Laparoendosc Adv Surg Tech A. 2009;19:87–91.
13. Binenbaum SJ, Teixeira JA, Forrester GJ, Harvey EJ, Afthinos J, Kim GJ, et al. Single-incision laparoscopic cholecystectomy using a flexible endoscope. Arch Surg. 2009;144:734–8.
14. Hodgett SE, Hernandez JM, Morton CA, Ross SB, Albrink M, Rosemurgy AS. Laparoendoscopic single site (LESS) cholecystectomy. J Gastrointest Surg. 2009;13:188–92.
15. Hong TH, Kim HL, Lee YS, Kim JJ, Lee KH, You YK, et al. Transumbilical single-port laparoscopic appen-dectomy (TUSPLA): scarless intracorporeal appendectomy. J Laparoendosc Adv Surg Tech A. 2009;19:75–8.
16. Fagotti A, Fanfani F, Marocco F, Rossitto C, Gallotta V, Scambia G. Laparoendoscopic single-site surgery (LESS) for ovarian cyst enucleation: report of first 3 cases. Fertil Steril. 2009;92:1168.e13–6.
17. Fader AN, Escobar PF. Laparoendoscopic single-site sur-gery (LESS) in gynecologic oncology: technique and initial report. Gynecol Oncol. 2009;114:157–61.

Pancreatic Surgery

6

Abstract

Pancreatic surgery is an extremely challenging field, partly owing to the retroperitoneal location of the pancreas, the wide range and influence of operation, numerous postoperative complications and so on. The application of laparoscopic surgery for the treatments of pancreatic diseases is only recently gaining widespread popularity. These included diagnostic explorative laparoscopy for cancer staging (Kim et al., Curr Probl Surg 44(4):228–269, 2007; Ahmed et al., J Laparoendosc Adv Surg Tech A 16:458–463, 2006) pancreatic drainage (Hauters et al., Surg Endosc 18:1645–1648, 2004), enucleation (Toniato et al., World J Surg 30:1916–1919, 2006), distal pancreatectomy (Melotti et al., Ann Surg 246:77–82, 2007; Uranues et al., Am J Surg 192:257–261, 2006), and even pancreaticoduodenectomy (Palanivelu et al., J Am Coll Surg 205:222–230, 2007). Among these different laparoscopic procedures, laparoscopic distal pancreatectomy (LDP) is the most widely used, possibly because of its acceptable technical feasibility without the necessity for anastomoses (Park et al., Am J Surg 177:158–163, 1999).

Distal pancreatectomy has been performed since early twentieth century (Finney, Ann Surg 51:818–829, 1910). In 1994, the laparoscopic distal pancreatectomy (LDP) was first reported to be feasible and safe in a porcine model (Soper et al., Surg Endosc 8:57–60, 1994). Then, the LDP was quickly attempted to perform in humans (Cuschieri et al., Ann Surg 223:280–285, 1996; Gagner et al., Surgery 120:1051–1054, 1996; Sussman et al., Aust N Z J Surg 66(6):414–416, 1996). With better improvement of technologies, like ultrasonography, staplers, and other instrumentations, the multiple incision laparoscopic distal pancreatectomy (LDP) rapidly gained popularity, and is becoming a more widely used approach. Multiple prospective studies have shown the feasibility and safety of LDP in single-center and multicenter settings (Kooby et al., Ann Surg 248:438–446, 2008; Røsok et al., Br J Surg 97:902–909, 2010; Kneuertz et al., J Am Coll Surg 215:167–176, 2012). Now, the application of laparoscopic surgery for the distal pancreatectomy seems to become a trend in surgical technique, and might be considered as the first approach for distal pancreatectomy in the near future (Jin et al., HPB (Oxford) 14:711–724, 2012).

For a more cosmetic result and further minimizing the surgical trauma, a new minimally invasive technique called "single-incision laparoscopic surgery" (SILS) has been rapidly developed recently, and until now this approach has been performed in a variety of organs. SILS performed on the pancreatic lesions has been reported only recently, and only five cases were reported in the literature (Barbaros et al., JSLS 14:566–570, 2010; Kuroki et al., Hepatogastroenterology 58(107–108):1022–1024, 2011; Chang et al., Minim Invasive Surg 2012:197429, 2012; Misawa et al., Asian J Endosc Surg 5:195–199, 2012). However, these data might still be able to suggest that the transumbilical single-incision laparoscopic distal pancreatectomy (TUSI-LDP) is feasible, as in these reports even for the patients that had previously undergone a nephrectomy which caused dense fibrosis in the retroperitoneal region (Barbaros et al., JSLS 14:566–570, 2010), or that had two previous laparoscopic

S. Wu et al. (eds.), *Atlas of Single-Incision Laparoscopic Operations in General Surgery*,
DOI 10.1007/978-94-007-6955-7_6, © Springer Science+Business Media Dordrecht 2013

procedures for pelvic inflammatory disease and excision of ovarian cyst (Chang et al., Minim Invasive Surg 2012:197429, 2012), a SILS pancreatectomy could also be smoothly performed, and the TUSI-LDP together with splenectomy or spleen and spleen vessels preserving distal pancreatectomy were all performed successfully (Barbaros et al., JSLS 14:566–570, 2010; Kuroki et al., Hepatogastroenterology 58(107–108):1022–1024, 2011; Chang et al., Minim Invasive Surg 2012:197429, 2012; Misawa et al., Asian J Endosc Surg 5:195–199, 2012).

Keywords
Distal pancreatectomy • Splenic vessels • Splenectomy • Pancreatic pseudocyst • Cystojejunal anastomosis

6.1 Laparoscopic Distal Pancreatectomy

6.1.1 Indications and Case Selection

1. Patients with chronic pancreatitis and benign tumors (including cystic tumors and solid tumors) in the tail or body of the pancreas.
2. Patients with pancreatic ductal strictures and a pseudocyst in the tail or body of the pancreas.

6.1.2 Contraindications

1. Patients with malignant tumors or adenocarcinoma of the pancreas were relative contraindications, since no data are currently available regarding long-term outcomes for single incision laparoscopic resection of pancreatic adenocarcinoma or malignant tumors.
2. Patients with relatively operative contraindications should also be ruled out.

6.1.3 Major Instruments or Energy Sources

1. Laparoscopy System.
2. Holding forceps.
3. Harmonic scalpel.
4. Endoscopic Linear Stapler.

6.1.4 Team Setup, Anesthesia and Position

Under general anesthesia, the patient was placed in supine position with the legs apart. The position of surgeon, assistants and nurses is shown in Fig. 6.1.

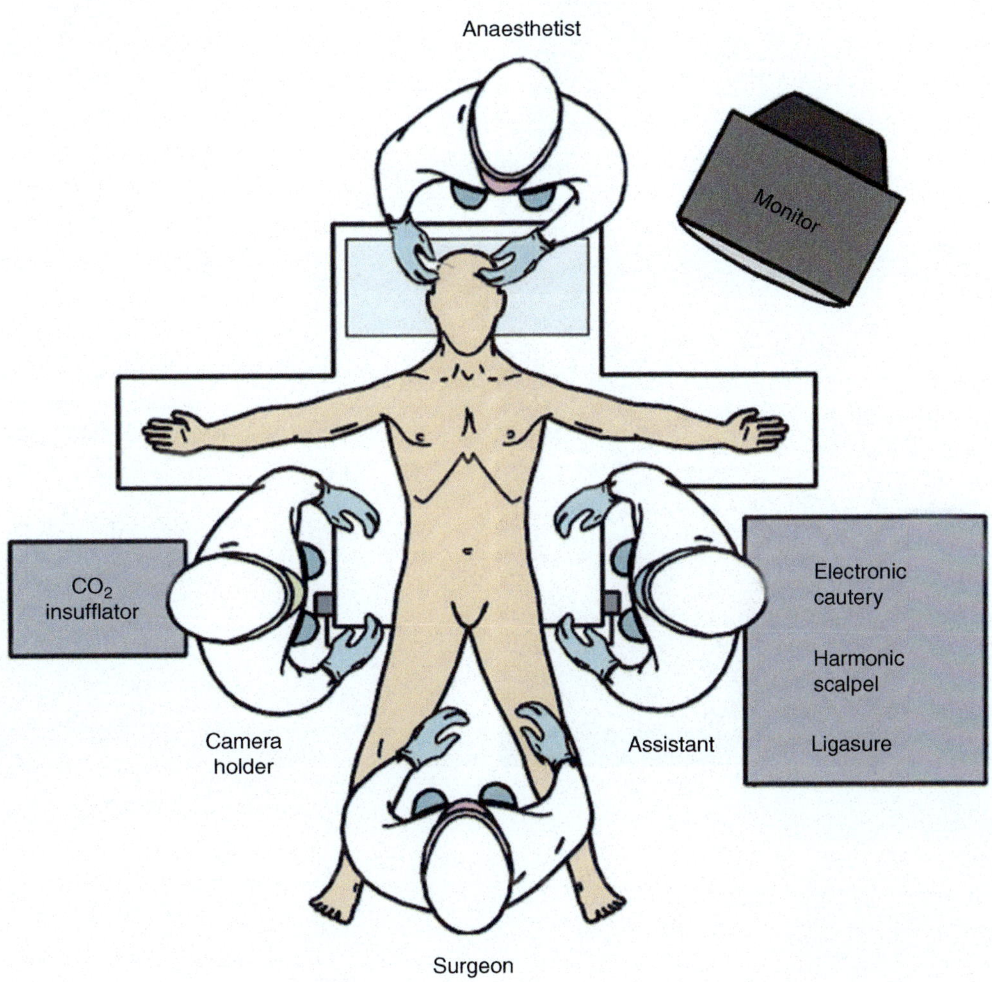

Fig. 6.1

6.1.5 Key Steps

1. Exploration of the abdominal cavity.
2. Exposure of pancreas.
3. Dissection of the pancreas.
4. Transection of pancreas.
5. Retrieval of the specimen and observation of the spleen.
6. Irrigation and drainage.

6.1.6 Surgical Techniques

1. Exploration of the abdominal cavity.
   A general exploration of the abdominal cavity was performed to rule out the possibility of an extrapancreatic lesion.
2. Exposure of pancreas.
   The patient was placed in a reverse Trendelenburg position. The operation began with the division of the gastrocolic ligament to expose the body and tail of pancreas and confirm the location and range of the lesion (Fig. 6.2a–e).

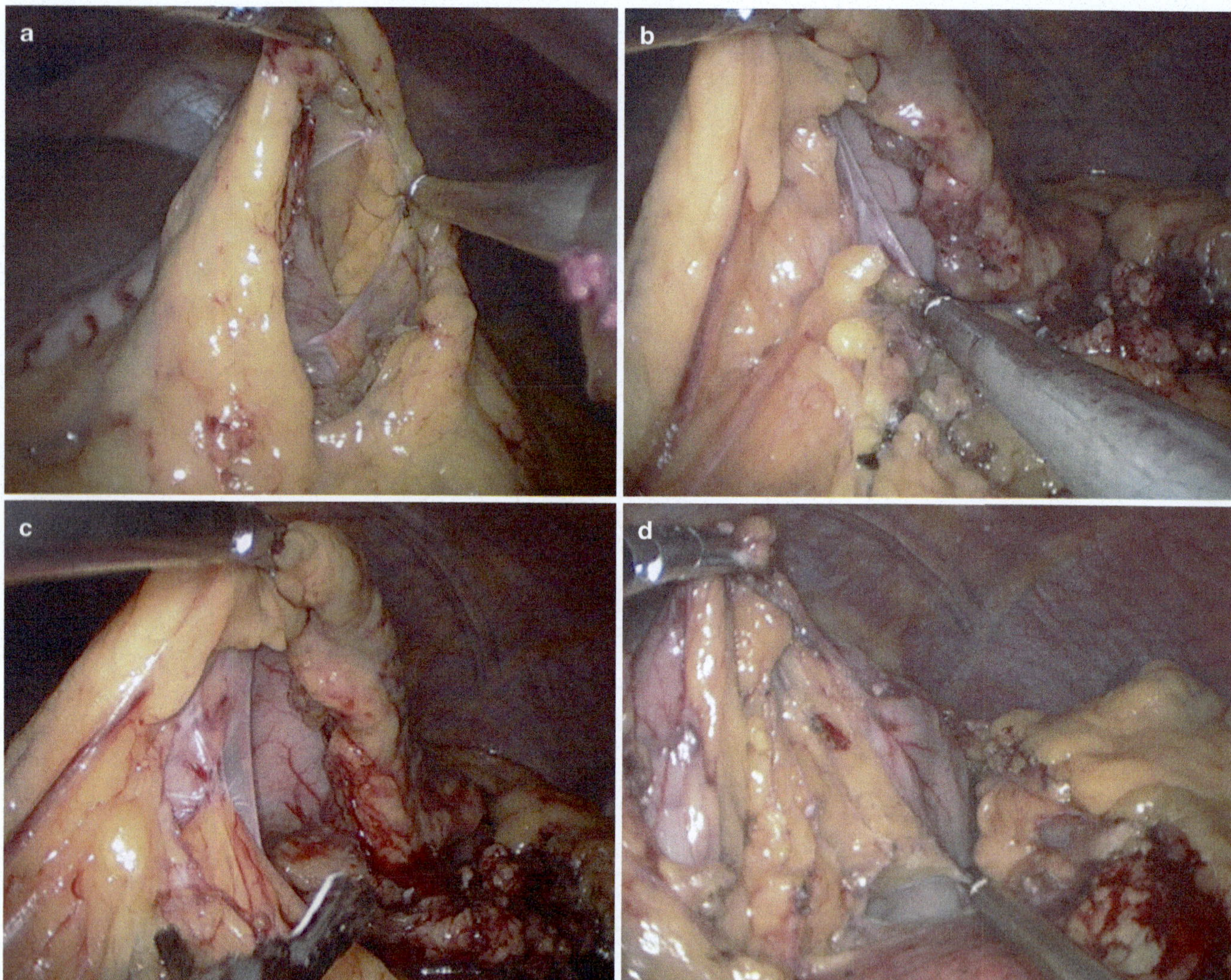

Fig. 6.2

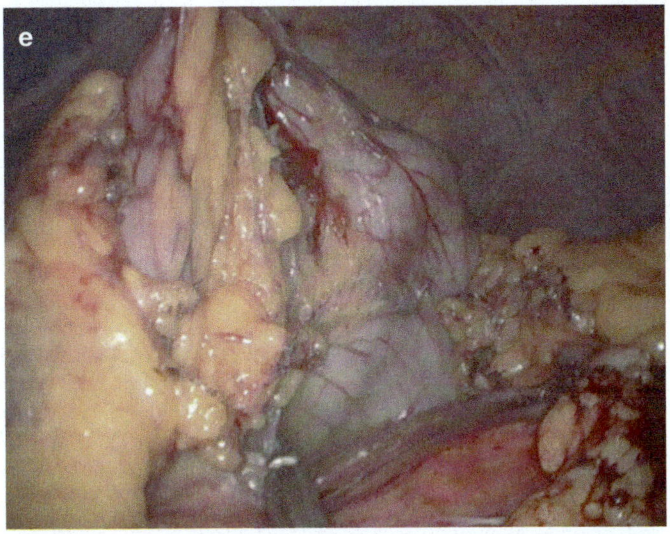

Fig. 6.2 (continued)

3. Dissection of the pancreas.

   The serous membrane was dissected along the lower edge of pancreas on the right of the lesion, to expose the lower edge of the pancreas (Fig. 6.3a–d).

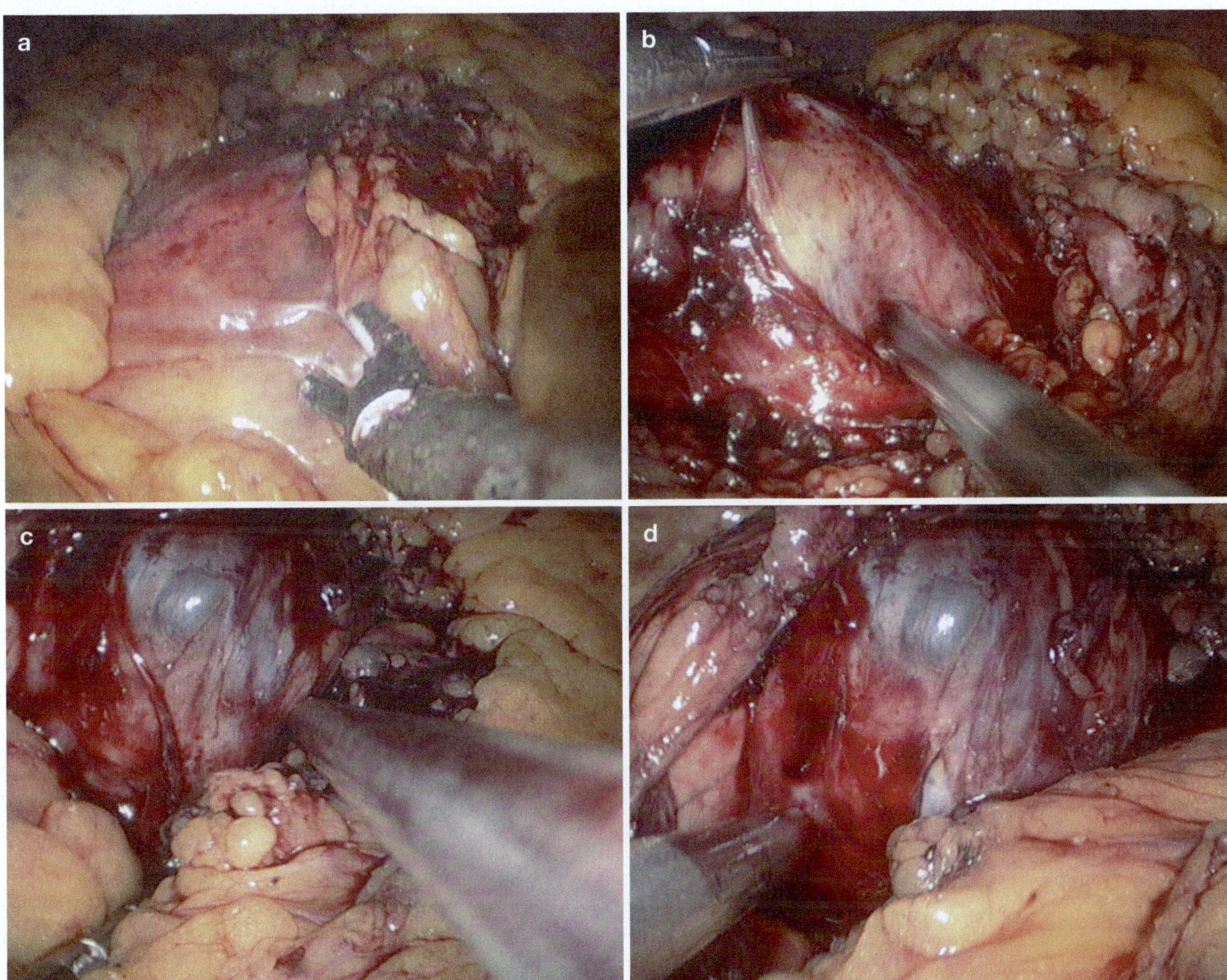

Fig. 6.3

Tunneling under the pancreatic neck was performed. Further dissection of the superior margin of the pancreas was done to facilitate tunneling beneath the pancreatic neck. Try not to injury the splenic vessels (Fig. 6.4a, b).

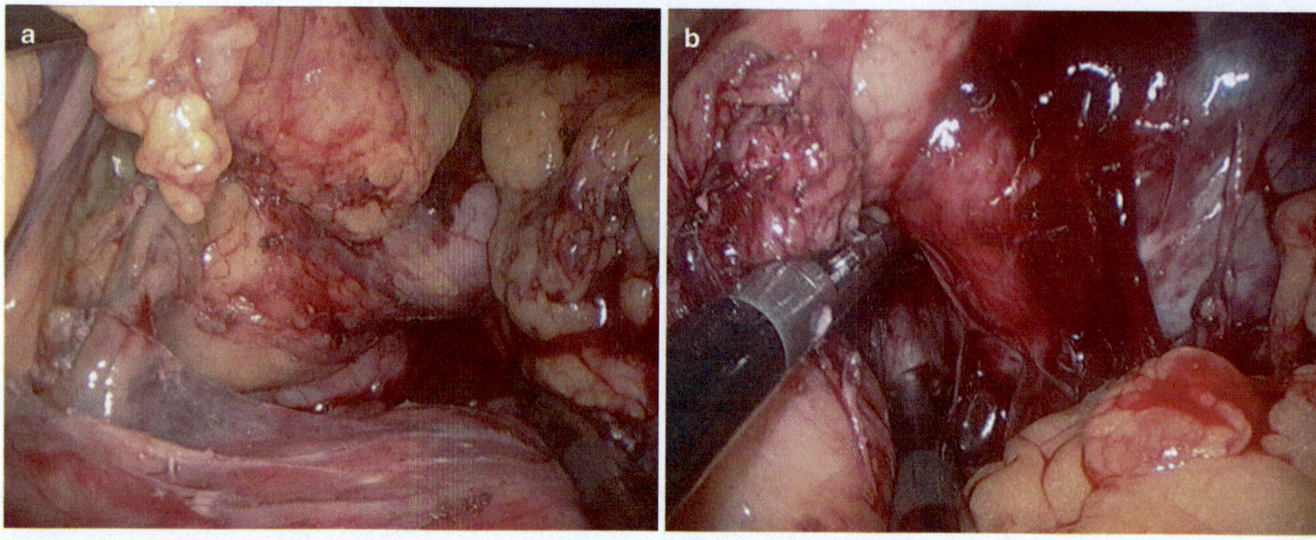

Fig. 6.4

4. Transection of distal pancreas.
   Transection of the pancreas along the neck was created using the endoscopic linear stapler. The splenic vessels were preserved carefully during the transection. Further dissection of the pancreas off the splenic vessels was carried on until the tail was reached. At the superior margin of the pancreas, care was taken to preserve the splenic vessels. The dissection was continued until the whole body and tail of the pancreas were dissected (Fig. 6.5a–h).

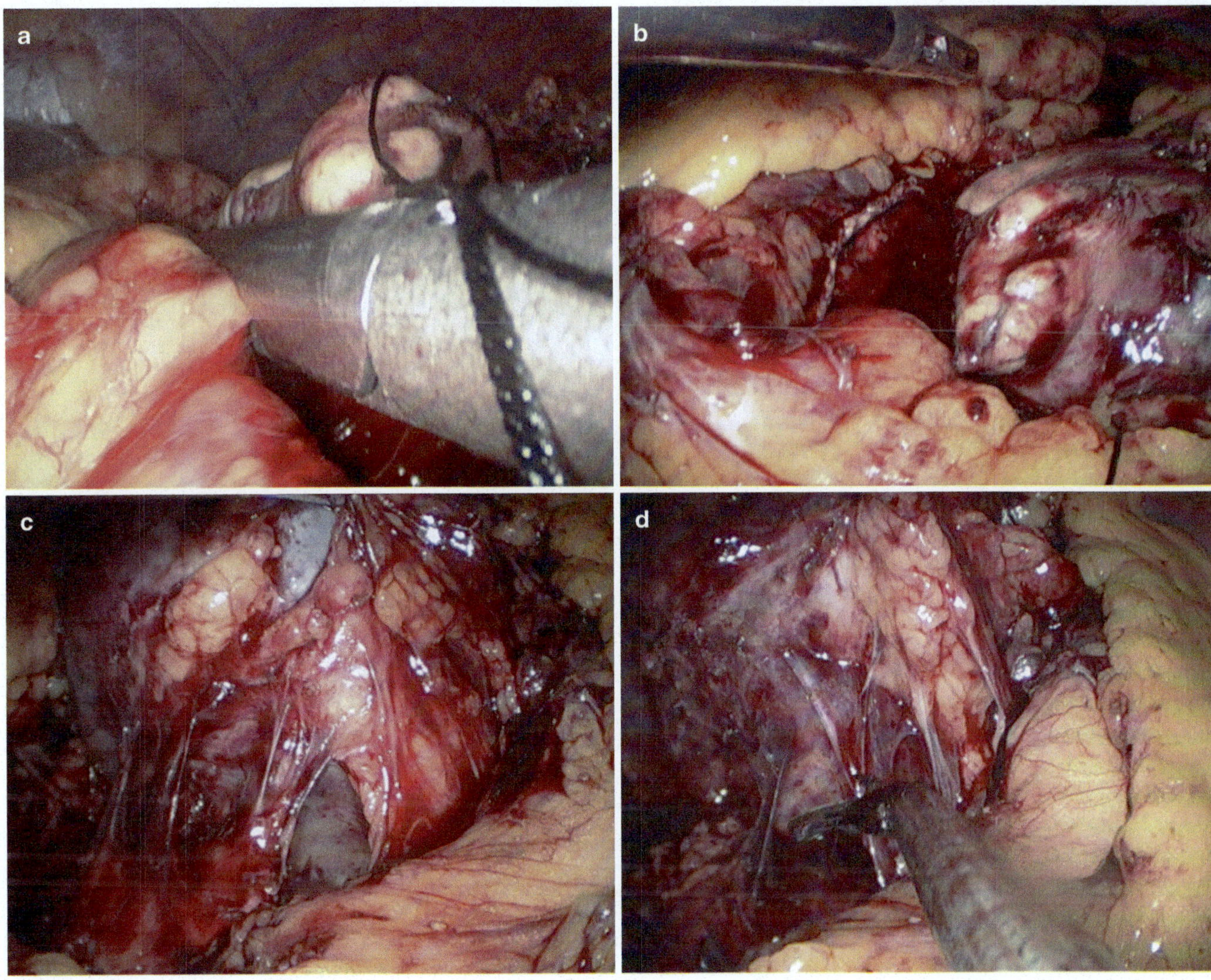

Fig. 6.5

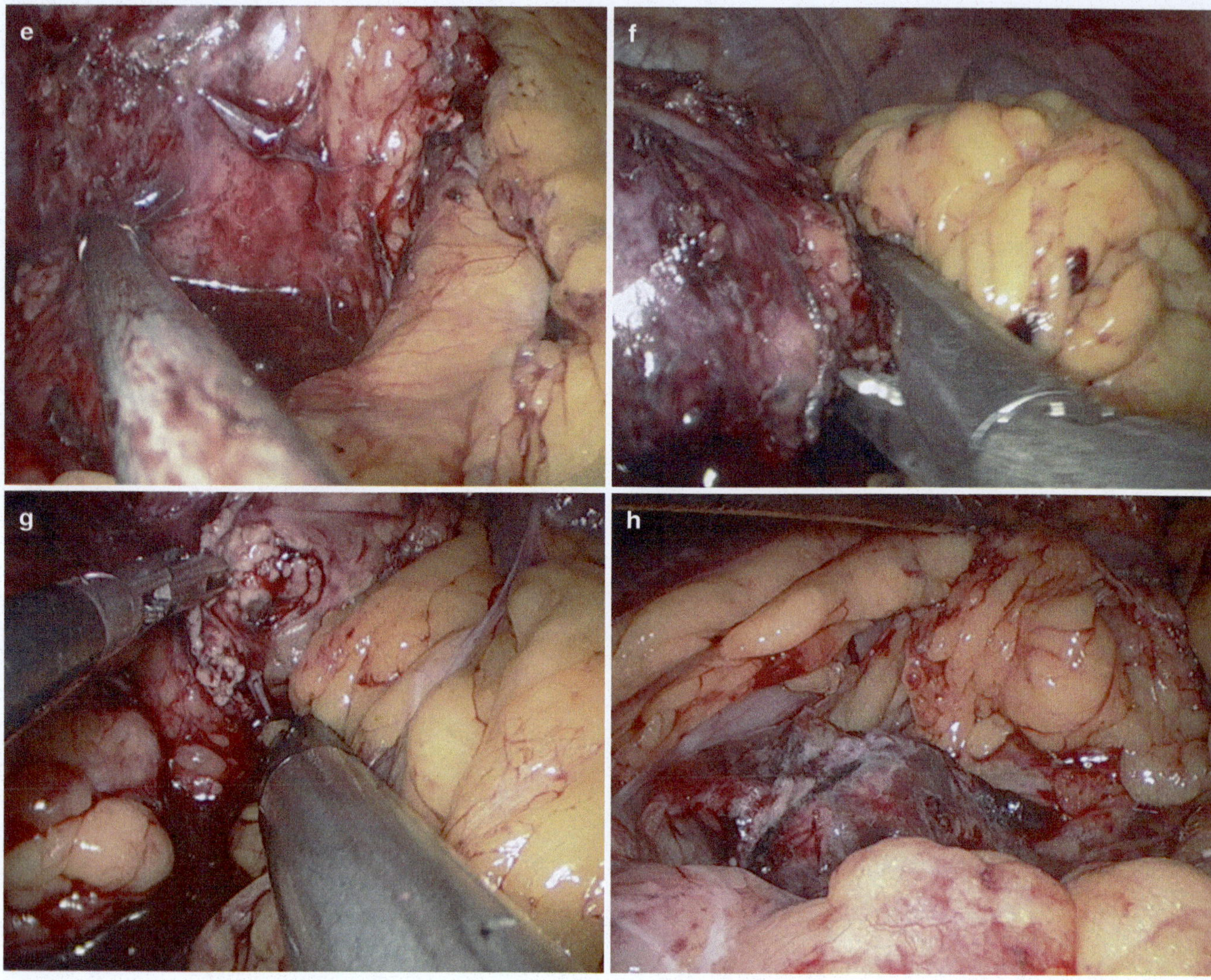

Fig. 6.5 (continued)

5. Retrieval of the specimen and observation of the spleen. The specimen was delivered out of the abdomen using a plastic bag. The viability of the spleen was assessed. No signs of infarct were detected (Fig. 6.6a, b).
6. Irrigation and drainage.
   After final inspection for the site of bleeding, aided by saline irrigation, the stump of the pancreas was reinforced with glue. The drainage tube was placed at the transected part of the pancreas.

6.1.7 Tips and Tricks

1. Several prolene straight needles stay sutures may be placed superficially to the posterior gastric wall and slinged to the anterior abdominal wall to expose the pancreas.
2. Intraoperative laparoscopic ultrasound may be used to confirm the lesion and exclude the presence of other lesions.
3. After the lesion has been identified and assessed to be operable, the inferior edge of the pancreatic capsule should be incised firstly. Then a tunnel should be created beneath the pancreatic neck from caudal to cephalad direction and freeing the pancreatic parenchyma from the splenic vessels for preserving the splenic vessels procedure.
4. A careful dissection of distal pancreas from medial to lateral approach should be carried out with preservation of the main splenic artery and veins.

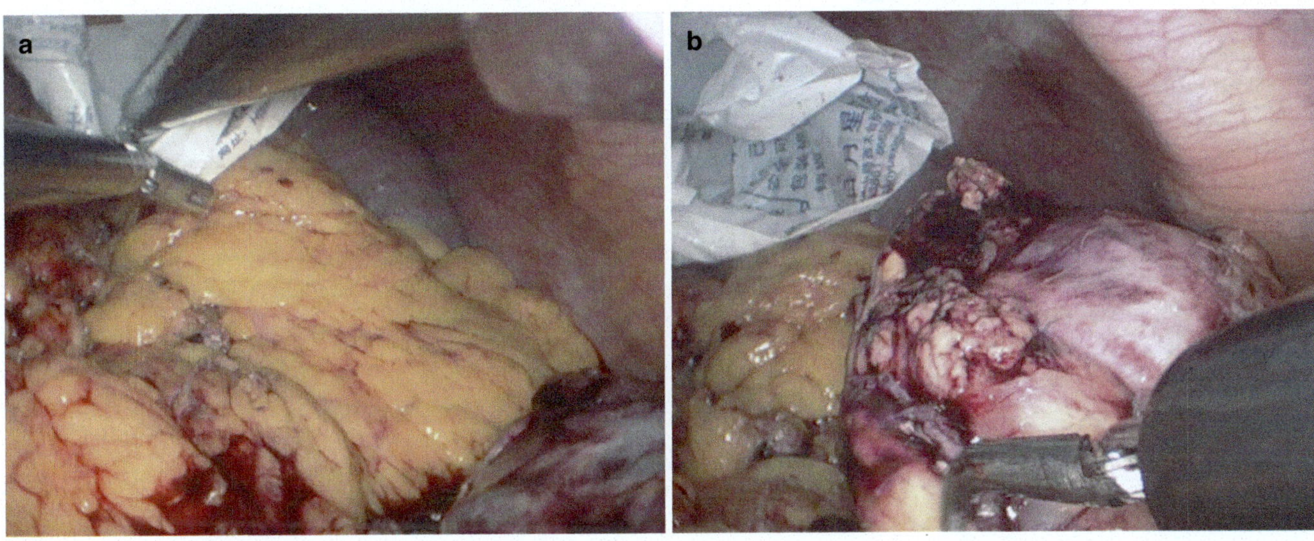

Fig. 6.6

6.2 Laparoscopic Distal Pancreatectomy Plus Splenectomy

6.2.1 Indications and Case Selection

Indications are similar with laparoscopic distal pancreatectomy, except the cases in which appropriate vascular inflow and outflow through splenic and /or short gastric vessels could not be preserved or was mandated by oncologic principles.

6.2.2 Contraindications

It's identical to Sect. 6.1.2.

6.2.3 Major Instruments or Energy Sources

1. Laparoscopy System.
2. Holding forceps.
3. Harmonic scalpel.
4. Endoscopic Linear Stapler.

6.2.4 Team Setup, Anesthesia and Position

It is the same as Sect. 6.1.4.

6.2.5 Key Steps

1. Exploration of the abdominal cavity.
2. Exposure of pancreas.
3. Dissection of the pancreas.
4. Dissection of distal pancreas and spleen.
5. Transection of the pancreas.
6. Retrieval of the specimen.
7. Irrigation and drainage.

6.2.6 Surgical Techniques

1. Exploration of the abdominal cavity.
   A general exploration of the abdominal cavity was performed to rule out the possibility of an extrapancreatic lesion.
2. Exposure of pancreas.
   The patient was placed in a reverse Trendelenburg position. The operation began with the division of the gastrocolic ligament and the lower part of gastrosplenic ligament, to expose the pancreas (Fig. 6.7a–l).

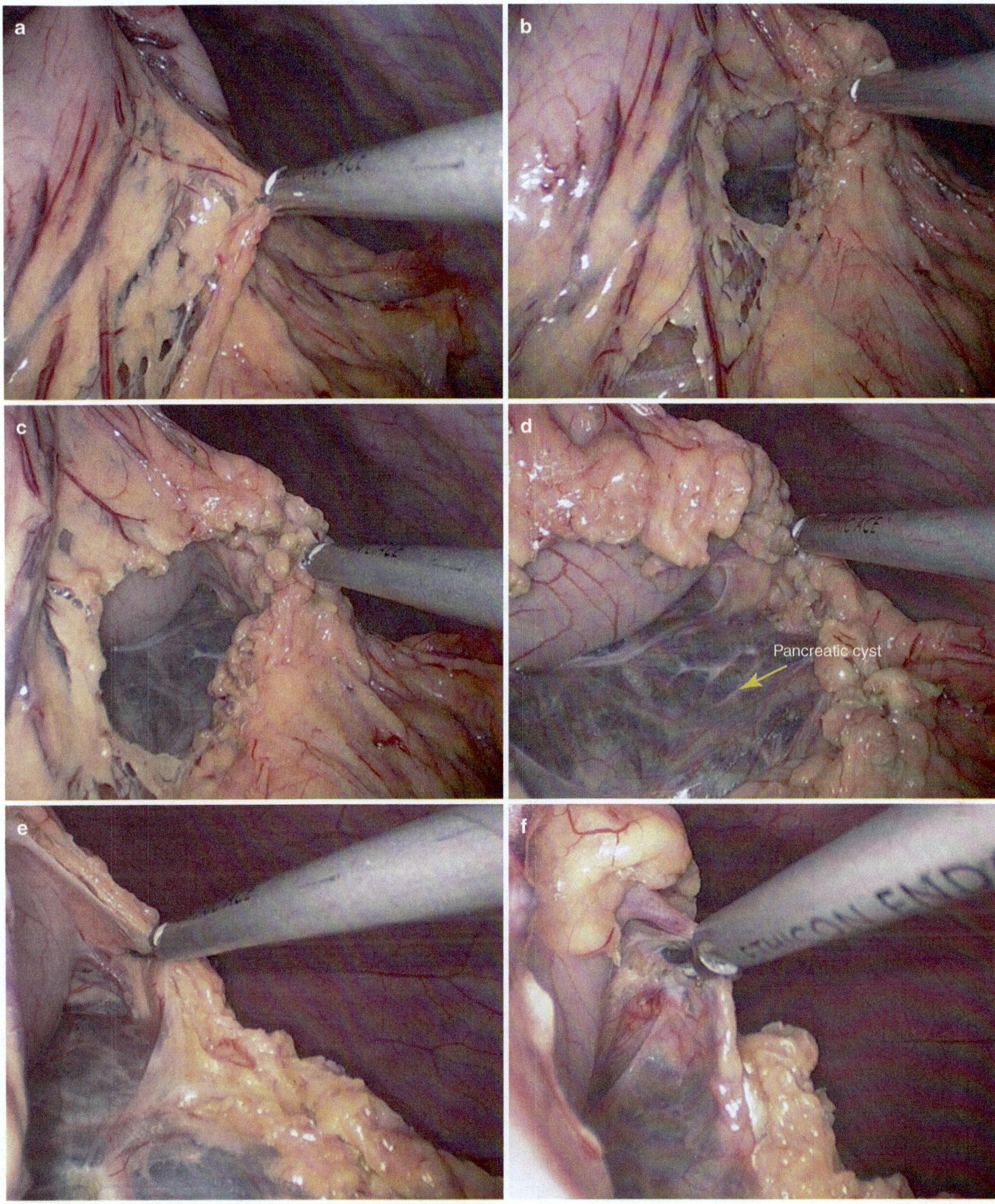

Fig. 6.7

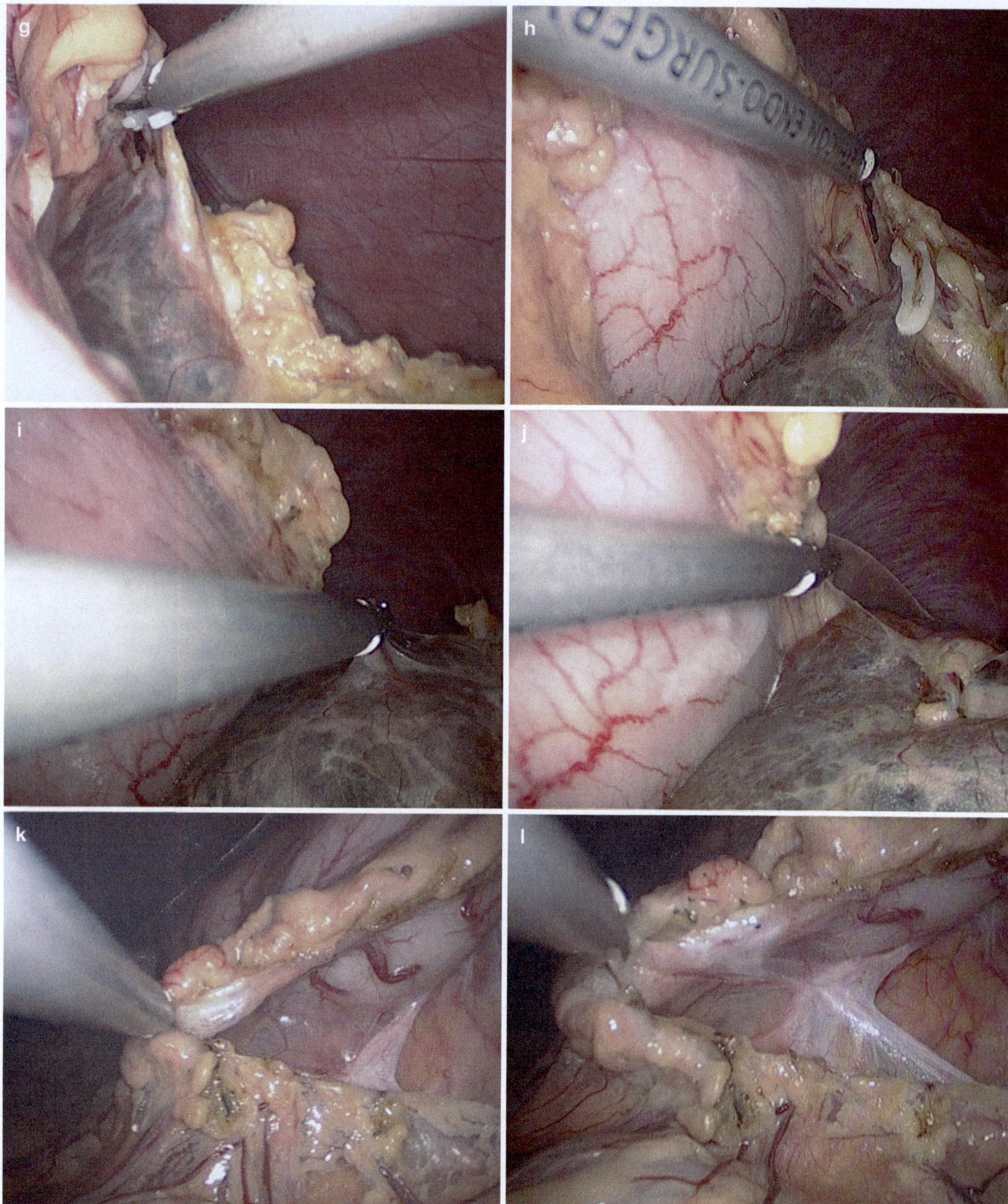

Fig. 6.7 (continued)

Continuous dissection of the adhesion between the superior margin of the pancreas and the posterior wall of the stomach was performed. The splenic vessels were exposed at the superior margin of the pancreas. In case of close relationship between the lesion and splenic vessels, combined splenectomy was scheduled (Fig. 6.8a–j).

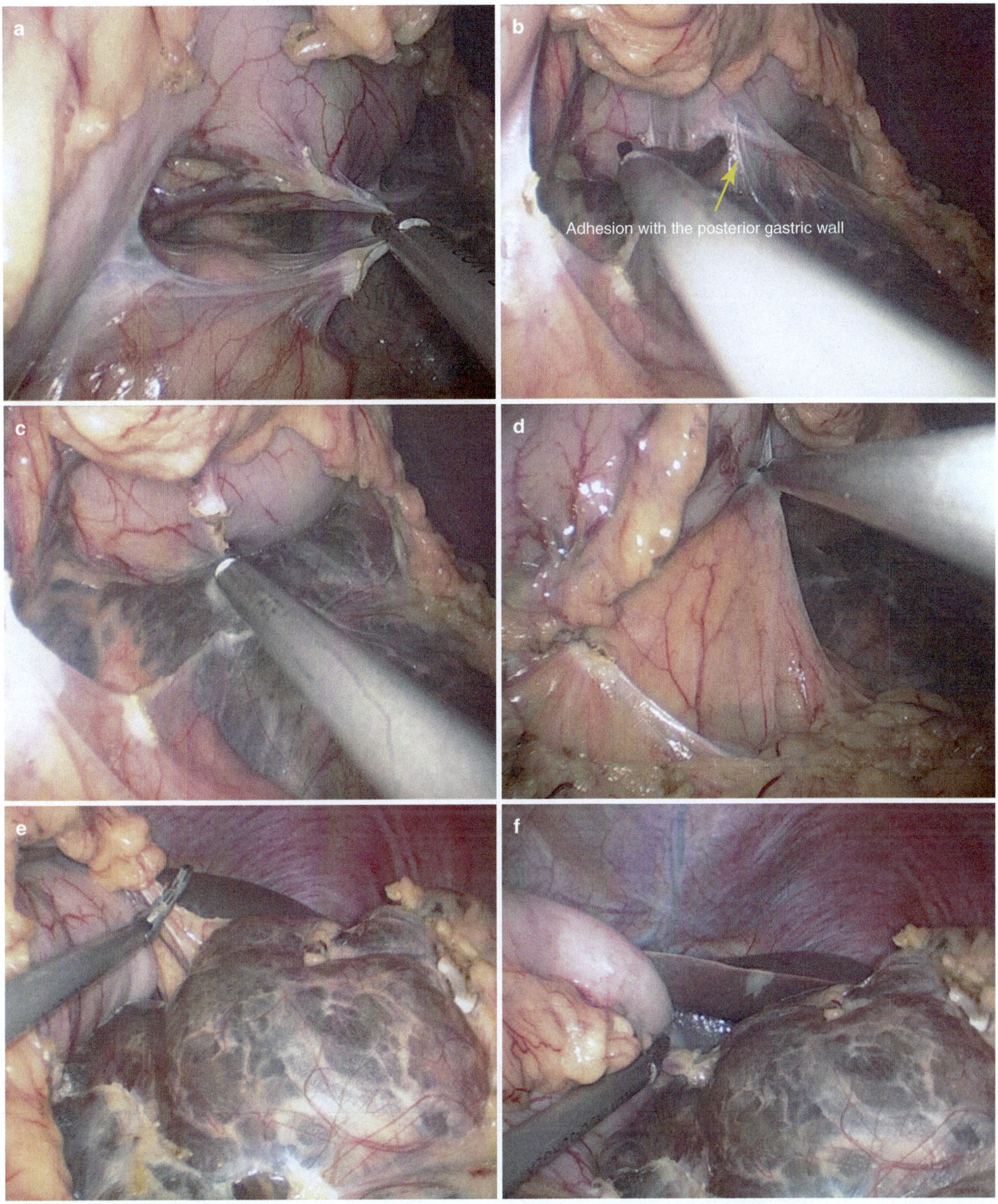

Fig. 6.8

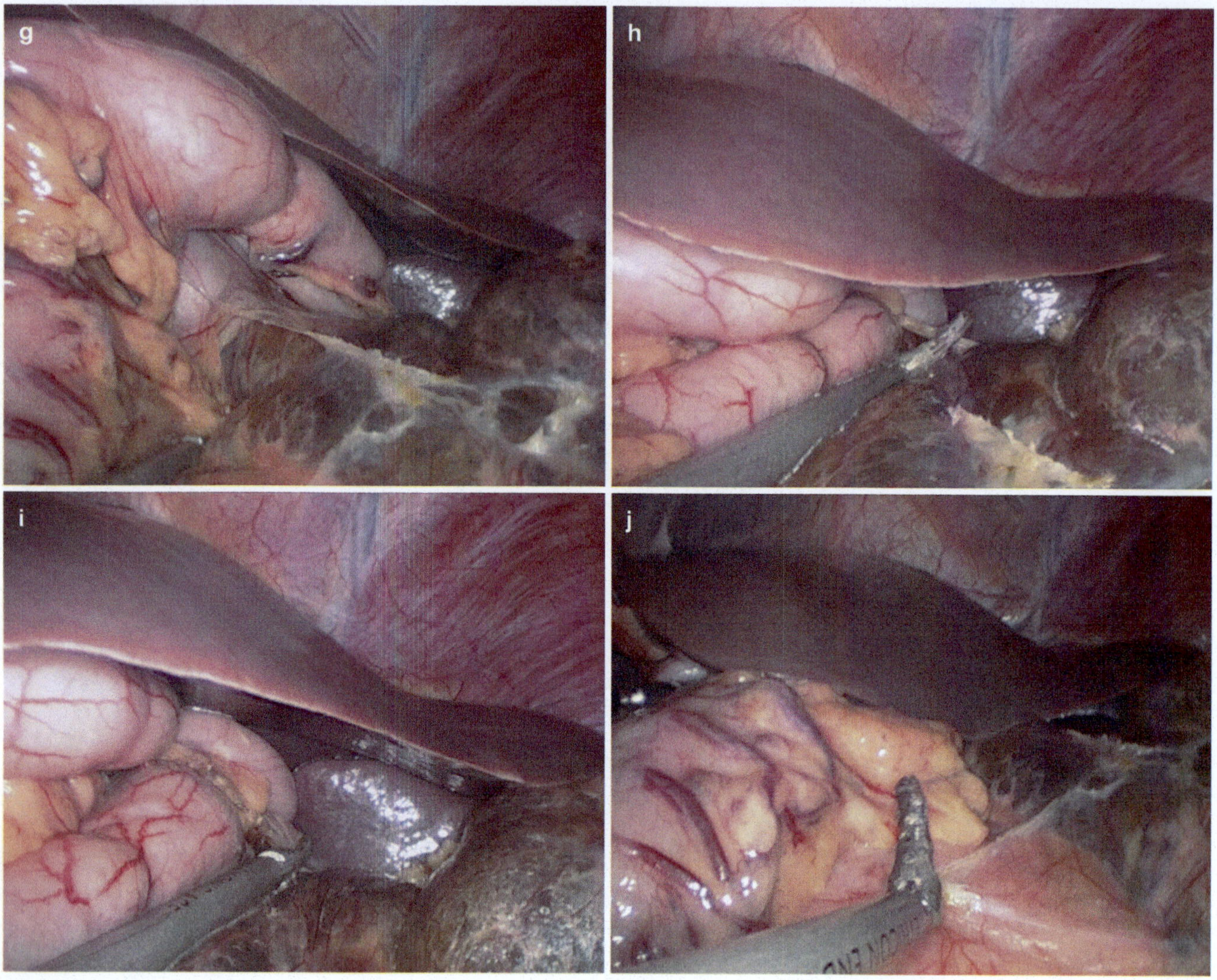

Fig. 6.8 (continued)

Mobilization of the superior margin of the pancreas was performed. Attention should be paid not to tear the splenic vessels (Fig. 6.9a–f).

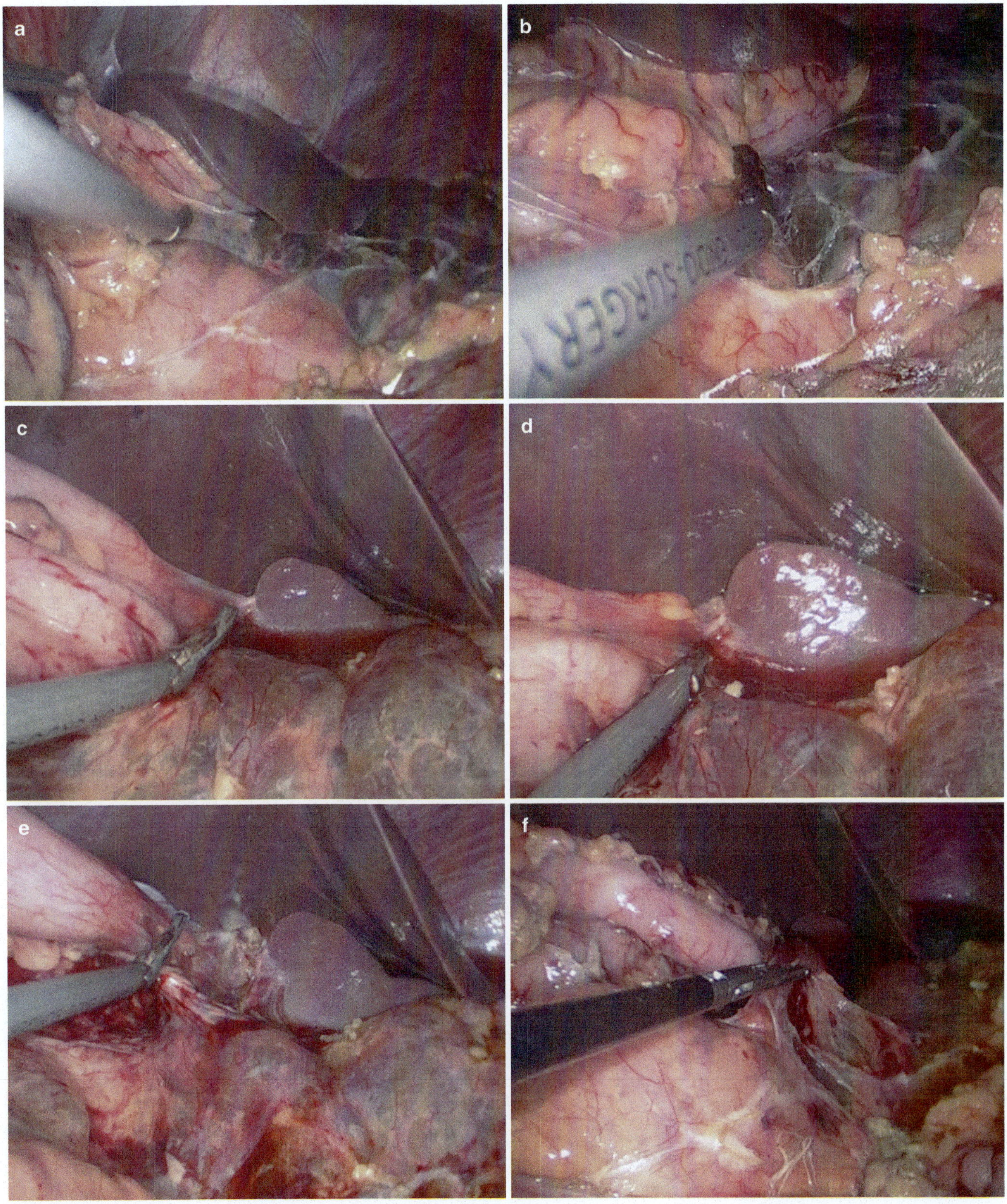

Fig. 6.9

3. Dissection of the pancreas.
   The transverse mesocolon was retracted downwards to fully expose the lower margin of the pancreas (Fig. 6.10a–g).

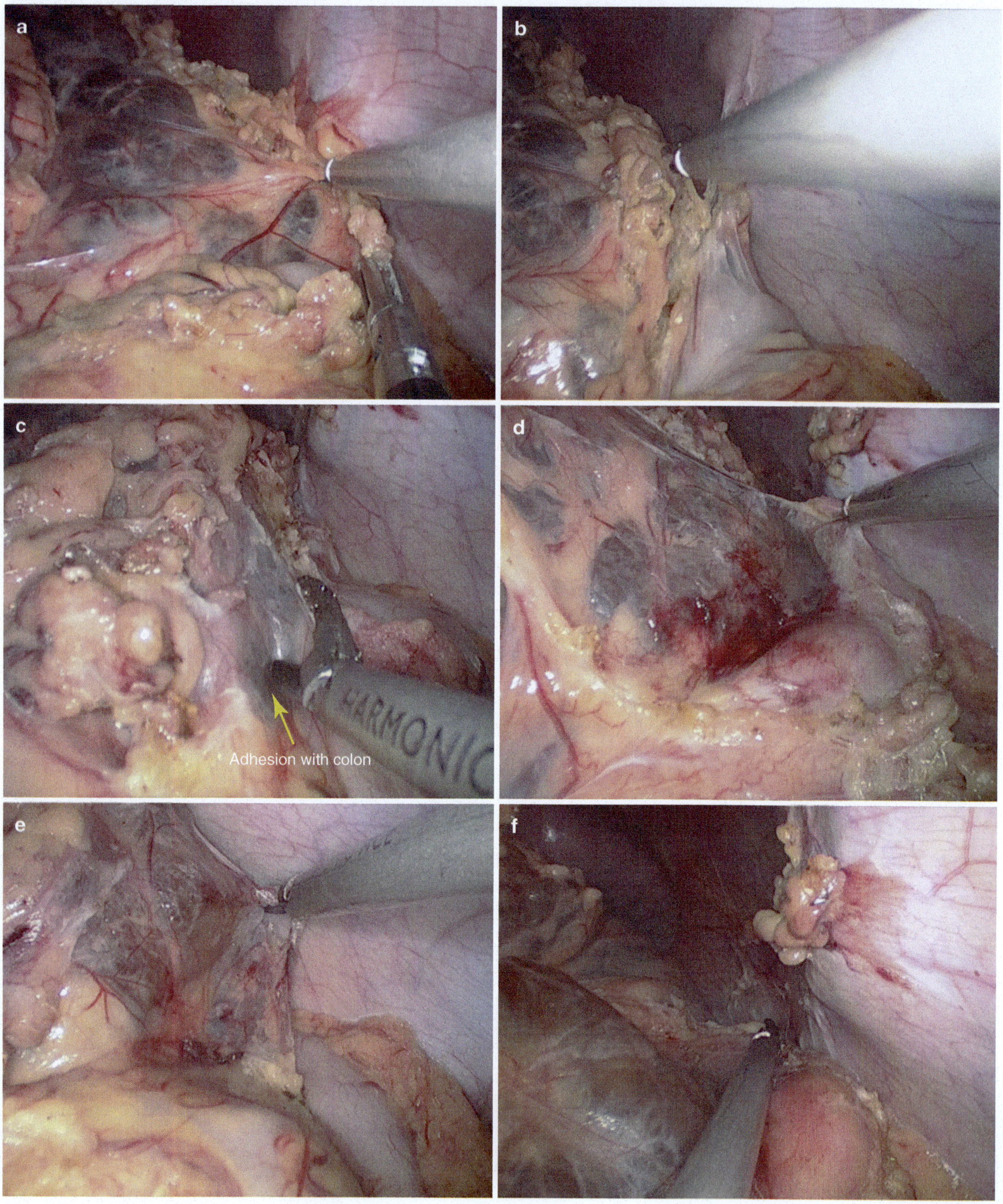

Fig. 6.10

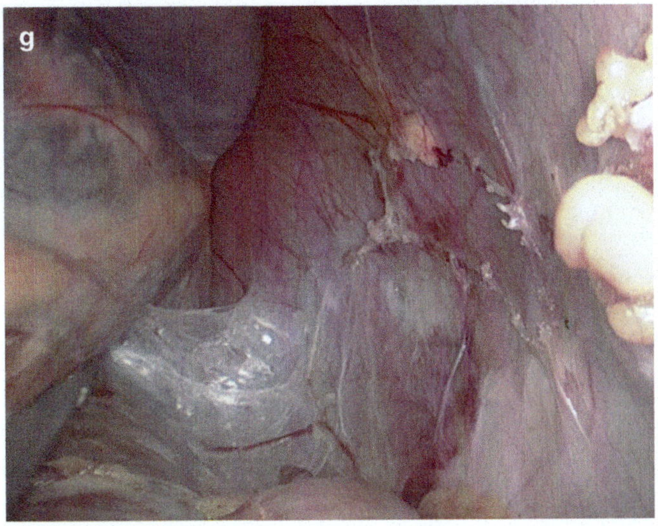

Fig. 6.10 (continued)

The loose connective tissues behind the pancreas was mobilized by using the harmonic scalpel to expand the posterior pancreatic space (Fig. 6.11a–h).

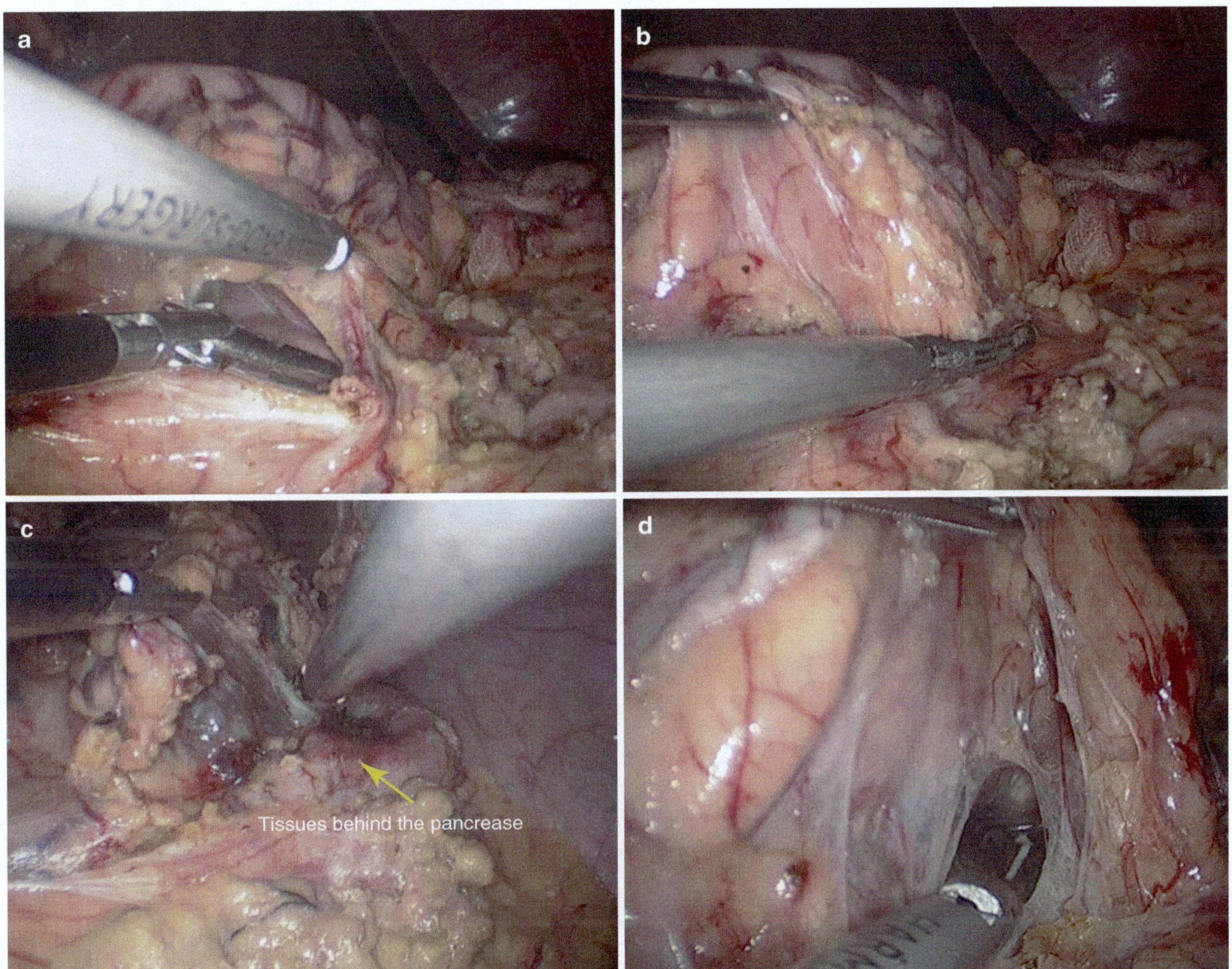

Fig. 6.11

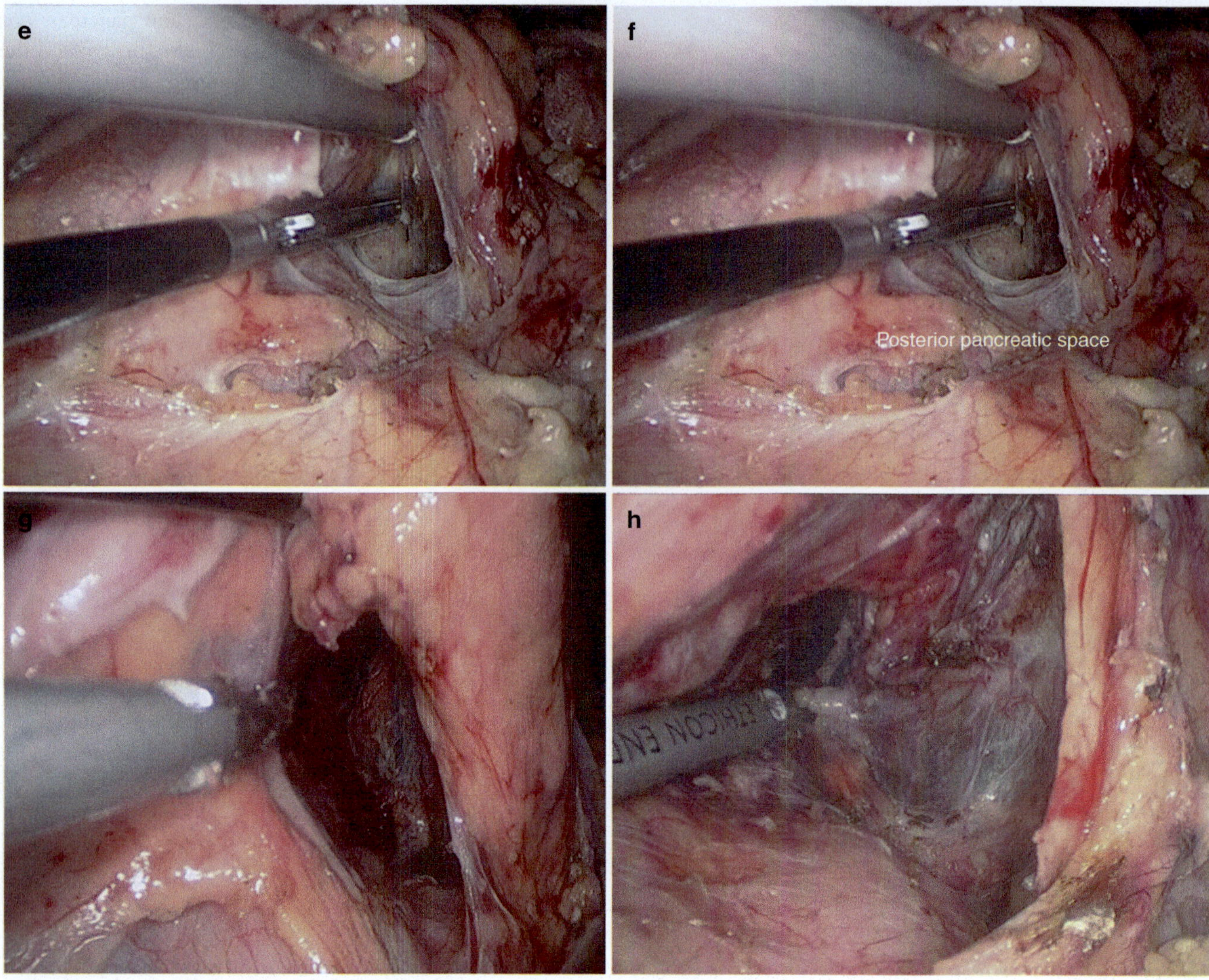

Fig. 6.11 (continued)

4. Dissection of distal pancreas and spleen.
   The division of the splenic artery was performed first so as to reduce the vascular supply at the level of the spleen, hence reducing its volume. The origin of the splenic vein was identified, and then ligated and dissected. After the superior part of gastrosplenic ligament, splenophrenic ligament and splenorenal ligament was respectively dissected, the spleen was freed (Fig. 6.12a–j).

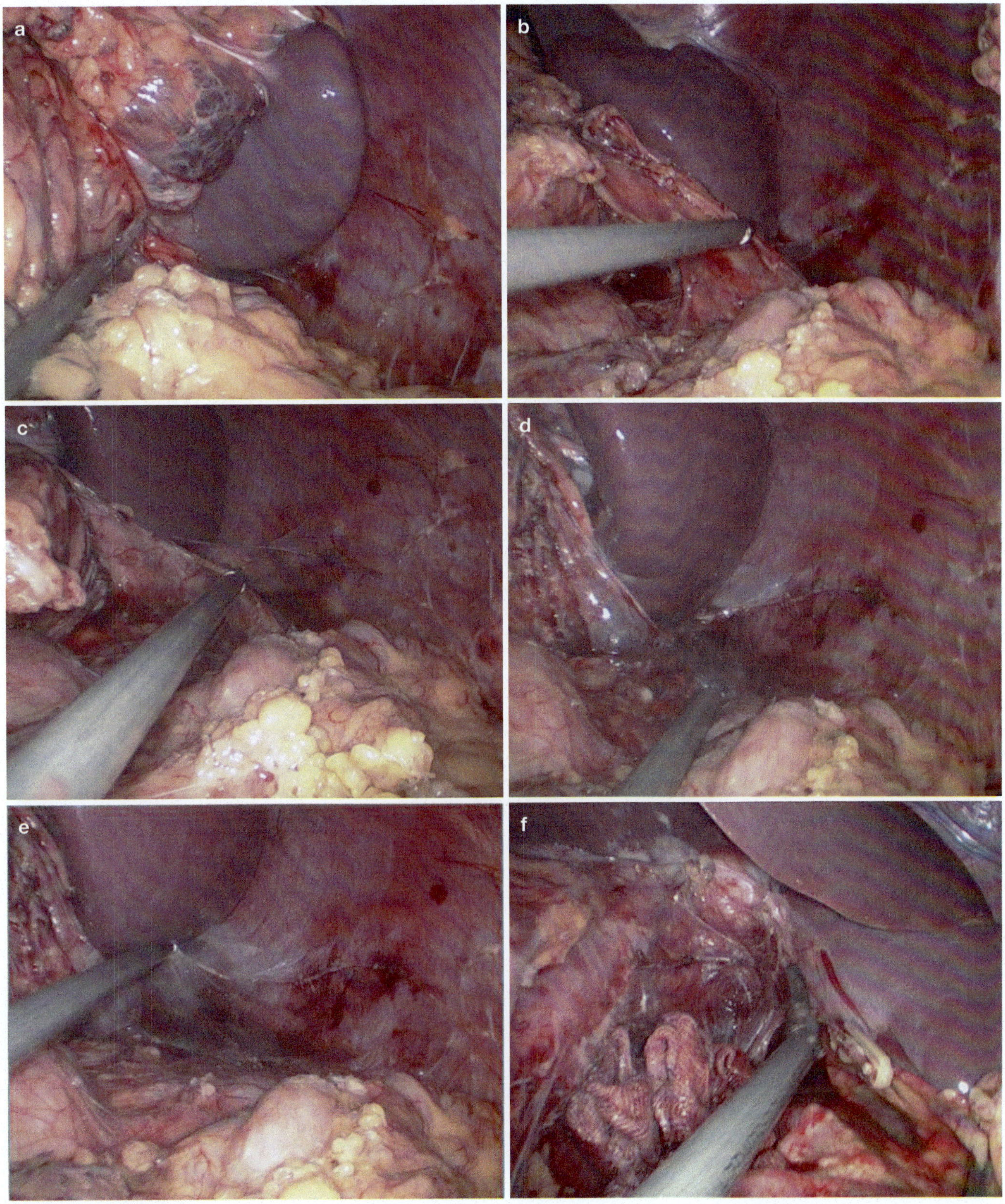

Fig. 6.12

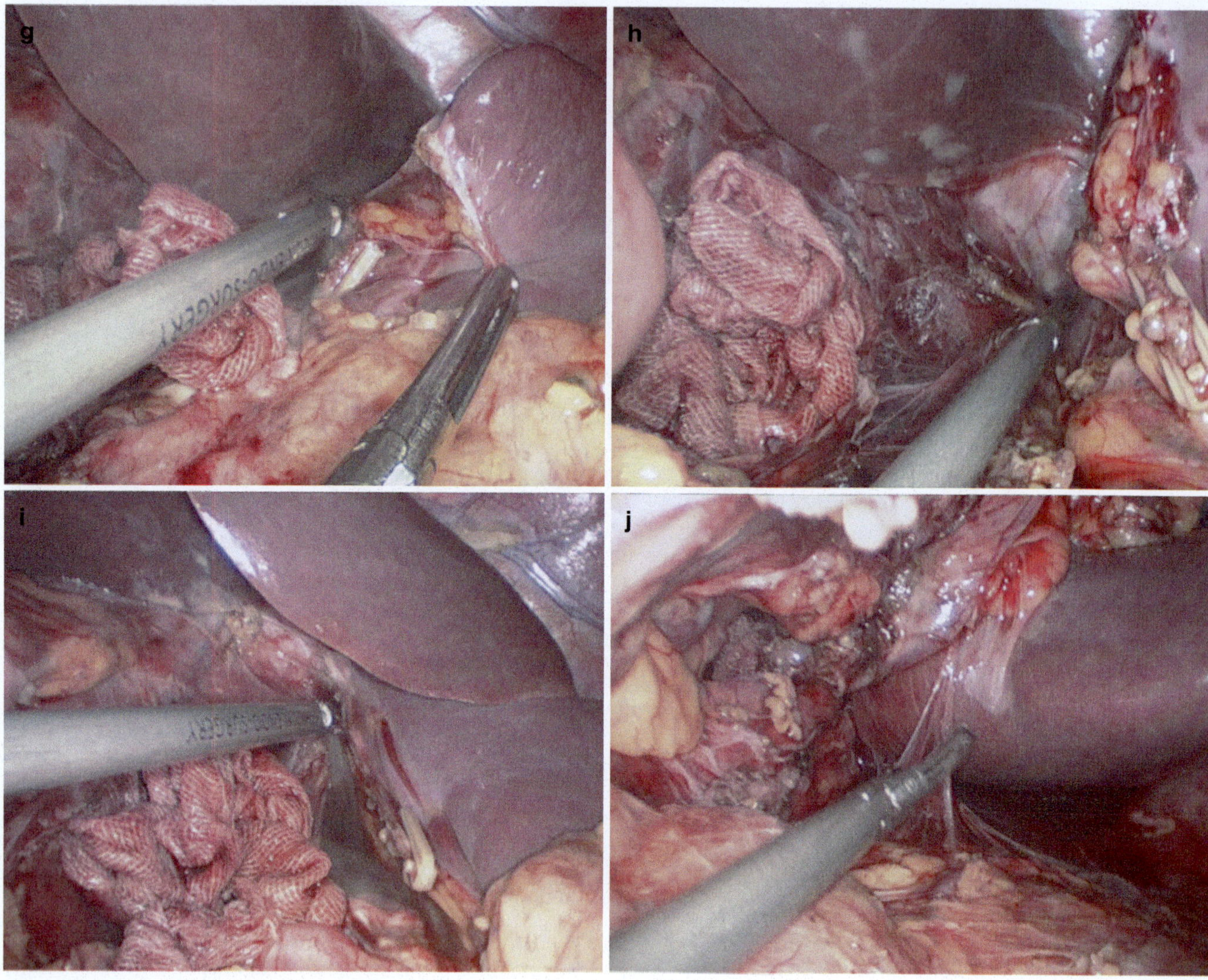

Fig. 6.12 (continued)

5. Transection of the pancreas.
Transection of the pancreas along the neck was created using the endoscopic linear stapler. The splenic vessels were transected simultaneously during the transection (Fig. 6.13a–h).

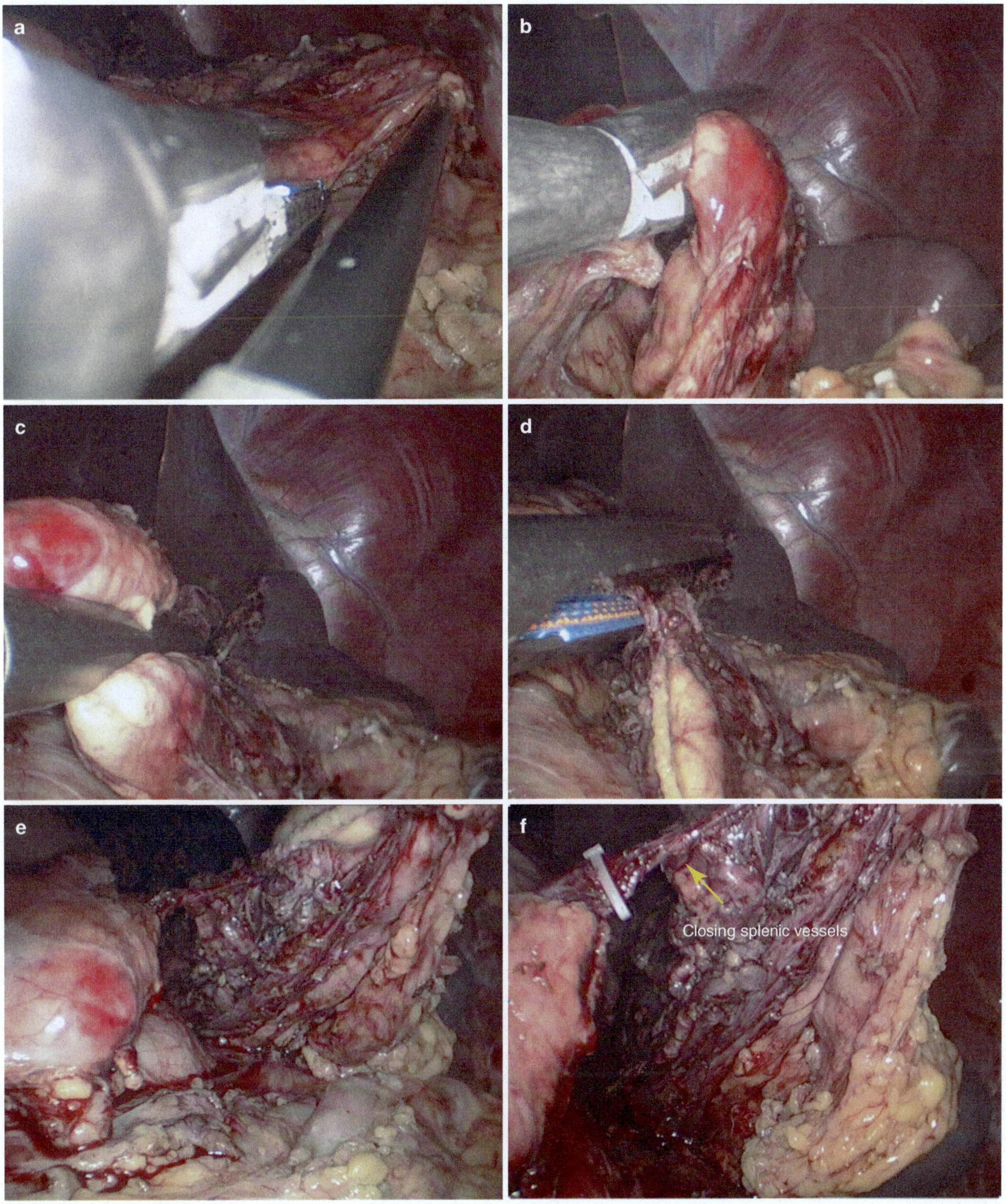

Fig. 6.13

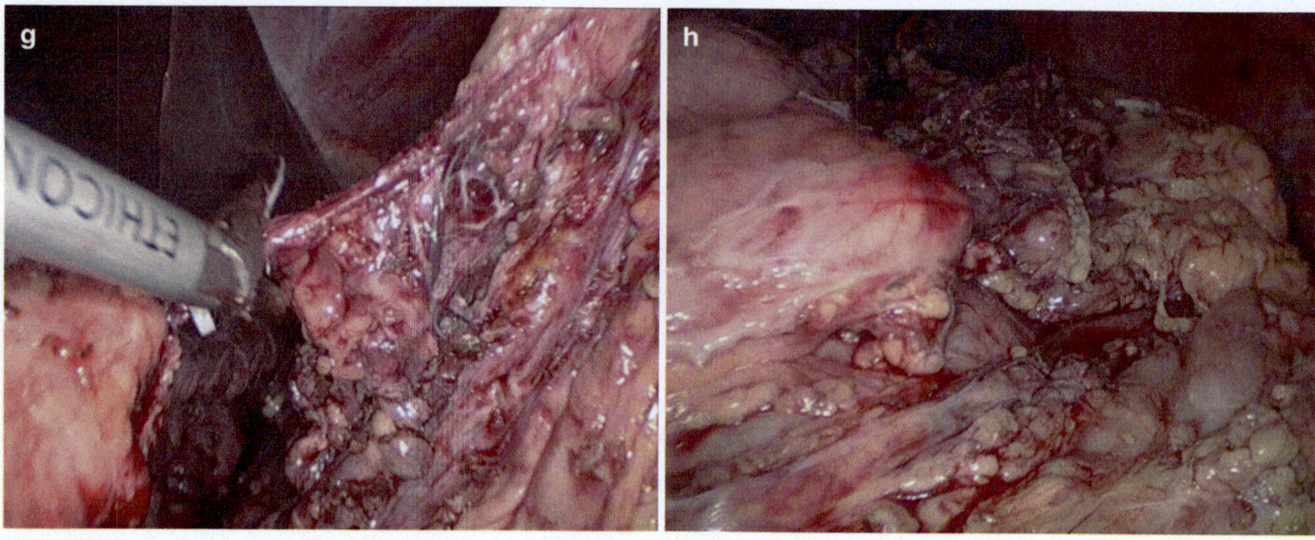

Fig. 6.13 (continued)

6. Retrieval of the specimen.
Once the distal pancreas was dissected in the way as formerly described, the specimen was removed in a plastic bag through the umbilical incision. A careful hemostatic control was performed at the level of the stump of the splenic artery and of the splenic vein (Fig. 6.14a, b).

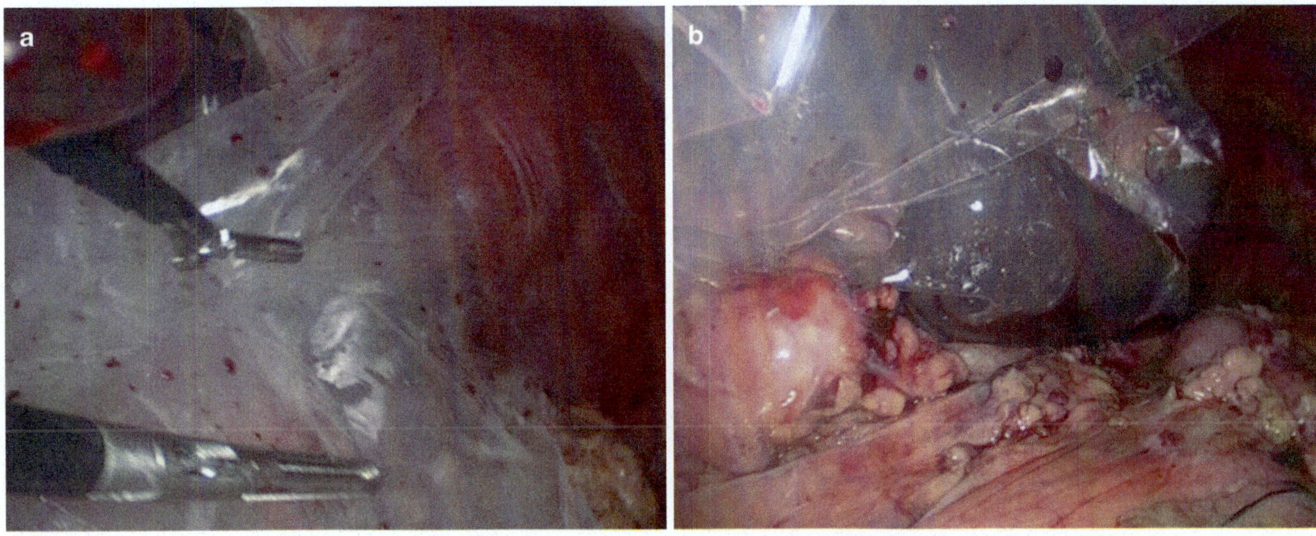

Fig. 6.14

7. Irrigation and drainage.
   After final inspection for the site of bleeding, aided by saline irrigation, the stump of the pancreas was reinforced with glue. The drainage tube was placed at the level of the splenic bed (Fig. 6.15a–d).

6.2.7 Tips and Tricks

1. Several prolene straight needles stay sutures may be placed superficially to the posterior gastric wall and slinged to the anterior abdominal wall to expose the pancreas.
2. Intraoperative laparoscopic ultrasound may be used to confirm the lesion and that no other lesion was present.

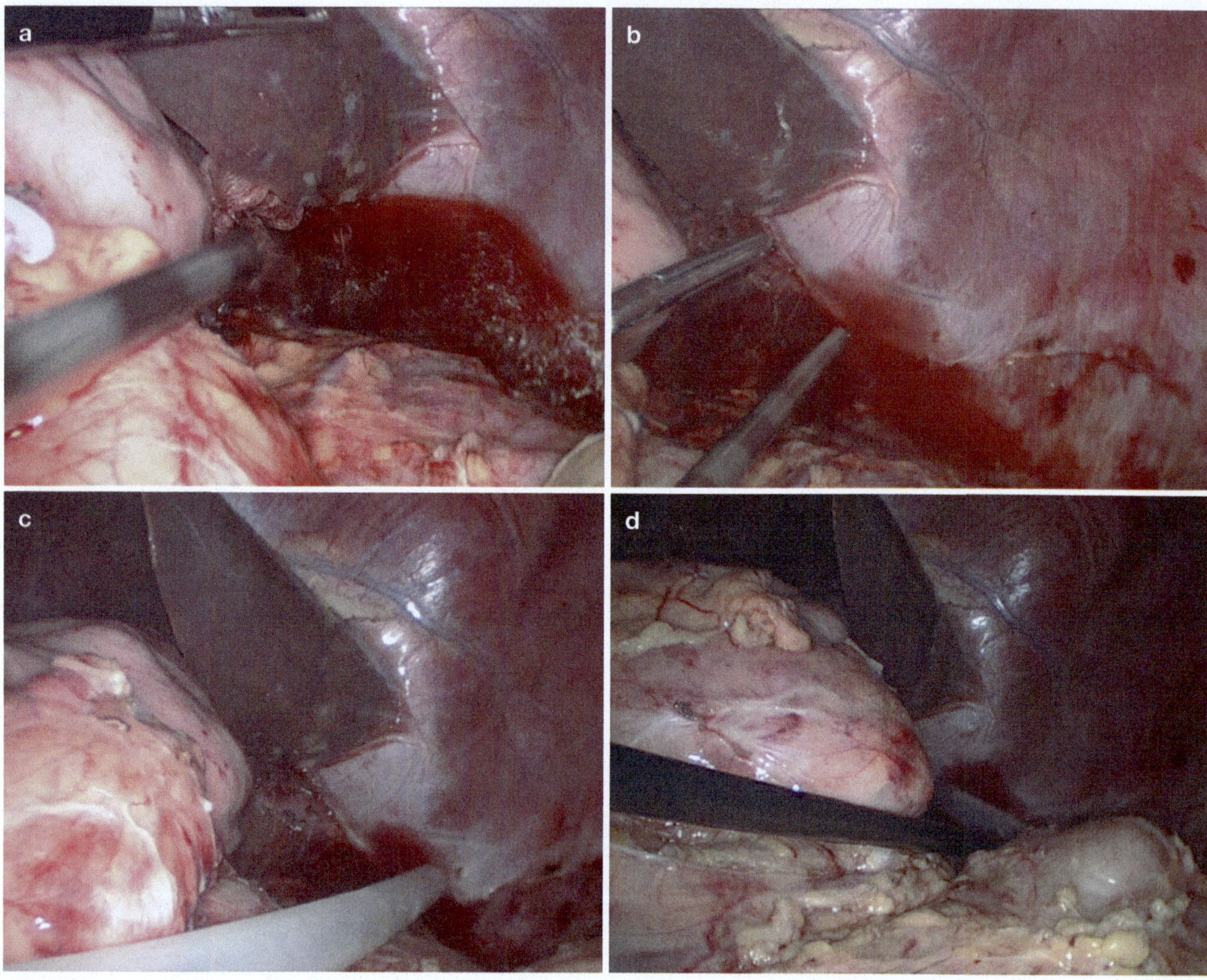

Fig. 6.15

6.3 Laparoscopic Surgery for Pancreatic Pseudocyst

6.3.1 Indications and Case Selection

1. Symptomatic pseudocyst greater than 6 cm in size that have been present for more than 6 weeks.
2. Pseudocyst with complications such as infection, hemorrhage, rupture, obstruction.
3. Suspicion of carcinoma requires biopsy and inspection of the pseudocyst wall.
4. Consideration for an easier reoperation when attempting more extensive debridement or subtotal pancreatic resection due to its minimally invasion to other intra-abdominal tissue.

6.3.2 Contraindications

1. Communication of the pseudocyst with the main pancreatic duct is not a contraindication to laparoscopic drainage, except in patients with multiple pancreatic duct strictures.
2. Patients with relatively operative contraindications should also be ruled out.

6.3.3 Major Instruments or Energy Sources

1. Laparoscopy System.
2. Holding forceps.
3. Harmonic scalpel.
4. Endoscopic Linear Stapler.

6.3.4 Team Setup, Anesthesia and Position

It is the same as Sect. 6.1.4.

6.3.5 Key Steps

1. Exploration of the abdominal cavity.
2. Exposure of pancreatic pseudocyst.
3. Dissection of loop of jejunum .
4. Cystojejunal anastomosis.
5. Anastomosis of jejunum and jejunum extracorporeally.
6. Irrigation and drainage.

6.3.6 Surgical Techniques

1. Exploration of the abdominal cavity.
   Pancreatic pseudocyst is usually secondary to acute pancreatitis that leads to abdominal adhesions. So a thorough abdominal exploration is needed to find out the size and the thickness of the cyst as well as its relationship with neighboring organs.
2. Exposure of the pancreatic pseudocyst.
   The patient was placed in reverse Trendlenburg position. The gastrocolic ligament was divided to expose pancreatic pseudocyst (Fig. 6.16a–d).

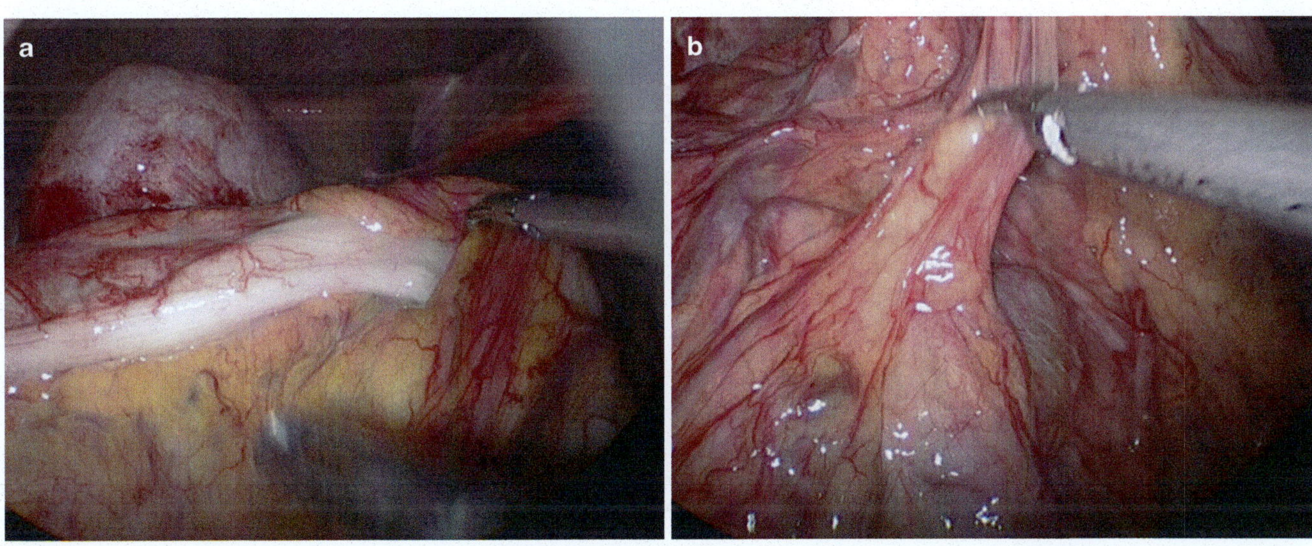

Fig. 6.16

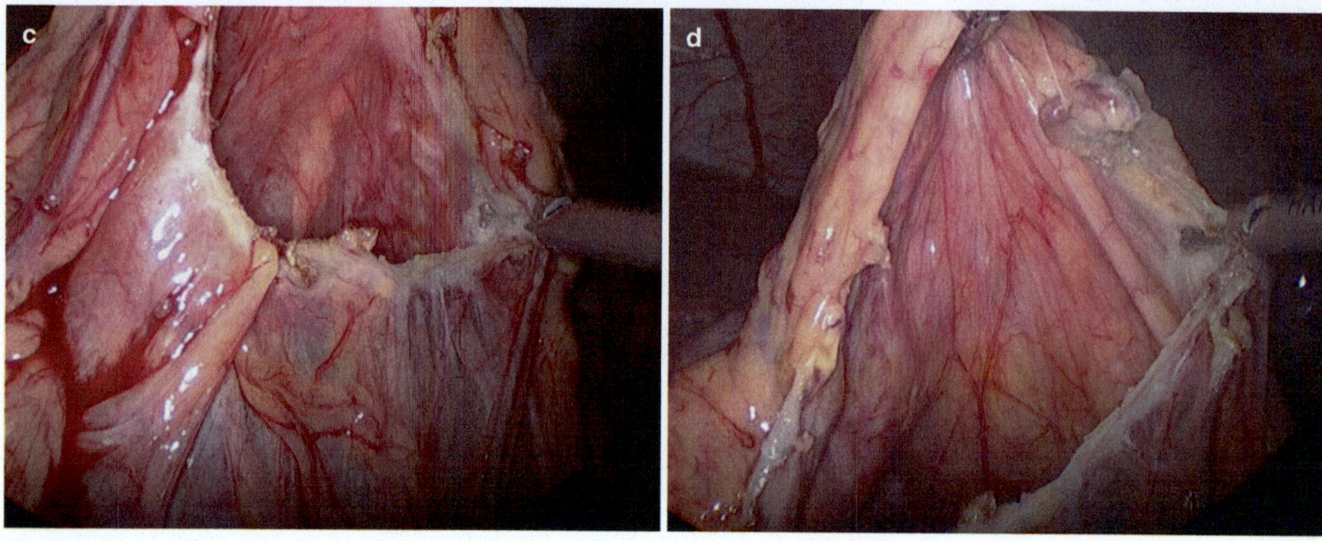

Fig. 6.16 (continued)

A puncture needle was used to extract the hydatid fluid. Once a cystojejunal anastomosis was decided, the cyst was opened with the hydatid fluid thoroughly drained out (Fig. 6.17a–e).

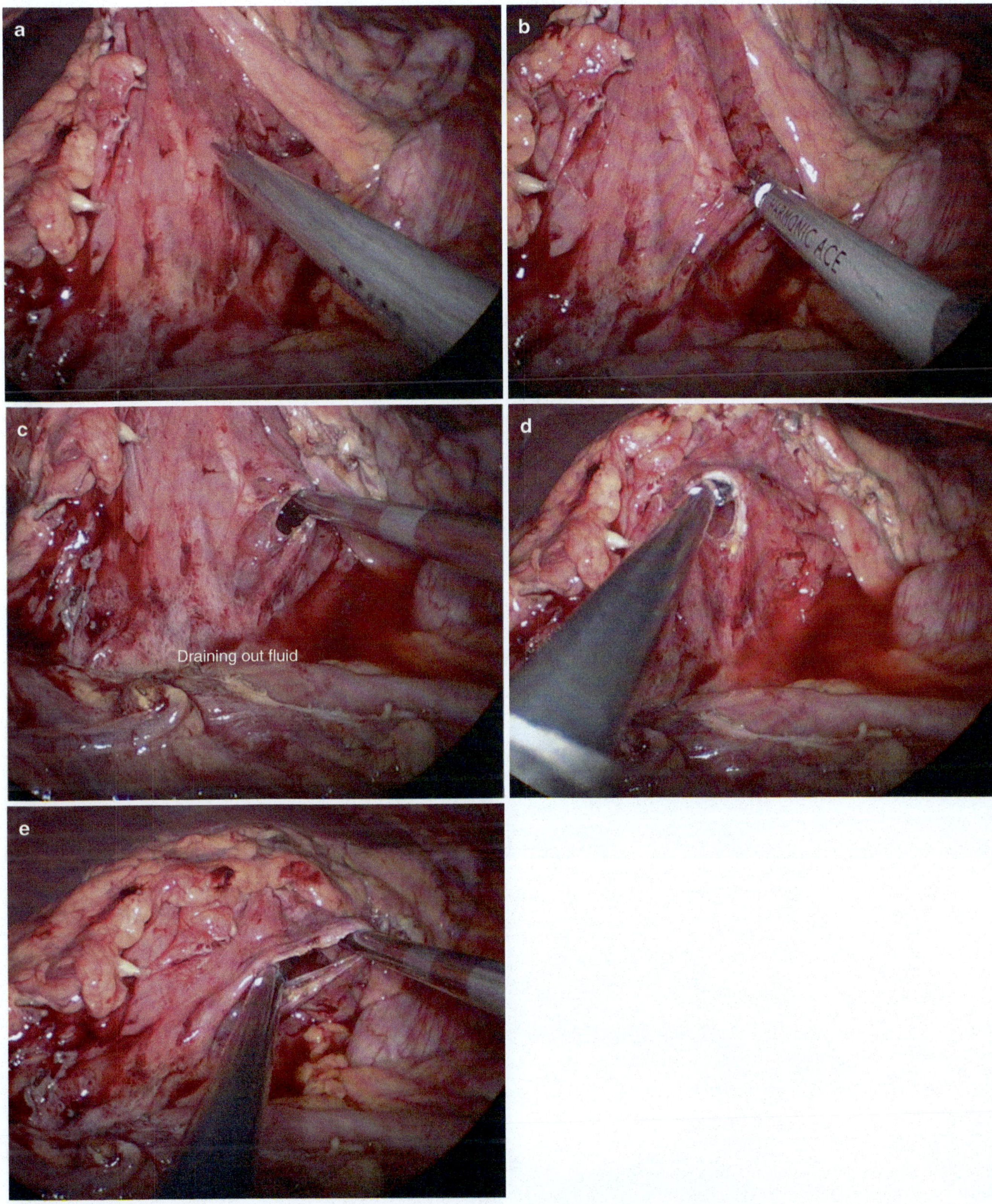

Fig. 6.17

3. Dissection of loop of jejunum.
   The proximal mesojejunum was dissociated. The proximal jejunum was disconnected by an endoscopic stapler with the distal stump lifted towards the cyst for anastomosis (Fig. 6.18a–h).

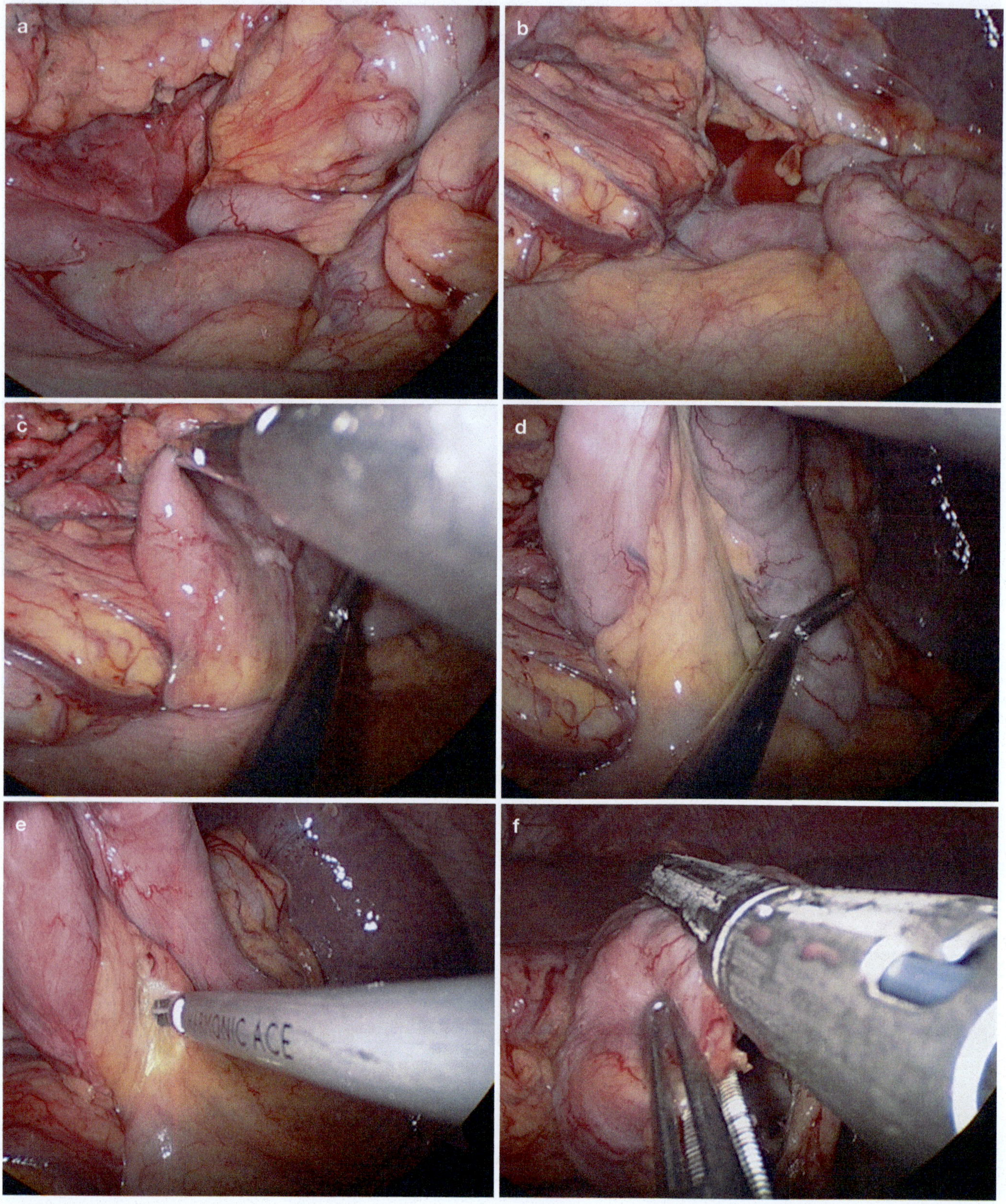

Fig. 6.18

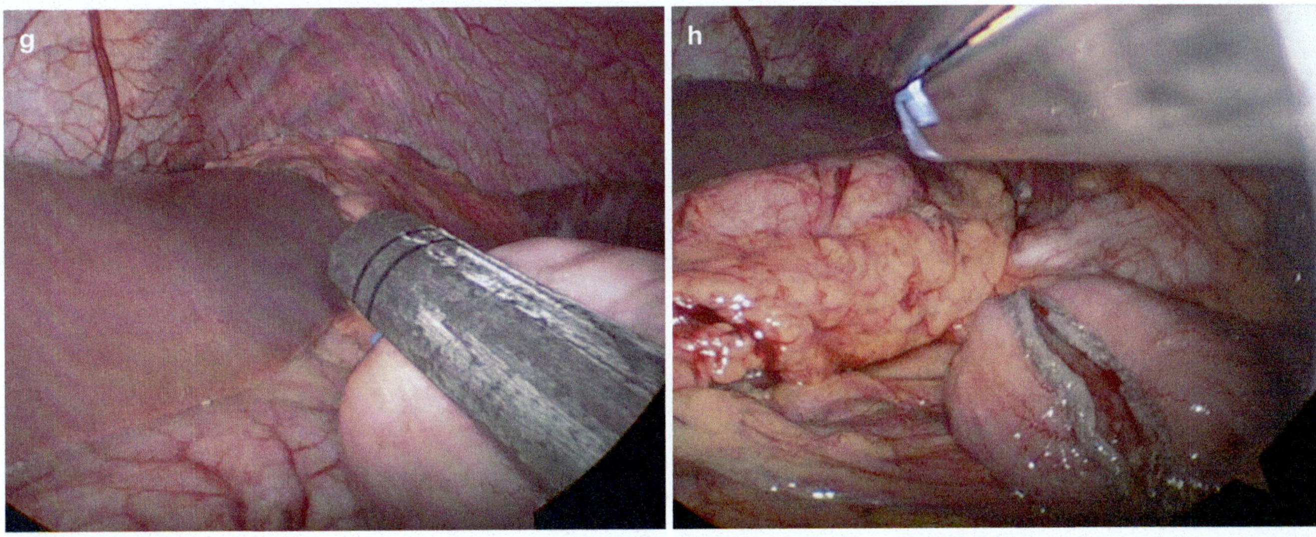

Fig. 6.18 (continued)

4. Cystojejunal anastomosis.

The distal jejunum was lifted towards the cyst with the enteric cavity opened by harmonic scalpel. In a step-by-step manner, an endoscopic stapler was inserted in both the incisions on the cyst and jejunum. The wall of the cyst and the anti-mesenteric side of the jejunum were put together. Then the endoscopic stapler was closed and fired (Fig. 6.19a–h).

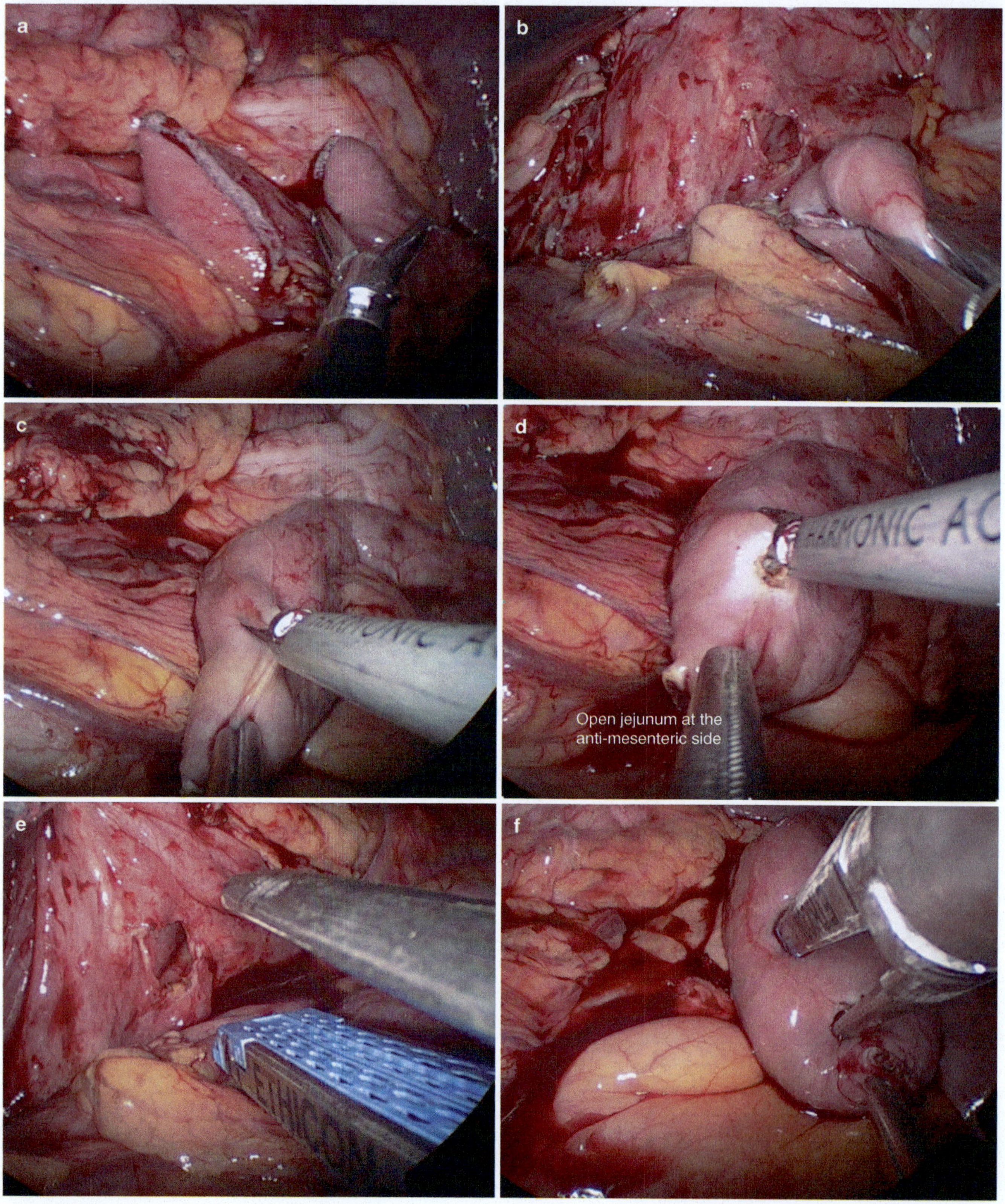

Fig. 6.19

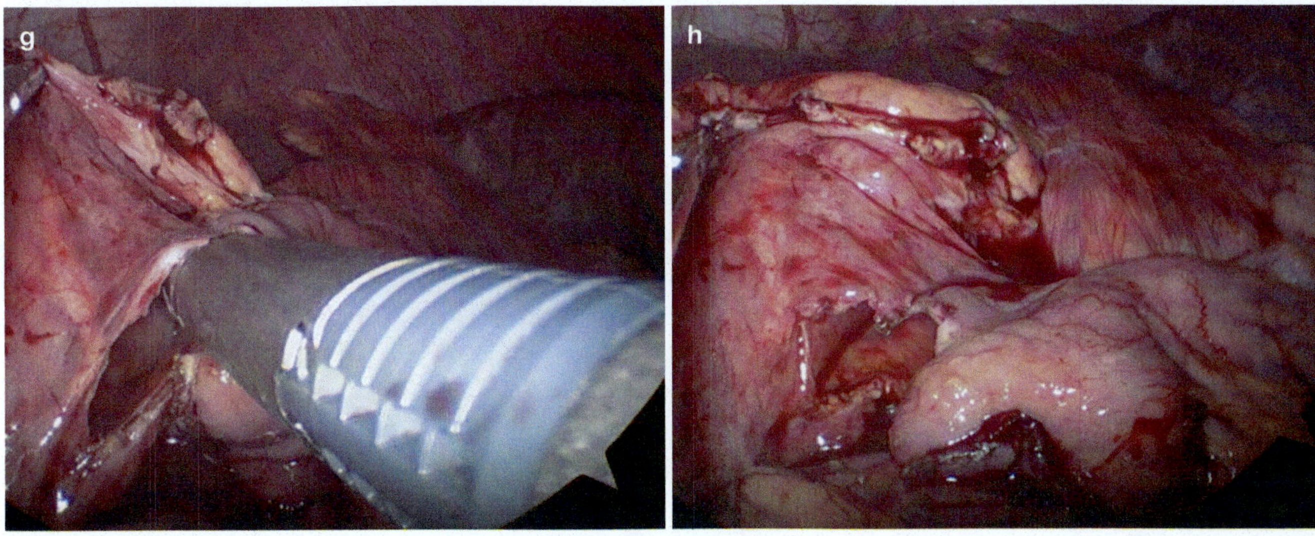

Fig. 6.19 (continued)

The common incisions were joined together and closed by running suture with 3/0 absorbable suture (Fig. 6.20a–e).

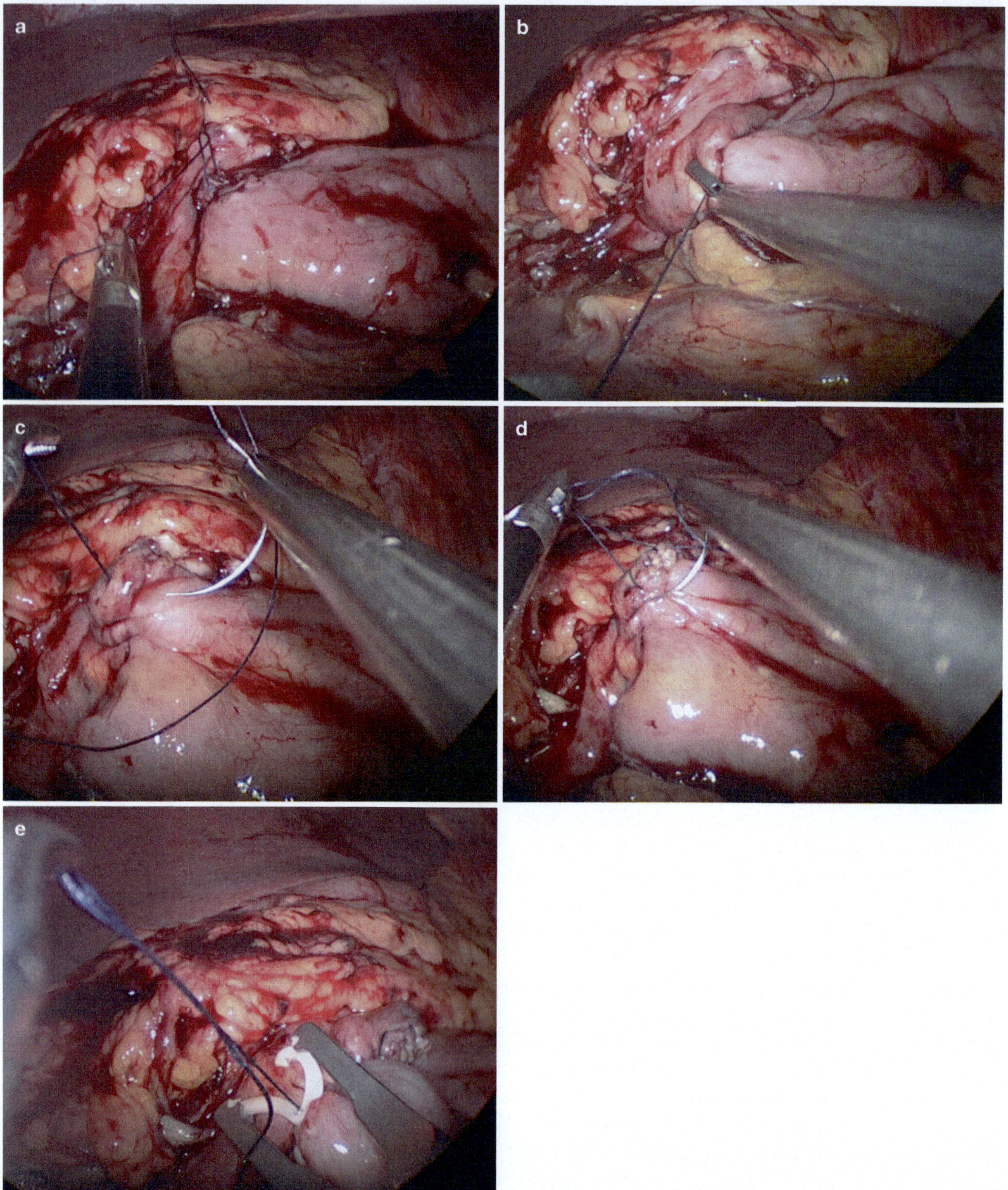

Fig. 6.20

5. Anastomosis of jejunum and jejunum extracorporeally. The proximal jejunum and intended anastomotic distal jejunum were marked by laparoscopic suture. Both were lifted out of the enlarged umbilical incision and then an extracorporeal intestinal anastomosis was performed. The intestine was then put back into the abdominal cavity and the peritoneum incision was closed (Fig. 6.21a–f).

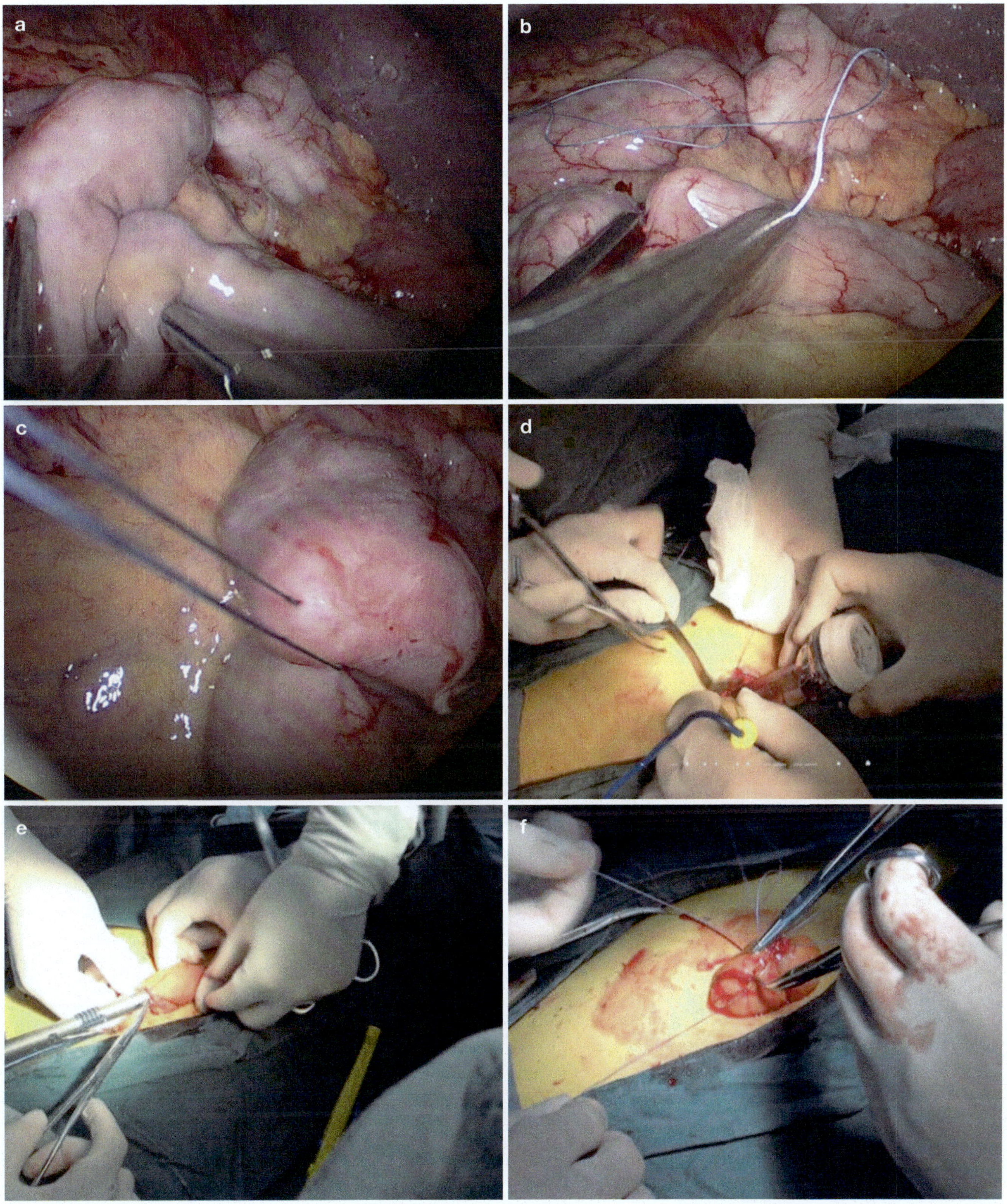

Fig. 6.21

6. Irrigation and drainage.
   The abdominal cavity was suctioned and a closed suction drain was placed beside the anastomotic stoma through the incision at umbilicus (Fig. 6.22a–d).

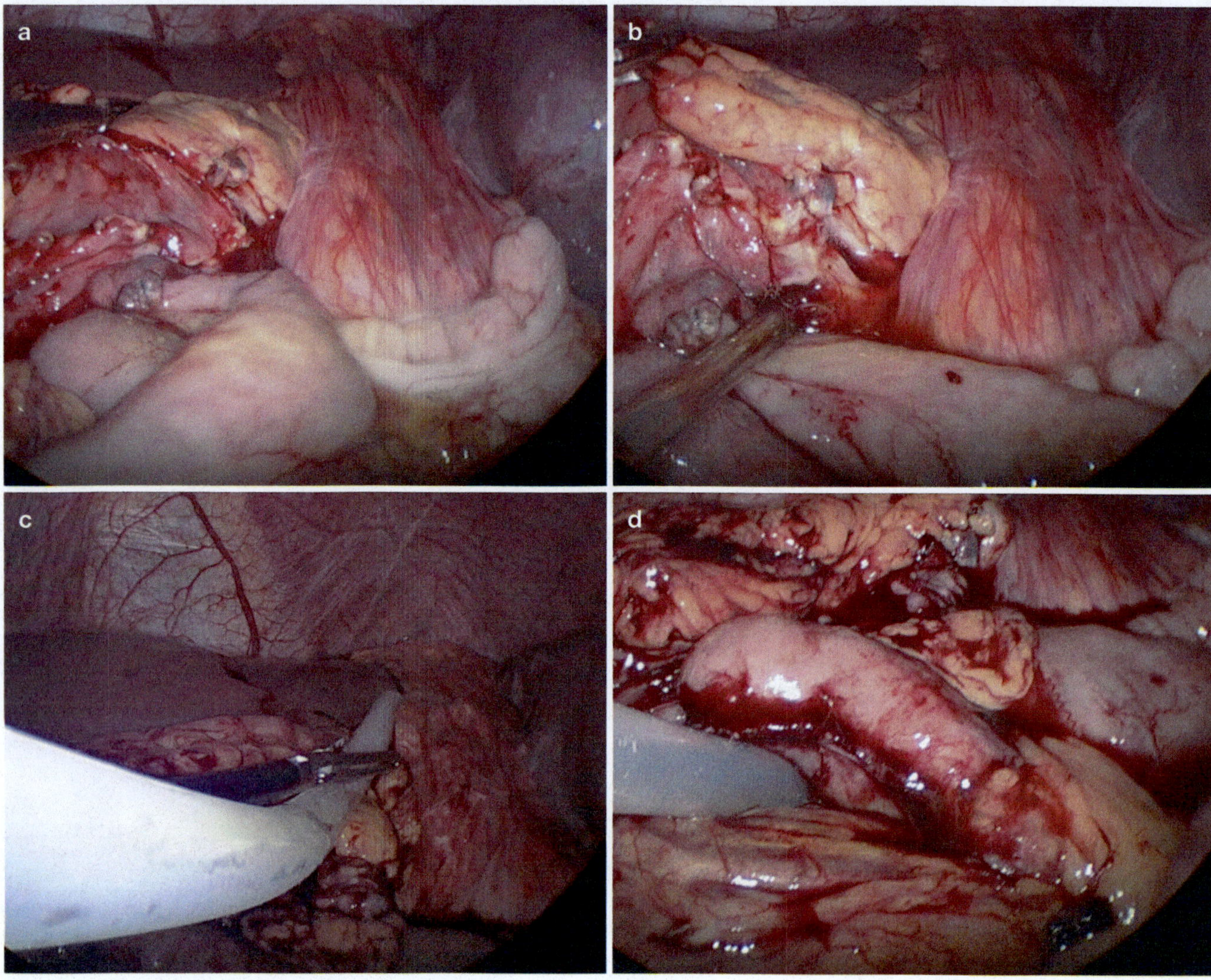

Fig. 6.22

6.4 Complications Analysis and Management

6.4.1 Haemorrhage

Intraoperative bleeding can be induced by the wrong treatment of peripancreatic vessels. Massive bleeding is commonly caused by the injury of splenic vessels during the dissection of the back of pancreas due to the lacking of essential assistant retraction in SILS. If the splenectomy is simultaneous, firstly, the splenic artery should be dissected and controlled to reduce the volume of spleen, which can decrease the haemorrhage in spleen dissection. The position of splenic artery is fixed, so it is not difficult to be handled. However, for spleen-preserving surgery, the key is the treatment of splenic vein. The texture of pancreas is crisp and has abundant blood supply, so the intraopertive hemostasis must be definite. The liner stapler is a nice choice for dissecting the splenic vessels and pancreas with excellent hemostatic effect of pancreatic stump.

In internal drainage of pancreatic cyst, anastomotic bleeding is common in the anastomosis of pancreatic cyst and intestinal wall. Therefore, after sealing, the anastomotic stoma should be examined carefully. Active bleeding can be stopped by absorbed suture.

6.4.2 Pancreatic Leakage

In SILS pancreatic procedure, stapler entering the abdomen via umbilical Trocar and being vertical to the direction of pancreas makes it suitable to dissect the pancreas. This is the advantage of SILS. But the vertical position to pancreas should be carefully kept to prevent the tearing of pancreas. And in internal drainage of pancreatic cyst, the residual incision of anastomosis must be closely sutured. Somatostation and a smooth drainage are necessary for pancreatic leakage.

6.4.3 Anastomotic Leakage

In SILS internal drainage of pancreatic cyst, if the formation of cyst is less than 6 weeks, the wall of pancreatic cyst is not mature. In addition, if the thickness of it is less than 0.5cm and inflammatory edema around pancreas is severe, the anastomotic leakage will be possible. The length of anastomotic stoma should be moderate and only a single bite should be enough.

6.4.4 Splenic Infarction

In SILS pancreatic spleen-preserving surgery, because of the limitation of surgical field vision and lacking of assistant help, the vessels of hilus lienis may be injured when dissecting the distal pancreas. In the procedure, the splenic vessels should be carefully dissected and protected to avoid blindly clamping the splenic vessels, which may induce ischemic splenic infarction.

References

1. Kim HJ, D'Angelica M, Hiotis SP, Shoup M, Weber SM. Laparoscopic staging for liver, biliary, pancreas, and gastric cancer. Curr Probl Surg. 2007;44(4):228–69.
2. Ahmed SI, Bochkarev V, Oleynikov D, Sasson AR. Patients with pancreatic adenocarcinoma benefit from staging laparoscopy. J Laparoendosc Adv Surg Tech A. 2006;16:458–63.
3. Hauters P, Weerts J, Navez B, Champault G, Peillon C, Totte E, Barthelemy R, Siriser F. Laparoscopic treatment of pancreatic pseudocysts. Surg Endosc. 2004;18:1645–8.
4. Toniato A, Meduri F, Foletto M, Avogaro A, Pelizzo M. Laparoscopic treatment of benign insulinomas localized in the body and tail of the pancreas: a single-center experience. World J Surg. 2006;30:1916–9.
5. Melotti G, Butturini G, Piccoli M, Casetti L, Bassi C, Mullineris B, Lazzaretti MG, Pederzoli P. Laparoscopic distal pancreatectomy: results on a consecutive series of 58 patients. Ann Surg. 2007;246:77–82.
6. Uranues S, Alimoglu O, Todoric B, Toprak N, Auer T, Rondon L, Sauseng G, Pfeifer J. Laparoscopic resection of the pancreatic tail with splenic preservation. Am J Surg. 2006;192:257–61.
7. Palanivelu C, Jani K, Senthilnathan P, Parthasarathi R, Rajapandian S, Madhankumar MV. Laparoscopic pancreaticoduodenectomy: technique and outcomes. J Am Coll Surg. 2007;205:222–30.
8. Park A, Schwartz R, Tandan V, Anvari M. Laparoscopic pancreatic surgery. Am J Surg. 1999;177:158–63.
9. Finney JM. VII. Resection of the pancreas: report of a case. Ann Surg. 1910;51:818–29.
10. Soper NJ, Brunt LM, Dunnegan DL, Meininger TA. Laparoscopic distal pancreatectomy in the porcine model. Surg Endosc. 1994;8:57–60.
11. Cuschieri A, Jakimowicz JJ, van Spreeuwel J. Laparoscopic distal 70 % pancreatectomy and splenectomy for chronic pancreatitis. Ann Surg. 1996;223:280–5.
12. Gagner M, Pomp A, Herrera MF. Early experience with laparoscopic resections of islet cell tumors. Surgery. 1996;120:1051–4.
13. Sussman LA, Christie R, Whittle DE. Laparoscopic excision of distal pancreas including insulinoma. Aust N Z J Surg. 1996;66(6):414–6.
14. Kooby DA, Gillespie T, Bentrem D, Nakeeb A, Schmidt MC, Merchant NB, Parikh AA, Martin 2nd RC, Scoggins CR, Ahmad S, Kim HJ, Park J, Johnston F, Strouch MJ, Menze A, Rymer J, McClaine R, Strasberg SM, Talamonti MS, Staley CA, McMasters KM, Lowy AM, Byrd-Sellers J, Wood WC, Hawkins WG. Left-sided pancreatectomy: a multicenter comparison of laparoscopic and open approaches. Ann Surg. 2008;248:438–46.
15. Røsok BI, Marangos IP, Kazaryan AM, Rosseland AR, Buanes T, Mathisen O, Edwin B. Single-centre experience of laparoscopic pancreatic surgery. Br J Surg. 2010;97:902–9.
16. Kneuertz PJ, Patel SH, Chu CK, Fisher SB, Maithel SK, Sarmiento JM, Weber SM, Staley CA, Kooby DA. Laparoscopic distal pancreatectomy: trends and lessons learned through an 11-year experience. J Am Coll Surg. 2012;215:167–76.
17. Jin T, Altaf K, Xiong JJ, Huang W, Javed MA, Mai G, Liu XB, Hu WM, Xia Q. A systematic review and meta-analysis of studies comparing laparoscopic and open distal pancreatectomy. HPB (Oxford). 2012;14:711–24.

18. Barbaros U, Sümer A, Demirel T, Karakullukçu N, Batman B, Içscan Y, Sarıçam G, Serin K, Loh WL, Dinççağ A, Mercan S. Single incision laparoscopic pancreas resection for pancreatic metastasis of renal cell carcinoma. JSLS. 2010;14:566–70.
19. Kuroki T, Adachi T, Okamoto T, Kanematsu T. Single-incision laparoscopic distal pancreatectomy. Hepatogastroenterology. 2011;58(107–108):1022–4.
20. Chang SK, Lomanto D, Mayasari M. Single-port laparoscopic spleen preserving distal pancreatectomy. Minim Invasive Surg. 2012;2012:197429.
21. Misawa T, Ito R, Futagawa Y, Fujiwara Y, Kitamura H, Tsutsui N, Shiba H, Wakiyama S, Ishida Y, Yanaga K. Single-incision laparoscopic distal pancreatectomy with or without splenic preservation: how we do it. Asian J Endosc Surg. 2012;5:195–9.

Splenic Surgery

7

Abstract

Splenectomy is a very common surgical procedure. Indications for splenectomy vary, therefore the operative steps, difficulty and post-operative results differ. With the development of laparoscopic surgical technique and improvement of surgical instruments, single-incision laparoscopic splenectomy has been used in clinic. Barbaros U et al. reported the index case of laparoendoscopic single-site splenectomy in 2009 (Barbaros and Dinççağ, Gastrointest Surg 13:1520–1523, 2009). Thereafter, this procedure has been adapted in clinical practice by some institutions (Vatansev and Ece, Surg Laparosc Endosc Percutan Tech 19:e225–e227, 2009; Malladi et al., JSLS 13:601–604, 2009; Lagrand and Kehdy, Am Surg 76:E158–E159, 2010; Barbaros et al., Surg Laparosc Endosc Percutan Tech 20:306–311, 2010; Colon et al., JSLS 15:384–386, 2011; Bell et al., J Pediatr Surg 47:898–903, 2012; Dapri et al., Surg Endosc 25:3419–3422, 2011). We have reported the first case of laparoendoscopic single-site splenectomy in the treatment of traumatic rupture of the spleen in 2011 (Fan et al., Surg Innov 18:185–188, 2011) and hypersplenism secondary to portal hypertension in 2012 (Jing et al., Surg Innov, 2012).

We believe, in early series of highly selected patients, laparoendoscopic single-site splenectomy appears to be feasible and safe when performed by experienced laparoscopic surgeons. Despite technical difficulties, there may be potential benefits associated with single-incision over multiple-incision laparoscopic splenectomy but it is yet to be proven objectively.

Keywords

Splenectomy • Gastrocolic ligament • Splenogastric ligament • Splenocolic ligament • Splenorenal ligament • Phrenosplenic ligament • Spleen pedicle • Pericardial devascularization • Gastric coronary vein

S. Wu et al. (eds.), *Atlas of Single-Incision Laparoscopic Operations in General Surgery*,
DOI 10.1007/978-94-007-6955-7_7,

7.1 Laparoscopic Splenectomy

7.1.1 Indications and Case Selection

1. Patients with haematological systemic disorder, including idiopathic thrombocytopenia purpura (ITP), thalassemia, hereditary spherocytosis, hairy cell leukemia, myelofibrosis, or hereditary elliptocytosis, etc.
2. Patients with benign occupying lesion, including splenic haematoma, splenic multilocular cysts, etc.
3. Patients undergoing splenic trauma with stable blood pressure.

7.1.2 Contraindications

1. Absolute contraindications:
   (a) severe cardiorespiratory dysfunction.
   (b) inability to tolerate general anesthesia or pneumoperitoneum.
   (c) severe refractory coagulopathy.
2. Relative contraindications:
   (a) morbid obesity.
   (b) pregnancy.
   (c) patients with "frozen upper abdomen" due to previous surgery or peritonitis.
   (d) patients with megalosplenia (>30 cm in diameter).
   (e) arteriosteogenesis.

7.1.3 Major Instruments or Energy Sources

1. Laparoscopy System.
2. Holding forceps.
3. Harmonic scalpel.
4. Endoscopic Linear Stapler.

7.1.4 Team Setup, Anesthesia and Position

Under general anesthesia, the patient was placed in supine position with the legs apart. The position of surgeon, assistants and nurses is shown in Fig. 7.1.

Fig. 7.1

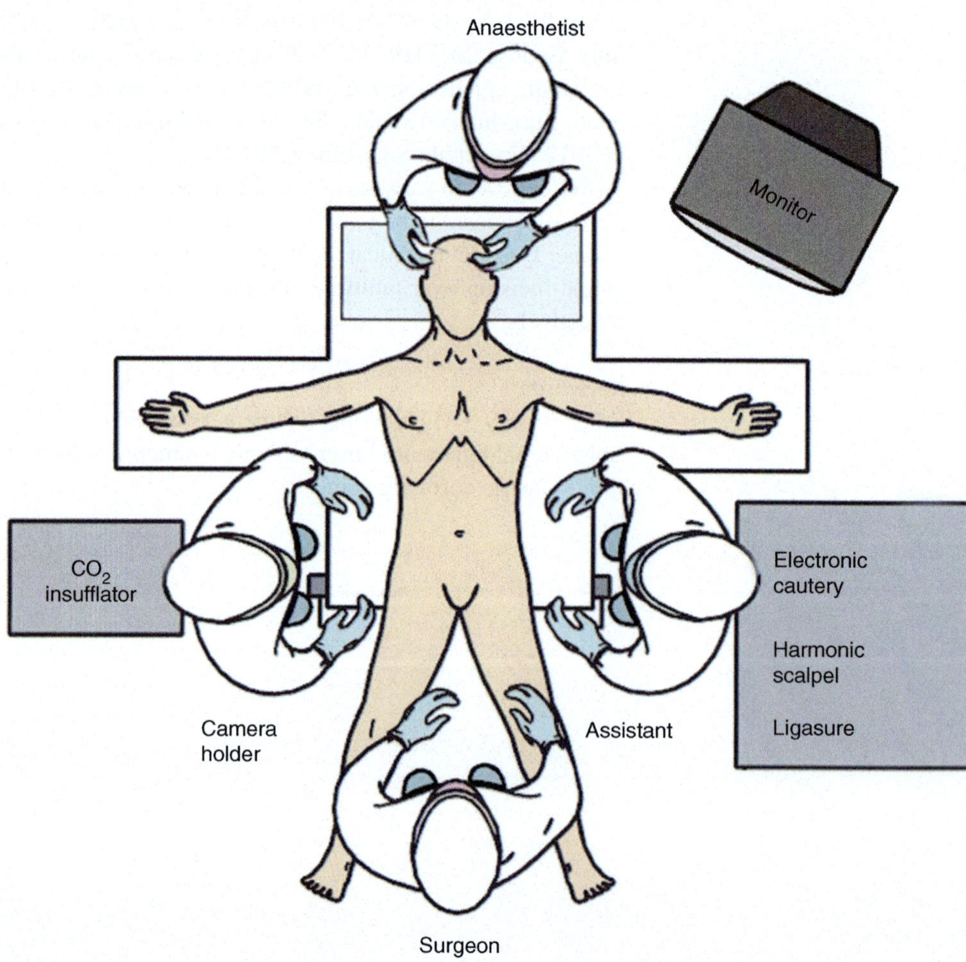

7.1.5 Key Steps

1. Dissection of gastrocolic ligament.
2. Dissection of splenogastric ligament.
3. Dissection of splenocolic ligament.
4. Dissection of splenorenal ligament.
5. Dissection of phrenosplenic ligament.
6. Dissection of splenic hilum and tail of pancreas.
7. Transection of spleen pedicle.
8. Retrieval of spleen.
9. Irrigation and drainage.

7.1.6 Surgical Techniques

1. Dissection of gastrocolic ligament.
   The patient was placed in reverse Trendlenburg position with a little tilt to the right in order to expose the spleen. The gastrocolic ligament was dissected with harmonic scalpel to expose the pancreas (Fig. 7.2a–d).

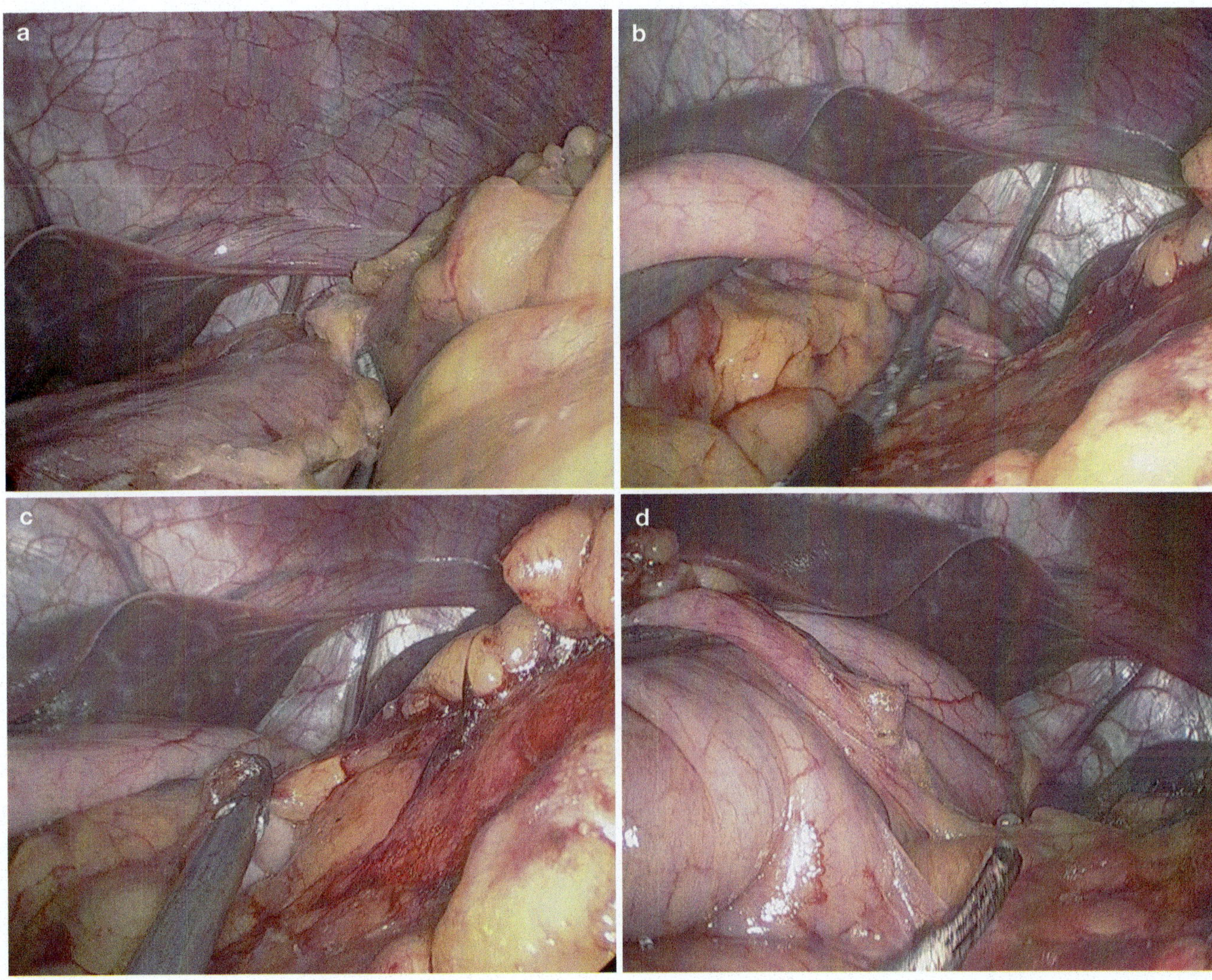

Fig. 7.2

2. Dissection of splenogastric ligament.
   The splenogastric ligament and short gastric vessels were divided with harmonic scalpel (Fig. 7.3a, b).

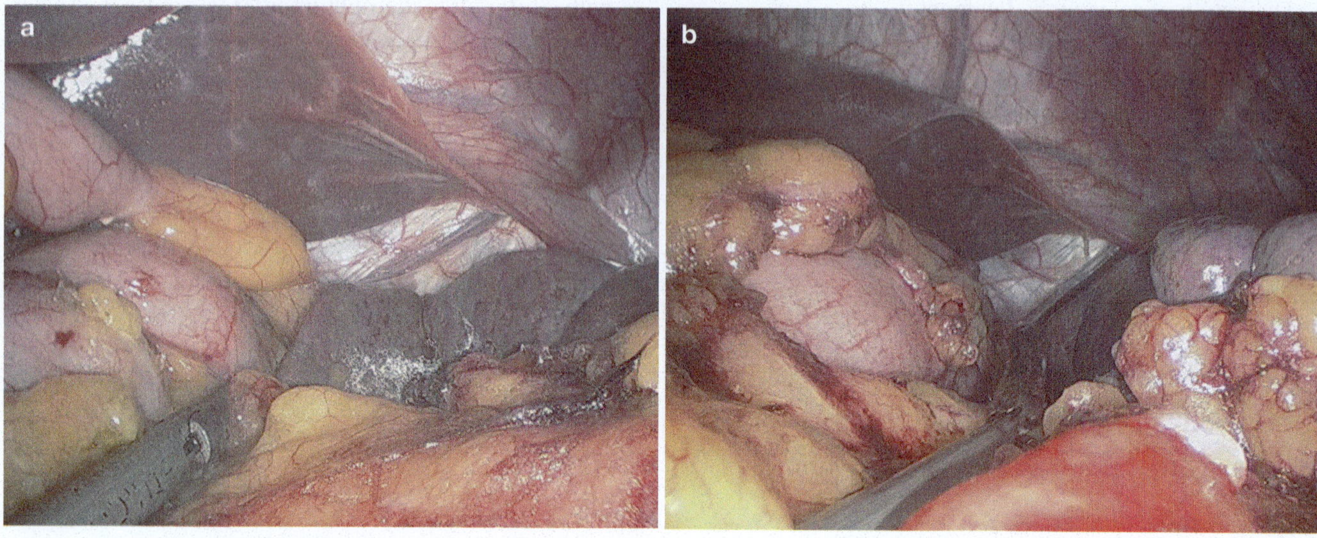

Fig. 7.3

3. Dissection of splenocolic ligament.
   The splenocolic ligament was divided and attention was paid not to injure the transverse colon (Fig. 7.4a–d).

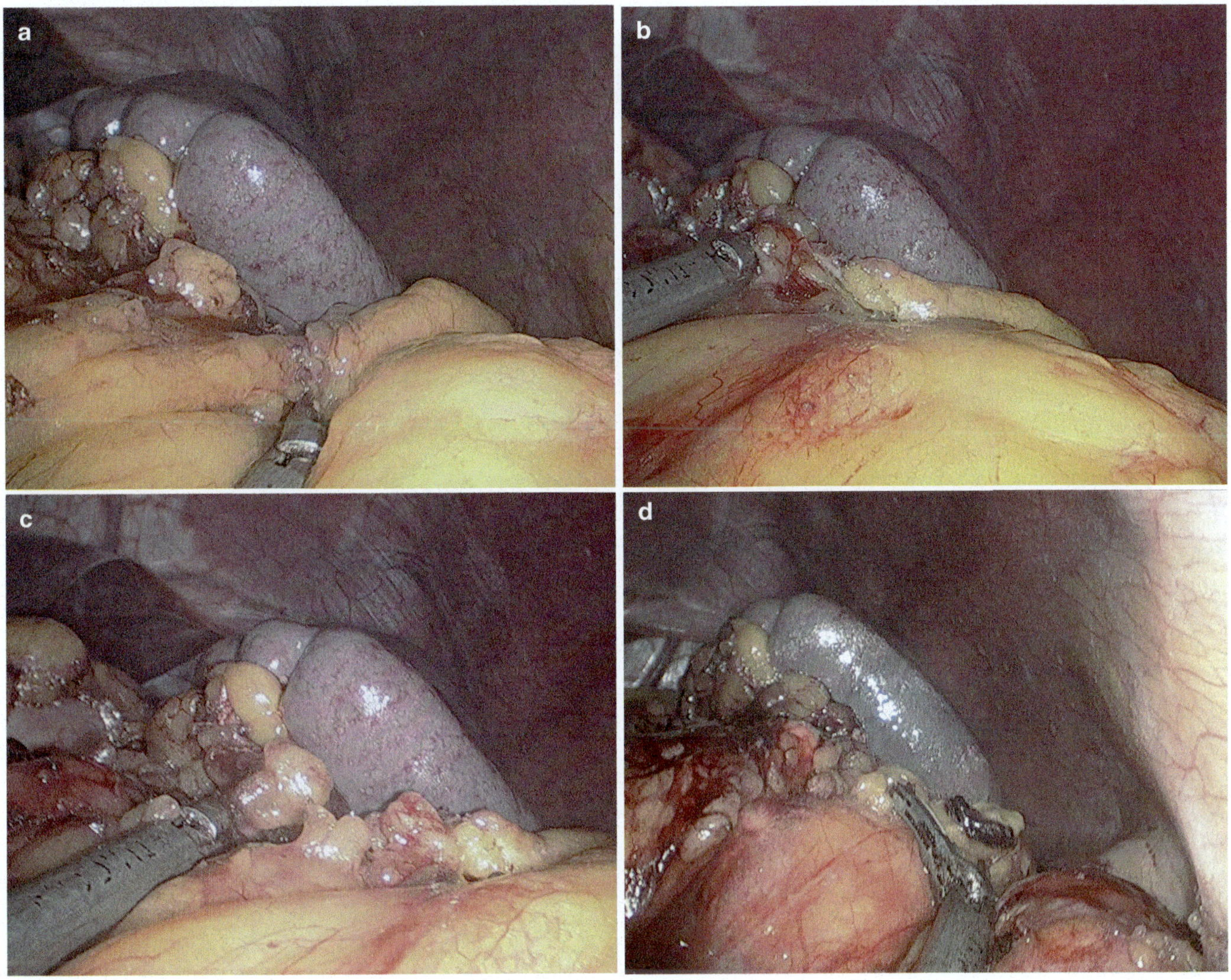

Fig. 7.4

4. Dissection of splenorenal ligament.
   The splenocolic ligament was divided and the splenorenal ligament was exposed by lifting the lower pole of the spleen (Fig. 7.5a, b).

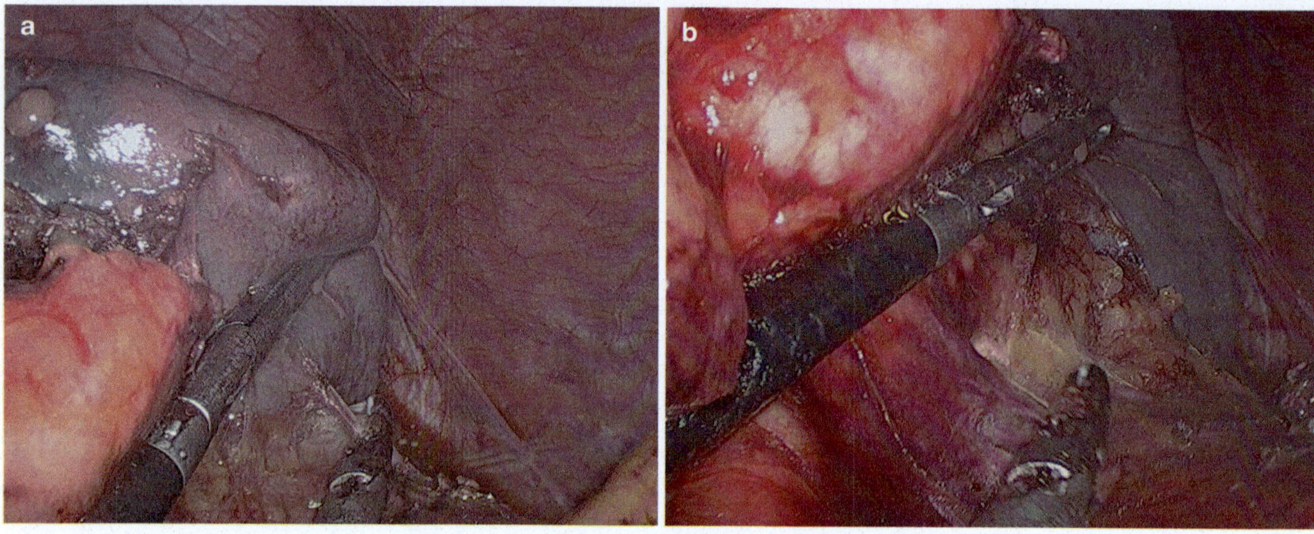

Fig. 7.5

5. Dissection of phrenosplenic ligament.
   The division was continued upwardly to the phrenosplenic ligament (Fig. 7.6a–d).

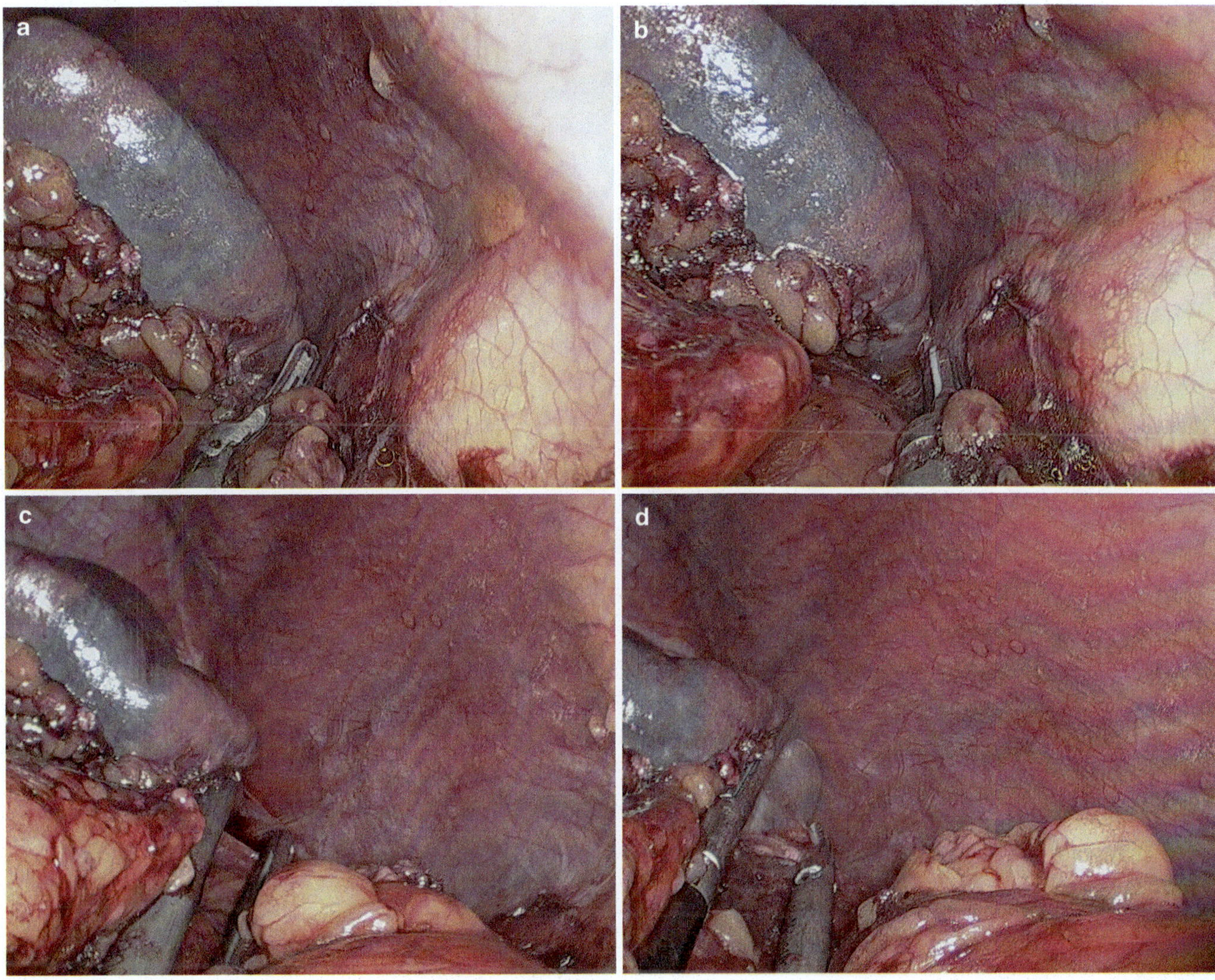

Fig. 7.6

6. Dissection of splenic hilum and tail of pancreas.
   The pancreatic tail was exposed by dissecting the peritoneum on the splenic hilum with harmonic scalpel (Fig. 7.7a–d).

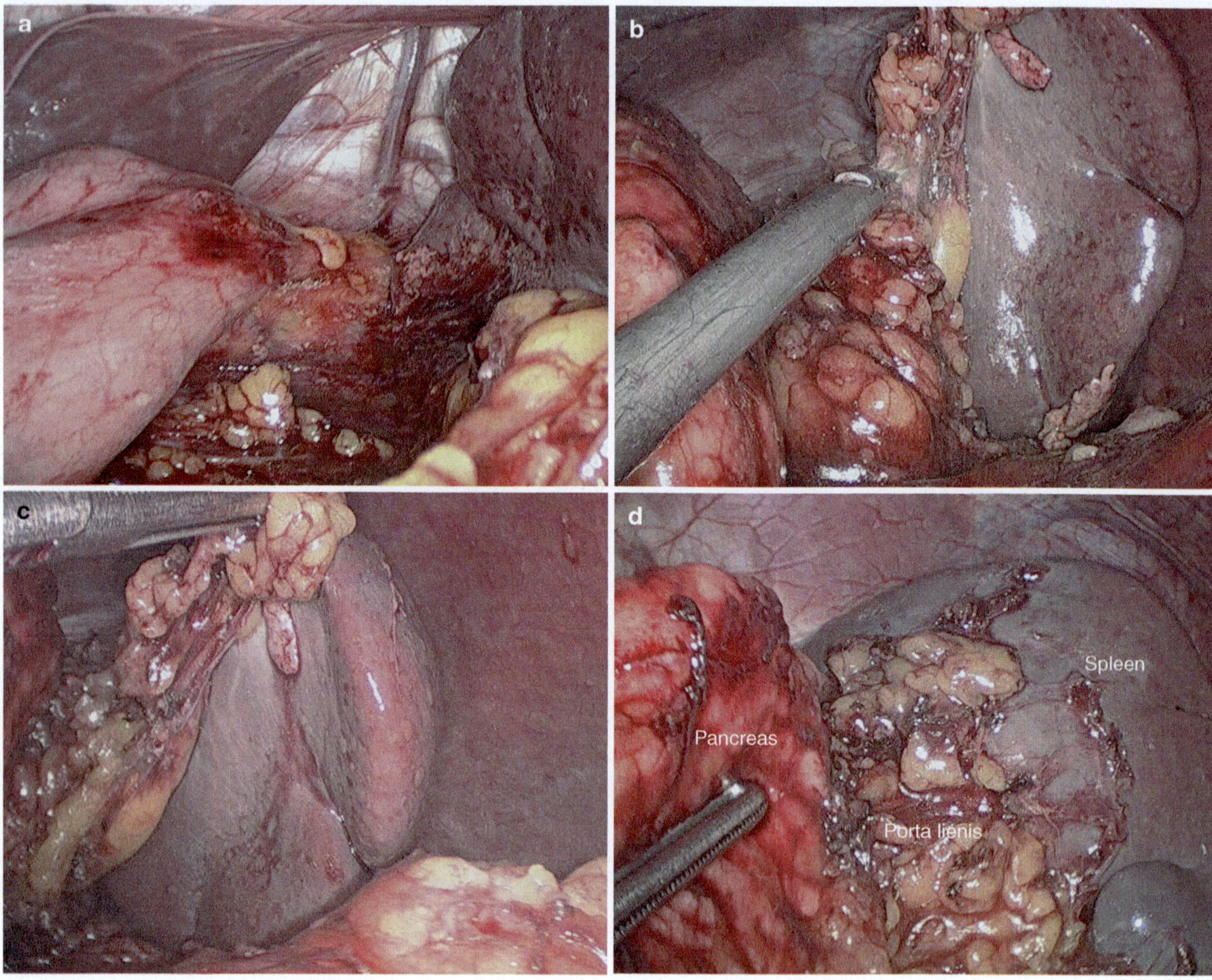

Fig. 7.7

7. Transection of spleen pedicle.
   The splenic pedicle was dissected and divided by a 60-mm endoscopic stapler inserted through the 12-mm trocar. The entire spleen was completely resected (Fig. 7.8a–f).

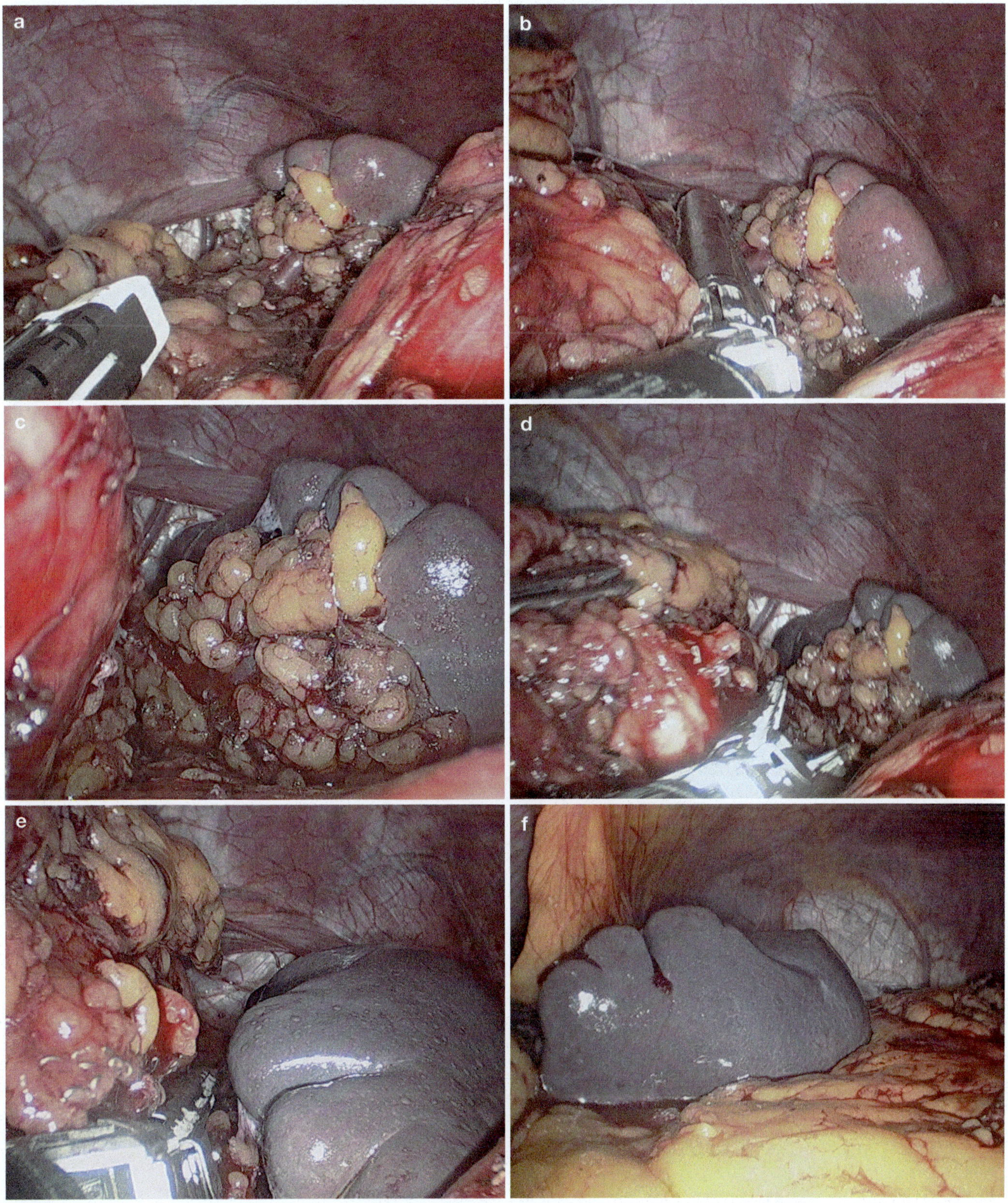

Fig. 7.8

8. Retrieval of spleen.
   The freely mobile spleen was put into a specimen bag placed through the 12 mm Trocar. Then the lura of the bag was dragged out of the abdominal cavity through the umbilical incision; the specimen was taken out in pieces by oval forceps (Fig. 7.9a–d).

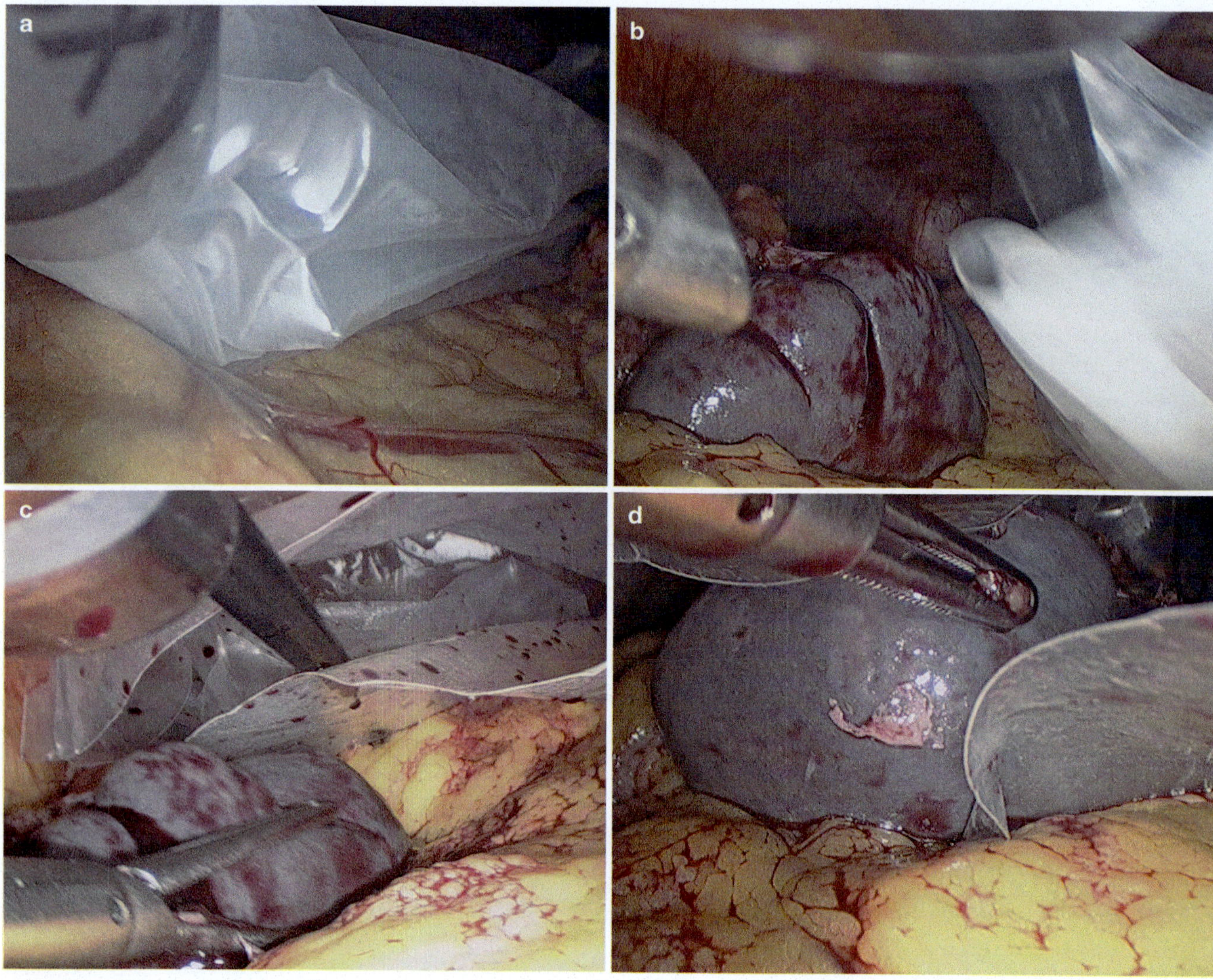

Fig. 7.9

9. Irrigation and drainage.
   The abdominal cavity was suctioned and a closed suction drain was placed into the splenic fossa through the incision at umbilicus (Fig. 7.10a–d).

7.1.7 Tips and Tricks

1. Difficulty with retraction can be solved with external traction suture placement. For example, the stomach may be retracted with a 2-0 polydioxanone traction suture placed percutaneously through the anterior gastric wall to facilitate exposure of the short gastric vessels.
2. Once the splenic hilum was exposed, one of the 5-mm ports was upsized to 12 mm to admit a reticulating vascular endostapler (Ethicon Endosurgery, Cincinnati, OH).
3. The hilar vessels were divided, taking care to avoid the tail of pancreas.
4. The spleen was placed within an endobag then morcellated within the bag using a finger fracture technique and subsequently removed in a piecemeal fashion.

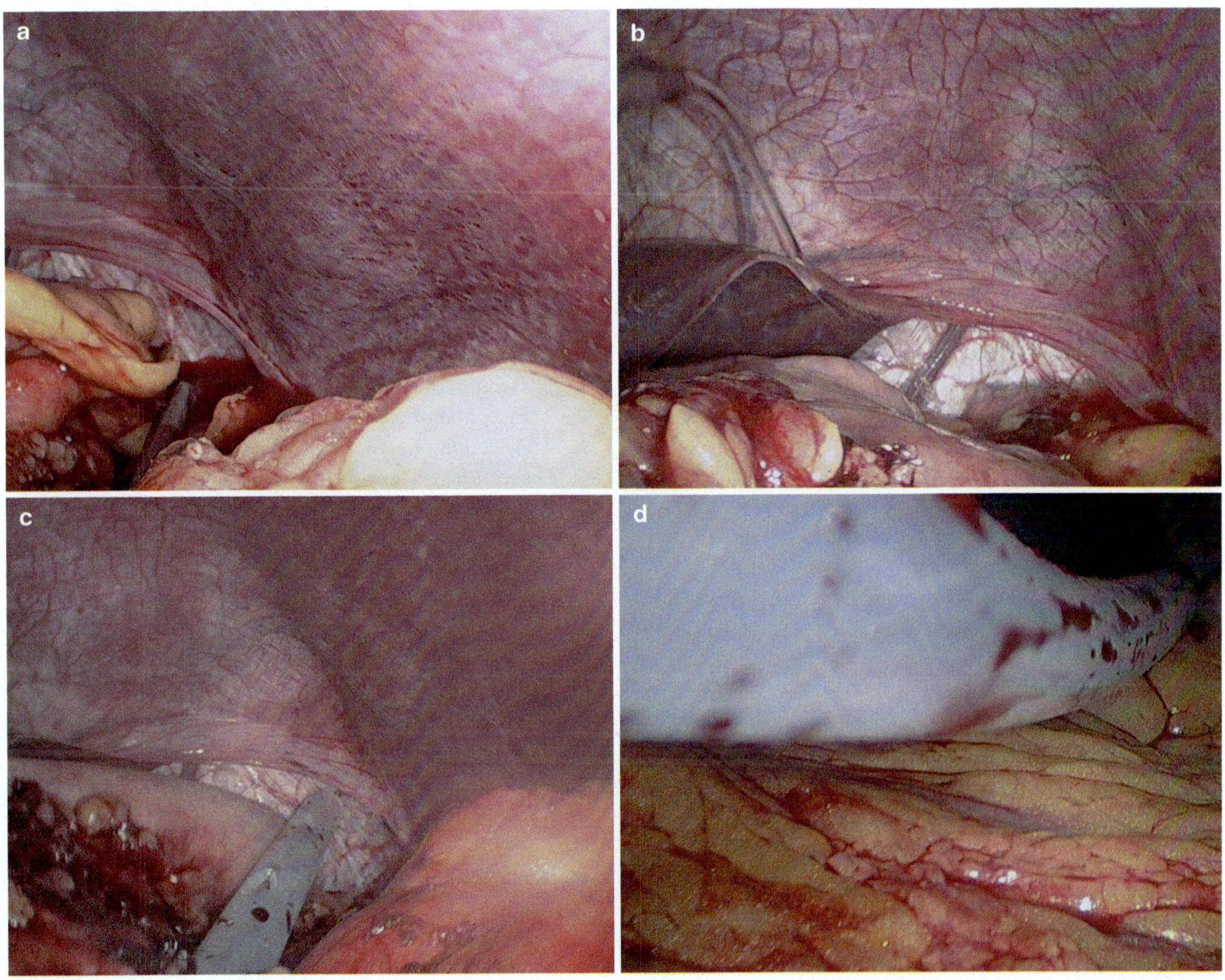

Fig. 7.10

7.2 Laparoscopic Splenectomy Plus Pericardial Devascularization

7.2.1 Indications and Case Selection

1. Patients suffer from hepatic cirrhosis complicated with portal hypertension, who have the history of upper gastrointestinal hemorrhage, and the hepatic function should be corrected to Child A or B.
2. Patients suffer from enlargement of spleen and hypersplenism with varicose veins in the middle or inferior segment of esophagus, who have the history of hematemesis or the possibility of uncontrolled hemorrhea due to phleborrhexis in the inferior segment of esophagus.
3. Patients with above indications suffering from non-severe ascites or icterus, or above symptoms worsened after medical treatment.

7.2.2 Contraindications

1. Absolute contraindications:
   (a) severe cardiorespiratory dysfunction.
   (b) inability to tolerate general anesthesia or pneumoperitoneum.
   (c) severe refractory coagulopathy.
2. Relative contraindications:
   (a) morbid obesity.
   (b) pregnancy.
   (c) patients with "frozen upper abdomen" due to previous surgery or peritonitis.

Laparoscopic splenectomy with pericardial devascularization performed for patients with icterus, large amount of ascites, or severe damage of liver function (Child C) have a high death rate.

7.2.3 Major Instruments or Energy Sources

1. Laparoscopy System.
2. Holding forceps.
3. Harmonic scalpel.
4. Endoscopic Linear Stapler.

7.2.4 Team Setup, Anesthesia and Position

It is the same as Sect. 7.1.4.

7.2.5 Key Steps

1. Dissection of gastrocolic ligament.
2. Dissection of varices around the spleen pedicle.
3. Dissection of splenorenal ligament.
4. Dissection of phrenosplenic ligament.
5. Dissection of splenogastric ligament.
6. Dissection of splenic hilum and tail of pancreas.
7. Transection of spleen pedicle.
8. Transection of posterior vein of stomach.
9. Dissection of esophagus and transection of varices around the esophagus.
10. Transaction of gastric coronary vein.
11. Retrieval of spleen.
12. Irrigation and drainage.

7.2.6 Surgical Techniques

1. Dissection of gastrocolic ligament.
   The patient was placed in reverse Trendlenburg position to expose the spleen. The splenocolic ligament was dissected with harmonic scalpel or Ligasure (Fig. 7.11a–d).

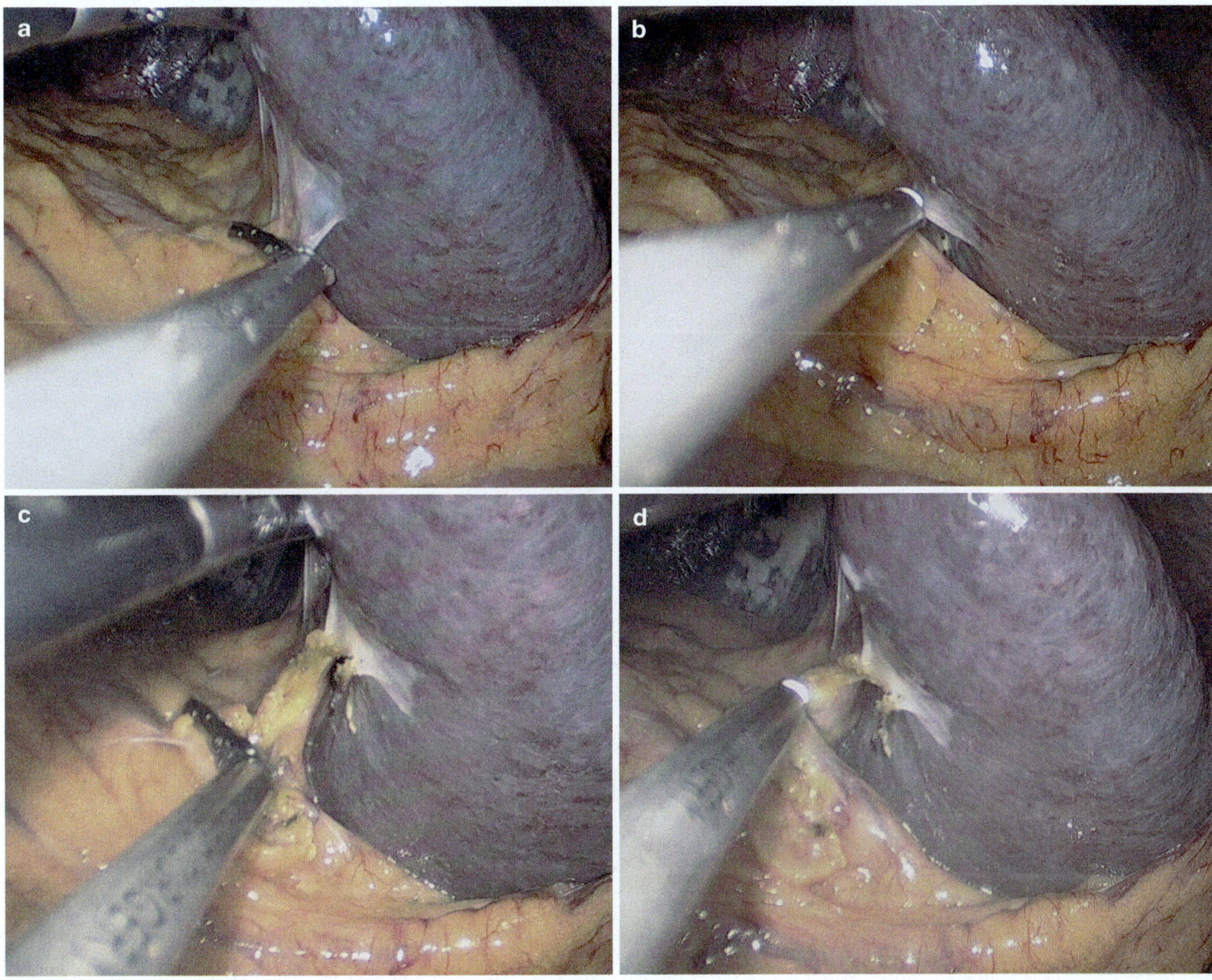

Fig. 7.11

2. Dissection of varices around the spleen pedicle. Peritoneum on the splenic hilum was divided with harmonic scalpel and secondary splenic pedicle exposed. Small vessels were coagulated with Ligasure and larger ones divided between clips (Fig. 7.12a–p).

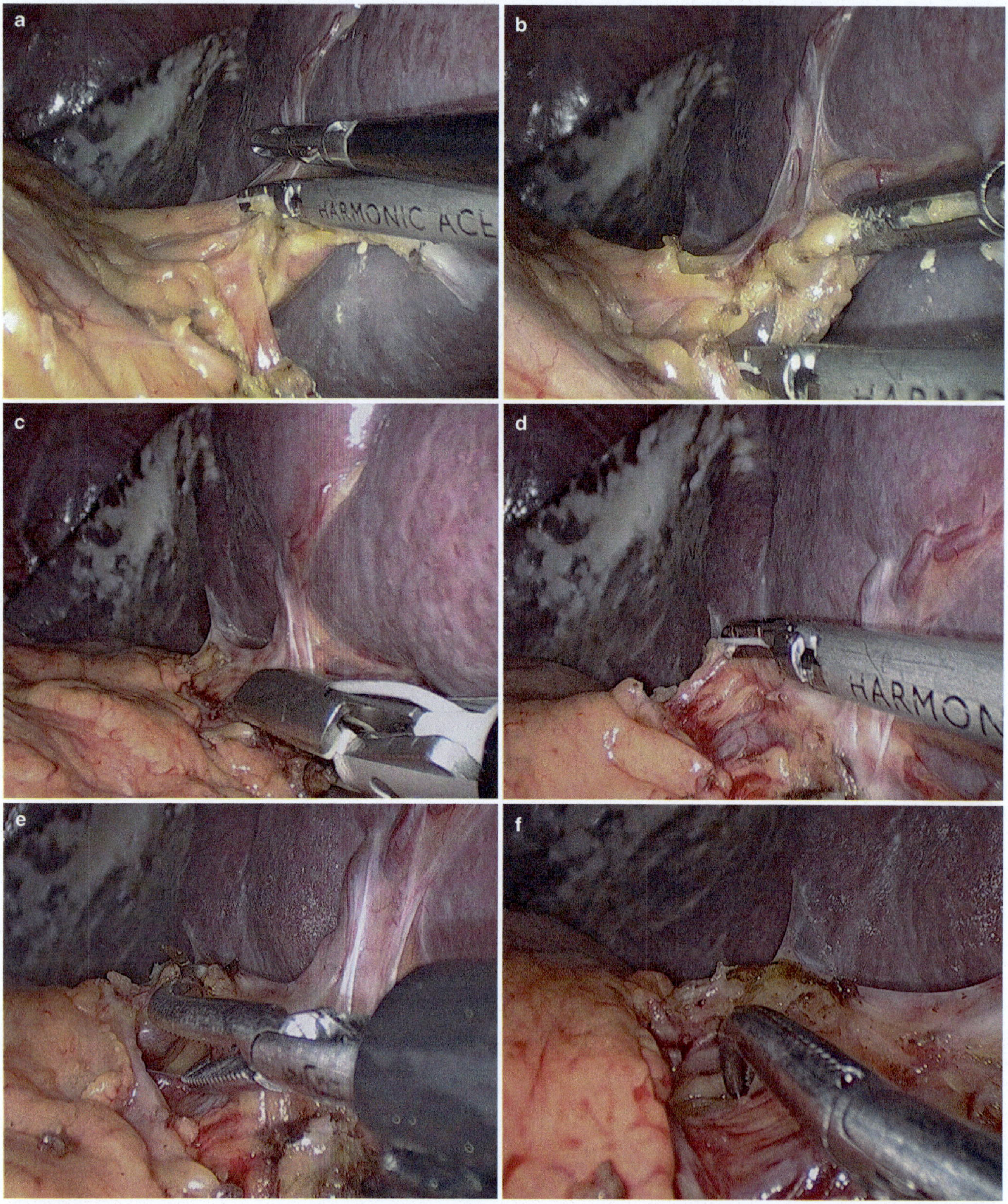

Fig. 7.12

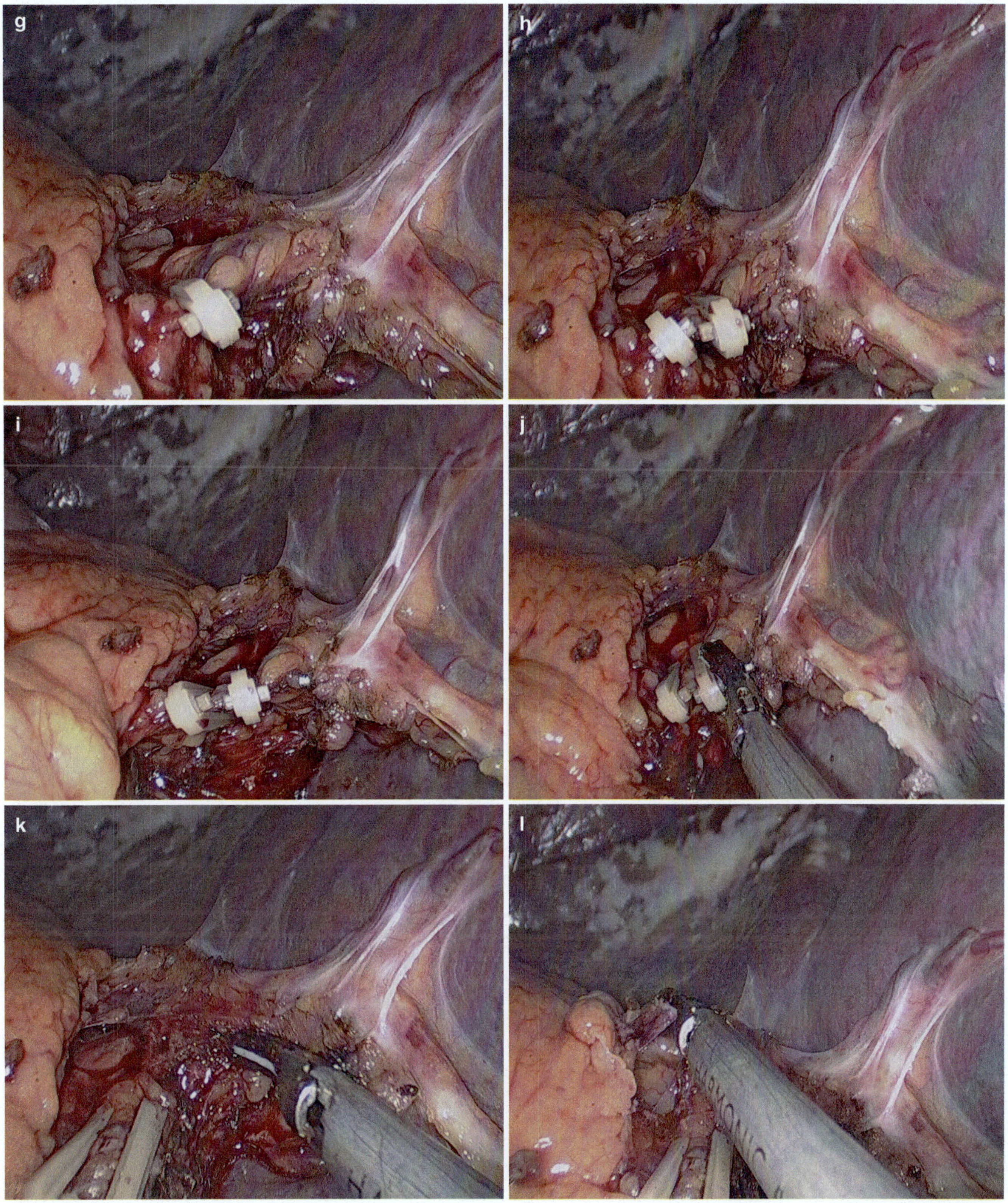

Fig. 7.12 (continued)

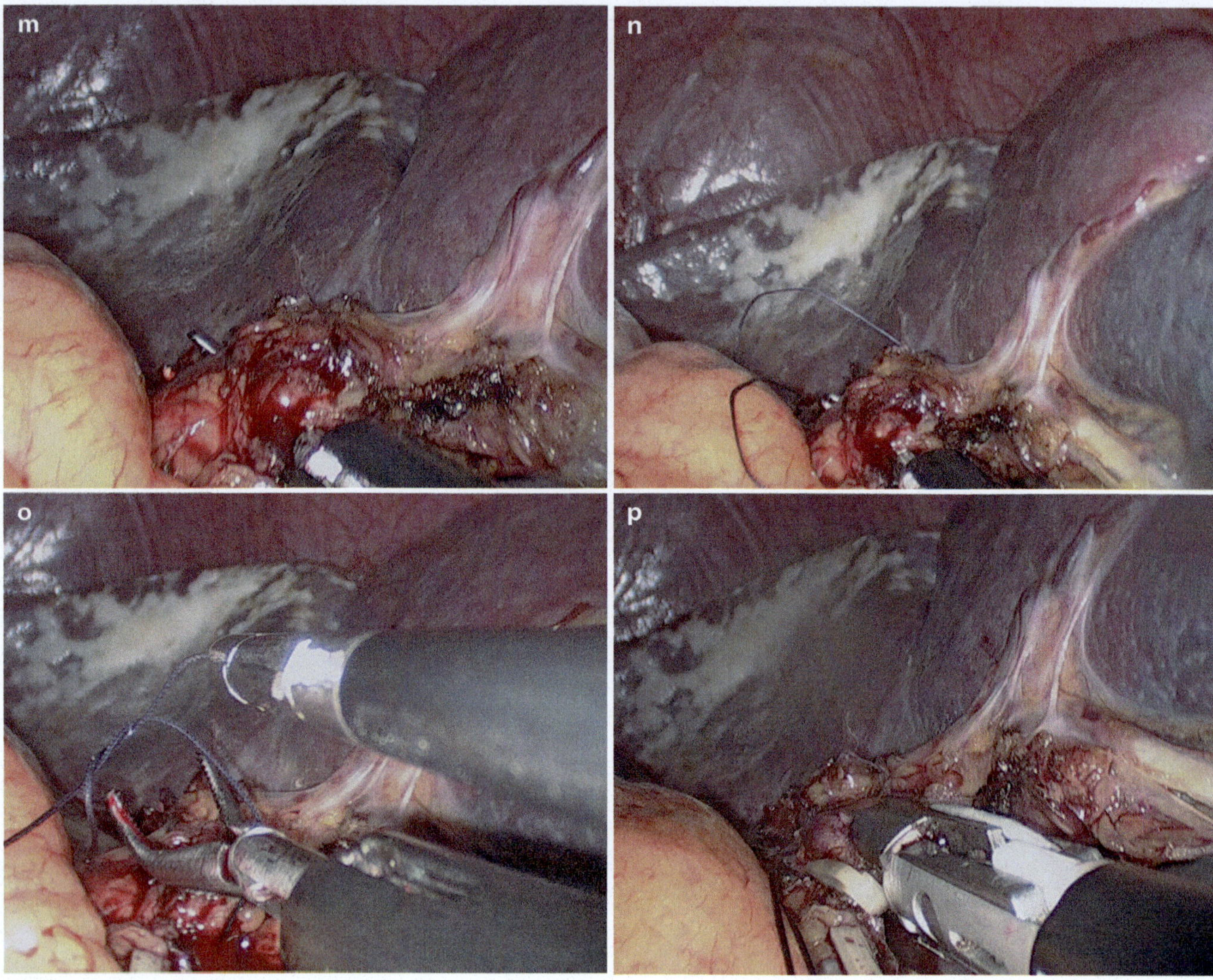

Fig. 7.12 (continued)

3. Dissection of splenorenal ligament.
   The division was further continued towards the splenorenal ligament. The exposure was assisted by lifting the spleen or by postural adjustment of the patient (Fig. 7.13a, b).

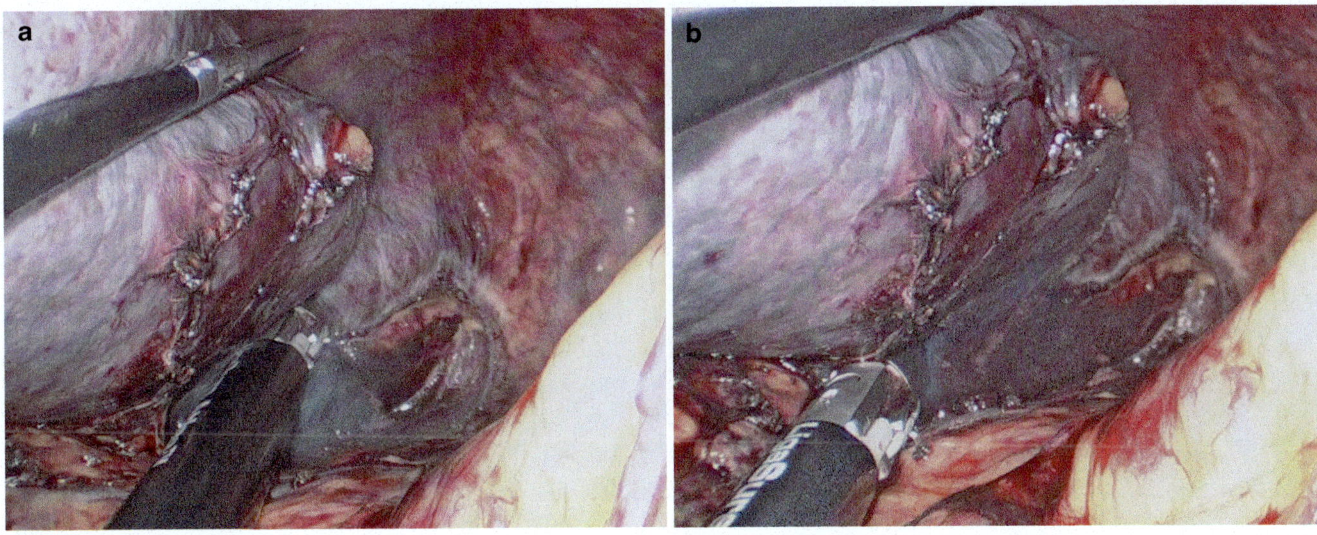

Fig. 7.13

4. Dissection of phrenosplenic ligament.
   The division was continued upwardly towards the phrenosplenic ligament (Fig. 7.14a–d).

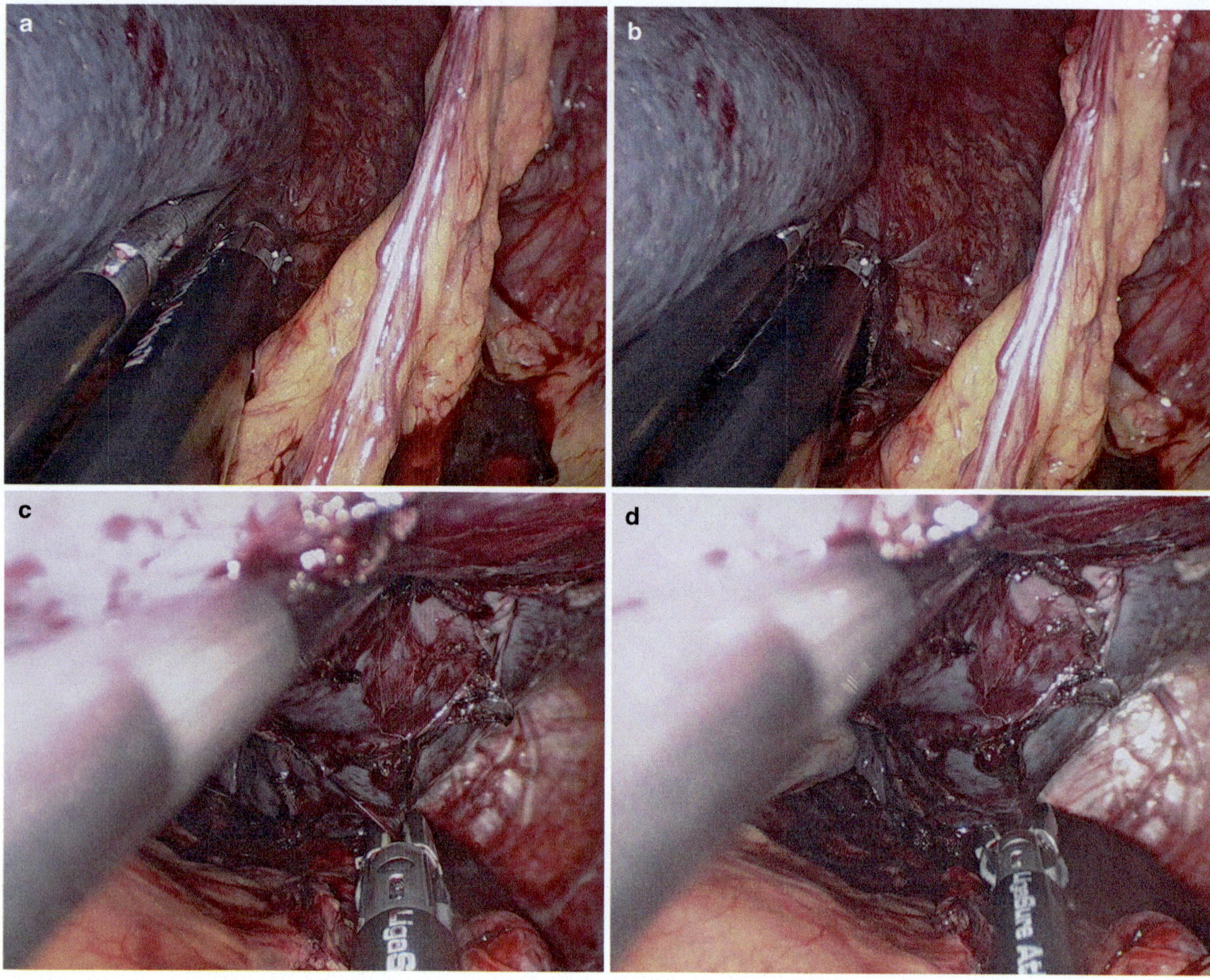

Fig. 7.14

5. Dissection of splenogastric ligament.
   The greater curvature of stomach was lifted and splenogastric ligament exposed. The splenogastric ligament and short gastric vessels were divided with harmonic scalpel or Ligasure (Fig. 7.15a–c).

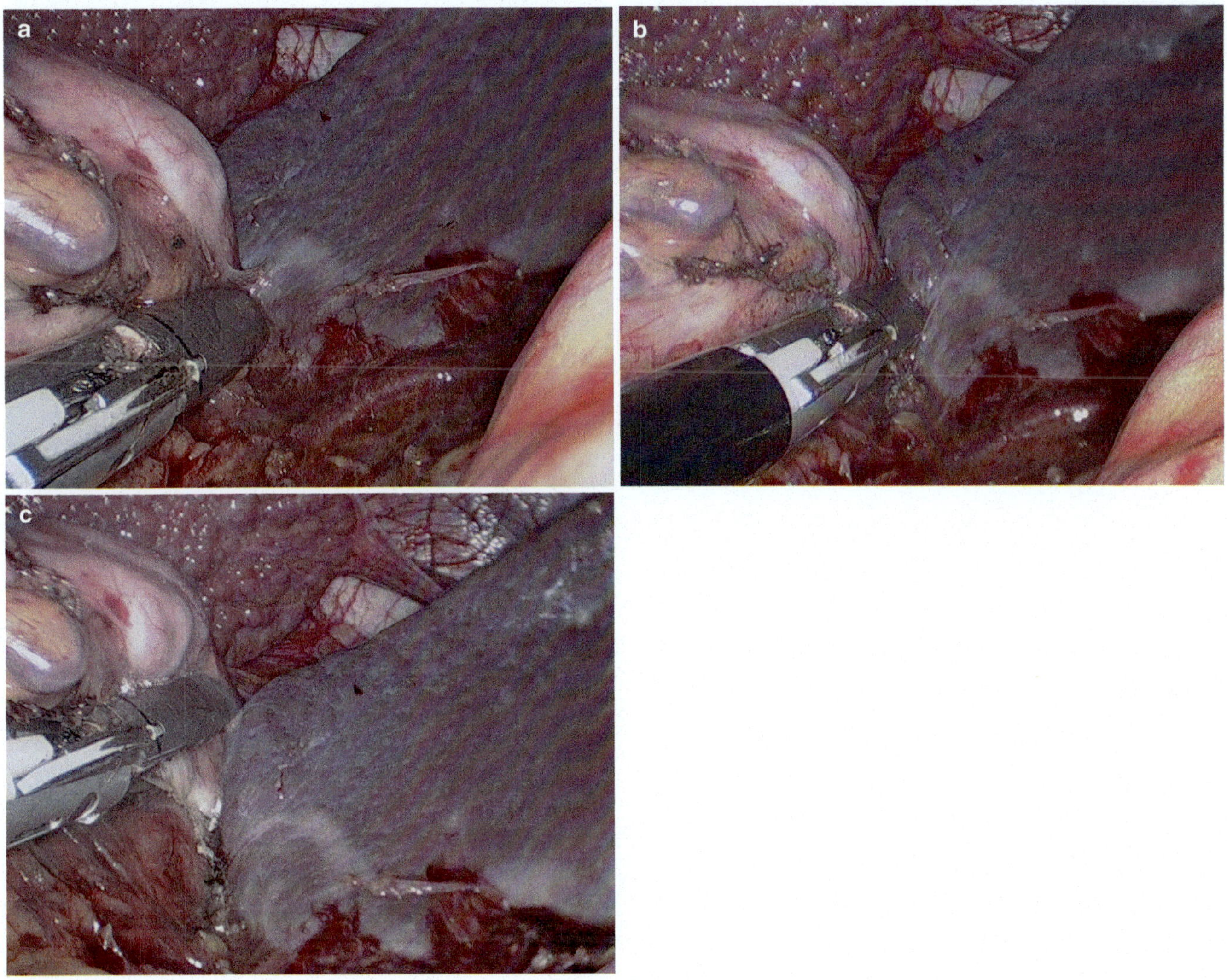

Fig. 7.15

6. Dissection of splenic hilum and tail of pancreas.
   The pancreatic tail was exposed by dissecting the peritoneum on the splenic hilum with the arteries and veins divided. The vessels were divided by harmonic scalpel with proximal ends double clipped (Fig. 7.16a, b).

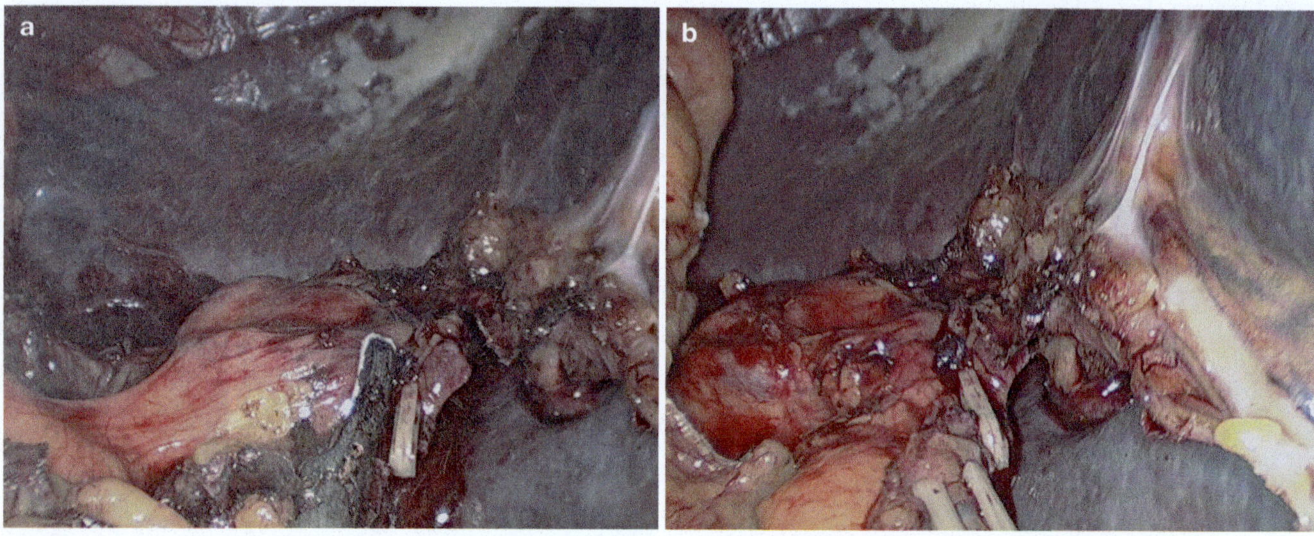

Fig. 7.16

7. Transection of spleen pedicle.
   The pancreatic tail was separated from the splenic pedicle. The splenic pedicle was dissected and divided by a 60-mm endoscopic stapler inserted through the 12-mm trocar (Fig. 7.17a–d).

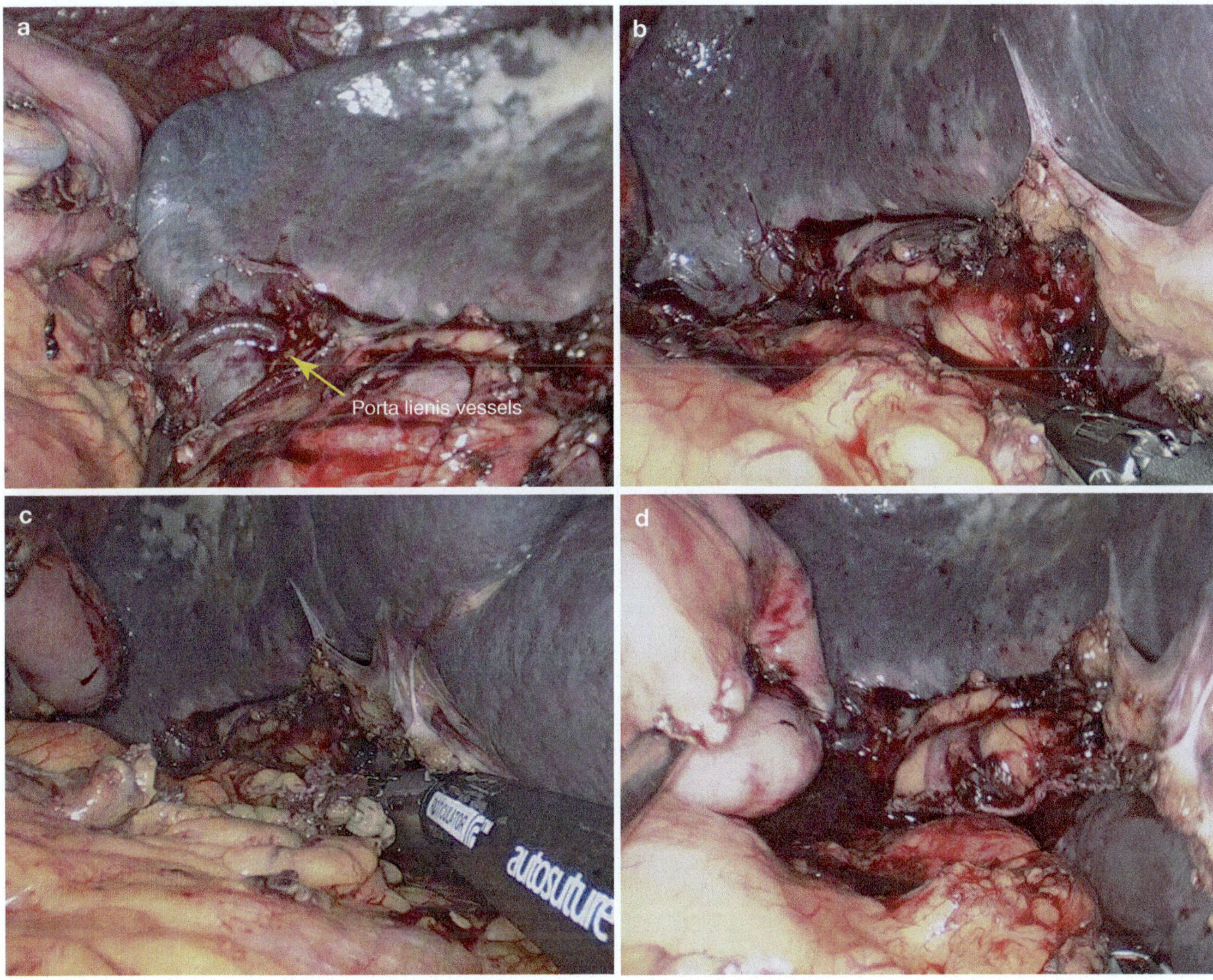

Fig. 7.17

8. Transection of posterior vein of stomach.
   The greater curvature was lifted upwardly and vena gastrica posterior was divided by Ligasure (Fig. 7.18a–d).

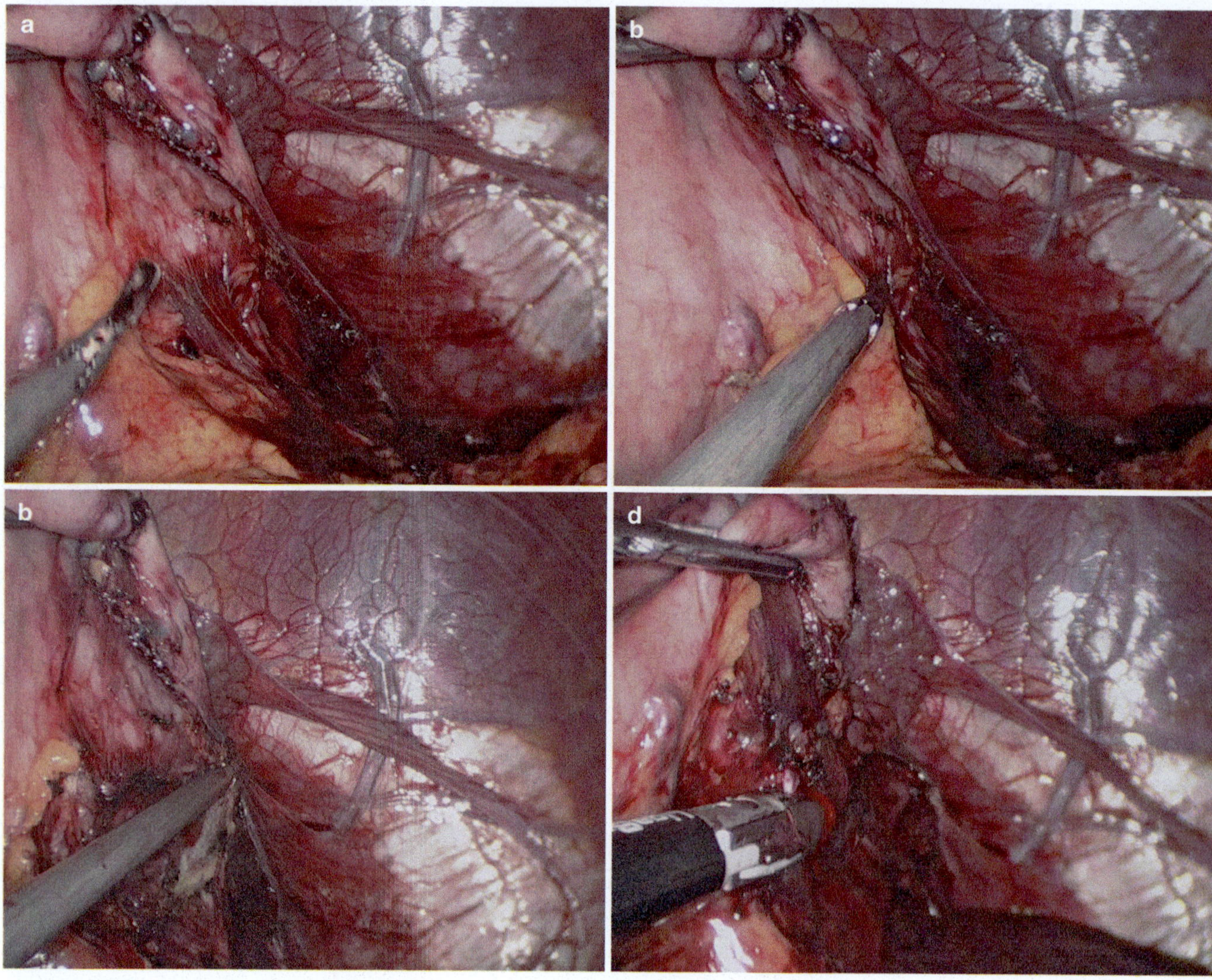

Fig. 7.18

9. Dissection of esophagus and transection of varices around the esophagus.

   The serosa on the esophagus was opened. The esophagus was pulled downward. Vessels around the lower esophagus were dissected superior to a point 6 cm away from the esophageal cardia junction. Small vessels were coagulated with Ligasure and larger ones divided between clips (Fig. 7.19a–j).

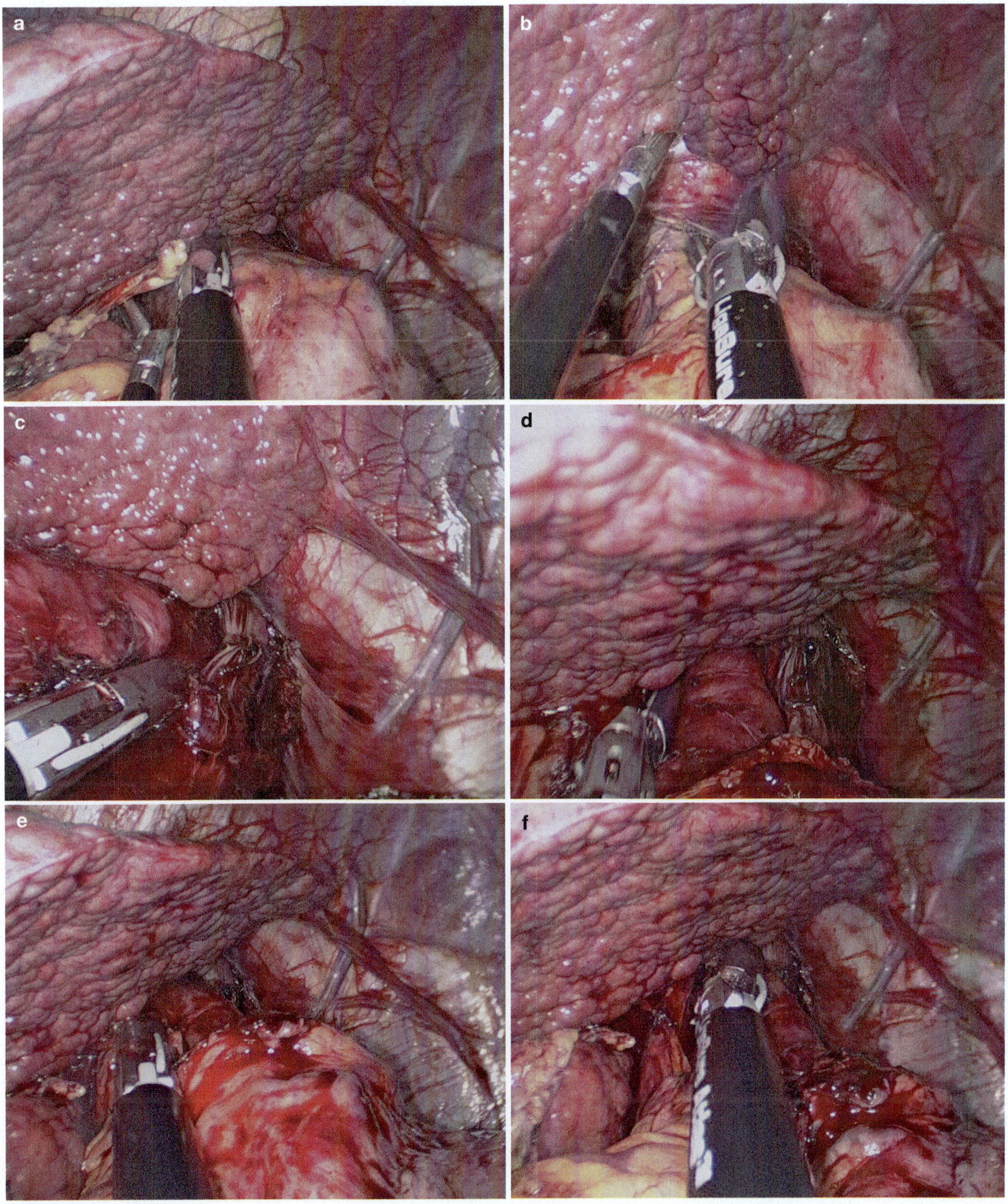

Fig. 7.19

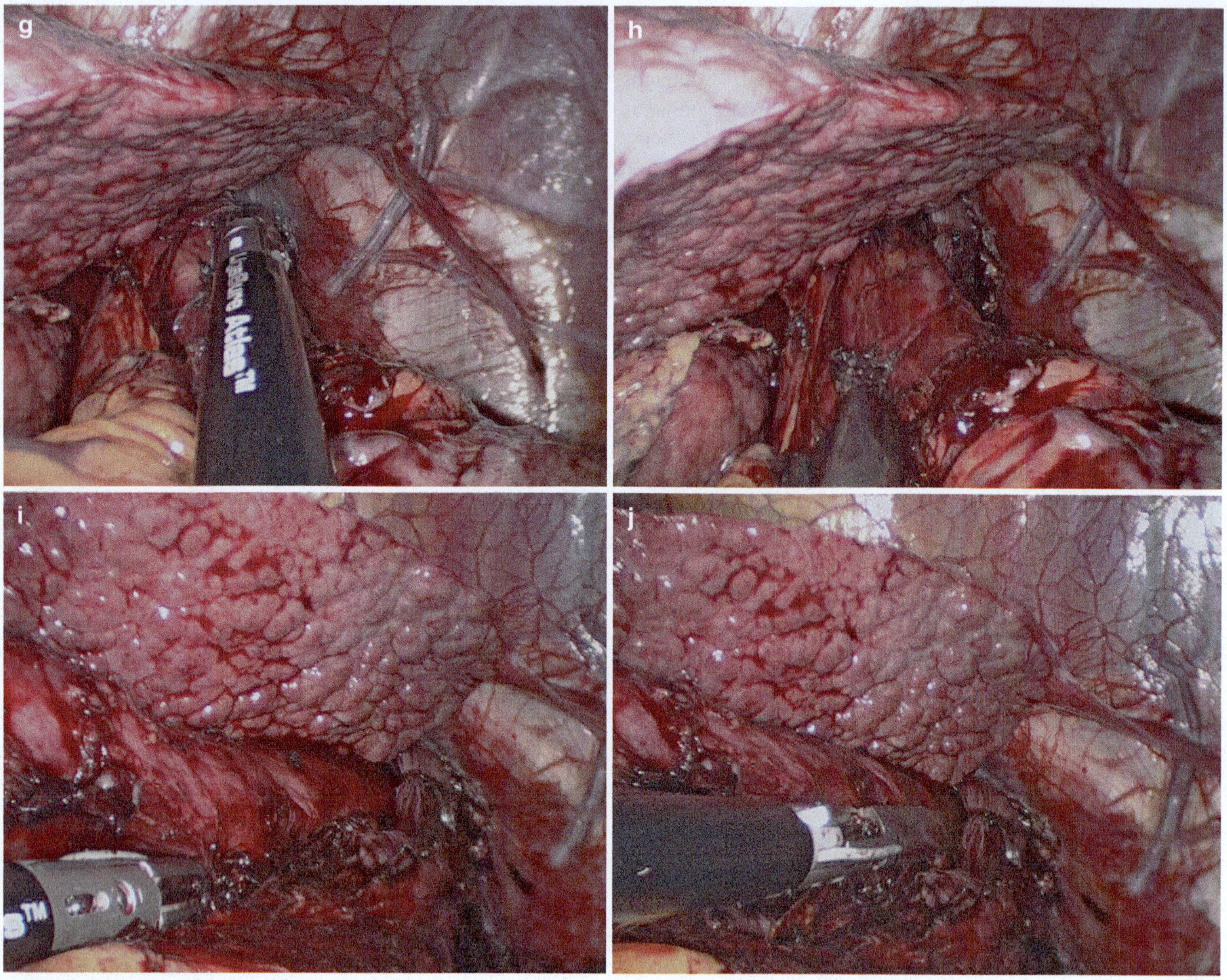

Fig. 7.19 (continued)

10. Transaction of gastric coronary vein.
    The gastrohepatic ligament was opened and devascularization of the lesser curvature was performed by the same way. With the use of Ligasure, this procedure can be performed without significant bleeding. A large draining vein left gastric vessel was ligated with an Endo-GIA stapler (Fig. 7.20a–f).

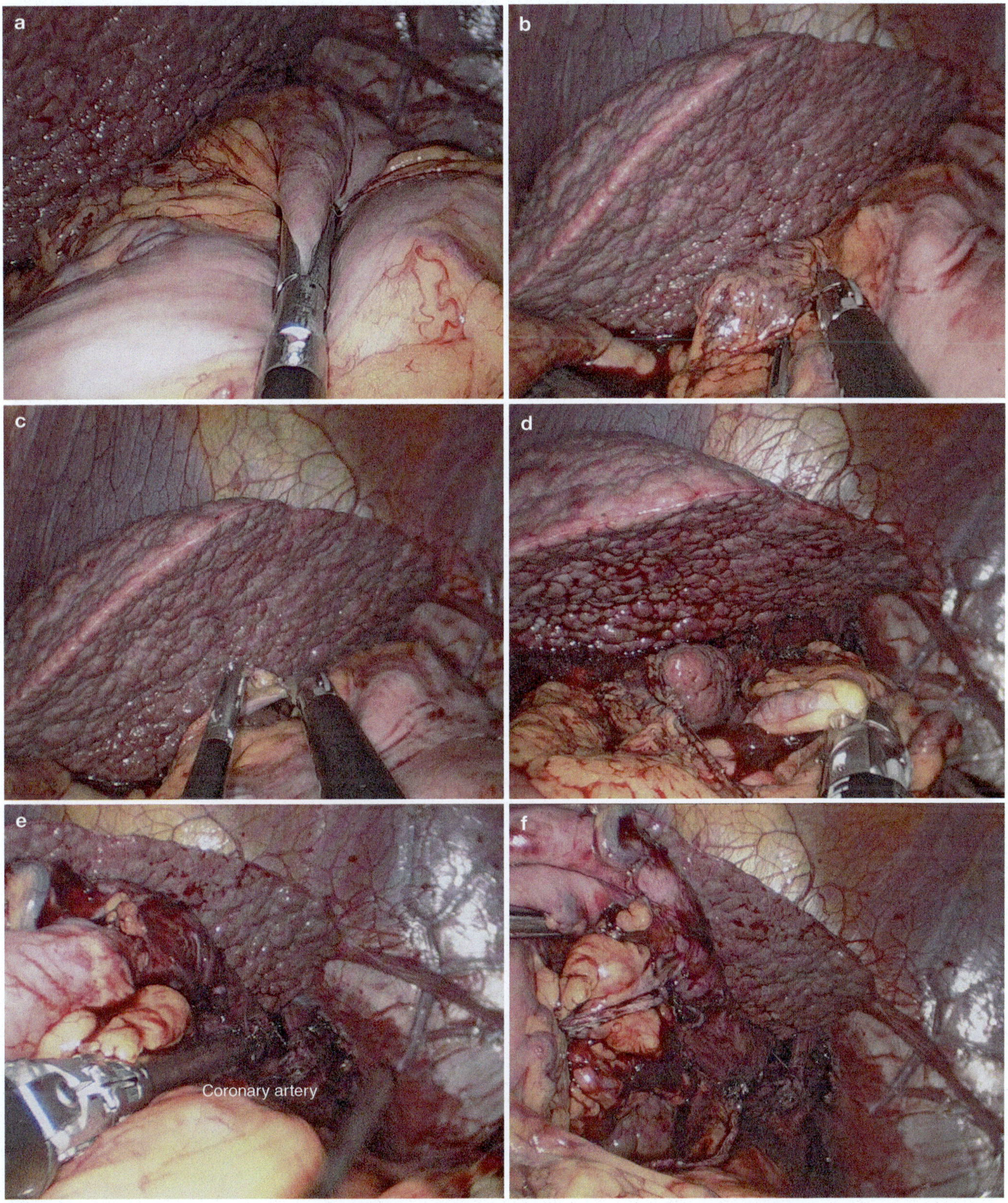

Fig. 7.20

11. Retrieval of spleen.
    The freely mobile spleen was put into a specimen bag placed through the 12 mm Trocar. Then the lura of the bag was dragged out of the abdominal cavity through the umbilical incision; the specimen was taken out in pieces by oval forceps (Fig. 7.21a, b).

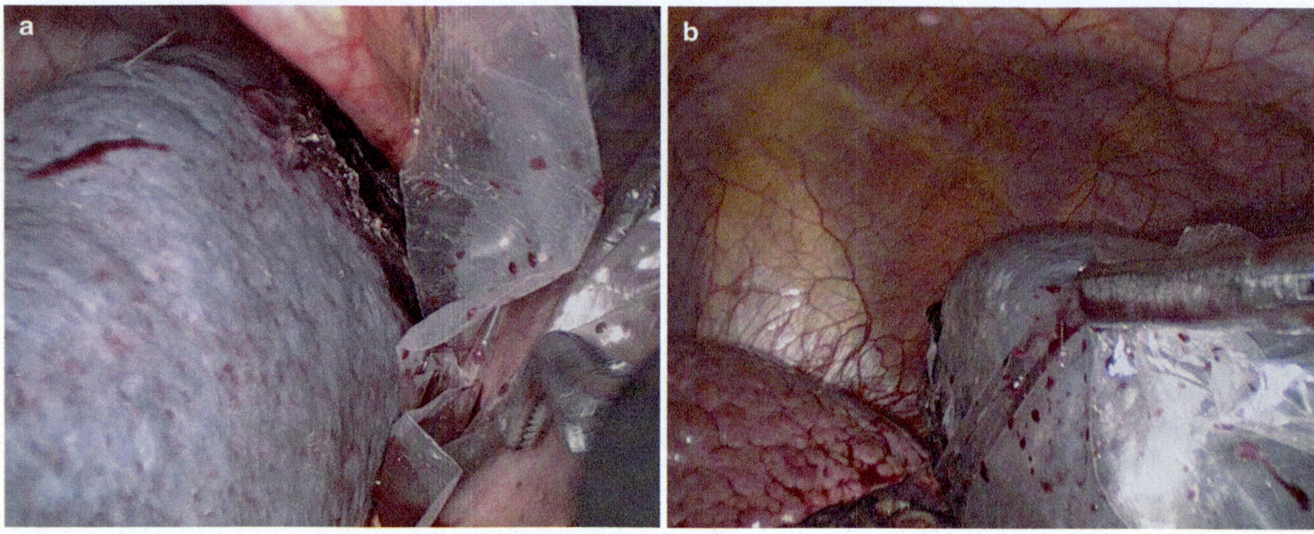

Fig. 7.21

12. Irrigation and drainage.
    The abdominal cavity was suctioned and a closed suction drain was placed into the splenic fossa through the incision at umbilicus (Fig. 7.22a–c). Tissue glue was sprayed if there was minor errhysis.

7.2.7 Tips and Tricks

1. The laparoscopic splenectomy should be performed by a lateral approach with the left side of the patient elevated 30–45°.
2. The dissection of spleen should begin with division of the splenocolic and gastrocolic ligament with a 5-mm Harmonic scalpel or a Ligasure. Then, the spleen was elevated properly by the assistant hand, while the Ligasure held by the dominant hand was used to divide and dissect the splenorenal ligament. Then, the splenophrenic ligament attached to the upper pole of the spleen was freed with the Ligasure, leaving the spleen hanging only on its pedicle.
3. When an endoscopic stapler through the trocar was used to dissect the pedicle, the position should be reversed in order to stretch the pedicle.
4. Vessels around the lower esophagus should be dissected superior to a point 6 cm away from the esophageal cardia junction.
5. With the use of a Ligasure, this procedure can be performed without significant bleeding.

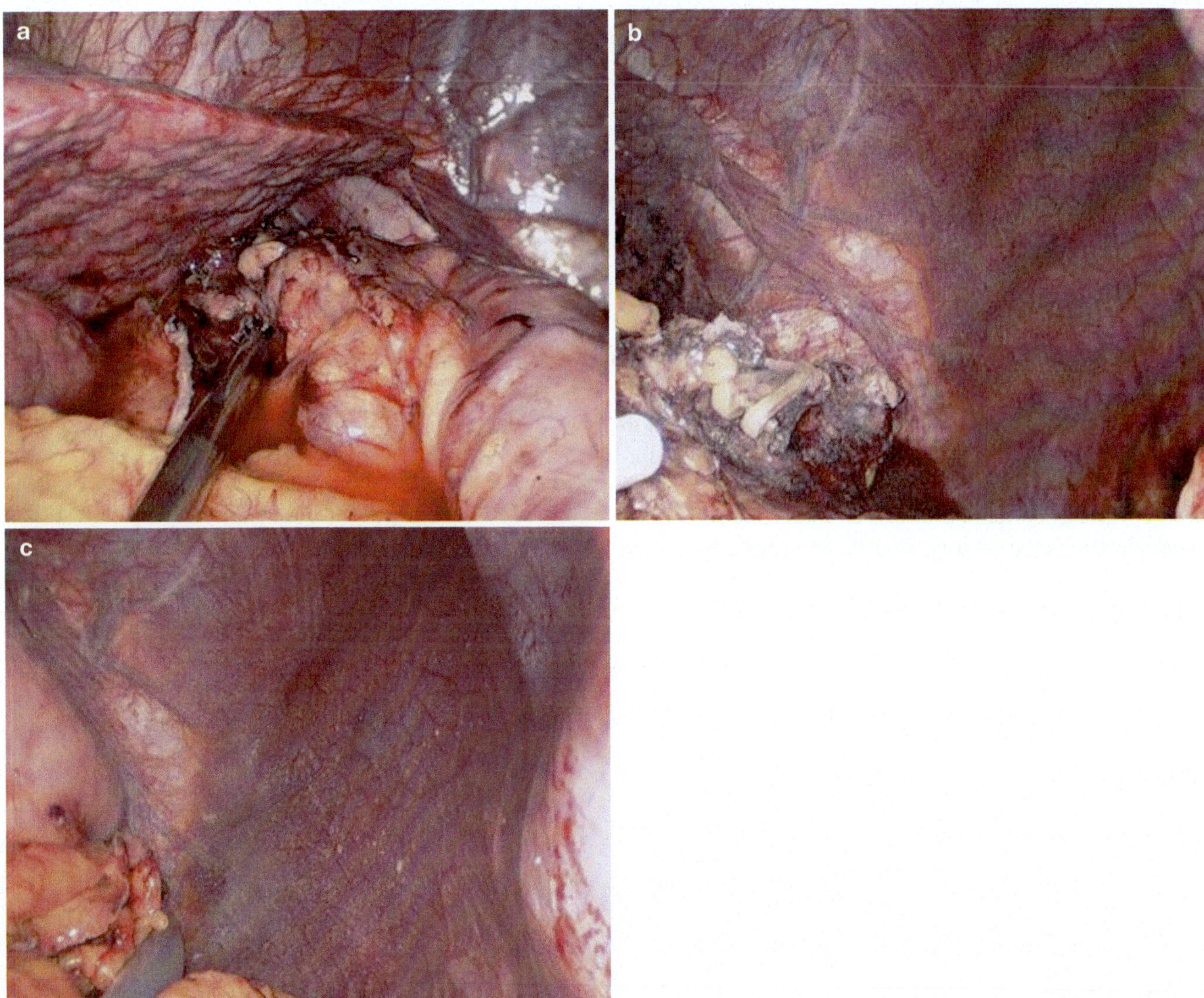

Fig. 7.22

7.3 Complications Analysis and Management

7.3.1 Haemorrhage

In SILS splenic surgery, triangle relationship is lack and the length of operational instruments is limited. When the superior part of spleen is dissected, the umbilical operational point is far from the surgical field. So the haemorrhage is common. Changing the body position and making it in anti-Trendelenburg position may assist the exposure of superior part of spleen. In SILS surgery, excessive retraction of spleen and tearing of splenic peripheral vessels may induce haemorrhage. So, violent retraction for exposure is forbidden in SILS splenic surgery. For larger spleen, changing body position may assist to expose the surgical field and splenic movement. And dissecting the splenic peripheral ligaments from the near to the distance may increase the activity of spleen and effectively prevent splenic haemorrhage. The key to preventing haemorrhage is correcting coagulation disorders preoperatively and definite hemostasis in the operation. If the bleeding is massive, it should be converted to conventional laparoscope or open surgery as soon as possible.

7.3.2 Esophageal Leak and Distal Pancreatic Injury

It is similar to the SILS Heller myotomy, the possibility of esophageal leak is existent. In addition to paying attention to dissecting area of pericardial vessels, which can prevent the formation of lower part esophageal necrosis and leak, the injury caused by energy devices should also be noticed. Persistent gastrointestinal decompression and smooth abdominal drainage can prevent the leak. Reoperation should be considered if abdominal abscess is formed.

When the splenic hilum is dissected, the distal pancreas may be injured, forming pancreatic leakage. Due to the lack of necessary assistance, hurried clamping of the spleen pedicle in obscure vision may injure the distal pancreas when the splenic hilum is dissected.

References

1. Barbaros U, Dinççağ A. Single incision laparoscopic splenectomy: the first two cases. J Gastrointest Surg. 2009;13:1520–3.
2. Vatansev C, Ece Jr I. Single incision laparoscopic splenectomy with double port. Surg Laparosc Endosc Percutan Tech. 2009;19: e225–7.
3. Malladi P, Hungness E, Nagle A. Single access laparoscopic splenectomy. JSLS. 2009;13:601–4.
4. Lagrand R, Kehdy F. Laparoendoscopic single site splenectomy. Am Surg. 2010;76:E158–9.
5. Barbaros U, Sümer A, Tunca F, Gözkün O, Demirel T, Bilge O, et al. Our early experiences with single-incision laparoscopic surgery: the first 32 patients. Surg Laparosc Endosc Percutan Tech. 2010;20:306–11.
6. Colon MJ, Telem D, Chan E, Midulla P, Divino C, Chin EH. Laparoendoscopic single site (LESS) splenectomy with a conventional laparoscope and instruments. JSLS. 2011;15:384–6.
7. Bell R, Boswell T, Hui T, Su W. Single-incision laparoscopic splenectomy in children. J Pediatr Surg. 2012;47:898–903.
8. Dapri G, Bron D, Himpens J, Casali L, Carnevali P, Koustas P, et al. Single-access transumbilical laparoscopic splenectomy using curved reusable instruments. Surg Endosc. 2011;25:3419–22.
9. Fan Y, Wu SD, Siwo EA. Emergency transumbilical single-incision laparoscopic splenectomy for the treatment of traumatic rupture of the spleen: report of the first case and literature review. Surg Innov. 2011;18:185–8.
10. Jing K, Shuo-Dong W, Ying F. Transumbilical single-incision laparoscopy surgery splenectomy plus pericaudial devascularization in one case with portal hypertension: the first report. Surg Innov. 2012 (Epub ahead of print).

Hernia Surgery

8

Abstract

Although described by Kelling G in 1901, the field of laparoscopic or minimally invasive surgery did not gain wide spread use until the advent of the transistor chip and a video camera attached to the end of the laparoscope was invented. As video imaging systems and new instruments continue to develop, single-incision laparoscopic surgery (SILS) has recently been a focus for active investigation in the surgical field. Potential advantages over conventional laparoscopic surgery include better cosmetic results, less postoperative wound pain, and less port site complications, which have yet to be validated by prospective comparative studies. Transumbilical single-incision laparoscopic cholecystectomy and appendectomy are among the most commonly described SILS procedures with various techniques having been reported in the literature. More recently, herniorrhaphy for inguinal hernia by SILS approach has also been reported in both adult and pediatric patients (Tai et al., Surg Endosc 25:2879–2883, 2011; Cugura et al., J Endourol 26:63–66, 2012; Muensterer and Georgeson, Surg Endosc 25:3438–3439, 2011; Kim et al., J Korean Surg Soc 81:339–343, 2011). The initial experience shows that SILS herniorrhaphy for inguinal hernia is technically feasible with satisfied outcomes. Technical challenges, including triangulation, inline vision, and clashing of instruments, were the most salient and frustrating aspect during the procedure. The short-term results have shown that in experienced hands, inguinal hernia repair with SILS technique could be as safe as the standard technique. However, long-term follow-up with larger trials and more sensitive evaluation tools are needed to confirm the initial experience.

Keywords

Totally extraperitoneal hernioplasty (TEP) • Cooper's ligament • Inferior epigastric artery • Transabdominal preperitoneal approach for hernia repair (TAPP) • Umbilical hernia repair • Doom triangle • Pain triangle

S. Wu et al. (eds.), *Atlas of Single-Incision Laparoscopic Operations in General Surgery*,
DOI 10.1007/978-94-007-6955-7_8, © Springer Science+Business Media Dordrecht 2013

8.1 Laparoscopic Totally Extraperitoneal Hernioplasty (TEP)

8.1.1 Indications and Case Selection

TEP is indicated for adults with type I/II/III/IV inguinal hernia, direct hernia, or femoral hernia, and the hernial sacs should be not too large, in which bilateral hernias are also indicated.

8.1.2 Contraindications

1. Inability to tolerate general anesthesia or pneumoperitoneum.
2. Refractory coagulopathy.
3. Irreducible hernia, sliding hernia, incarcerated hernia, strangulated hernia.
4. Extensive previous surgery of lower abdomen.
5. Pregnancy.

8.1.3 Major Instruments or Energy Sources

1. Laparoscopy System
2. Holding forceps
3. Harmonic scalpel

8.1.4 Team Setup, Anesthesia and Position

Under general anesthesia, the patient was placed in supine position with the arms adducted along the side. The position of surgeon, assistants and nurses is shown in Fig. 8.1.

8.1.5 Key Steps

1. Establishment of the extraperitoneum space
2. Dissection and handle of hernia cyst
3. Placement of the mesh
4. Closure of the incision

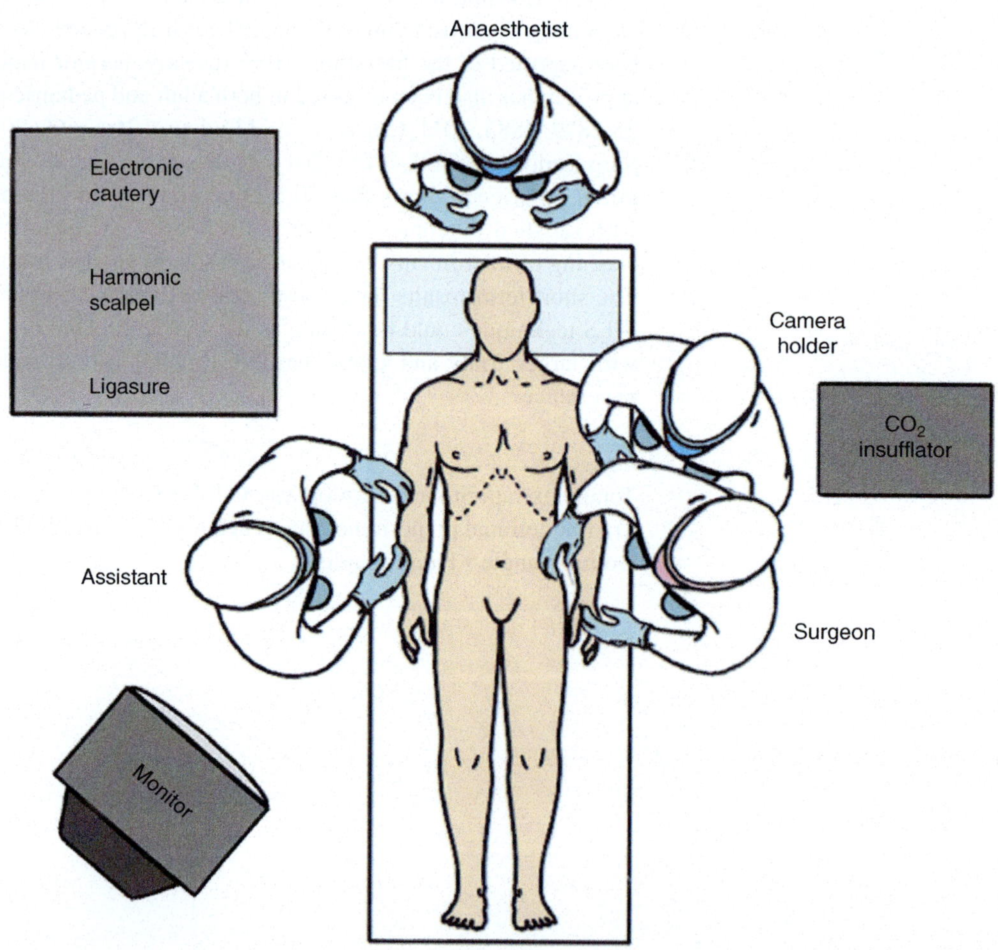

Fig. 8.1

8.1.6 Surgical Techniques

1. Establishment of the extraperitoneum space

   A longitudinal skin incision approximately 20 mm in length was made in the area immediately below the umbilicus, and the anterior rectus sheath of rectus abdominis muscle was opened. A small tunnel was made between rectus muscle and the posterior sheath. The pre-peritoneal space was entered with a 30° laparoscope, and CO_2 gas was added until it reaches 7–8 mmHg. A suture fixation was needed when there was air leakage (Fig. 8.2a, b).

   Conventional trocars were used, including two 5-mm and a 10-mm standard trocar. All three trocars were introduced through the same incision at different fascial sites. entry sites were approximately 10-mm apart in a reverse triangular arrangement (Fig. 8.3).

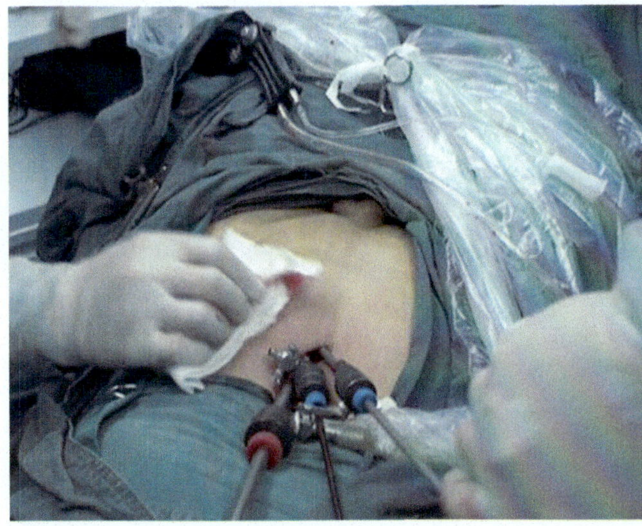

Fig. 8.3

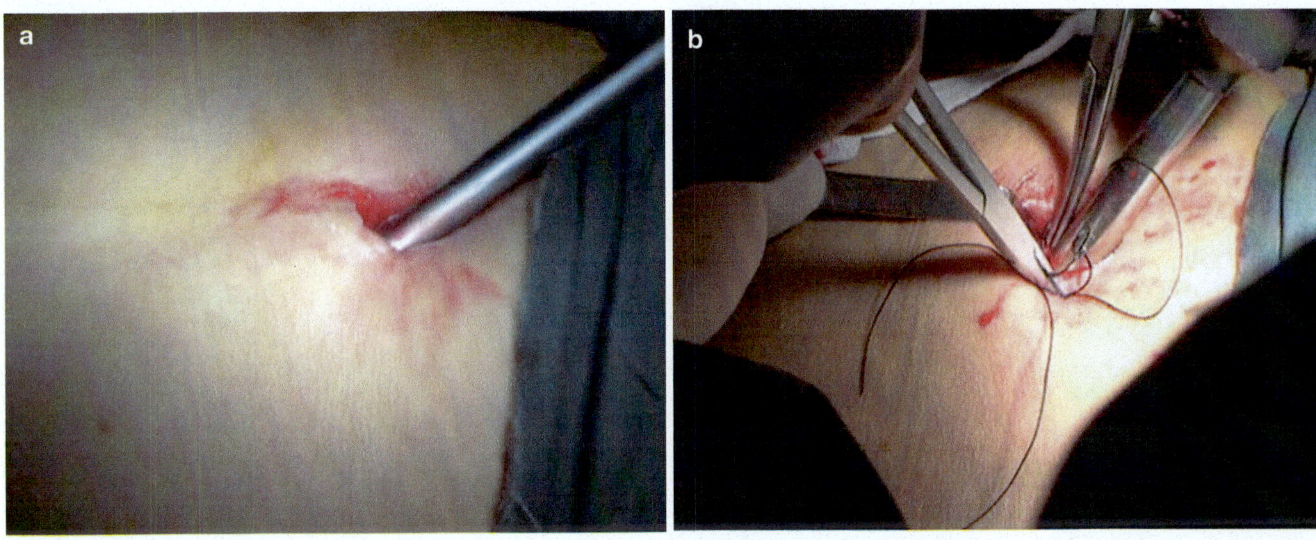

Fig. 8.2

The pre-peritoneal space was sufficiently expanded with Harmonic scalpel, downwards to Cooper's ligament and symphysis pubis (Fig. 8.4a–j).

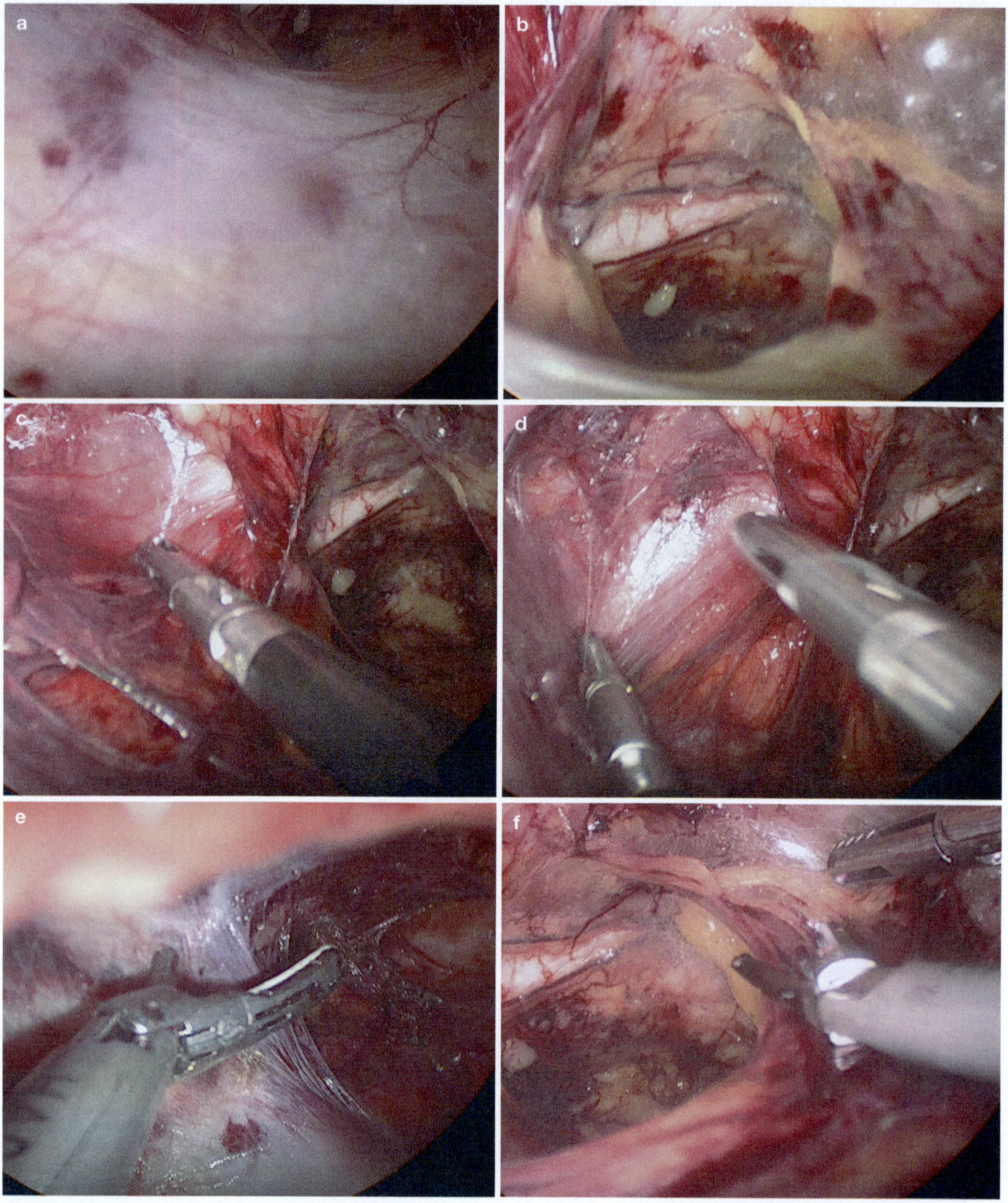

Fig. 8.4

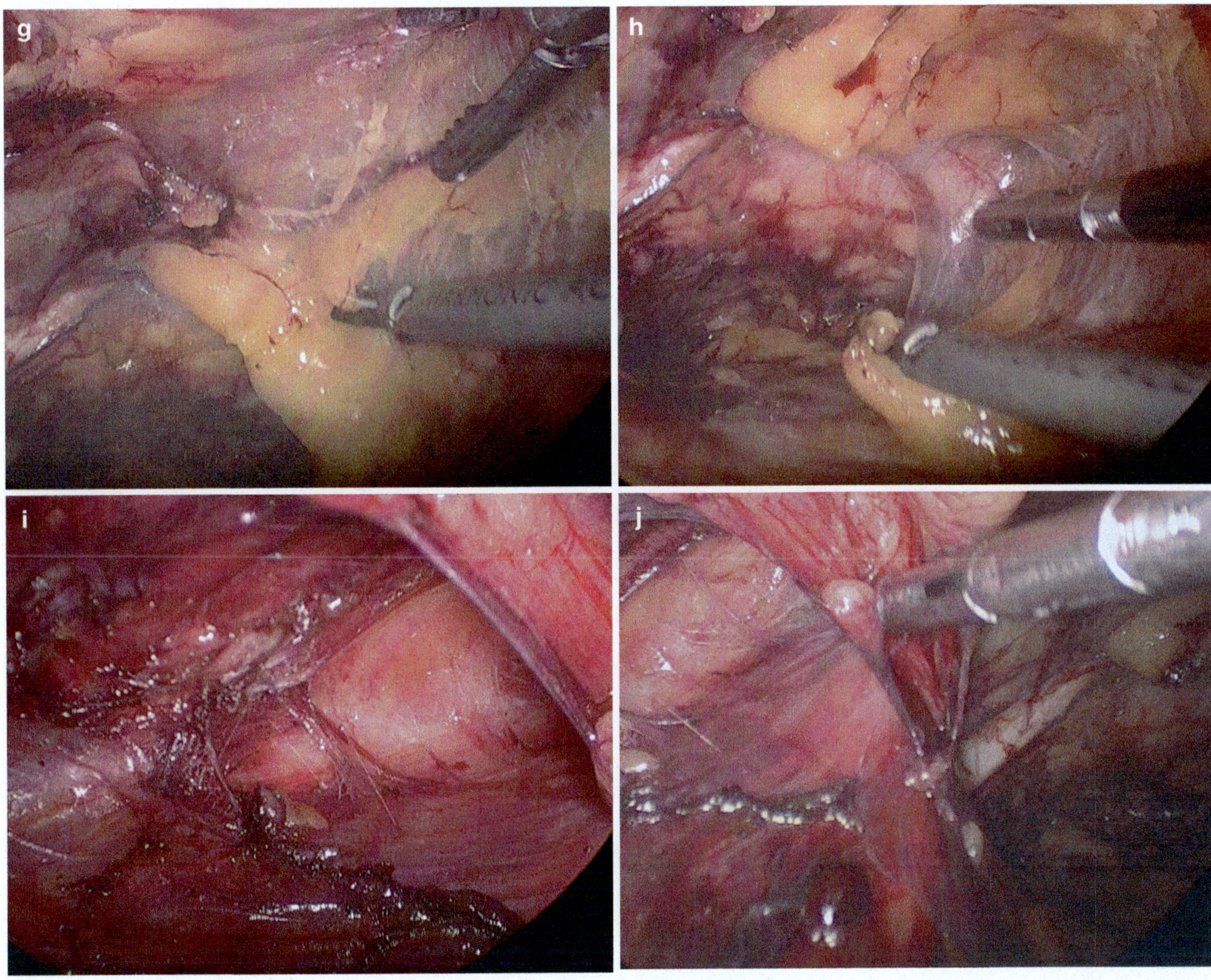

Fig. 8.4 (continued)

2. Dissection and handle of hernia cyst
   Continue expansion of the pre-peritoneal space, middle to the midline, lateral to the anterior superior iliac spine, inferior to the area 2 cm below the Cooper's ligament (Fig. 8.5a–n).

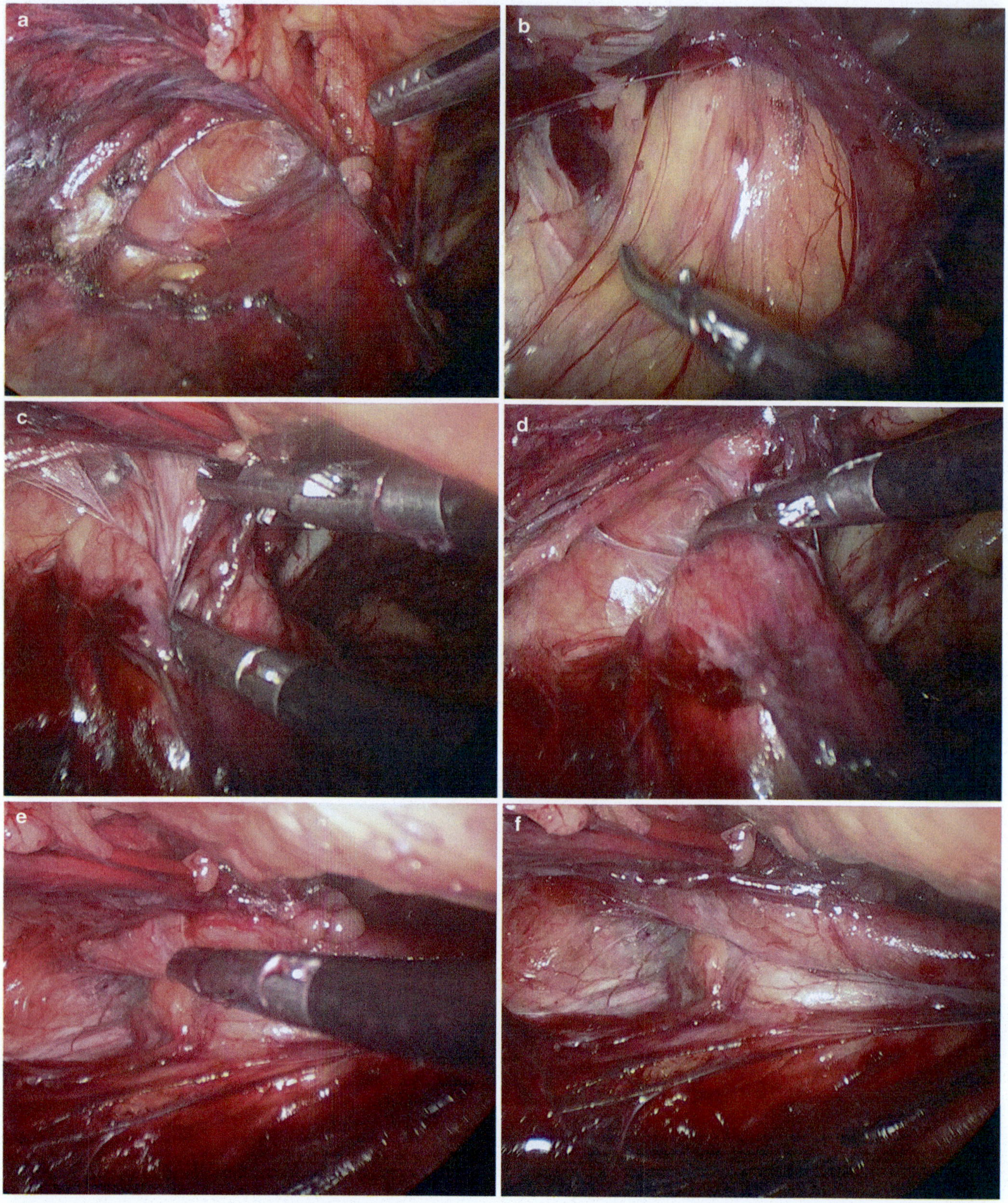

Fig. 8.5

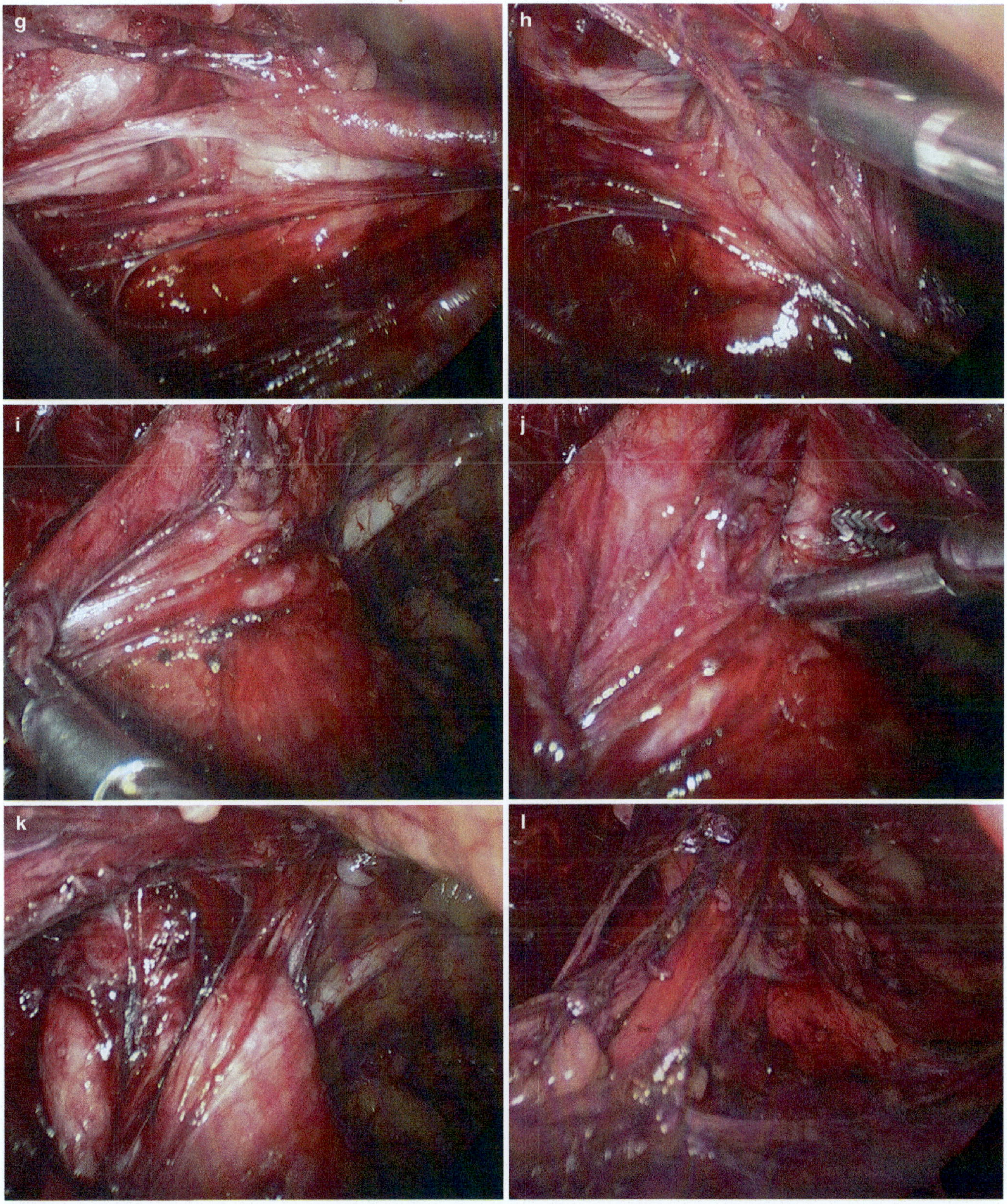

Fig. 8.5 (continued)

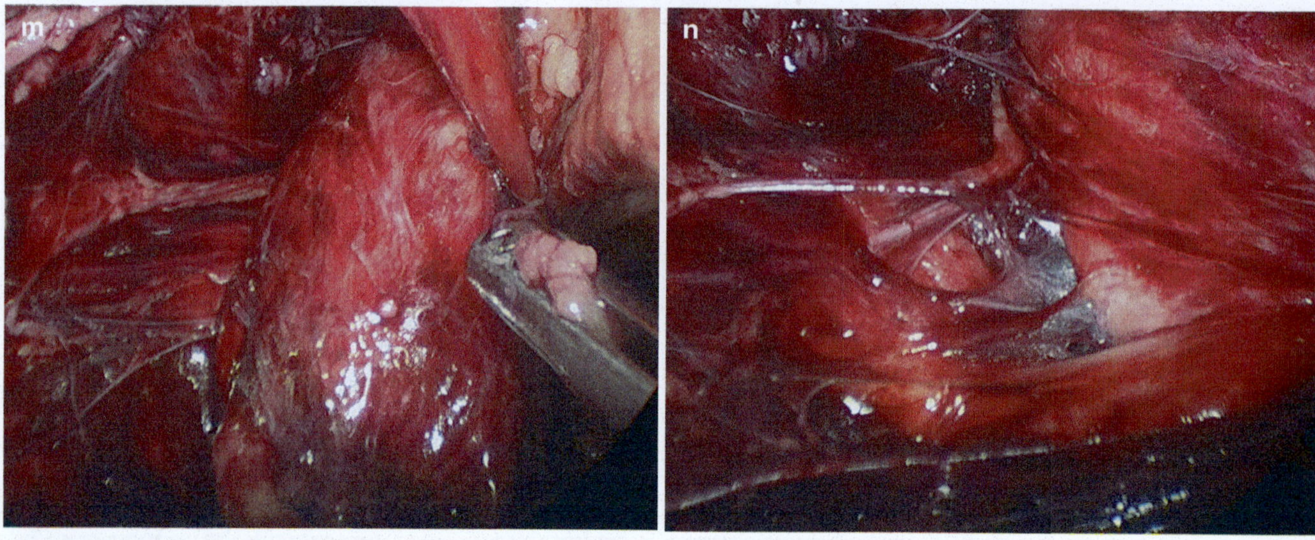

Fig. 8.5 (continued)

The inferior epigastric artery and spermatic cord were exposed (Fig. 8.6a–d).

Expose the hernial sac and reduce its contents. Larger hernial sac was exposed to the neck, which was transected and clipped (Fig. 8.7a–h).

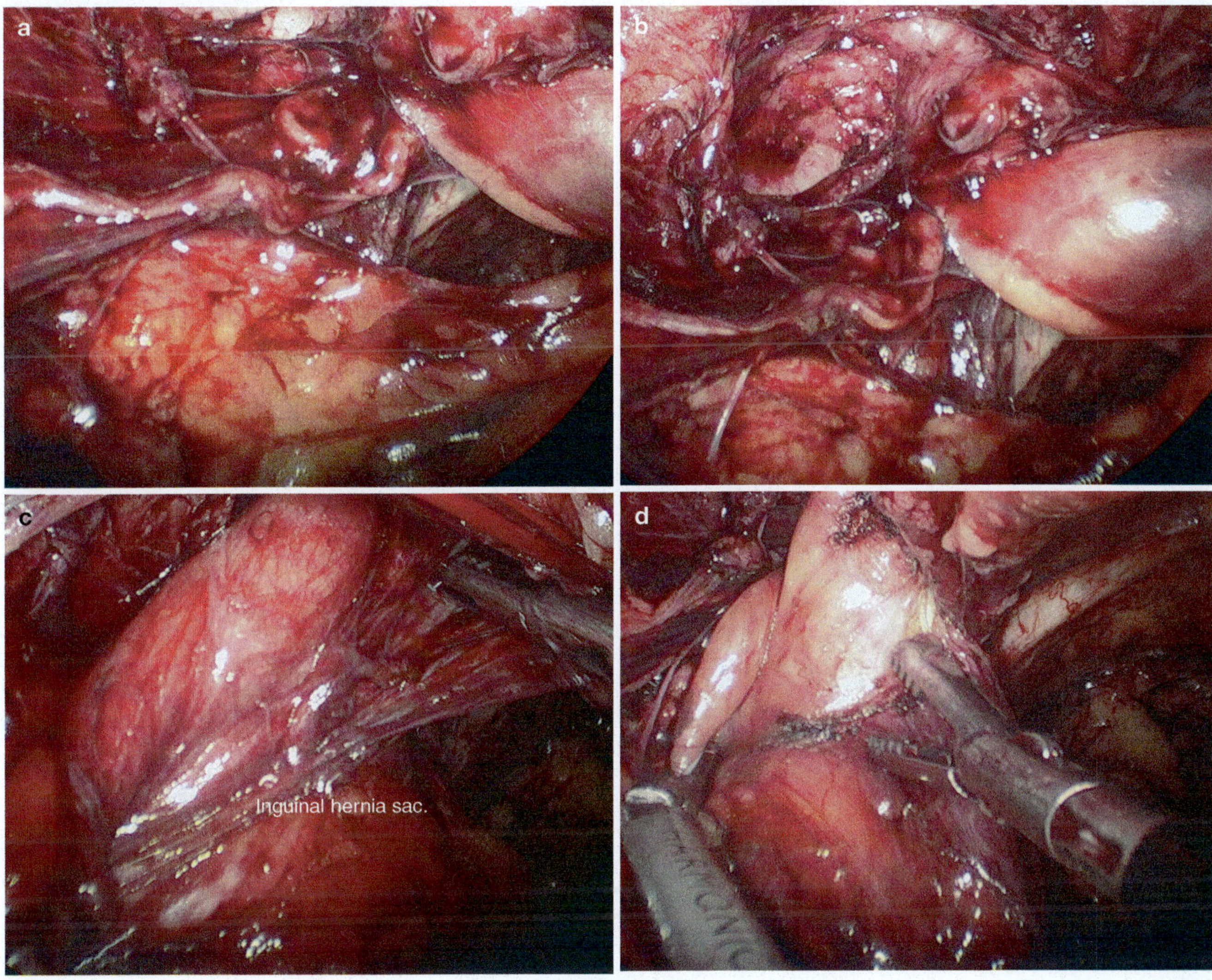

Fig. 8.6

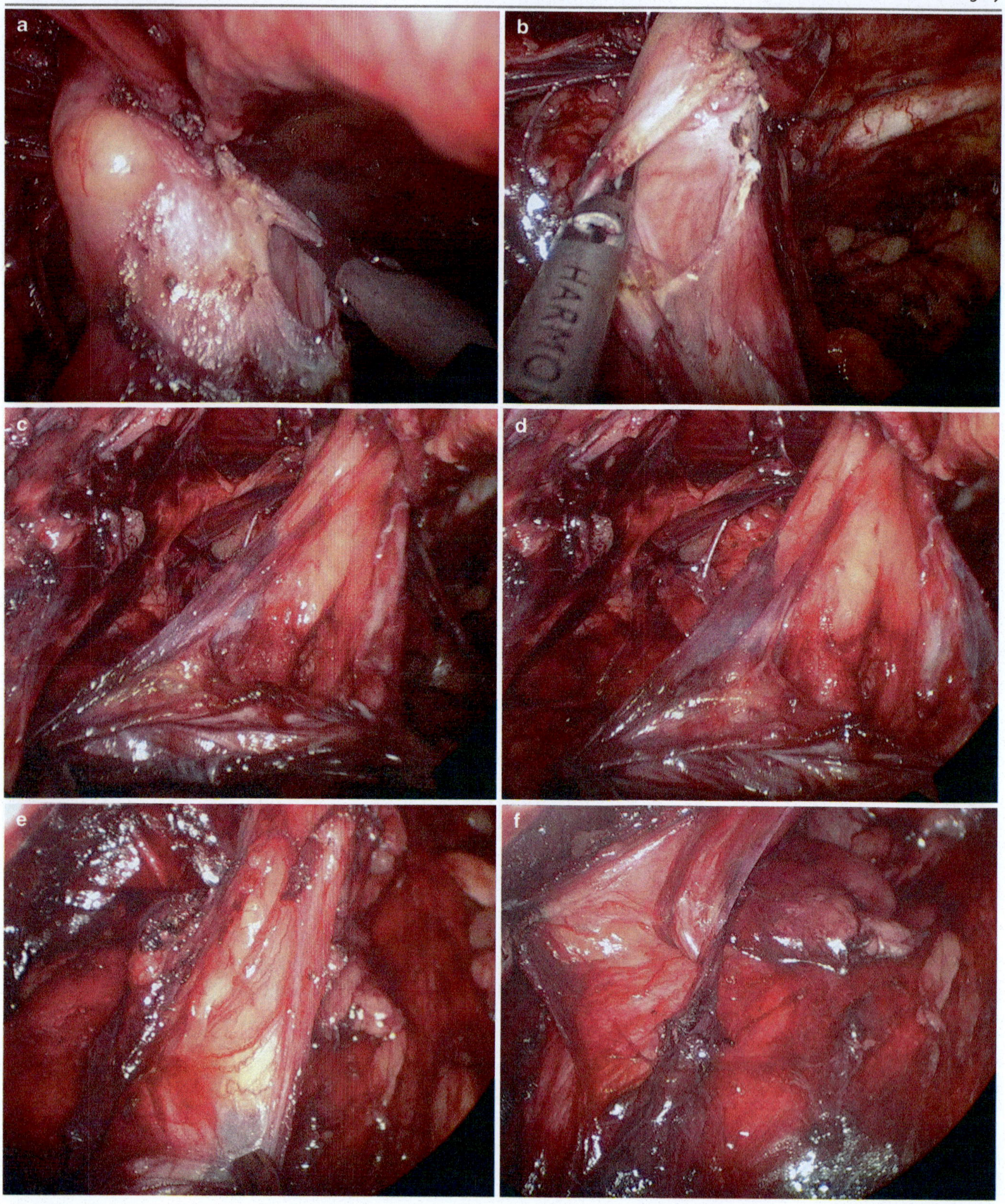

Fig. 8.7

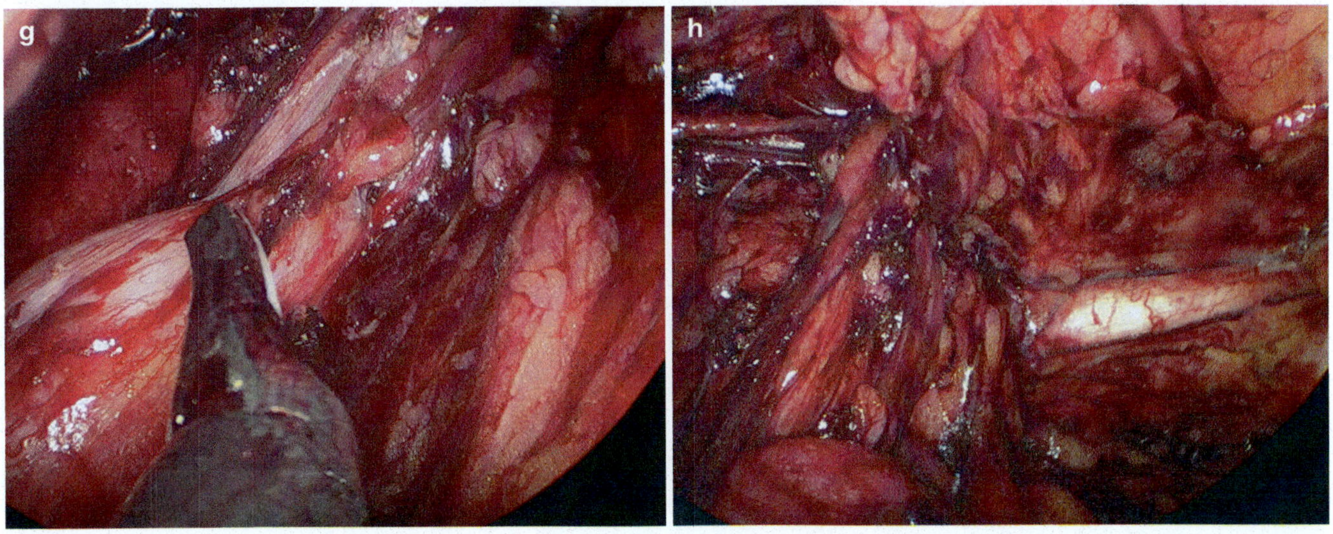

Fig. 8.7 (continued)

3. Placement of the mesh
   The mesh was put into the pre-peritoneal space through the 10 mm Trocar. The inner and outer rings were covered by the mesh so as to strengthen the posterior wall (Fig. 8.8a–f).

4. Closure of the incision
   The inferior umbilical incision was closed and the operation was thus completed.

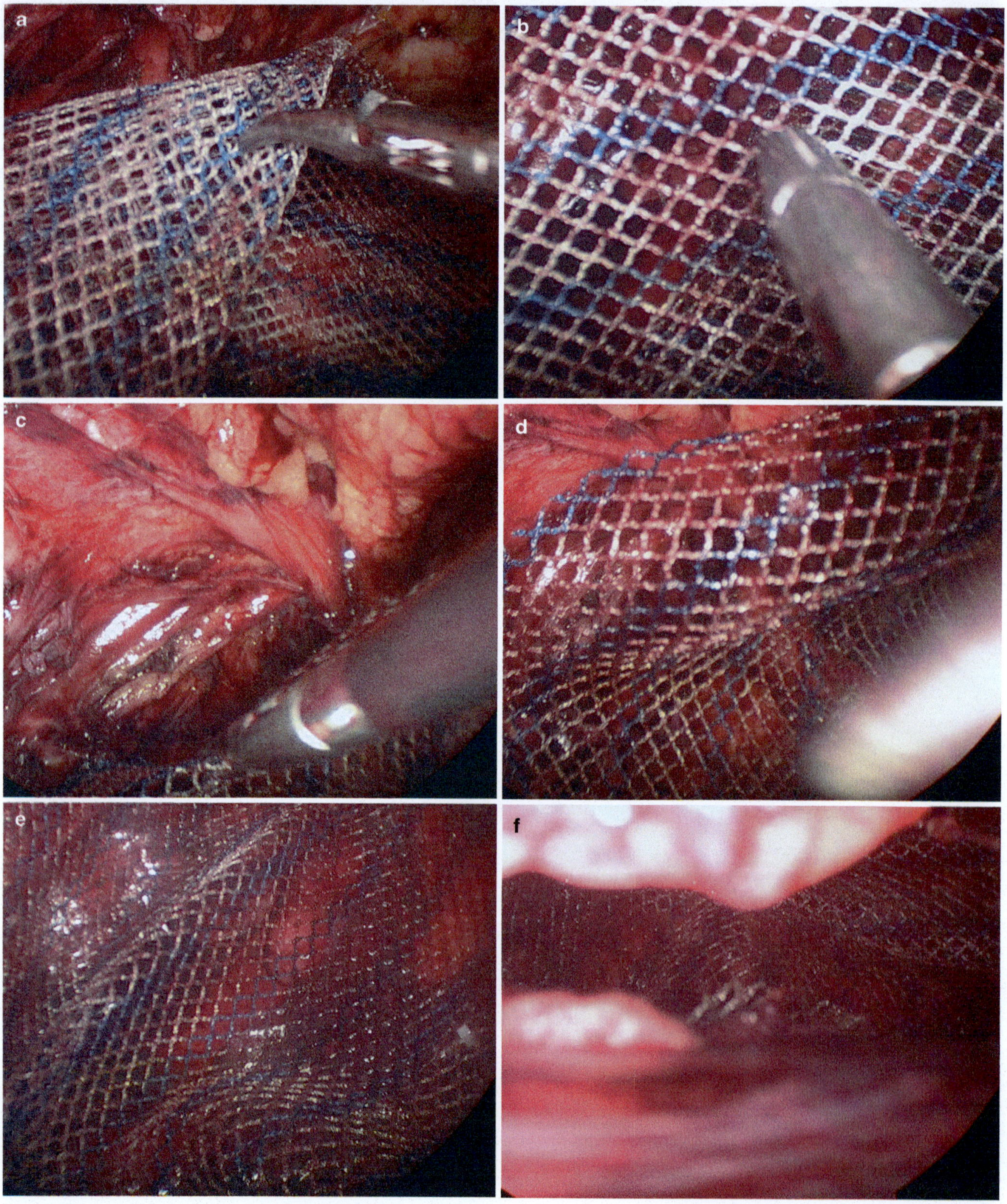

Fig. 8.8

8.1.7 Tips and Tricks

1. The bladder should be drained by a urethral catheter to maximize the working space.
2. A combination of sharp and blunt dissection defines and reduces the hernial sac.
3. In cases of indirect hernias, the spermatic cord should be carefully isolated and freed from the hernial sac.
4. It is important to ensure adequate lateral dissection to the level of the anterior superior iliac spine to allow placement of the mesh. A small cut is fashioned to accommodate the cord structures.
5. The mesh may be rolled up and tied with two stay sutures to allow easy insertion through the trocar. Once inside, the stay sutures are cut and the mesh unfurled. It is positioned in place around the spermatic cord from the pubic symphysis in the midline to the anterior iliac spine laterally.

8.2 Laparoscopic Transabdominal Preperitoneal Approach for Hernia Repair (TAPP)

8.2.1 Indications and Case Selection

TAPP is indicated for adults with type I/II/III/IV inguinal hernia, direct hernia, or femoral hernia, including irreducible hernia, recurrent hernia, postoperative recurrent hernia, sliding hernia, or if the hernial sac is large.

8.2.2 Contraindications

1. Inability to tolerate general anesthesia or pneumoperitoneum.
2. Refractory coagulopathy.
3. Irreducible hernia, sliding hernia, incarcerated hernia, strangulated hernia.
4. Extensive previous surgery of lower abdomen.
5. Pregnancy.

8.2.3 Major Instruments or Energy Sources

1. Laparoscopy System
2. Holding forceps
3. Harmonic scalpel

8.2.4 Team Setup, Anesthesia and Position

Under general anesthesia, the patient was placed in supine position with the arms adducted along the side. The position of surgeon, assistants and nurses is shown in Fig. 8.9.

8.2.5 Key Steps

1. Establishment of pneumopneutonium
2. Dissection of peritoneum around the hernia cyst
3. Dissection of sperm cord and ligature of the hernia cyst
4. Placement of the mesh
5. Closure of the incision

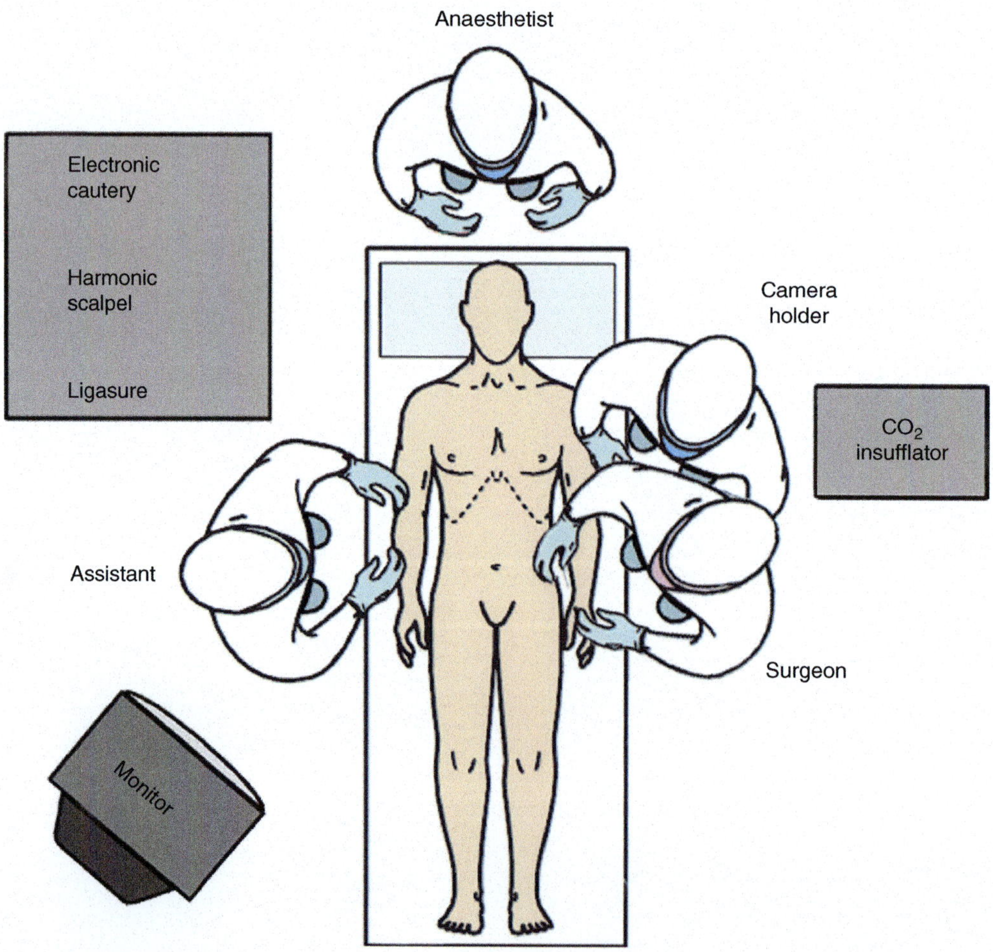

Fig. 8.9

8.2.6 Surgical Techniques

1. Establishment of pneumopneutonium
   Pneumoperitoneum was created with the closed method using a veress needle, and insufflations pressure maintained at 13 mmHg. A 2-cm periumbilical incision was made for trocar access. Conventional trocars were used, including two 5-mm trocars, a 10-mm standard trocar. An exploration of the abdomen was performed. The size of the hernia ring and hernial content were checked (Fig. 8.10a, b).

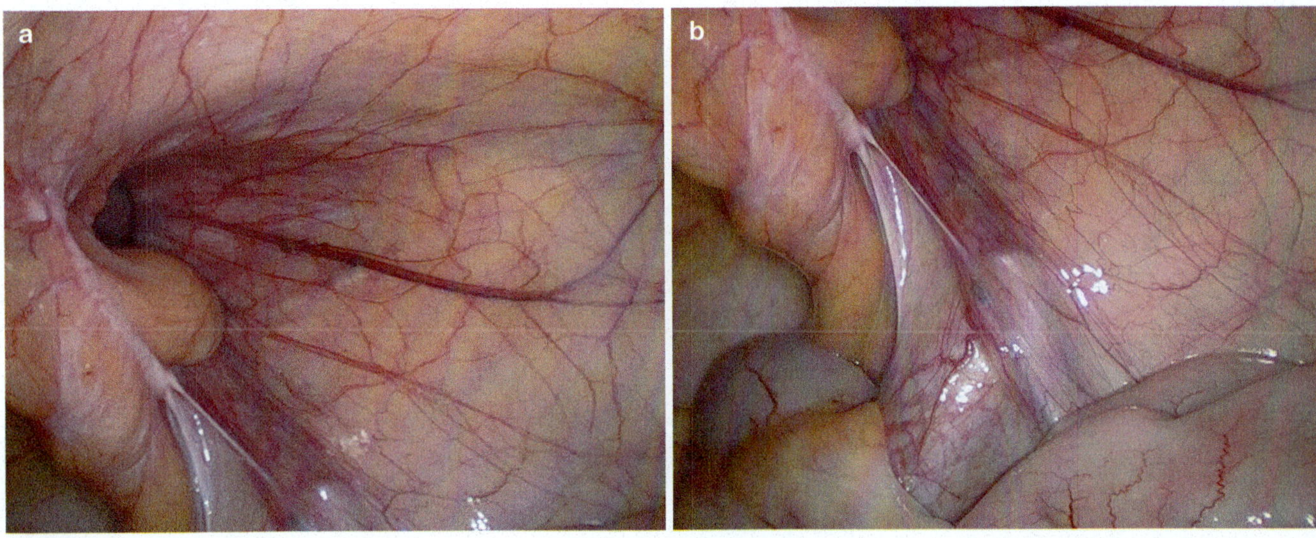

Fig. 8.10

2. Dissection of peritoneum around the hernia cyst
   The surrounding peritoneum of the hernia ring was lifted and opened with the Harmonic Scalpel, middle to the midline, lateral to the anterior superior iliac spine, inferior to the pectineal ligament (Fig. 8.11a–h).

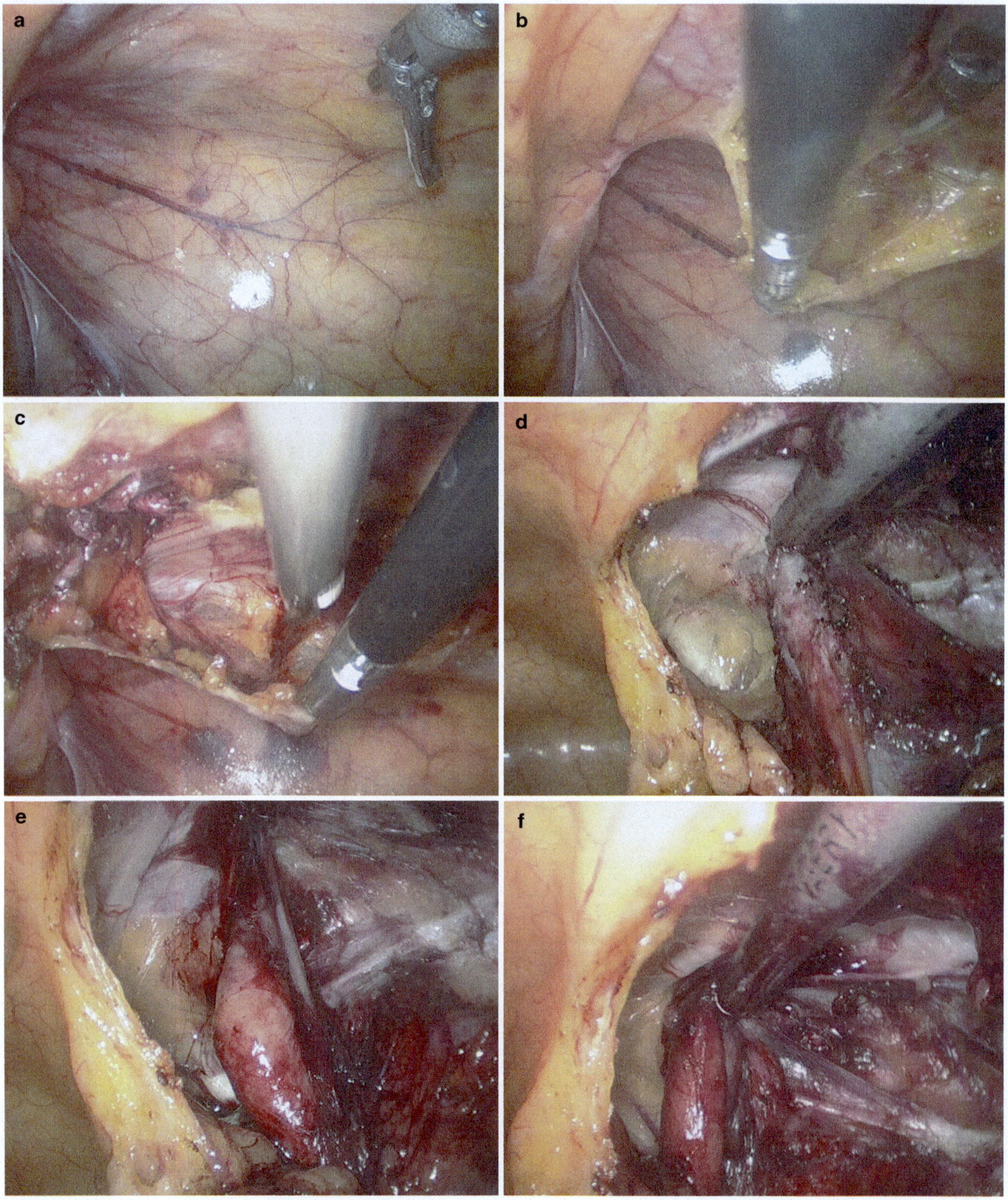

Fig. 8.11

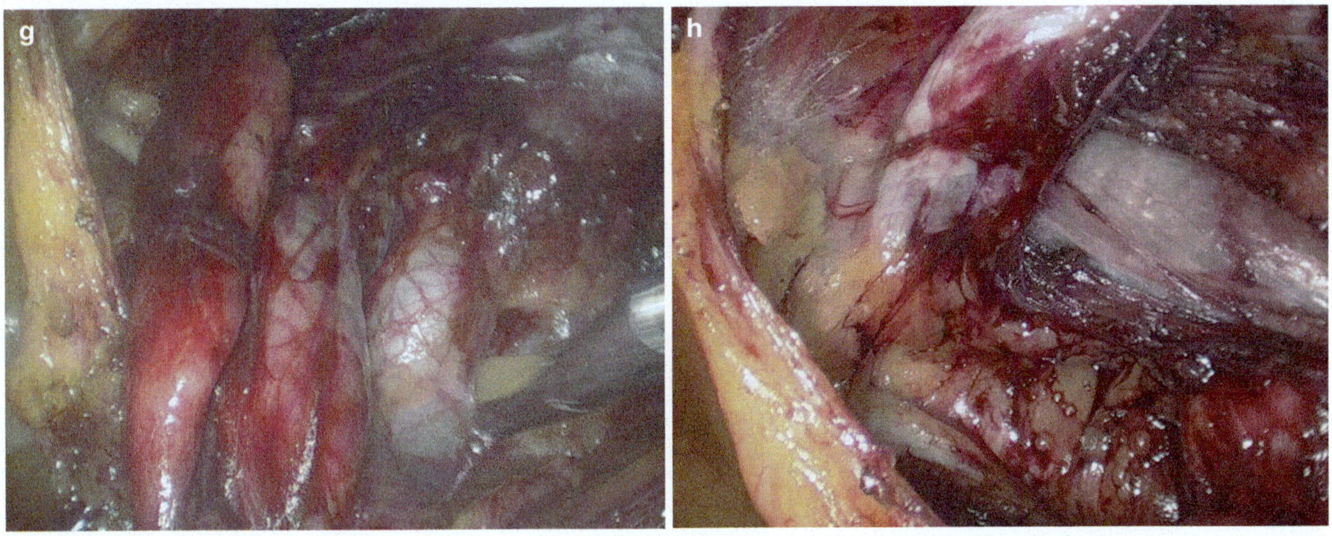

Fig. 8.11 (continued)

3. Dissection of spermatic cord and ligature of the hernia cyst
   Separate hernial sac from spermatic duct and spermatic vessels leaving the sac on the abdominal wall. Avoid damage to the spermatic vessels and iliac vessels (Fig. 8.12a–d).

The hernia sac was transected and ligated after fully mobilized. The hernia sac was pulled downwards with the peritoneum and the pre-peritoneal space was fully exposed (Fig. 8.13a–d).

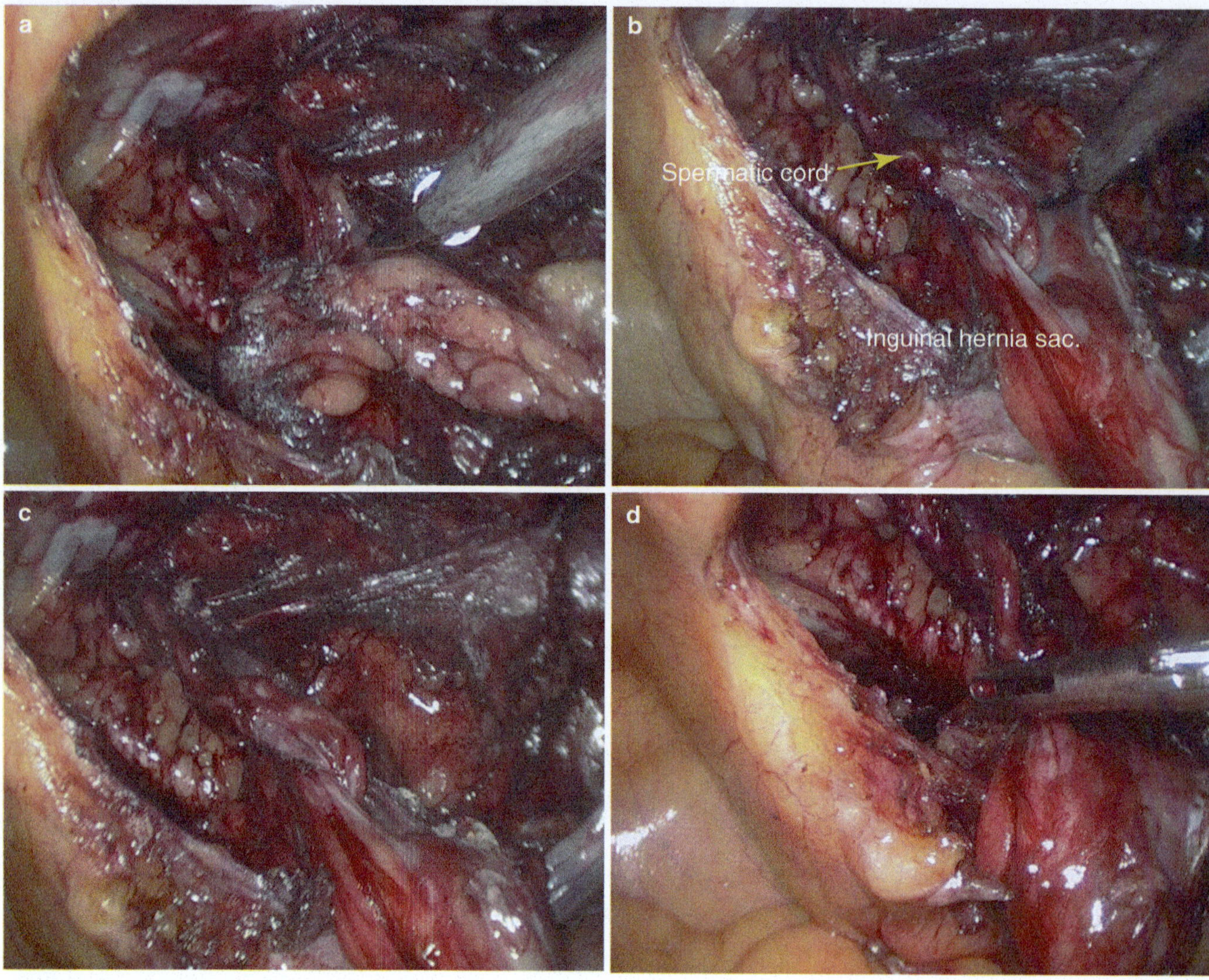

Fig. 8.12

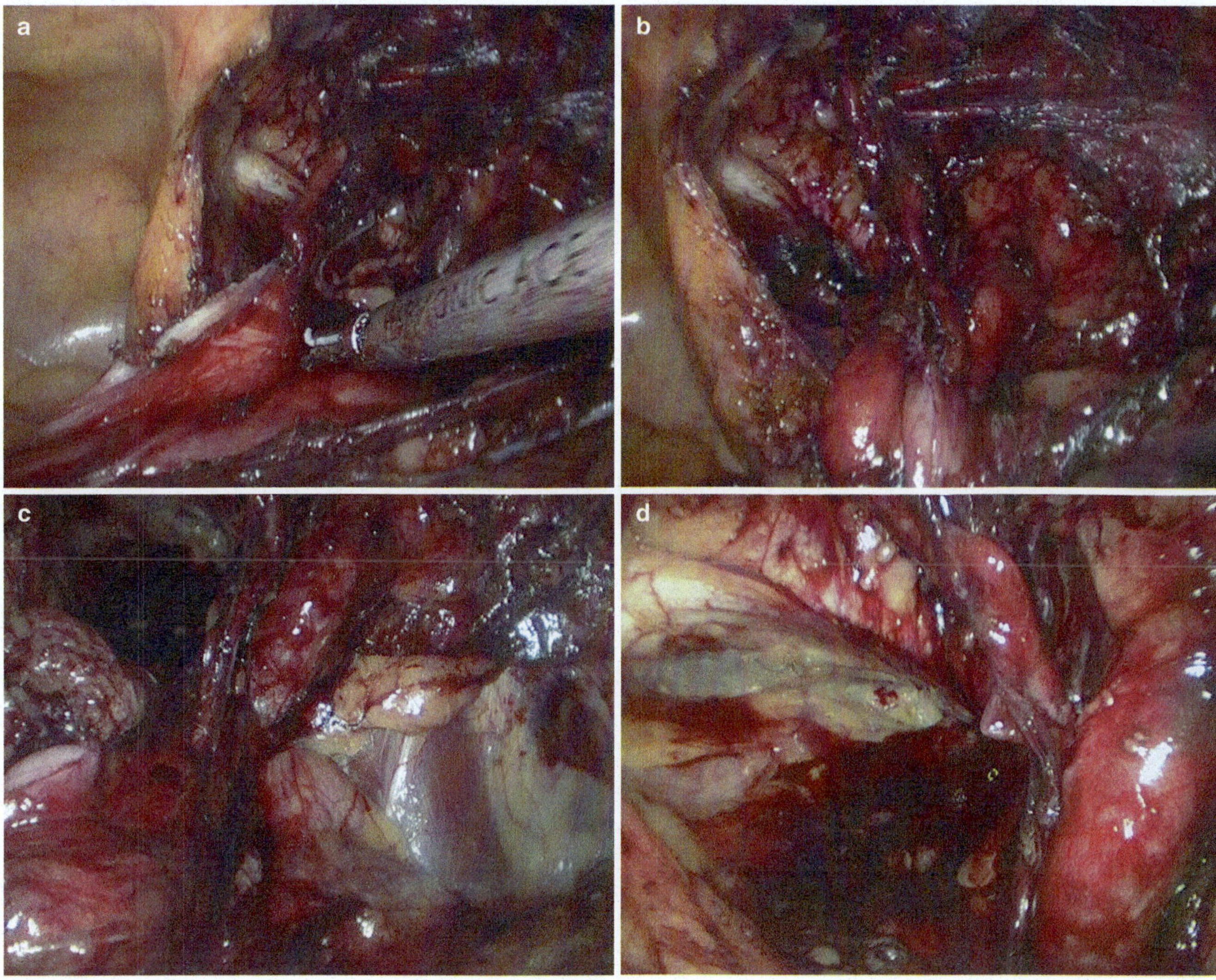

Fig. 8.13

4. Placement of the mesh
   The mesh was put into the pre-peritoneal space through the 10 mm Trocar and paved nicely to cover the inner ring. The spermatic duct was left intact in front of the mesh. The peritoneum was closed with 3/0 absorbable suture and overlay the mesh (Fig. 8.14a–h).

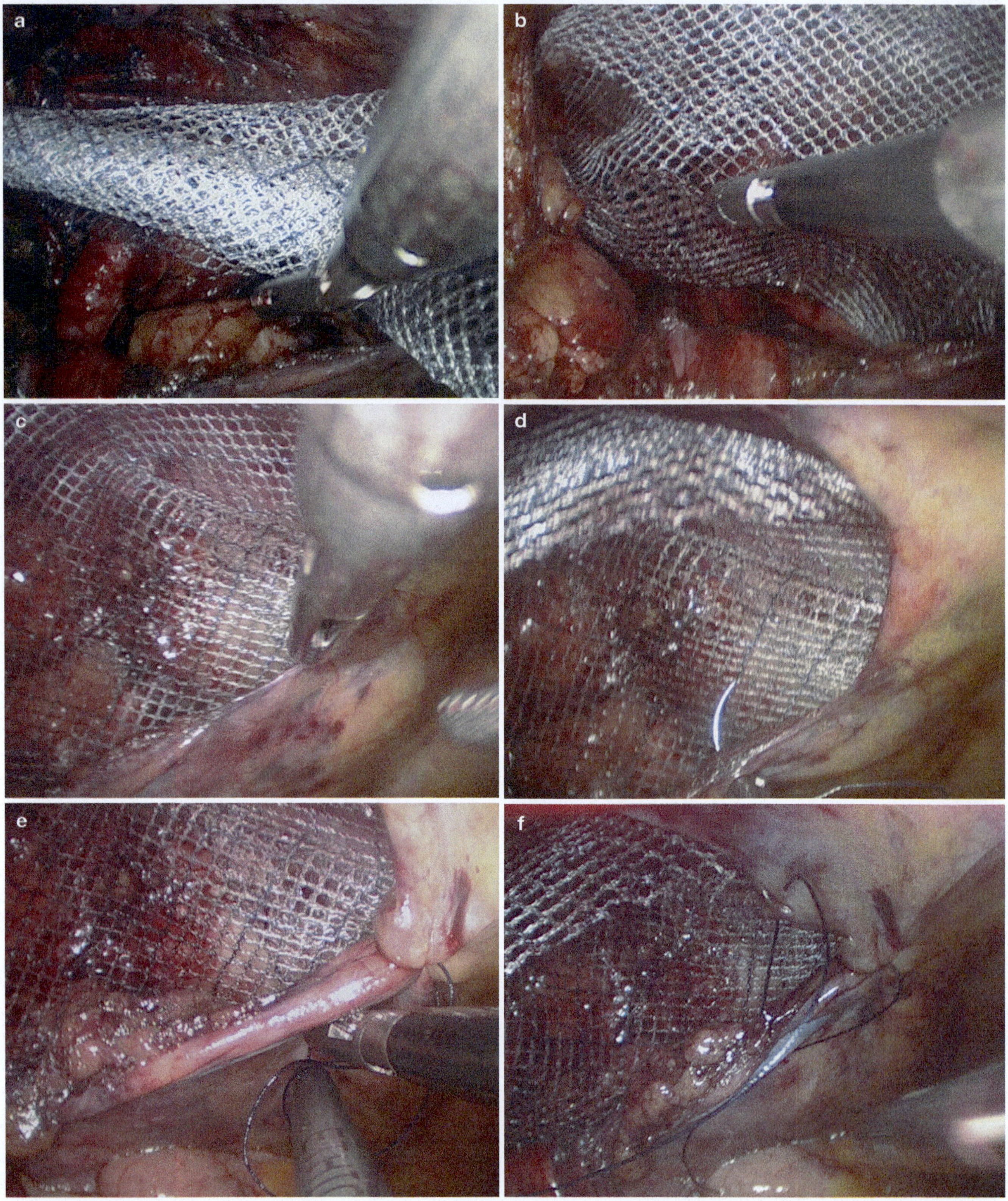

Fig. 8.14

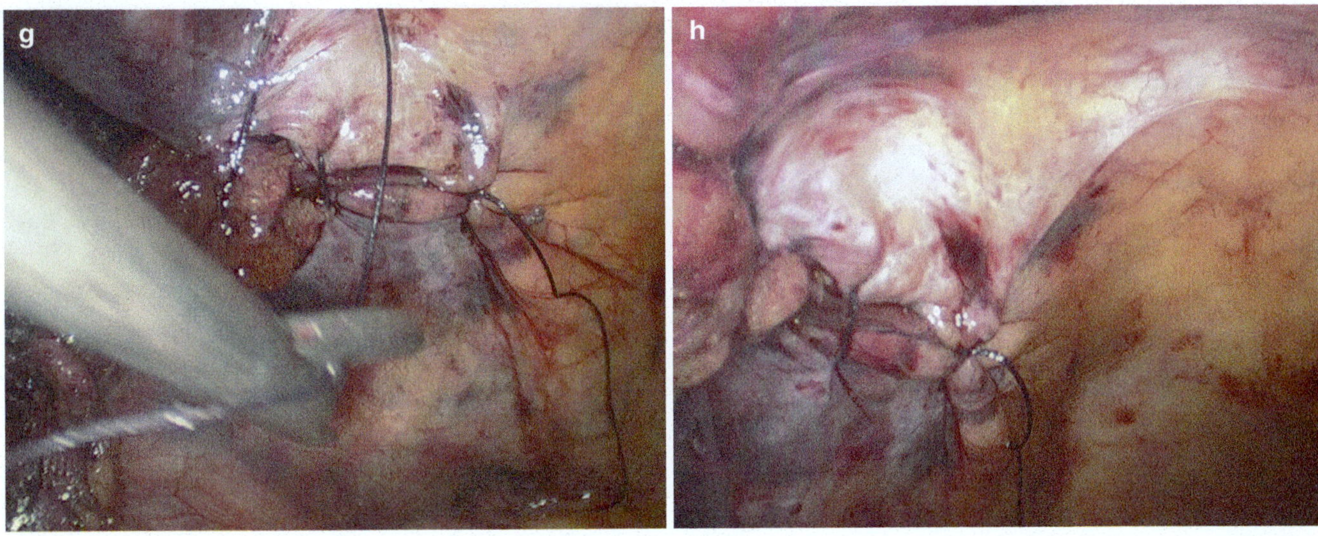

Fig. 8.14 (continued)

5. Closure of the incision
   The periumbilical incision was closed and the operation was thus completed (Fig. 8.15).

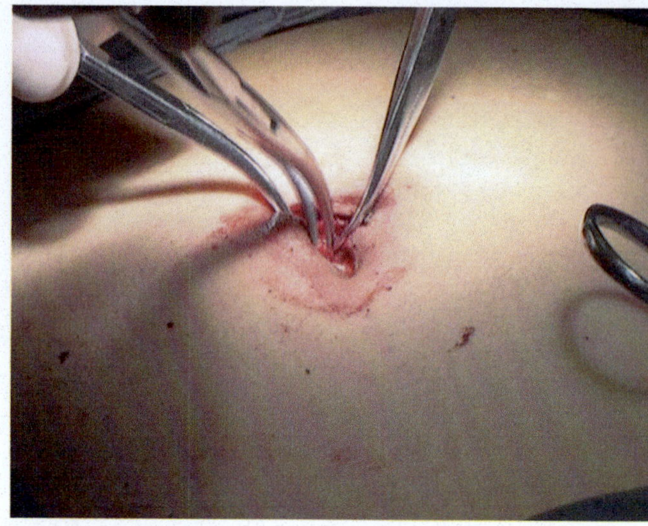

Fig. 8.15

8.2.7 Tips and Tricks

1. The patient should be put into a Trendelenburg position to allow the small bowel loops to fall back from the groin region.
2. The surgeon should stand on the opposite side of the hernia while the surgeon who was handling the camera should stand on the same side of hernia.
3. The peritoneal flap should be created with an incision extending from the medial umbilical ligament to the level of anterior superior iliac spine.
4. One endoscissors or endodissector and one rigid dissector or grasper was very helpful for tissue dissection.
5. The mesh should be positioned to cover the entire dissected area reinforcing the myopectineal orifice.
6. The peritoneal flap should be closed by continuous suturing with 2-0 vicryl sutures. The needle, along with the suture of the estimated required length, is dragged in with a needle holder, and suturing is started with a bite of the lower flap and then of the upper flap. The suturing is terminated with an intracorporeal knot.

8.3 Laparoscopic Approach for Umbilical Hernia Repair

8.3.1 Indications and Case Selection

Laparoscopic approach for umbilical hernia repair is indicated for patients with umbilical hernia, it's superior for patients with the requirements of reserving navel.

8.3.2 Contraindications

1. Inability to tolerate general anesthesia or pneumoperitoneum.
2. Refractory coagulopathy.
3. Acute incarcerated hernia, strangulated hernia.
4. Pregnancy.

8.3.3 Major Instruments or Energy Sources

1. Laparoscopy System
2. Holding forceps
3. Harmonic scalpel

8.3.4 Team Setup, Anesthesia and Position

Under general anesthesia, the patient was placed in supine position with the arms adducted along the side. The position of surgeon, assistants and nurses is shown in Fig. 8.16.

8.3.5 Key Steps

1. Establishment of pneumoperitonium
2. Reduction of content of hernia cyst
3. Cover the orifice of hernia cyst with mesh and fixation
4. Closure of the incision

8.3.6 Surgical Techniques

1. Establishment of pneumoperitonium
   Pneumoperitoneum was created using a veress needle, and insufflations pressure maintained at 15 mmHg. Conventional trocars were used, including two 5-mm standard trocars and an unbladed trocar. All three trocars were introduced through the same incision at different fascial sites. Entry sites were approximately

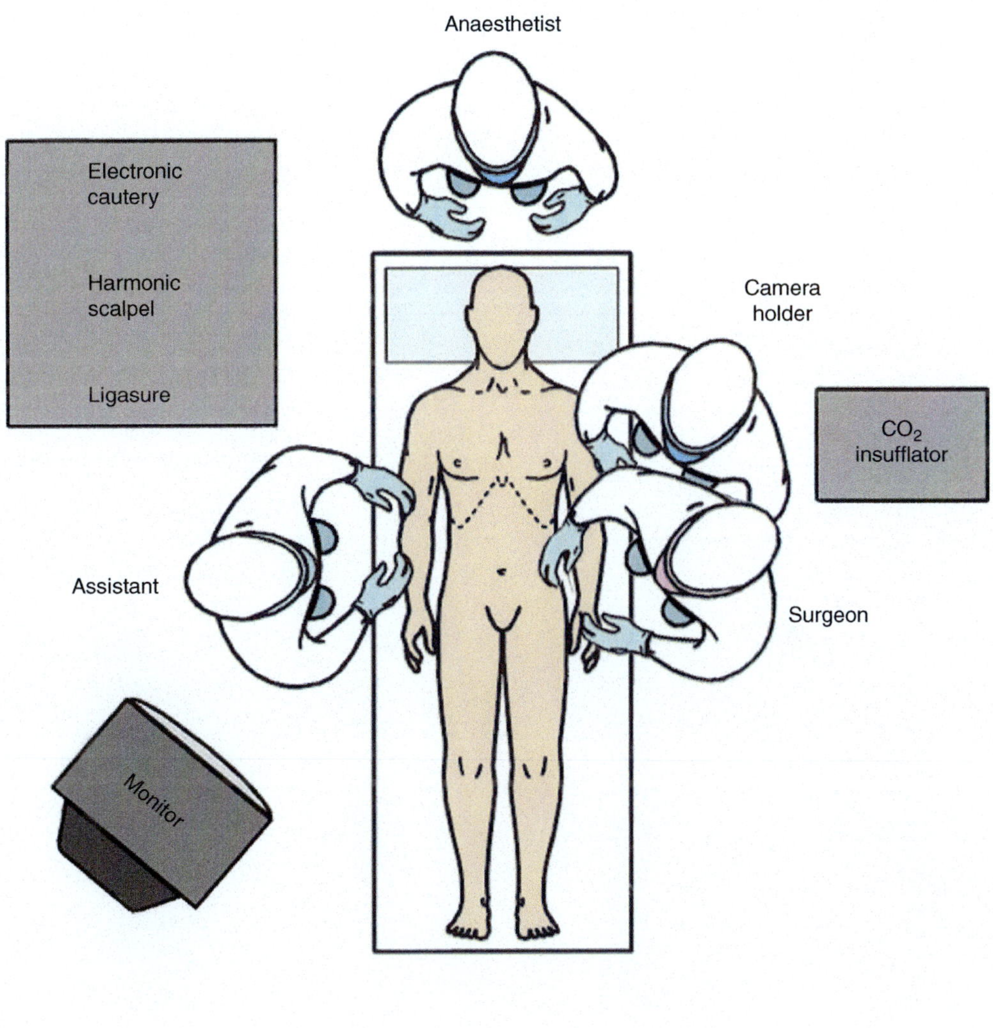

Fig. 8.16

10-mm apart in a reverse triangular arrangement. The umbilical hernial sac was found to be protruding outwards.

2. Reduction of content of hernia cyst
   The hernial contents were reduced with intestinal forceps (Fig. 8.17).

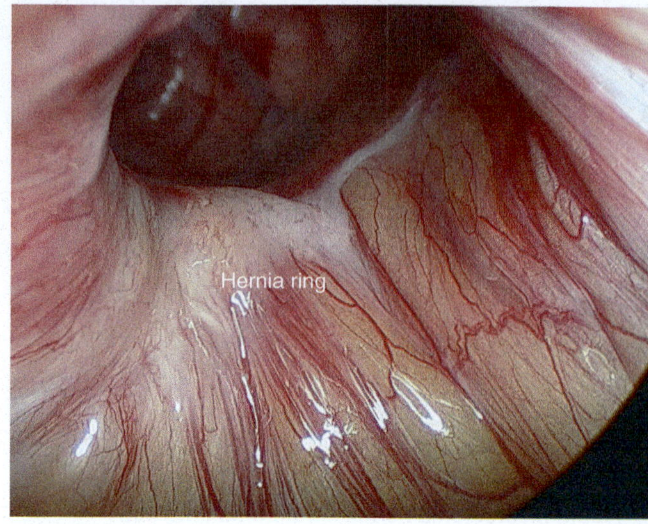

Fig. 8.17

3. Cover the orifice of hernia cyst with mesh and fixation
   The mesh was placed into the abdominal cavity, with anti-adhesion surface facing the intestines. The hernial sac was covered with the mesh, which was fixed to abdominal wall by laparoscopic staple (Fig. 8.18a–i).

4. Closure of the incision
   The incision was closed in two layers, and the operation was thus completed.

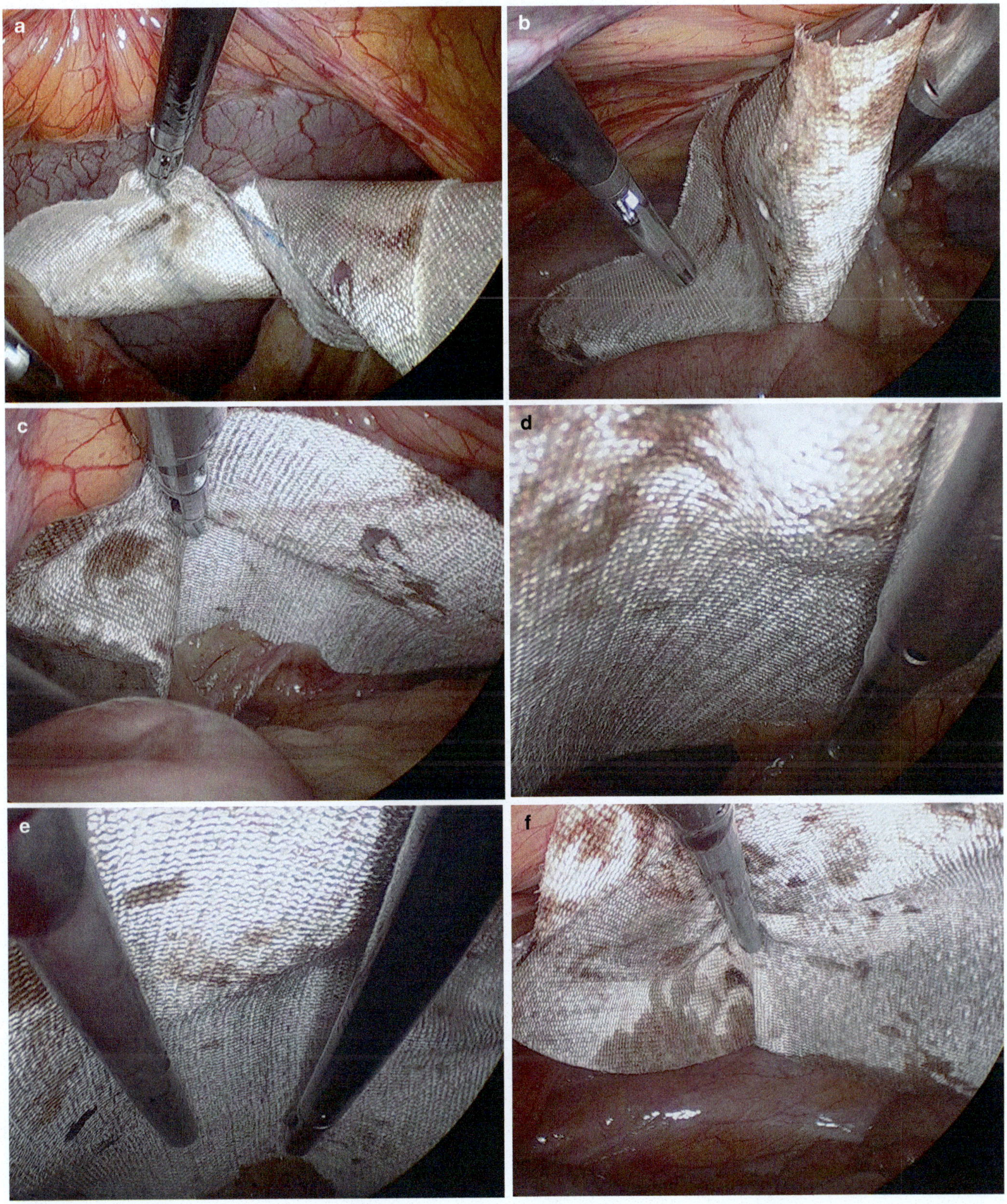

Fig. 8.18

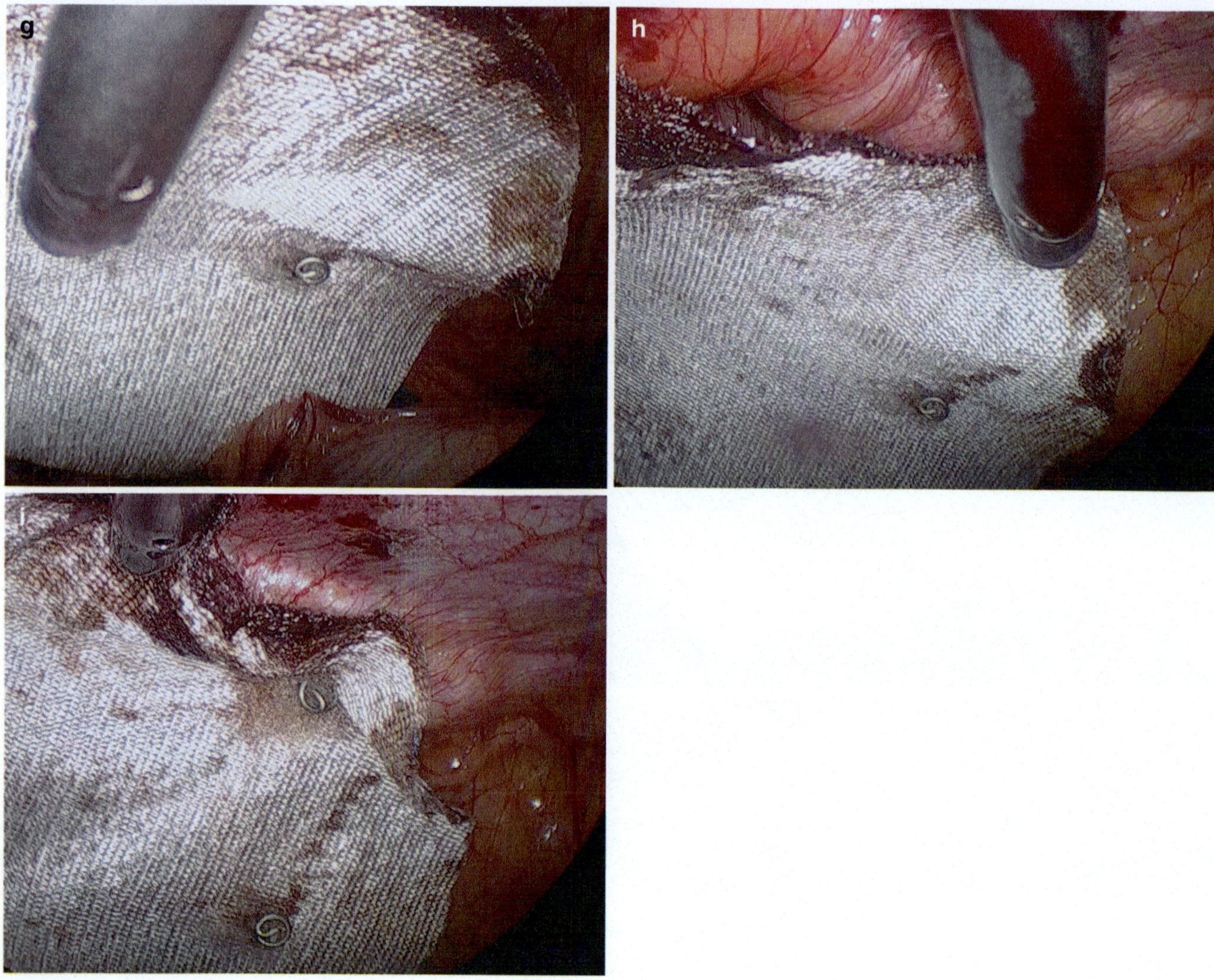

Fig. 8.18 (continued)

8.4 Complications Analysis and Management

8.4.1 Hematoma

Because the preperitoneal space is wildly dissected in the procedure, postoperative hematoma formation in this space is possible. The manifestations are skin swelling and ecchymosis formation. Local physical therapy or puncture may gradually absorb the hematoma. Postoperative local pressure dressing or pressed by sand bag can decrease the exudation and prevent the formation of hematoma.

8.4.2 Blood Vessels Injury

In SILS herniorrhaphy, the vessels that may be injured include spermatic vessels, external iliac vessels, and obturator muscle blood vessels. The injury of spermatic vessels is common and the result of external iliac vessels injury is the most severe. The area between seminiferous duct and spermatic vessels is called "doom triangle". The external iliac vessels are in this area and traumatic operation should be avoided in this area.

8.4.3 Nerve Injury

In SILS procedure, the risk of iliohypogastric and ilioinguinal nerve injury is lower than that in open procedure. However, the genital branch and femoral branch of genitofemoral nerve may be injured. In the procedure, these nerves are difficult to identify and the surgical operation should avoid the "pain triangle" (space between iliopubic tract and spermatic vessels), these nerves are within this area.

8.4.4 Hernia Recurrence

Hernia recurrence may occur post SILS herniorrhaphy. The risk of hernia recurrence is related to the surgeon's increasing operational experiences and the selection and fixation of hernia patch.

References

1. Tai HC, Lin CD, Chung SD, Chueh SC, Tsai YC, Yang SS. A comparative study of standard versus laparoendoscopic single-site surgery (LESS) totally extraperitoneal (TEP) inguinal hernia repair. Surg Endosc. 2011;25:2879–83.
2. Cugura JF, Kirac I, Kulis T, Sremac M, Ledinsky M, Beslin MB. Comparison of single incision laparoscopic totally extraperitoneal and laparoscopic totally extraperitoneal inguinal hernia repair: initial experience. J Endourol. 2012;26:63–6.
3. Muensterer OJ, Georgeson KE. Multimedia manuscript: inguinal hernia repair by single-incision pediatric endosurgery (SIPES) using the hydrodissection-lasso technique. Surg Endosc. 2011; 25:3438–9.
4. Kim JH, Park SM, Kim JJ, Lee YS. Initial experience of single port laparoscopic totally extraperitoneal hernia repair: nearly-scarless inguinal hernia repair. J Korean Surg Soc. 2011;81:339–43.

Breast Surgery: Breast Conserving Radical Mastectomy with Single-Incision Endoscopic Axillary Dissection

9

Abstract

Minimally invasive and functional therapy represents an inevitable trend in breast surgery. Although much progress has been made in the surgical approaches to the breast, little progress has been made in the surgical approach to the axilla. Improved surgical techniques for breast cancer would be to decrease the morbidity of the axillary dissection without necessarily sacrificing lymph node retrieval for accurate staging. Endoscopic surgery on breasts represents the developing trend in breast surgery toward the minimally invasive techniques, improving functional and cosmetic aspects of the procedure with great potential patient benefits (Chengyu et al., Surg Laparosc Endosc Percutan Tech 15:153–159, 2005). Because of an improved visualization and magnification of the operative field, laparoscopic-assisted axillary lymph node dissection provides a precise, gentle, and safe alternative to lymphadenectomy performed via a standard axillary incision (Lim and Lam, Am J Surg 90:641–643, 2005). As video imaging systems and new instruments continue to develop, single-incision laparoscopic surgery (SILS) has recently been a focus for active investigation in the surgical field. After attempts in the techniques of cholecystectomy and thyroid surgery with satisfied outcomes (Wu et al., Adv Surg Tech A 21:25–28, 2011), wide segmental excision and SILS axillary lymph node dissection was performed in our department. The initial results have shown that in experienced hands, this technique could be as safe as the standard technique. However, larger studies are required to confirm these findings and determine the true benefits of SILS axillary lymph node dissection.

Keywords

Mastectomy • Axillary dissection

S. Wu et al. (eds.), *Atlas of Single-Incision Laparoscopic Operations in General Surgery*,
DOI 10.1007/978-94-007-6955-7_9, © Springer Science+Business Media Dordrecht 2013

9.1 Indications and Case Selection

1. Patients with breast tumor no more than 3 cm, and have no adhesions with the skin and pectoral fascia.
2. Patients with no documented enlarged lymph nodes, or the diameter of lymph nodes is less than 1 cm in the homonymy axillary fossa.
3. Patients with no remote metastasis.

9.2 Contraindications

1. Patients with breast tumor larger than 5 cm, and have adhesions with the skin and chest wall.
2. Patients with documented enlarged lymph nodes larger than 1 cm, or with multiple lymph nodes mixed together.
3. Patients with the history of operation in axillary fossa, and have severe adhesion.
4. Patients have remote metastasis.
5. Patients with inability to tolerate general anesthesia.

9.3 Major Instruments or Energy Sources

1. Laparoscopy System.
2. Holding forceps.
3. Harmonic scalpel.

9.4 Team Setup, Anesthesia and Position

Under general anesthesia, the patient was placed in supine position. The arm on the lesion side was extended to expose the axilla. The position of surgeon, assistants and nurses is shown in Fig. 9.1a, b.

Fig. 9.1

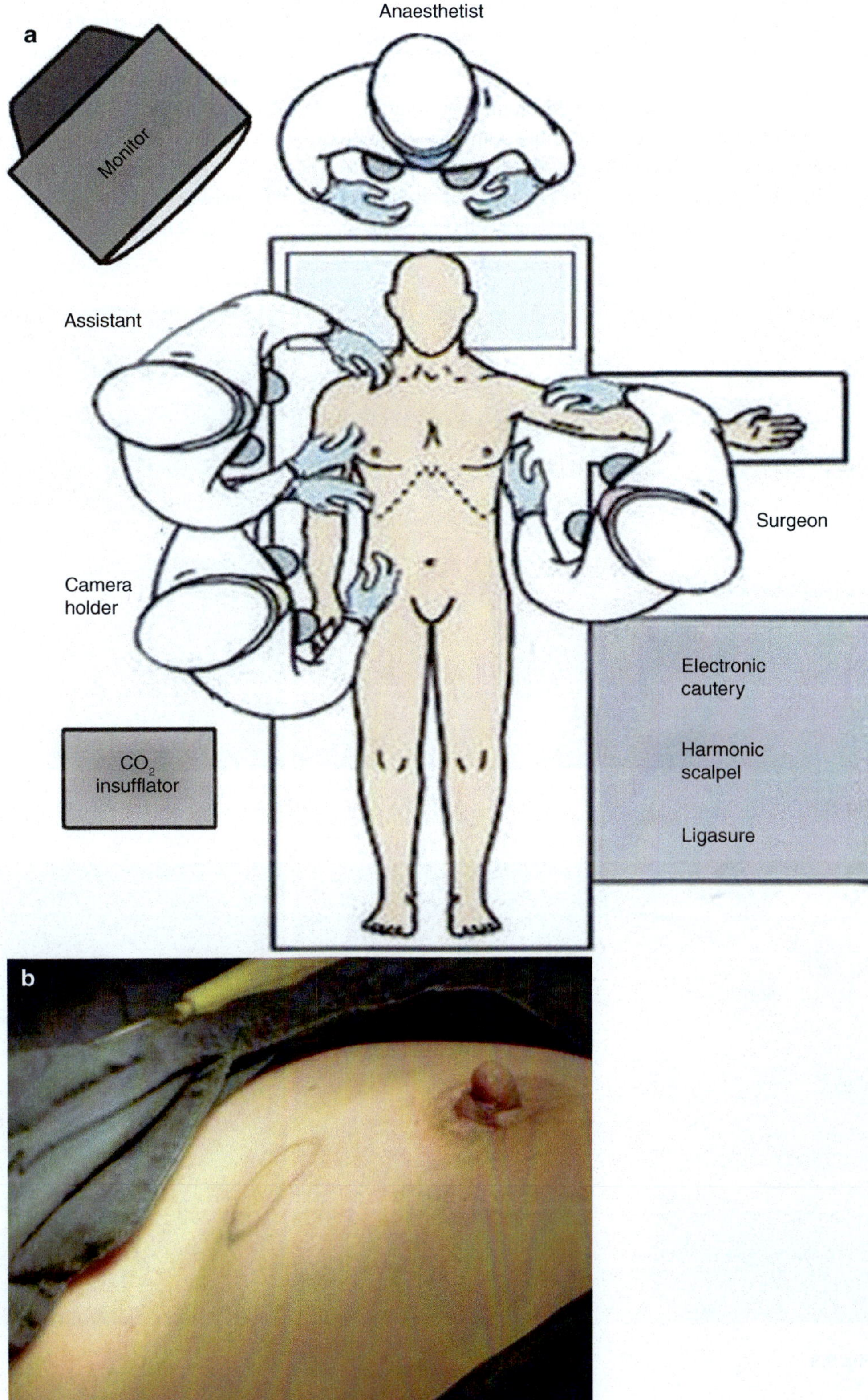

9.5 Key Steps

1. Resection of the tumor and pathologic examination
2. Establish the operation channel through the incision
3. Axillary lymph node dissection
4. Retrieval of the specimen
5. Irrigation and Drainage

9.6 Surgical Techniques

1. Resection of the tumor and pathologic examination
   A routine local excision of the tumor with surrounding tissue was performed. If it was diagnosed to be malignant by frozen pathology, a further excision was need until all the margins were reported to be negative for tumor cell (Fig. 9.2a, b).
2. Establish the operation channel through the incision
   The breast cavity was irrigated with lipolytic water (distilled water: physiological saline: adrenalin=300:90:0.1) and solute was suctioned out. Hemostasis was achieved before commencement of the axillary dissection (Fig. 9.3a, b).

   Triport was placed in the incision and CO_2 gas was insufflated until it reaches 6–8 mmHg. A 30° laparoscope, Harmonic scalpel and holding forceps were inserted through the triport (Fig. 9.4a, b).
3. Axillary lymph node dissection
   The fiber tissue was dissected. The lymph node groups of pectoralis muscles were dissected firstly. Pay attention to protect the long thoracic nerve (Fig. 9.5a–d).

   The dissection continues deep to the lymph nodes between the pectoralis major and pectoralis minor (Fig. 9.6a–d).

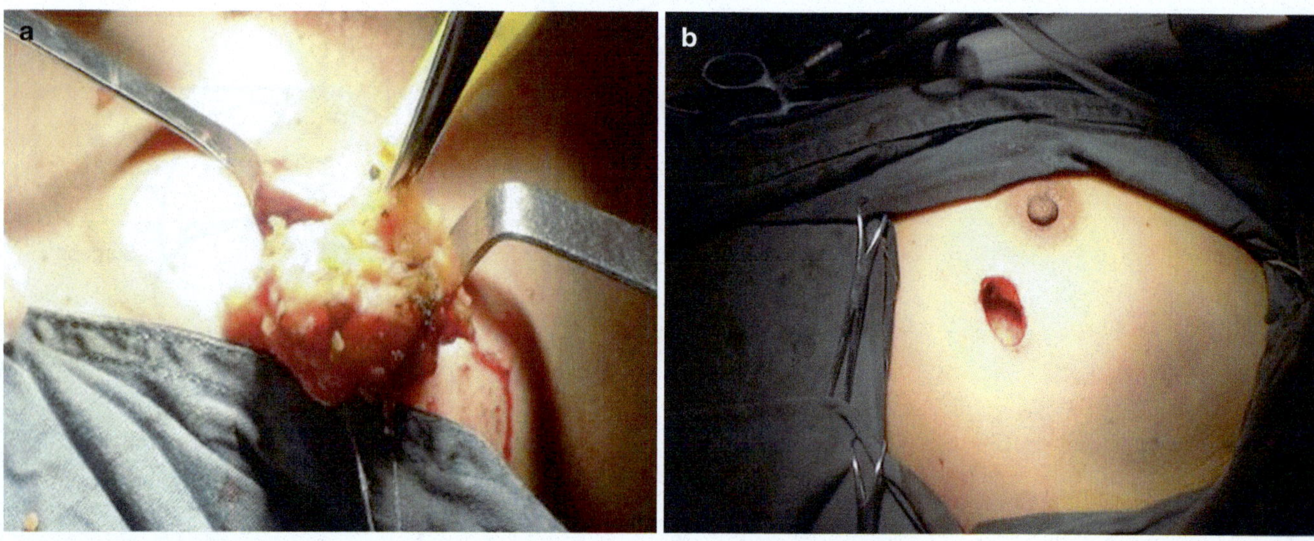

Fig. 9.2

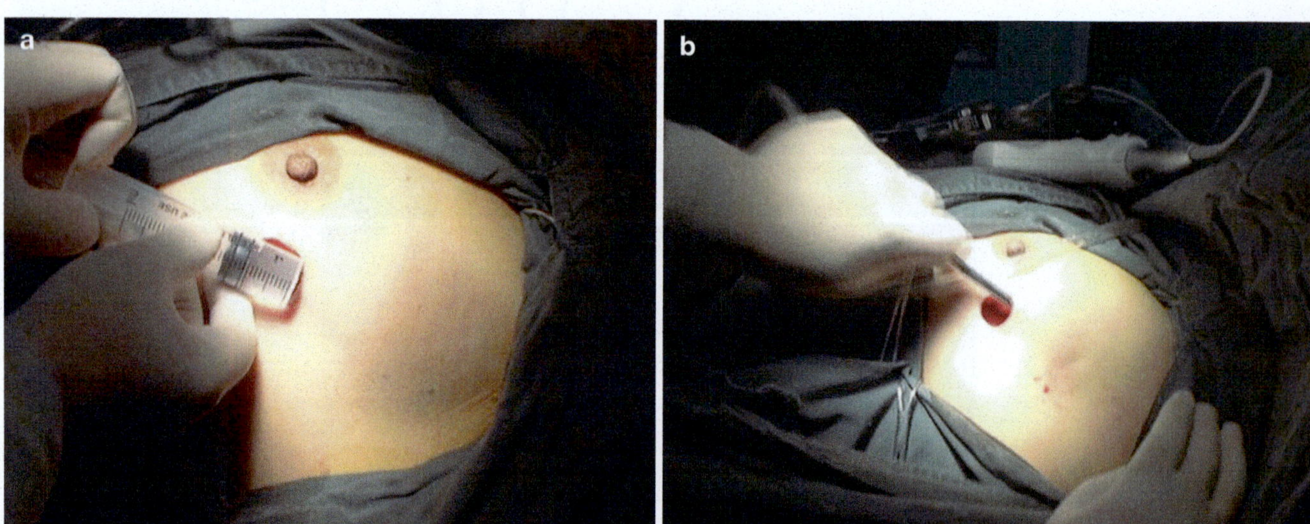

Fig. 9.3

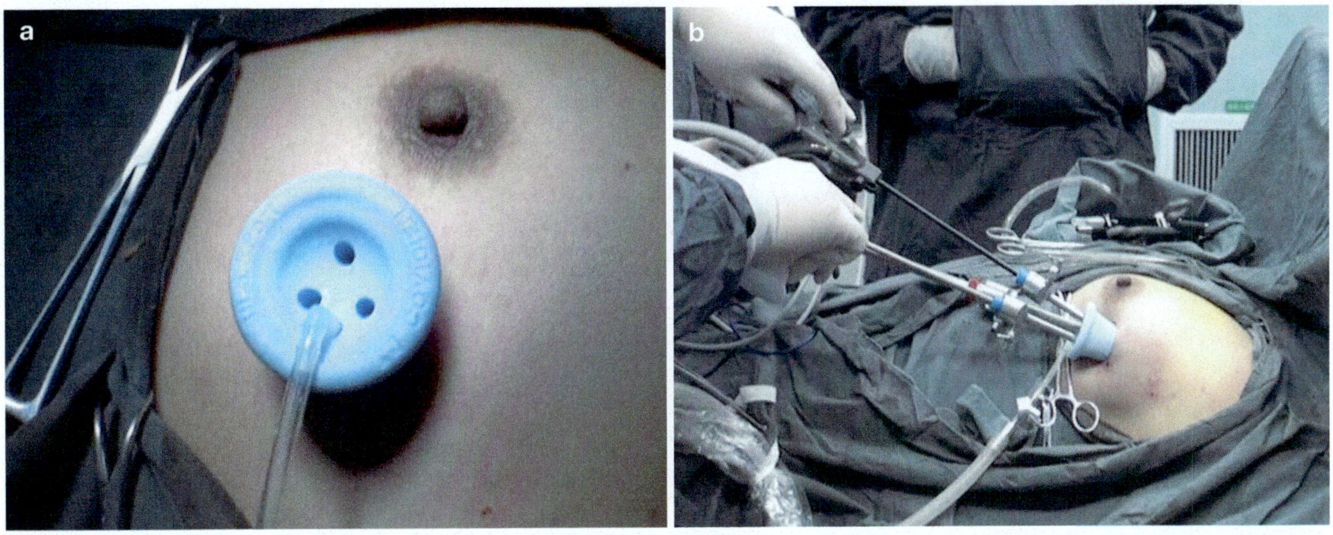

Fig. 9.4

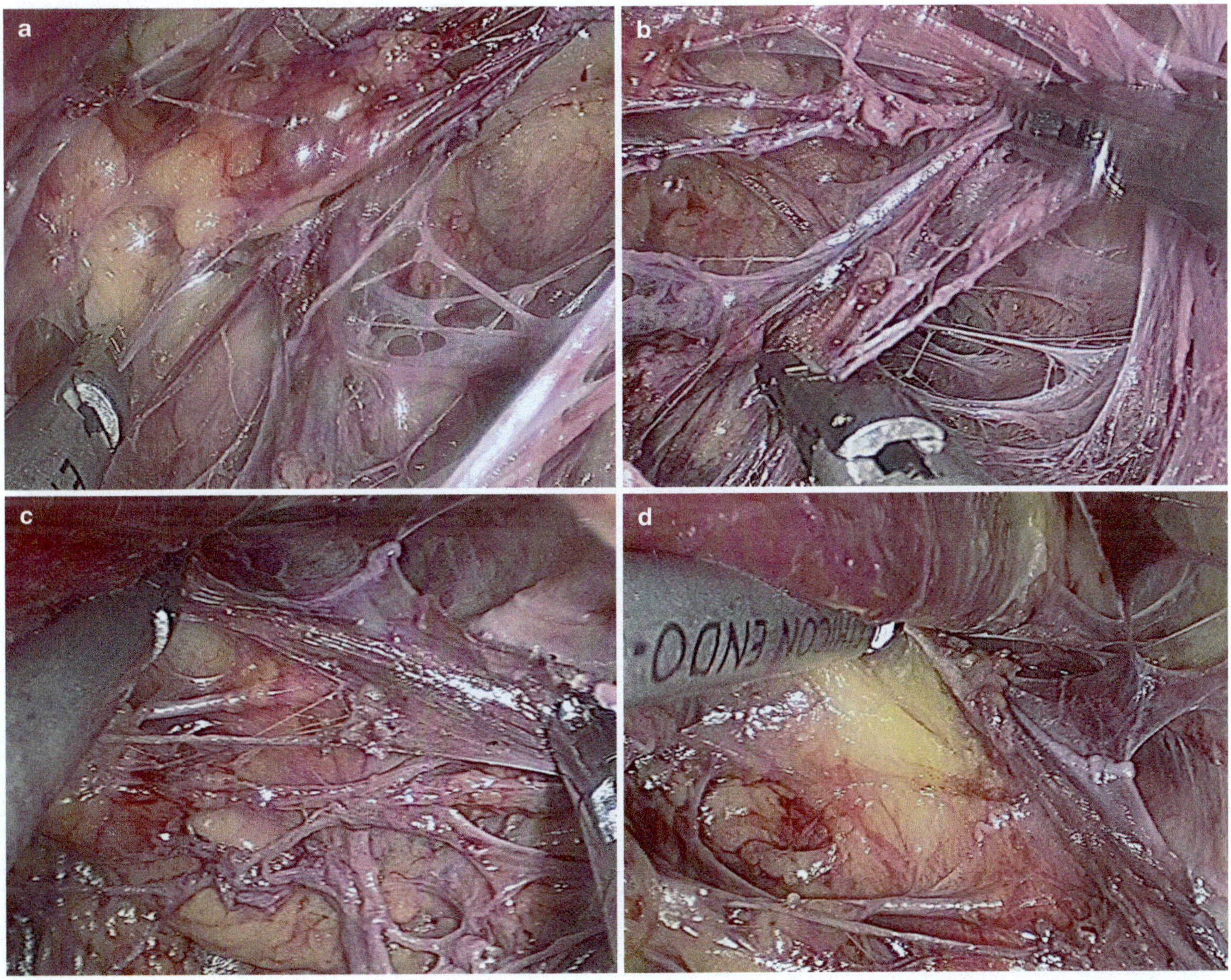

Fig. 9.5

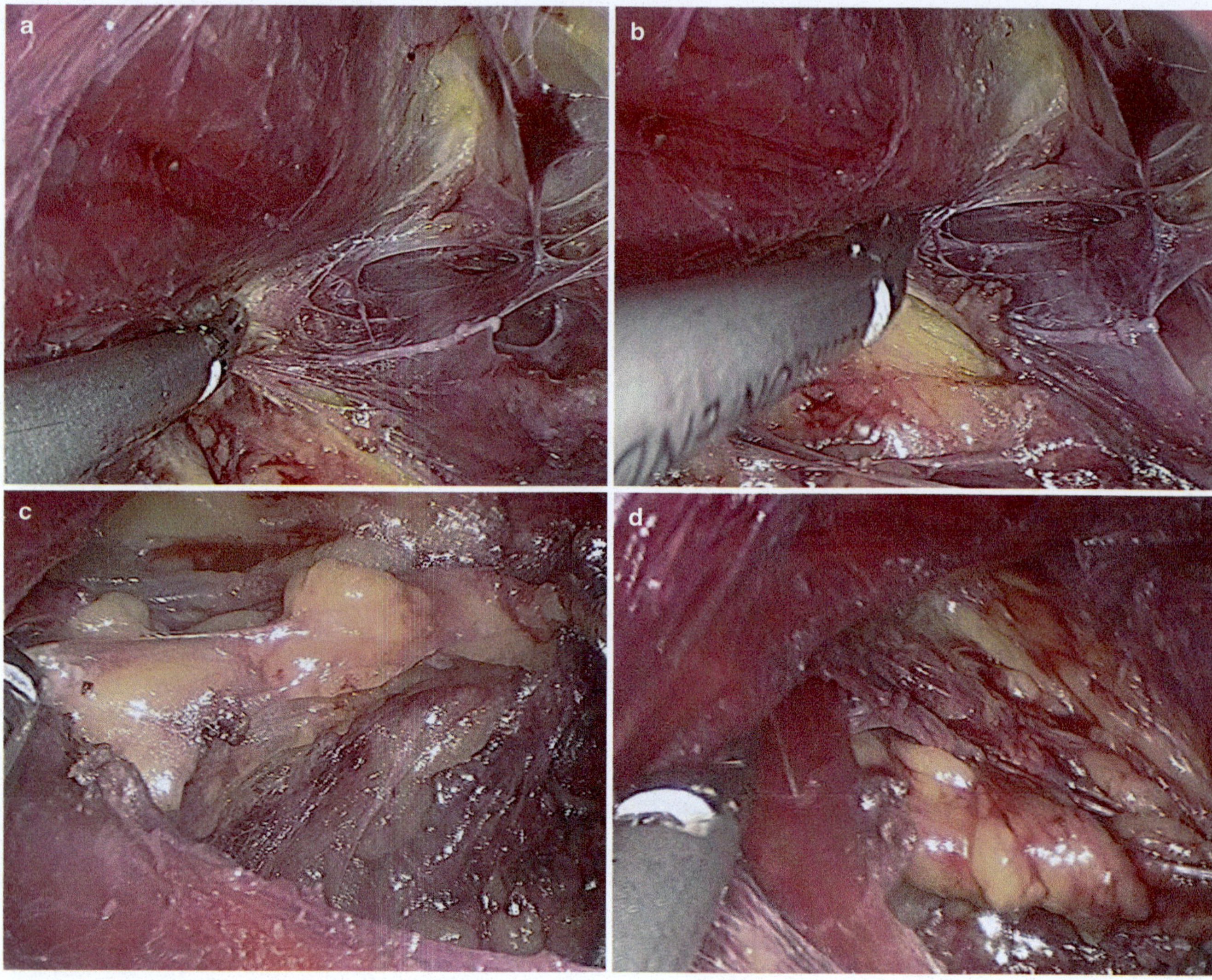

Fig. 9.6

Subscapular lymph nodes were dissected. The thoracodorsal nerve and subscapular artery and vein lying on the anterior surface of subscapularis muscle are identified and preserved (Fig. 9.7a–d).

Near the apex of the axilla, coracoclavicular fascia was opened and axillary vessels exposed. Apical, lateral and central lymph node groups were dissected (Fig. 9.8a–d).

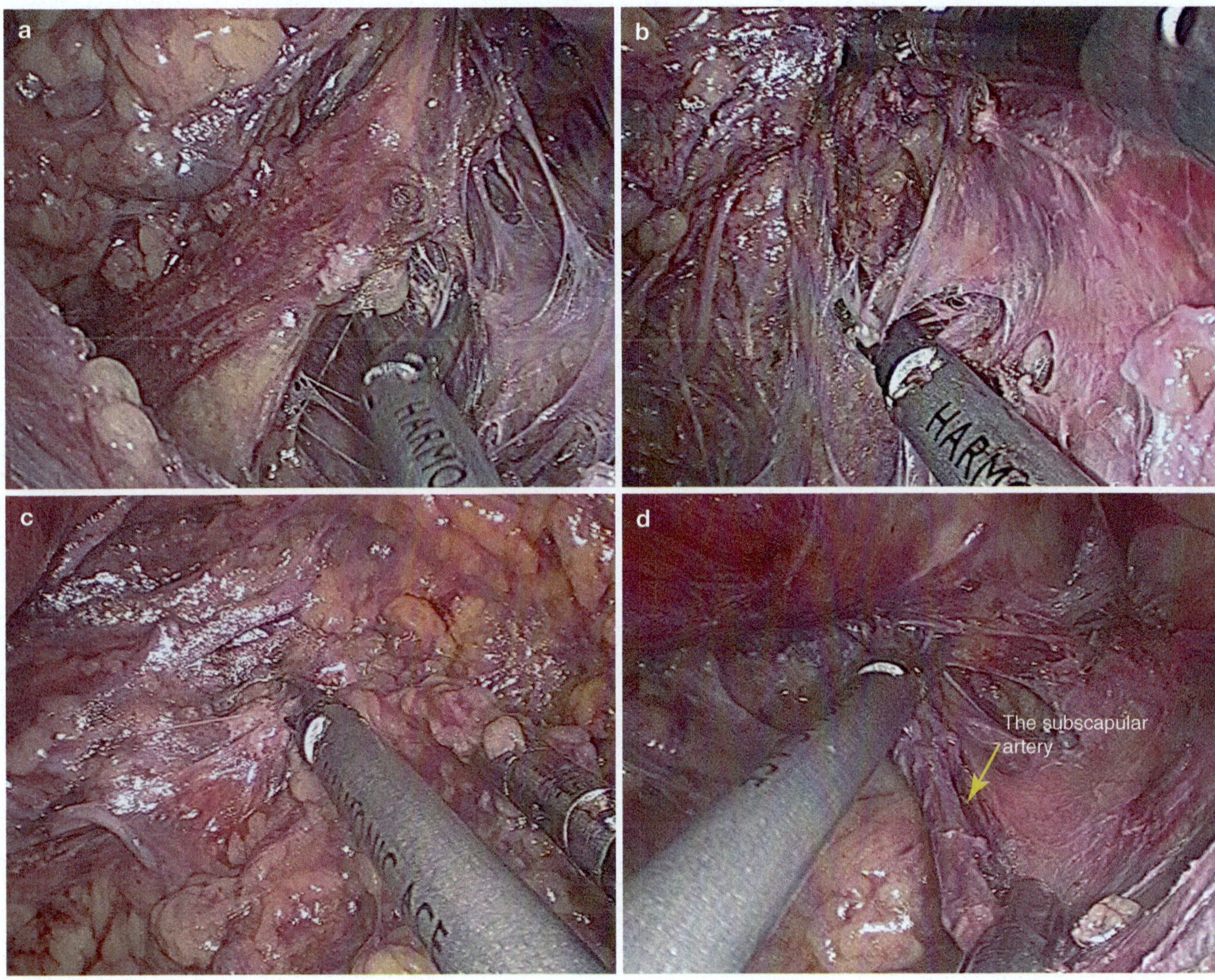

Fig. 9.7

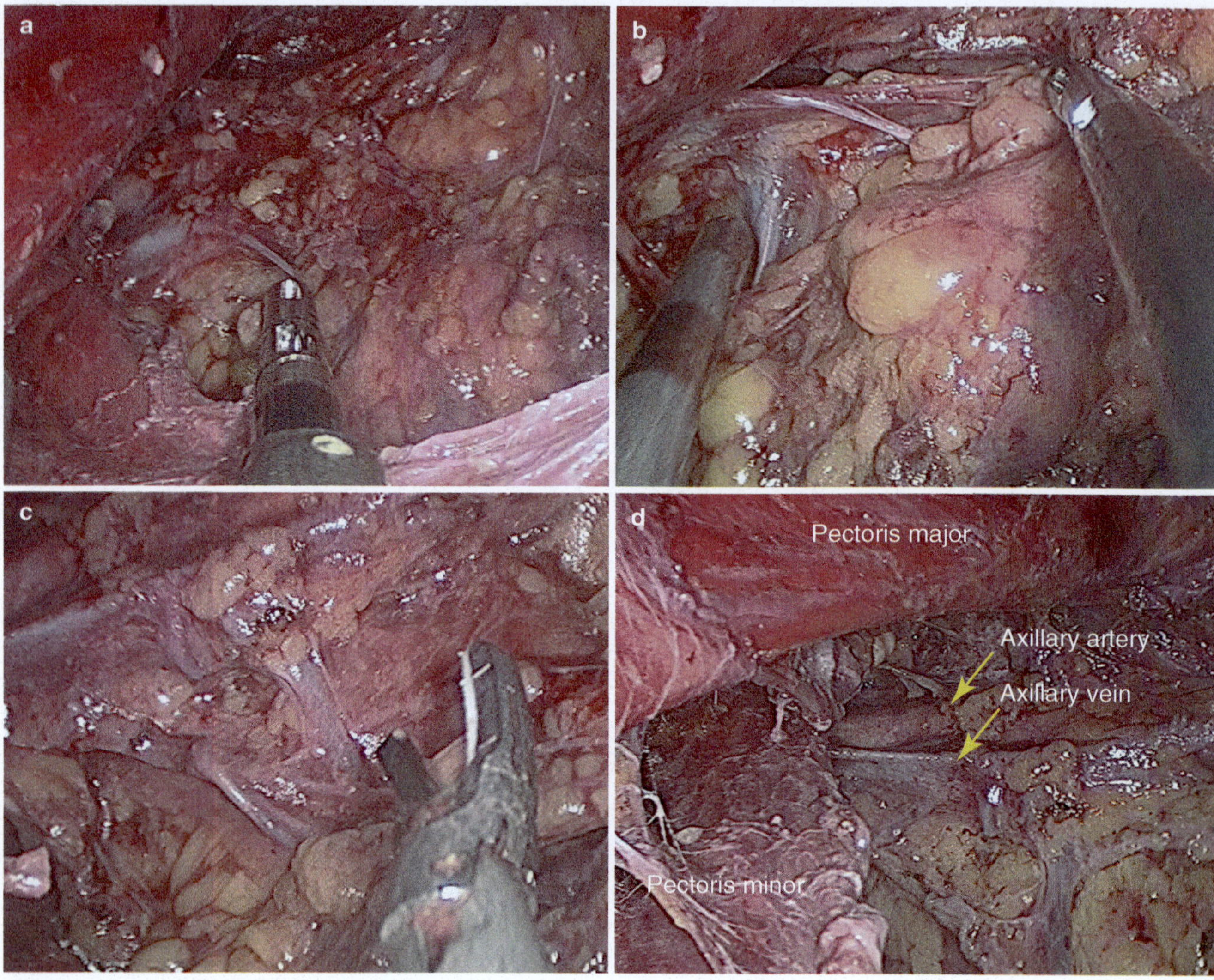
a
b
c
d
Pectoris major
Axillary artery
Axillary vein
Pectoris minor

Fig. 9.8

4. Retrieval of the specimen
   The specimen and lymph nodes contained within were extracted through the breast incision (Fig. 9.9a, b).
5. Irrigation and Drainage
   The cavity was suctioned and a closed suction drain was placed into the axillary fossa through the incision. The incision was closed and the operation was completed (Fig. 9.10a–c).

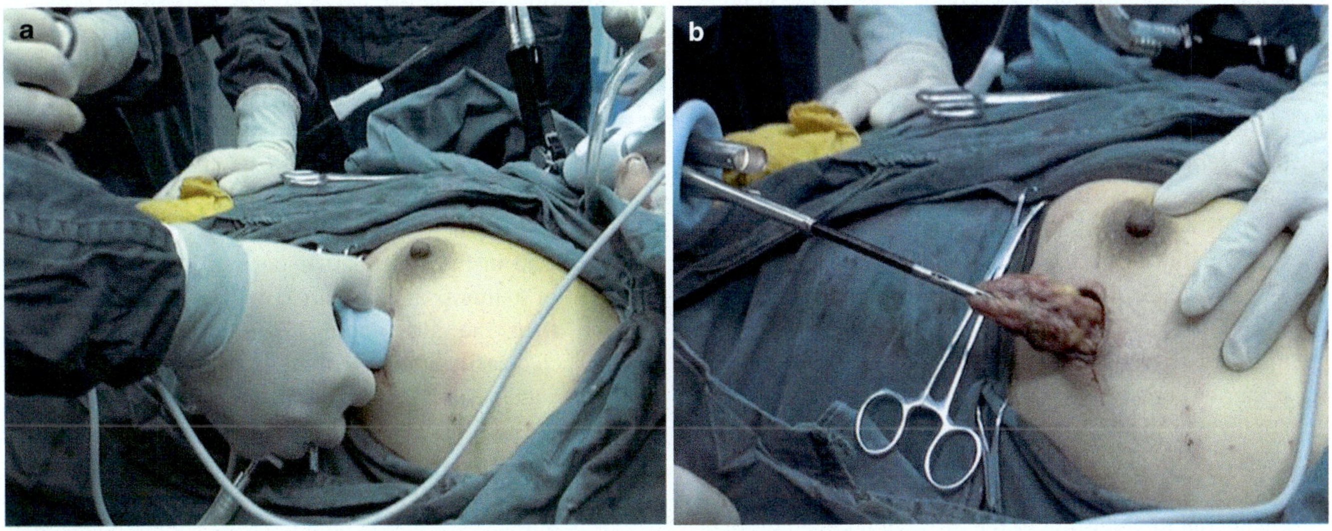

Fig. 9.9

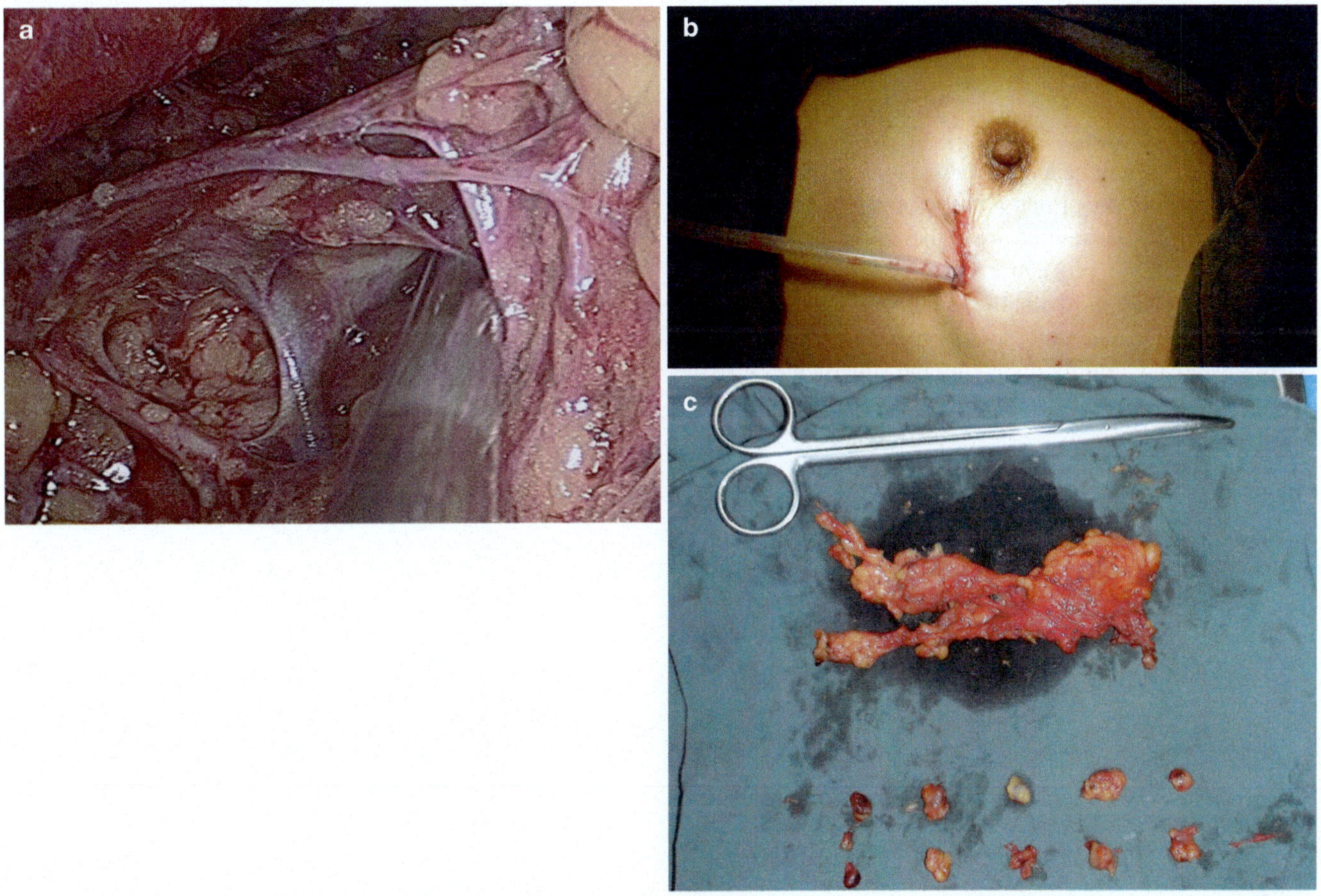

Fig. 9.10

9.7 Tips and Tricks

1. With the relative redundancy of the pectoralis major muscles and a more lateral angulation of the overtube, the interpectoral space could be found with relative ease. The primary anatomic landmark for the axilla with this approach was the lateral border of the pectoralis minor muscle.
2. Using harmonic ace, an incision was made down the lateral border of the pectoralis minor muscle, keeping close to the muscle itself dividing a thin fascial layer overlying the anterior aspect of the axilla and attaching to the pectoralis minor muscle. Once divided, the axillary fat was freed but remained attached to the chest wall, and the focus could be turned to exposure of the axillary vein using cephalad-directed dissection.
3. Blunt dissection enabled this inferior aspect of the axilla to be teased away from the latissimus dorsi muscle at the posterior border.
4. Division of the fat from the inferior border of the axillary vessels marked the completion of the excision.
5. The axillary fat was grasped and placed under tension to enable the final portion of the dissection to be completed more efficiently.

9.8 Complications Analysis and Management

1. Axillary vein injury
   Injury of axillary vein may induce massive bleeding and air embolism. The primary reason of injury is because the surgeon is not familiar with the axillary anastomotic structures. In the procedure, dissecting from the center of air space to top of axilla, the middle part of axillary vein locates the infra-anterior to the intercostobrachial nerve. In this area, carefully dissecting the superficial fat tissue and axillary vessel sheath along the direction of axillary vein may expose the vein. If the axillary vein is injured, it must be converted to open surgery as soon as possible.
2. Thoracodorsal nerve and long thoracic nerve injury
   The thoracodorsal nerve arises from the brachial plexus. It follows the course of the subscapular artery, along the posterior wall of the axilla to the Latissimus dorsi, in which it may be traced as far as the lower border of the muscle. It supplies latissimus dorsi on its deep surface. The long thoracic nerve descends behind the brachial plexus and the axillary vessels, resting on the outer surface of the serratus anterior. It extends along the side of the thorax to the lower border of that muscle, supplying filaments to each of its digitations. In SILS surgery, the fat tissue in the deep part under the junction of lateral inferior to thorax and bottom to axilla should be lifted up, and then the surrounding lymphoid tissue may be dissected easily along the tight long thoracic nerve.
3. Subcutaneous emphysema and hypercapnia
   Higher pressure in air space can induce the air to enter the subcutaneous layer or to be absorbed into blood. Proper pressure in axillary air space is 0.800–1.07 kPa (6–8 mmHg), excessive high pressure should be avoided. But lower pressure in air space may expand or collapse along with the respiratory movement, and interfere with the procedure.

References

1. Chengyu L, Yongqiao Z, Hua L, Xiaoxin J, Chen G, Jing L, Jian Z. A standardized surgical technique for mastoscopic axillary lymph node dissection. Surg Laparosc Endosc Percutan Tech. 2005;15:153–9.
2. Lim SM, Lam FL. Laparoscopic-assisted axillary dissection in breast cancer surgery. Am J Surg. 2005;90:641–3.
3. Wu SD, Han JY, Tian Y. Single-incision laparoscopic cholecystectomy versus conventional laparoscopic cholecystectomy: a retrospective comparative study. J Laparoendosc Adv Surg Tech A. 2011;21:25–8.

Thyroid Surgery: Single-Port Access Transaxillary Totally Endoscopic Thyroidectomy

10

Abstract

Since the first endoscopic thyroidectomy performed by Huscher et al. (Surg Endosc 11:877, 1997) in 1997, more than 20 different techniques of endoscopic thyroidectomy have been reported. Video-assisted minimal endoscopic thyroidectomy (Miccoli surgery) was first brought up by Miccoli et al. (J Endocrinol Invest 22:849–851, 1999), who accomplished the thyroidectomy through a 2–3 cm incision in neck with the help of endoscope. This surgery decreases the length of the incision in the neck with a better cosmetic result than traditional open surgery. After that, some different approaches of endoscopic thyroidectomy were reported. All of them shifted the incision from neck to more hidden or unexposed sites such as chest wall (Takami and Ikeda, ANZJ Surg 72:841–842, 2002), axillary (Ikeda et al., J Am Coll Surg 191:336–340, 2000) and breast (Ohgami et al., Surg Laparosc Endosc Percutan Tech 10:1–4, 2000) et al. The most obvious advantage of these surgeries is cosmesis. Although in experienced hands, the overall morbidity and mortality haven't increased, some special complications such as seroma, metastasis along the path of tunnel was reported. Furthermore, robotic assisted endoscopic thyroidectomy was reported (Kang et al., Surgery 146:1048–1055, 2009; Kang et al., J Am Coll Surg 209:e1–e7, 2009; Lee et al., J Oncol 2012:734541, 2012). More complicated surgery such as thyroid carcinoma resection can be performed under robotic assisted endoscope due to its better flexibility. Recently, laparoendoscopic single-site thyroidectomy was reported by some authors (Youben et al., Surg Laparosc Endosc Percutan Tech 21:e192–e196, 2011; Lee et al., J Laparoendosc Adv Surg Tech A 20:839–842, 2010; Fan et al., J Laparoendosc Adv Surg Tech A 21:243–247, 2011). The indications were limited to unilateral benign lesions, such as adenoma or nodule. The procedure was partial lobectomy. Laparoendoscopic single-site thyroidectomy decreased the dissection space, which decreased the postoperative discomfort and complication, at the same time; one incision can achieve the best cosmetic results. During the procedure, the axillary approach was thought the best way although some authors reported breast approach and even trans-oral approach (Nakajo et al., Surg Endosc 27:1105–1110, 2013).So far, we have performed single incision transaxillary endoscopic thyroid lobectomy in more than ten cases with good results.

Keywords

Single-port access • Transaxillary • Thyroidectomy • Strap muscle

S. Wu et al. (eds.), *Atlas of Single-Incision Laparoscopic Operations in General Surgery*,
DOI 10.1007/978-94-007-6955-7_10, © Springer Science+Business Media Dordrecht 2013

10.1 Indications and Case Selection

A single-port totally endoscopic thyroidectomy was offered to patients according to criteria specifying young female gender, unilateral thyroid benign lesion with lesion diameter of less than 3 cm and strong desire for cosmesis.

10.2 Contraindications

1. Patients with history of operation around the neck and proximal upper limbs.
2. Patients with history of thyroiditis or radiation therapy.
3. Patients suffer from malignancy with the thyroid.
4. A lesion located in the thyroid dorsal area (especially adjacent to the tracheoesophageal groove) owing to possible injury to the trachea, esophagus, or recurrent laryngeal nerve (RLN) was also excluded.
5. Patients with inability to tolerate general anesthesia.
6. Patients with relatively operative contraindications.

10.3 Major Instruments or Energy Sources

1. Laparoscopy System
2. SILS port
3. Harmonic scalpel

10.4 Team Setup, Anesthesia and Position

Under general anesthesia, the patient was placed in supine position with the neck slightly extended. The arm on the lesion side was extended to expose the axilla. The position of surgeon, assistants and nurses is shown in Fig. 10.1a, b.

Fig. 10.1

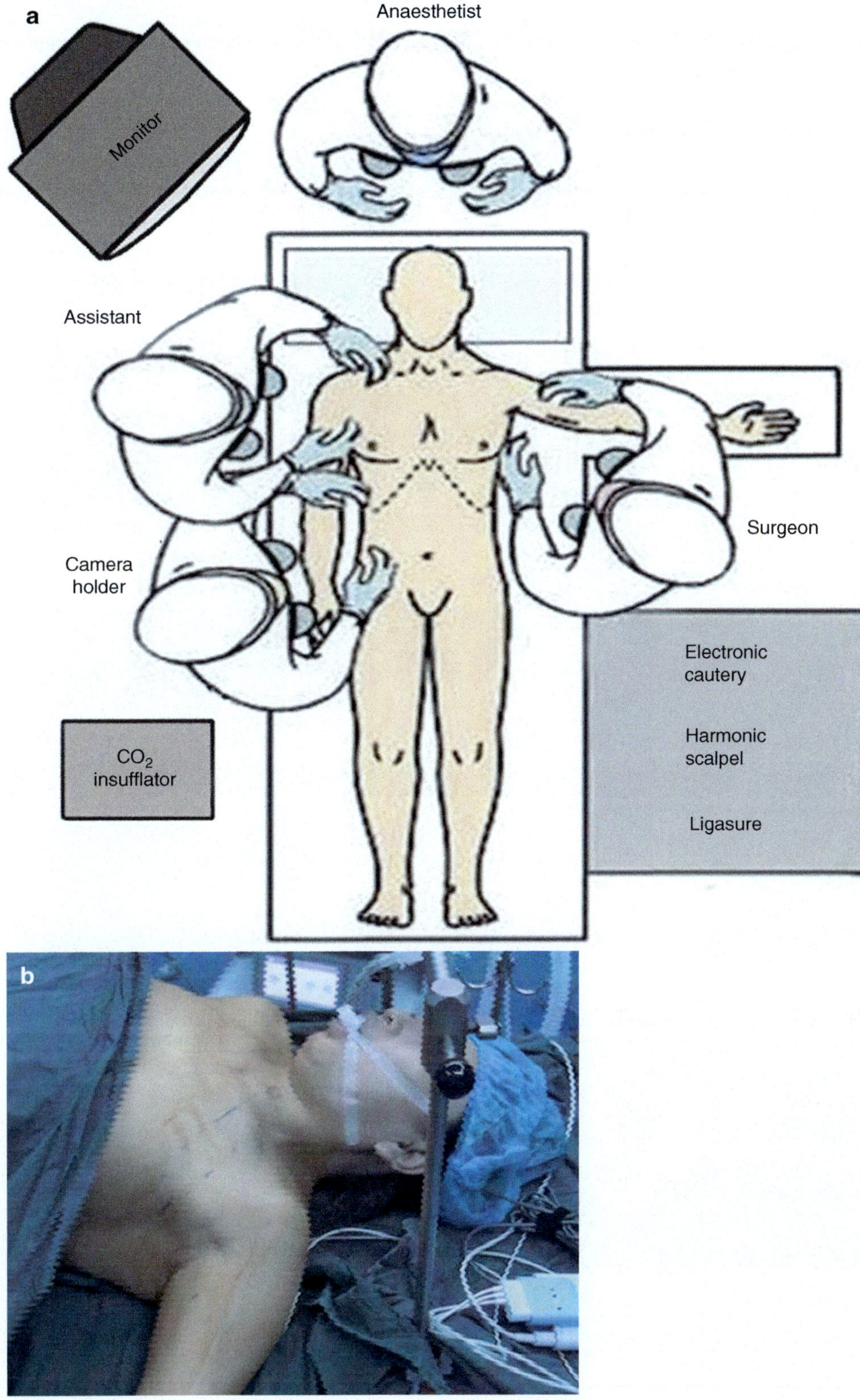
a
Anaesthetist
Monitor
Assistant
Camera
holder
Surgeon
Electronic
cautery
Harmonic
scalpel
Ligasure
CO_2
insufflator
b

10.5 Key Steps

1. Set up of the subcutaneous tunnel
2. Extension of working space
3. Division of Strap muscle
4. Removal of the lesion of the thyroid
5. Extraction of the specimen
6. Irrigation and suction of working space
7. The placement of drain

10.6 Surgical Techniques

1. Set up of the subcutaneous tunnel
   0.1 % epinephrine solution was injected subcutaneously along the operating area for vasoconstriction and hemostasis. A 3 cm incision was made along the skin fold in axilla. The working space was created subcutaneously by gentle dissection with blunt instrument. The dissection range is shown in Fig. 10.1b. Then the single-port was inserted. CO_2 was insufflated up to the pressure of 6 mmHg. The 10 mm 30° laparoscopy was inserted (Fig. 10.2a–f).

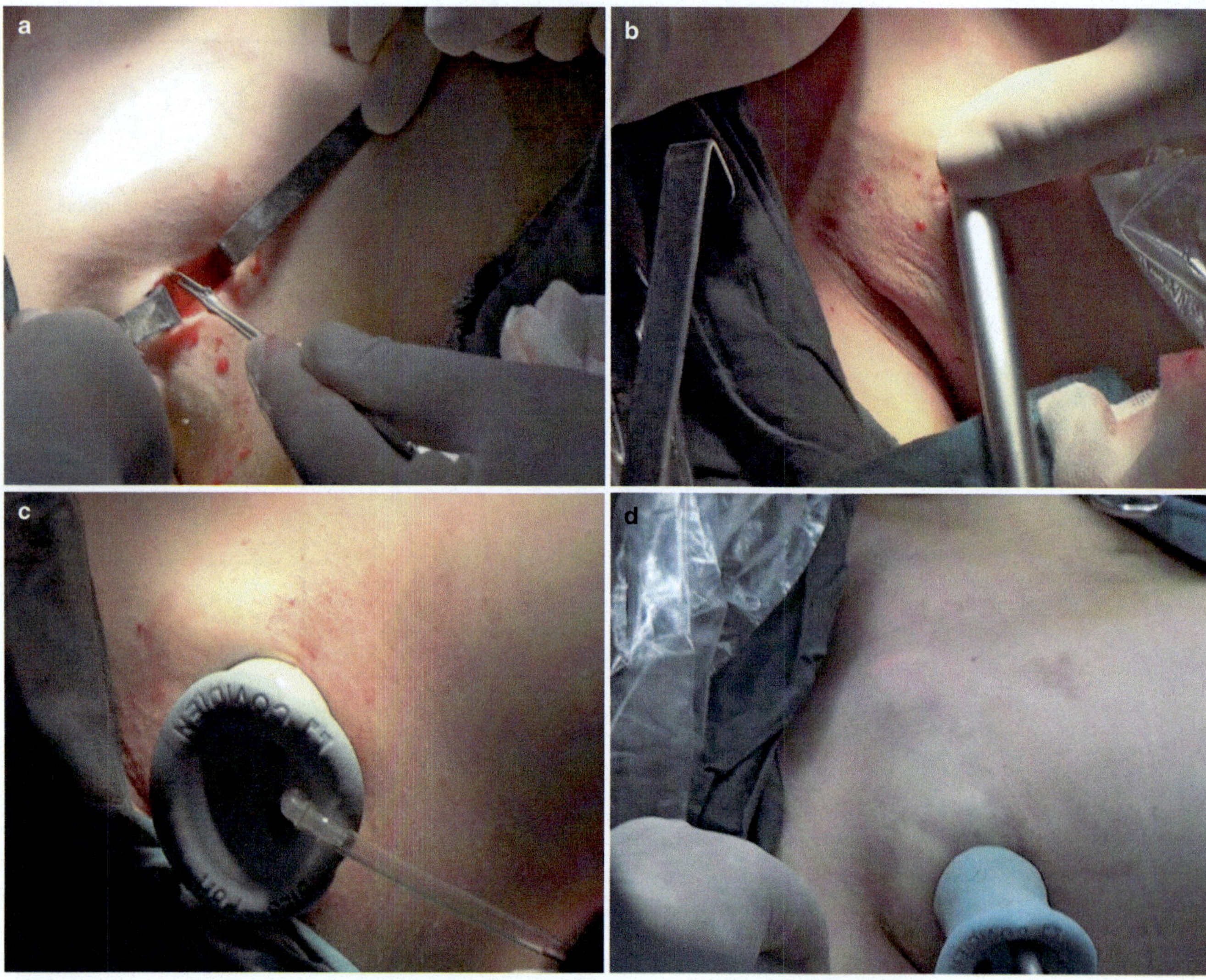

Fig. 10.2

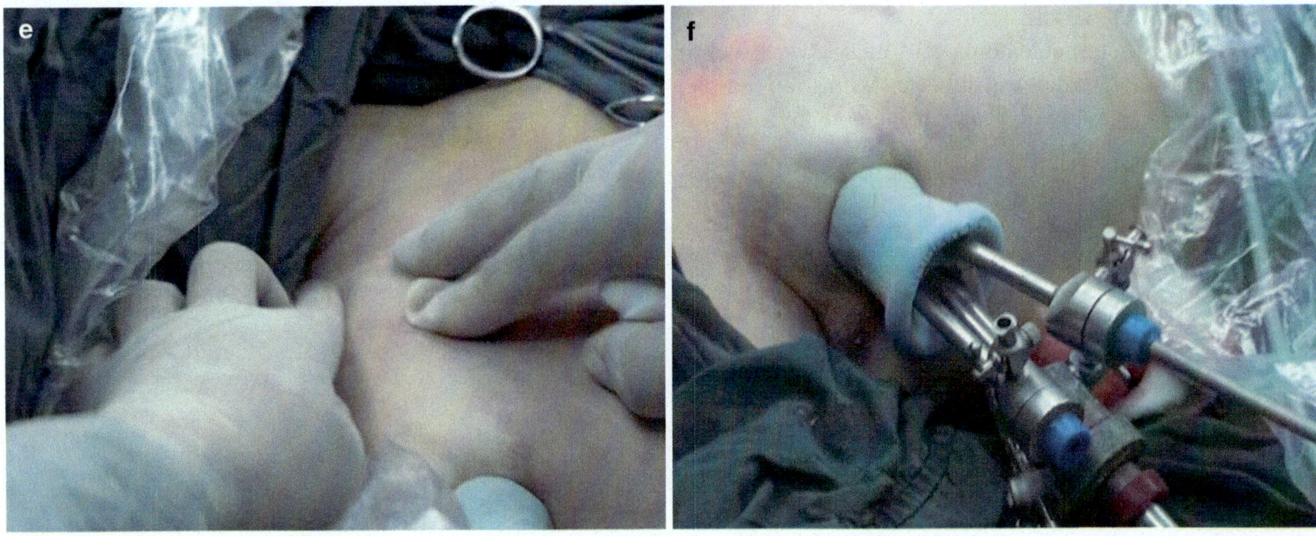

Fig. 10.2 (continued)

2. Extension of working space
   5 mm scalpel and grasp forceps were inserted through the 5 mm port. The connective tissue was sharply dissected using scalpel to extend the working space further (Fig. 10.3).

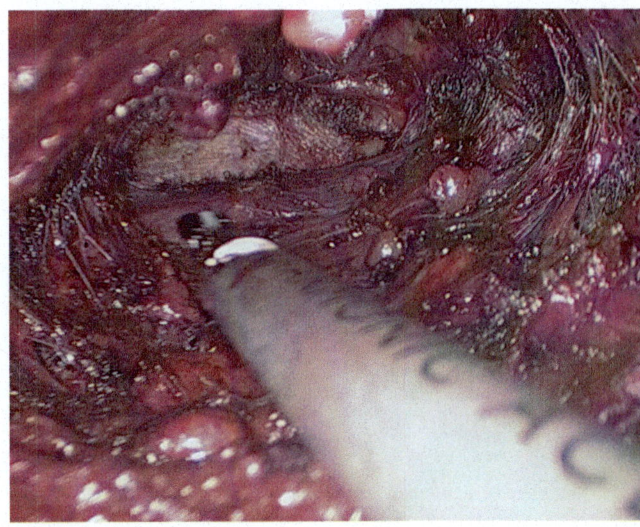

Fig. 10.3

3. Division of Strap muscle

   The ispilateral sternocleidomastoid muscle was identified. The medial border was dissected with strap muscle. Strap muscle was divided and ispilateral thyroid was exposed (Fig. 10.4a–d).

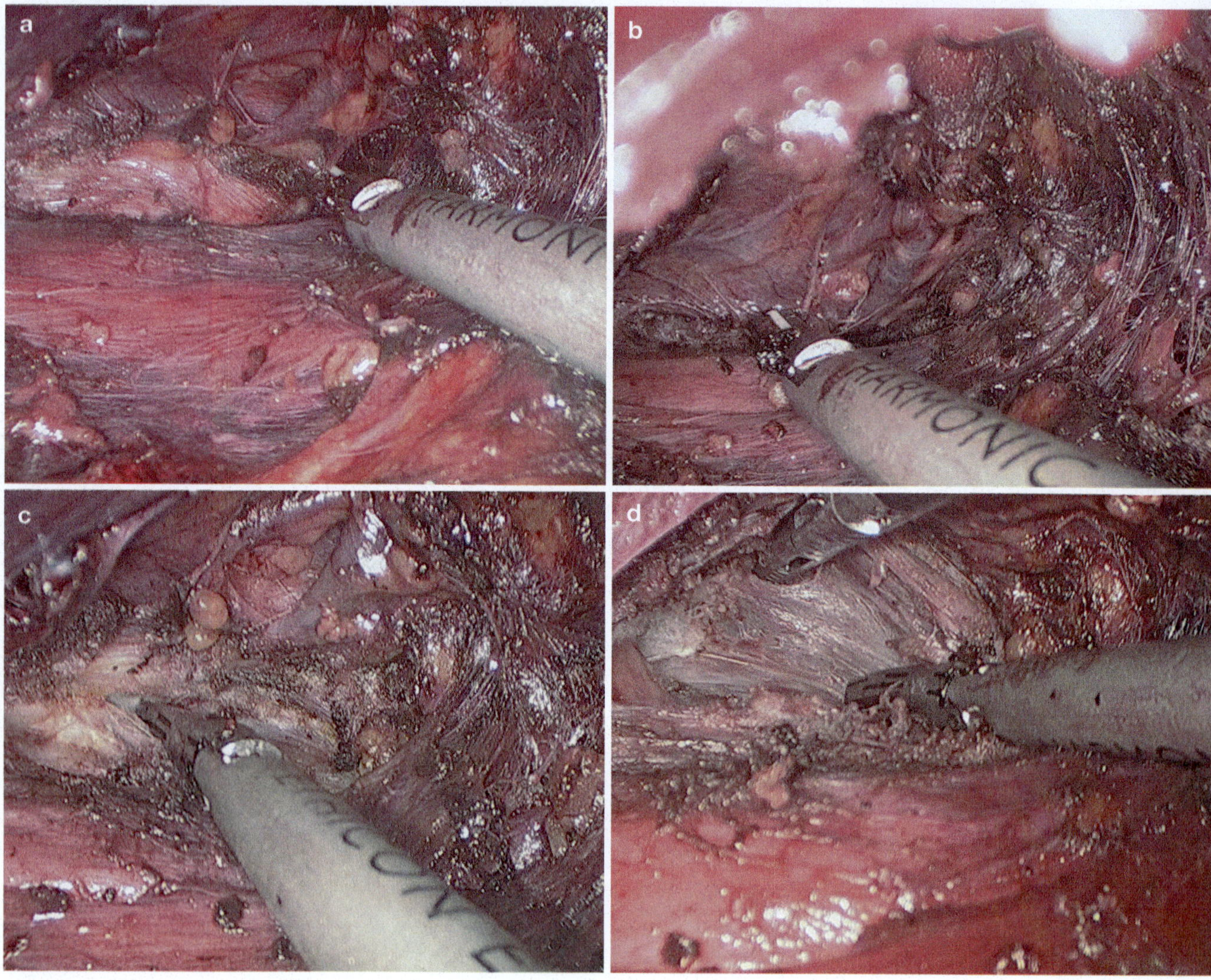

Fig. 10.4

4. Removal of the lesion of the thyroid
   The surface of the thyroid tissue was divided until the lesion was exposed. The lesion was removed with the capsule or with a little normal thyroid tissue (Fig. 10.5a–f).

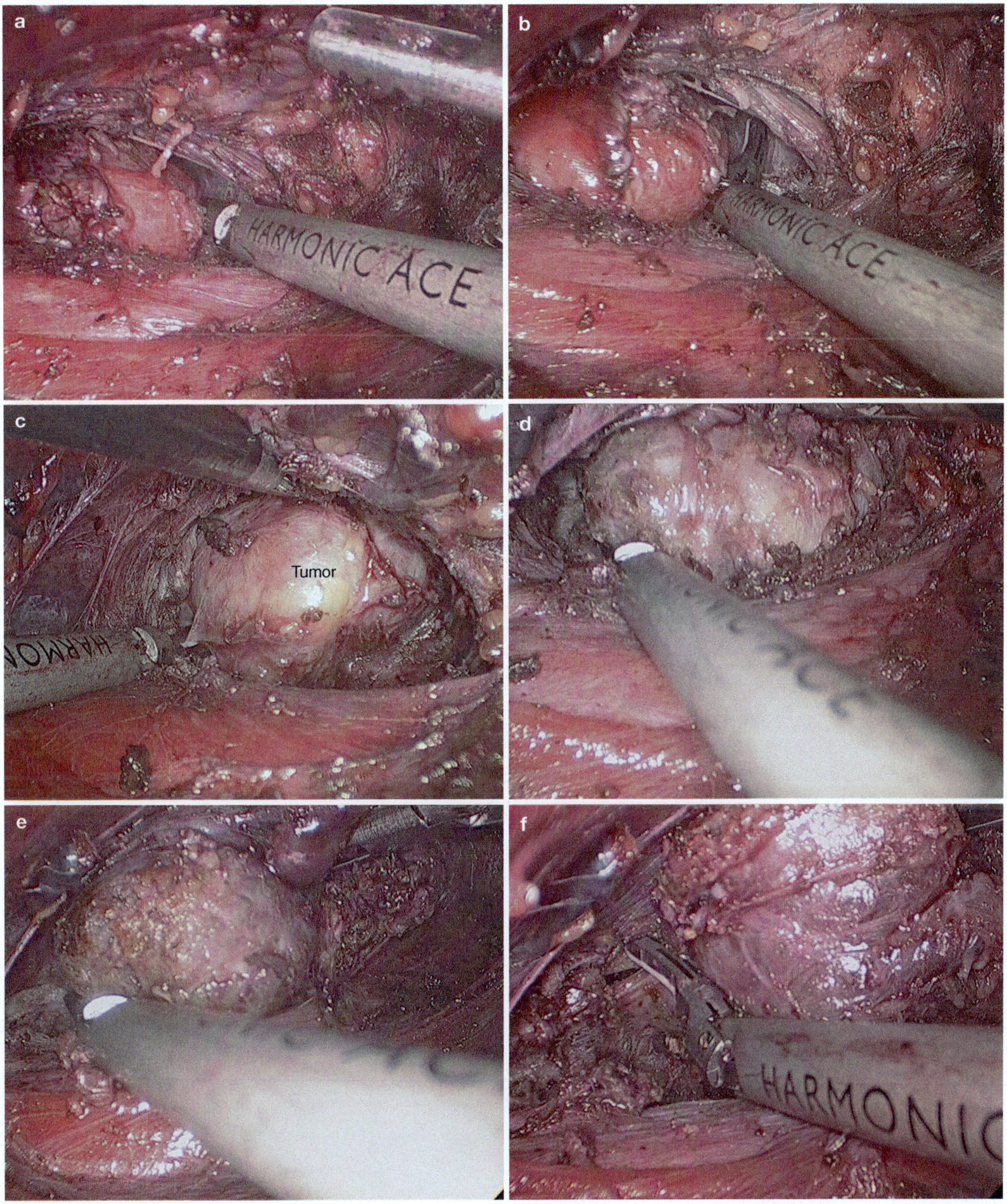

Fig. 10.5

5. Extraction of the specimen
   The specimen was extracted from the incision. Occasionally, the specimen was placed in the bag and extracted from the incision (Fig. 10.6a–c).

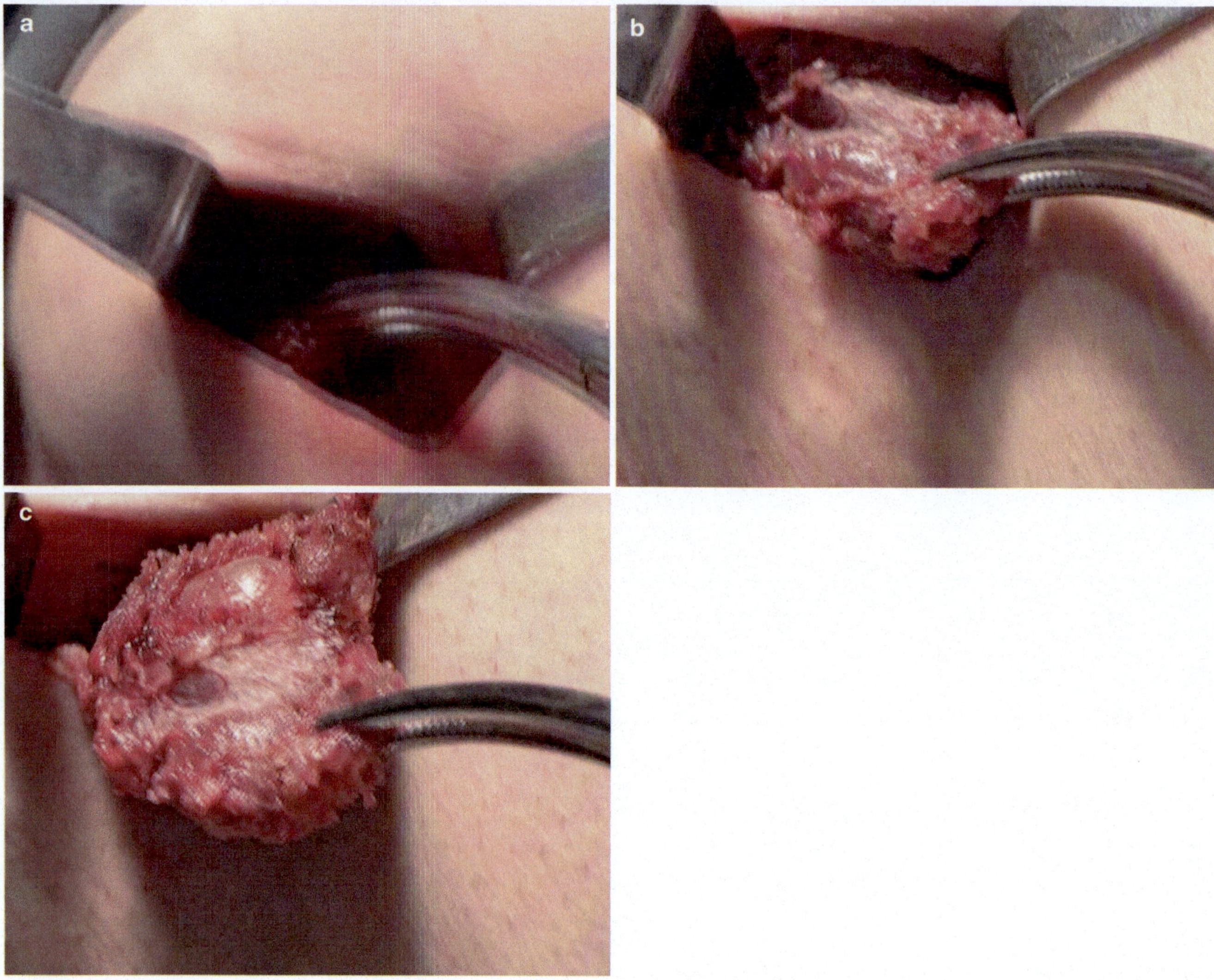

Fig. 10.6

6. Irrigation and suction of working space
   After complete hemostasis, the working space was irrigated and cleaned (Fig. 10.7).

7. The placement of drain
   A drain was placed and extracted from the incision (Fig. 10.8a, b).

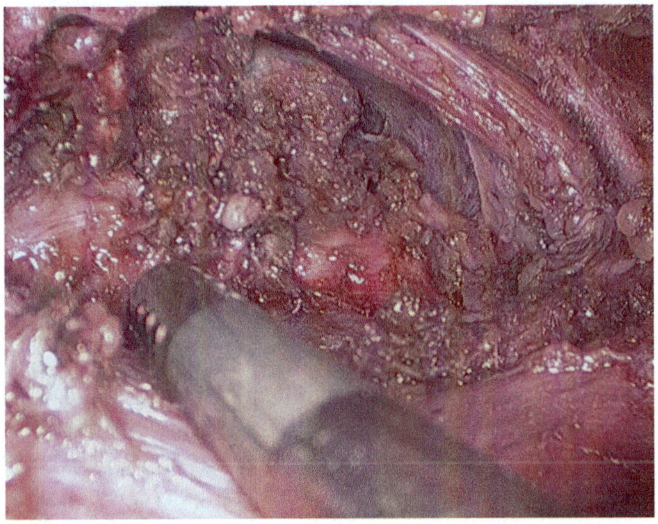

Fig. 10.7

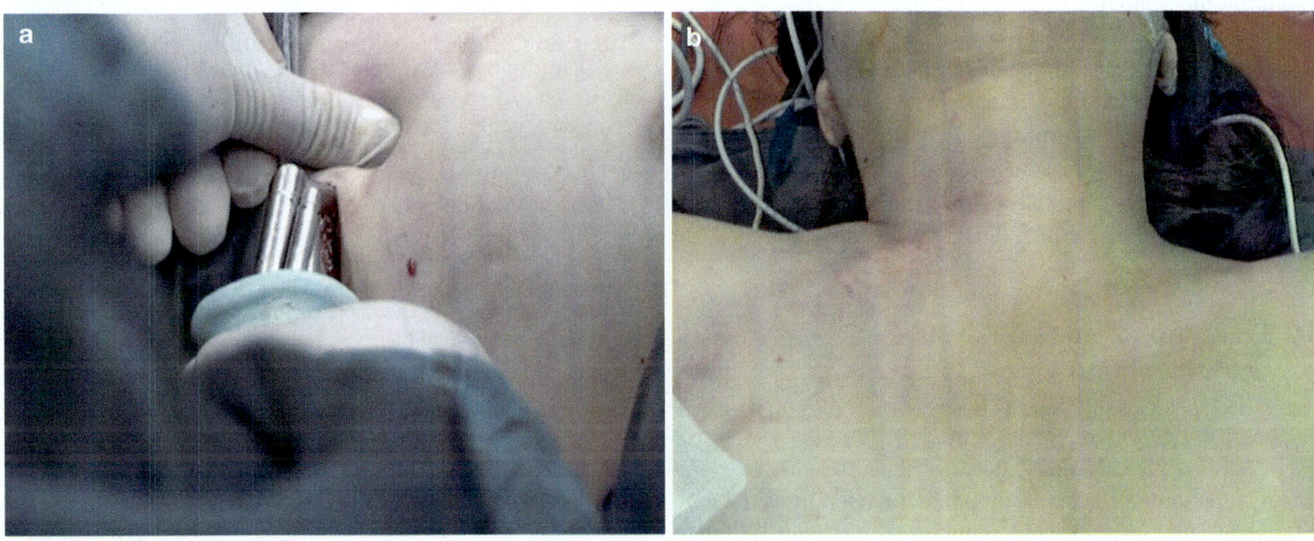

Fig. 10.8

10.7 Tips and Tricks

1. The neck is slightly extended and the lesion-side arm is stretched out at 90°.
2. A 2.5 cm long incision was made parallel to the skin folds on the anterior axillary line of the lesion side and a subcutaneous skin flap from the axilla to the anterior neck area is dissected over the anterior surface of the pectoralis major muscle and clavicle by electrical cautery under direct vision.
3. After exposing the medial border of the sternocleidomastoid muscle, the dissection is approached bluntly through the superficial space of the sternocleidomastoid muscle to reach the surface of the strap muscle above the ipsilateral lobe of the thyroid.
4. The lesion-side thyroid lobe was reached by vertical dissection of the strap muscle.
5. Under endoscopic guidance, the lower pole of the thyroid lobe was drawn upward and medially using the grasper forceps, and inferior thyroid vessels were identified and individually divided.
6. Careful dissection was performed to identify the middle thyroid vein, and individual division was performed by Harmonic scalpel.
7. The upper pole of the thyroid was drawn downward and medially using the forceps, and superior thyroid vessels were identified and individually divided close to the thyroid gland to avoid injuring the external branch of the superior laryngeal nerve using the Harmonic scalpel.
8. Usually, the thyroid tissue near the tracheoesophageal groove should be preserved to prevent injury to the RLN.

10.8 Complications Analysis and Management

1. Recurrent laryngeal nerve injury
   In SILS thyroid surgery, because the instruments, light and the tumor that was prepared to be removed were coaxial, the operator's judgment regarding depth and distance would be affected. Thus, the distal part near to the trachea cannot be seen clearly. So, the recurrent laryngeal nerve may be injured. When the tumor in inferior thyroid is larger than 3 cm, the occurrence of recurrent laryngeal nerve injury may increase. To avoid the recurrent laryngeal nerve injury, the operative point should be close to the tumor surface and keep far away from the paratracheal groove, when the side of tumor near to trachea is dissected.
2. Purple and broken skin of thorax and neck
   Establishing the operational space should be in strict accordance with the operation essentials to dissect the loose connective tissue between platysma and throat muscles. If the dissection is too deep, it may induce anterior superficial jugular bleeding and difficult construction of operative space. On the other hand, if the dissection is too shallow, it may form purple and broken skin of thorax and neck.
3. Subcutaneous fat liquefaction
   Subcutaneous fat liquefaction may be induced by situations such as the when the operational space is too shallow, large area of subcutaneous fat is destroyed, and too much tissue is coagulated by ultrasound scalpel. So, appropriate dissecting level and area may prevent this complication effectively
4. Haemorrhage
   Thyroid is abundant in blood. Intraoperative haemorrhage is major in thyroid gland and vessels bleeding, which are induced by incorrect use of ultrasound scalpel or large vessels injury. Low gear of ultrasound scalpel is appropriate for coagulating while cutting the thyroid gland. Do not violently tear the thyroid gland. Inferior thyroid gland vessels and middle thyroid vein can be cut off by ultrasound scalpel. But if the vessels are thicker, ligation is better.

References

1. Huscher CS, Chiodini S, Napolitano C, Recher A, et al. Endoscopic right thyroid lobectomy. Surg Endosc. 1997;11:877.
2. Miccoli P, Berti P, Conte M, Bendinelli C, Marcocci C. Minimally invasive surgery for thyroid small nodules: preliminary report. J Endocrinol Invest. 1999;22:849–51.
3. Takami H, Ikeda Y. Minimally invasive thyroidectomy. ANZ J Surg. 2002;72:841–2.
4. Ikeda Y, T akami H, Sasaki Y, Kan S, Niimi M, et al. Endoscopic neck surgery by the axillary approach. J Am Coll Surg. 2000;191:336–40.
5. Ohgami M, Ishii S, Arisawa Y, Ohmori T, Noga K, Furukawa T, Kitajima M. Scarless endoscopic thyroidectomy: breast approach for better cosmesis. Surg Laparosc Endosc Percutan Tech. 2000;10:1–4.
6. Kang SW, Lee SC, Lee SH, Lee KY, Jeong JJ, Lee YS, Nam KH, Chang HS, Chung WY, Park CS. Robotic thyroid surgery using a gasless, transaxillary approach and the da Vinci S system: the operative outcomes of 338 consecutive patients. Surgery. 2009;146:1048–55.
7. Kang SW, Jeong JJ, Nam KH, Chang HS, Chung WY, Park CS. Robot-assisted endoscopic thyroidectomy for thyroid malignancy using a gasless transaxillary approach. J Am Coll Surg. 2009;209:e1–7.
8. Lee J, Yun JH, Choi UJ, Kang SW, Jeong JJ, Chung WY. Robotic versus endoscopic thyroidectomy for thyroid cancers: a multi-institutional analysis of early postoperative outcomes and surgical learning curves. J Oncol. 2012;2012:734541.
9. Youben F, Bomin G, Bo W, Jie K, Fan Y, Wencai Q, Yuyao H, Qi Z. Trans-areola single-incision endoscopic thyroidectomy. Surg Laparosc Endosc Percutan Tech. 2011;21:192–6.
10. Lee D, Nam Y, Sung K. Single-incision endoscopic thyroidectomy by the axillary approach. J Laparoendosc Adv Surg Tech A. 2010;20:839–42.
11. Fan Y, Wu SD, Kong J. Single-port access transaxillary totally endoscopic thyroidectomy: a new approach for minimally invasive thyroid operation. J Laparoendosc Adv Surg Tech A. 2011;21:243–7.
12. Nakajo A, Arima H, Hirata M, Mizoguchi T, Kijima Y, Mori S, Ishigami S, Ueno S, Yoshinaka H, Natsugoe S. Trans-Oral Video-Assisted Neck Surgery (TOVANS). A new transoral technique of endoscopicthyroidectomy with gasless premandible approach. Surg Endosc. 2013;27:1105–10.

Single-Incision Laparoscopic Multivisceral Resection

11

Abstract

Since Philippe Mouret's first video-assisted cholecystectomy in 1987 (Kaiser and Corman, Surg Oncol Clin N Am 10:483–492, 2001), fundamental changes have occurred in laparoscopic surgery making it one of the most significant advances of twentieth century surgery. There is increasing evidence that laparoscopy provides better cosmetic results, less incision pain and shorter hospital stay when compared with open surgery. With the laparoscopic technique developing so fast in the last decade, surgeons are seeking a surgical method to reduce operative trauma. Single-incision laparoscopic surgery (SILS) has come into being on the base of this notion. This technique is well described in literature for appendectomy, nephrectomy, adrenalectomy, cholecystectomy, and colectomy (Ateş et al., J Pediatr Surg 42:1071–1074, 2007; Ponsky et al., J Endourol 22:663–665, 2008; Castellucci et al., J Endourol 22:1573–1576, 2008; Wu et al., J Laparoendosc Adv Surg Tech A 21:25–28, 2011; Tian et al., J Gastrointest Surg 14:1429–1433, 2010; Kaouk and Palmer, BJU Int 102:97–99, 2008). But there are only a few sporadic reports of SILS combined procedures (Mantke and Wicht, Surg Laparosc Endosc Percutan Tech 20:e28–e30, 2010; Cai et al., Hepatogastroenterology 59:986–989, 2012). Beginning in May 2009, we performed over 1,000 transumbilical single-incision cholecystectomies. During the period, SILS combined procedures were attempted using conventional instruments with satisfied outcomes. Combined SILS, based on combined laparoscopic surgery but not needing to add extra trocars, operates on two or more target organs in one anesthesia. Considering the procedure itself, SILS combined surgery brought no new advance to technique indeed. But with the fact that patients with coexisting pathologies at different sites are common clinically, this technique will be performed in a gradually widening field of application.

Keywords

Multivisceral resection • Sleeve gastric resection • Resection of transverse colon • Resection of pancreatic body and tail

S. Wu et al. (eds.), *Atlas of Single-Incision Laparoscopic Operations in General Surgery*,
DOI 10.1007/978-94-007-6955-7_11,

11.1 Indications and Case Selection

Patients have coexisting diseases that should and could be treated at the same time.

11.2 Contraindications

The contraindications of one-stage on multi-organ diseases consult the chapters of referred organs.

11.3 Major Instruments or Energy Sources

1. Laparoscopy System
2. Harmonic scalpel
3. Ligasure

11.4 Team Setup, Anesthesia and Position

Under general anesthesia, the patient was placed in supine position with the legs apart. The position of surgeon, assistants and nurses is shown in Fig. 11.1.

Fig. 11.1

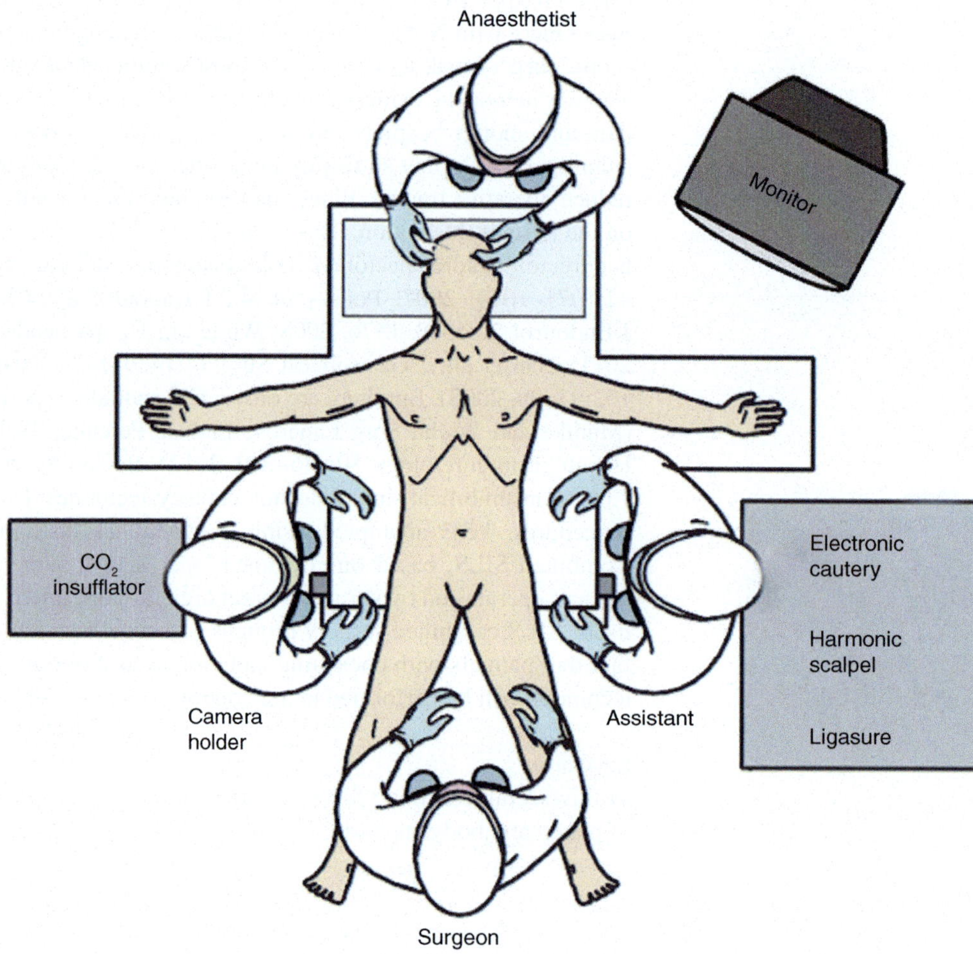

11.5 Key Steps

1. Abdominal exploration
2. Partial gastric resection
3. Dissection and resection of transverse colon
4. Resection of pancreatic body and tail
5. Rebuilding of transverse colon
6. Irrigation, drainage and closure of the incision

11.6 Surgical Techniques

1. Abdominal exploration
   The abdominal cavity was explored carefully to identify if there was remote metastasis or located involvement. The lesion was identified on the posterior wall of stomach and infiltrated to splenic flex of transverse colon and pancreatic tail (Fig. 11.2a–c).

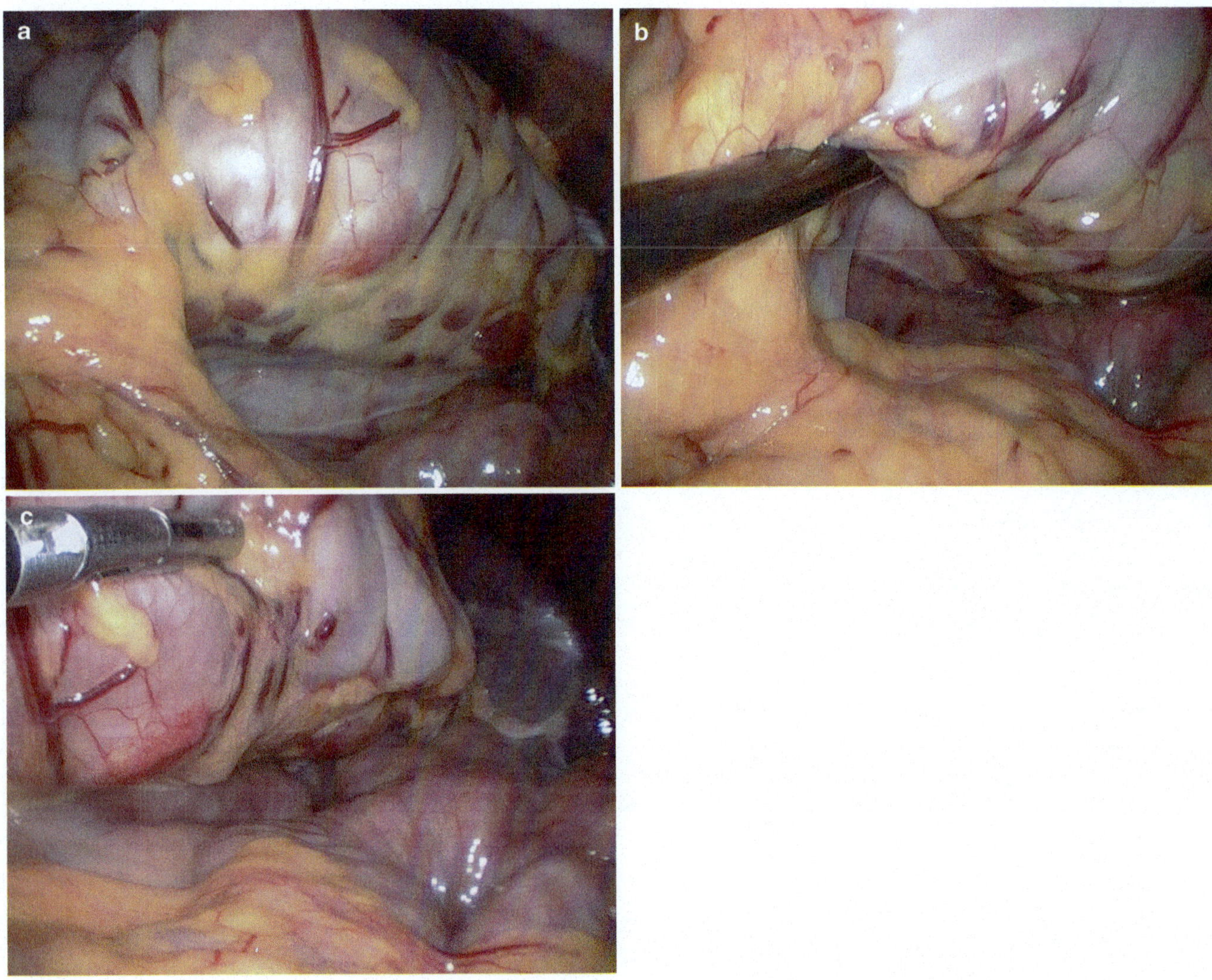

Fig. 11.2

2. Partial gastric resection

   The greater curvature was retracted with noninvasive forceps. The gastrocolic ligament and gastrosplenic ligament were divided cephalad to the fundus. The posterior wall was exposed and mobilized (Fig. 11.3a–d).

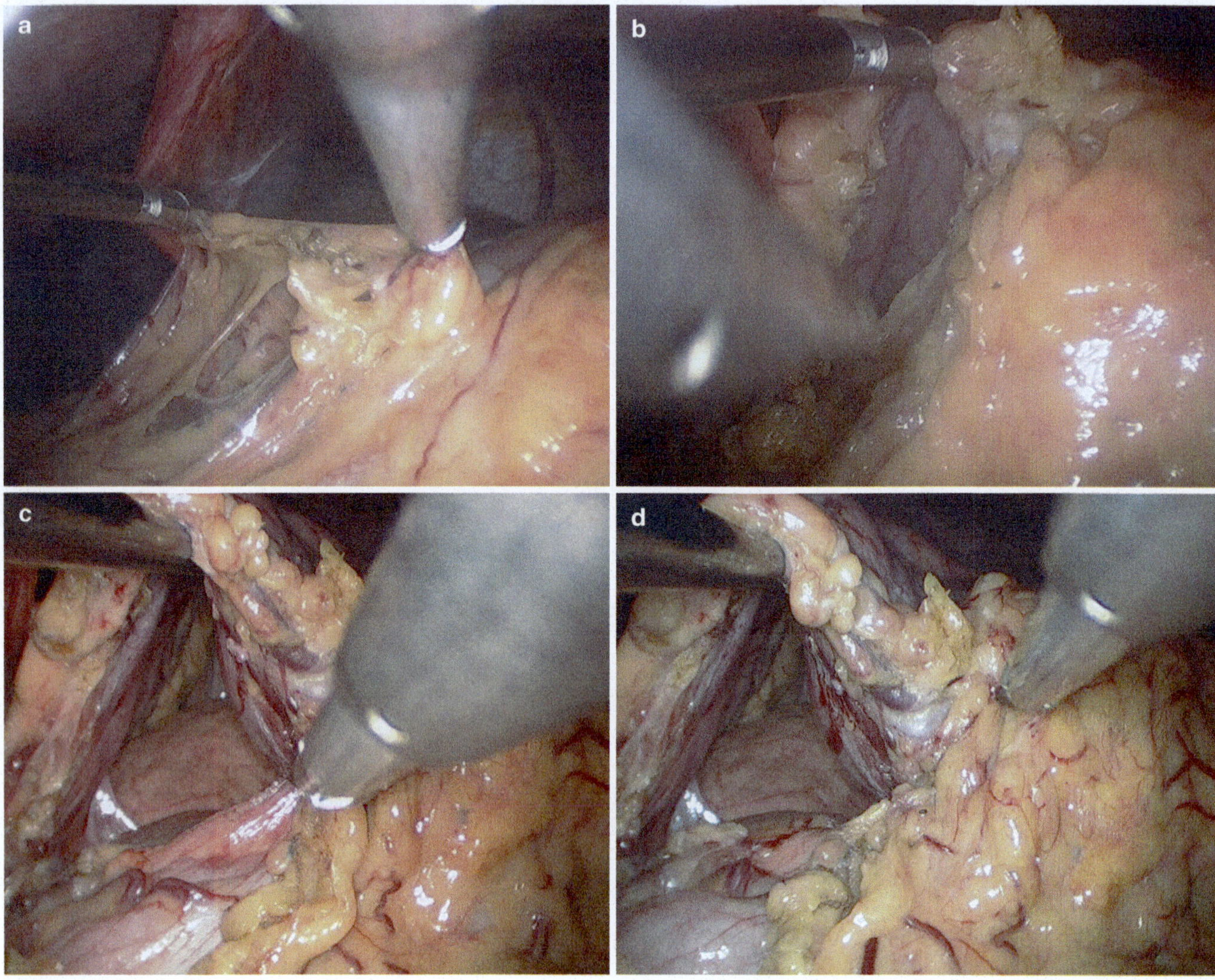

Fig. 11.3

The greater curvature was retracted and the connective tissue between posterior gastric wall and pancreas was divided using harmonic scalpel. The range of lesion was confirmed (Fig. 11.4a–d).

Gastric body was grasped with noninvasive forceps and held with a little tension. Sleeve gastric resection was performed along the greater curvature and fundus using a 60 mm endoscopic linear cutter. The gastric antrum remained complete with 3–4 cm wide residual less curvature (Fig. 11.5a–j).

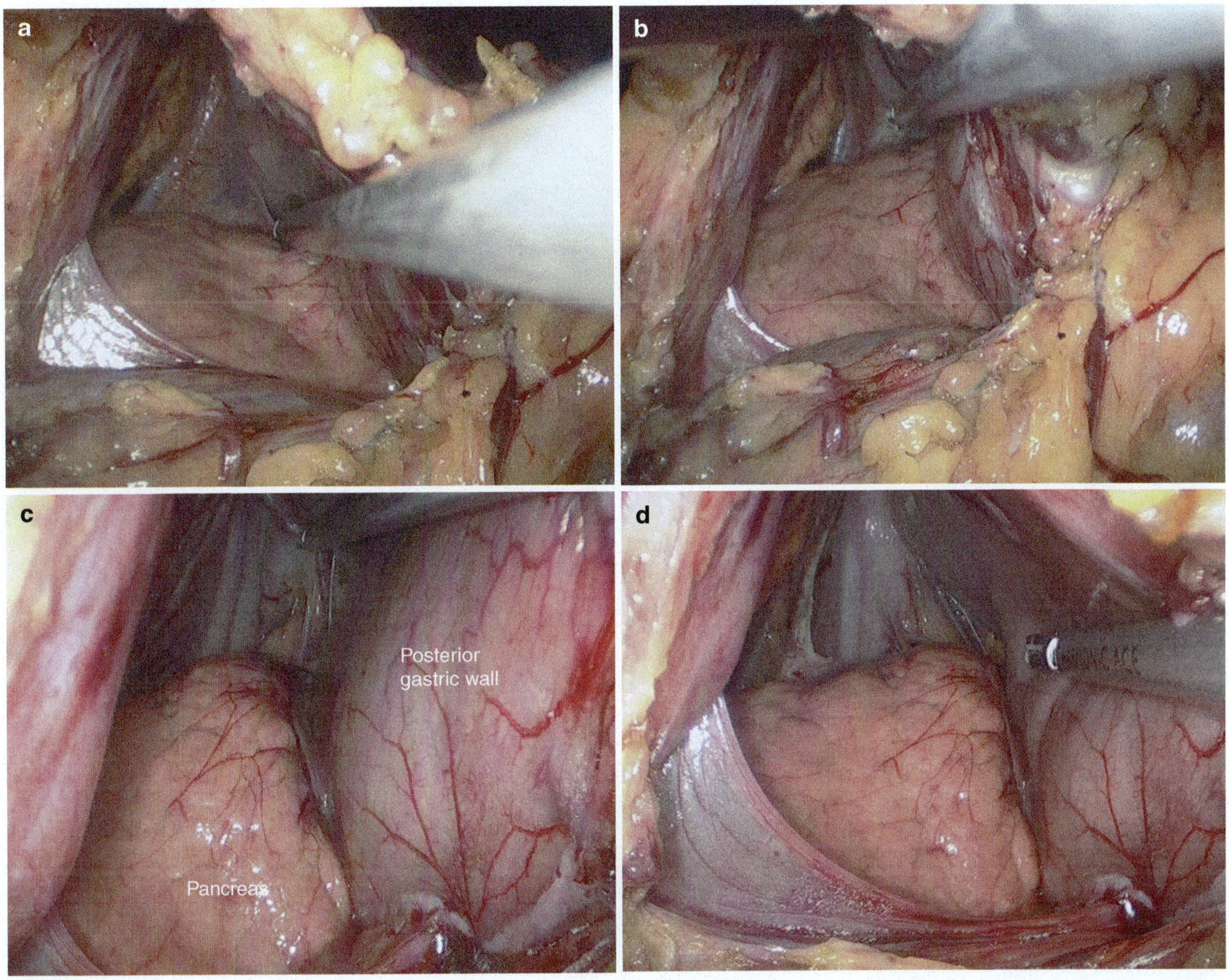

Fig. 11.4

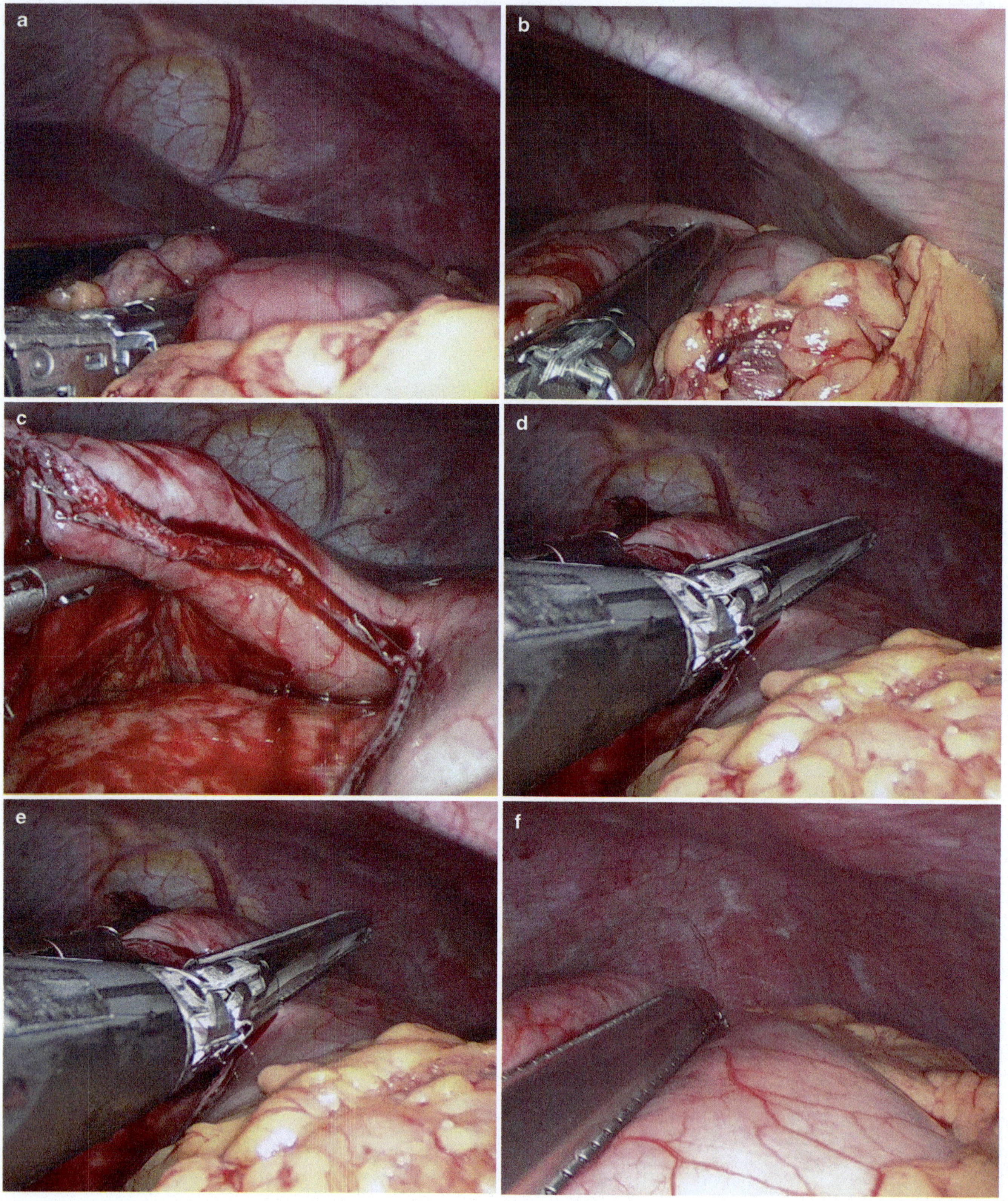

Fig. 11.5

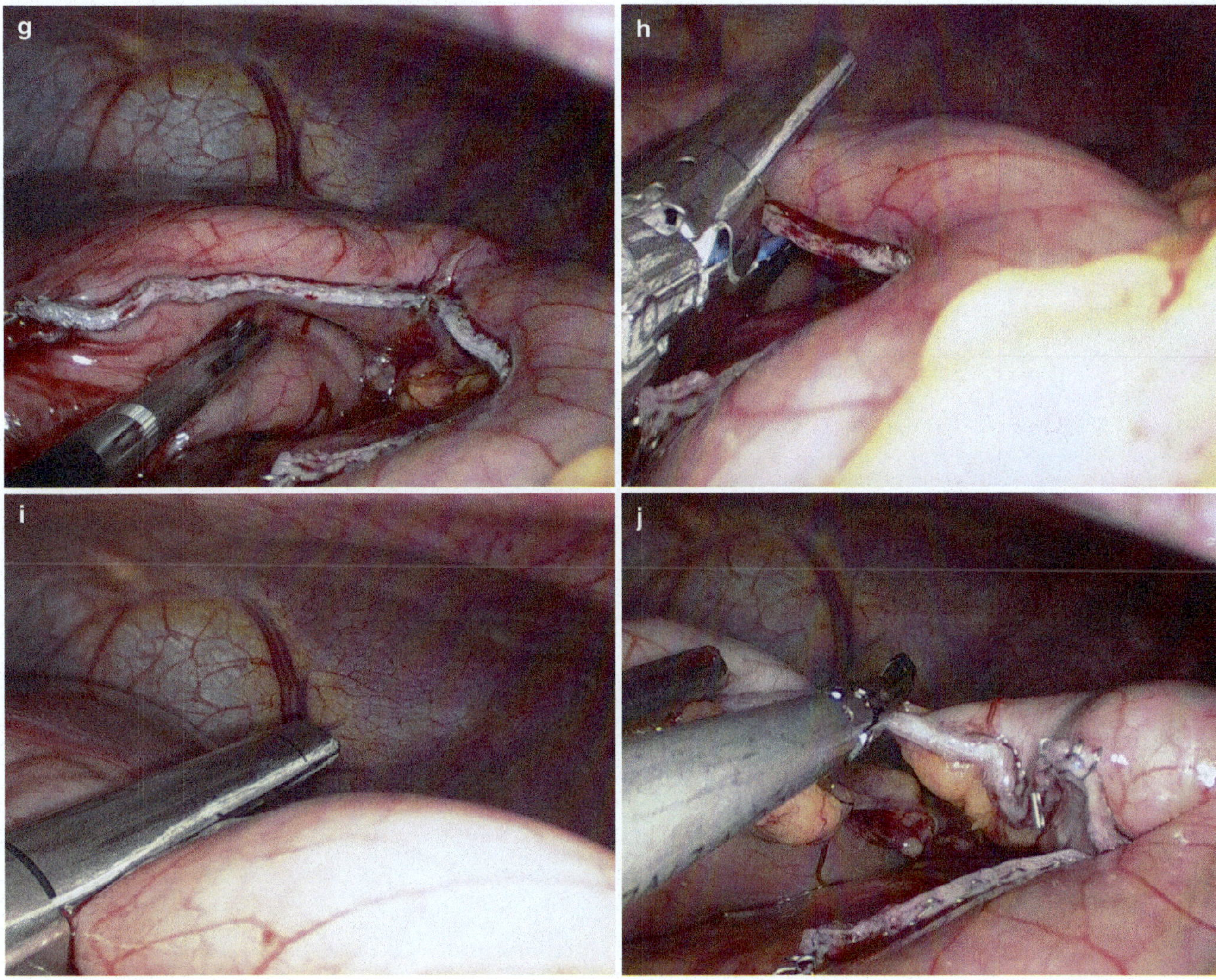

Fig. 11.5 (continued)

3. Dissection and resection of transverse colon
   Splenocolic ligament was divided using harmonic scalpel or Ligasure (Fig. 11.6a–d).

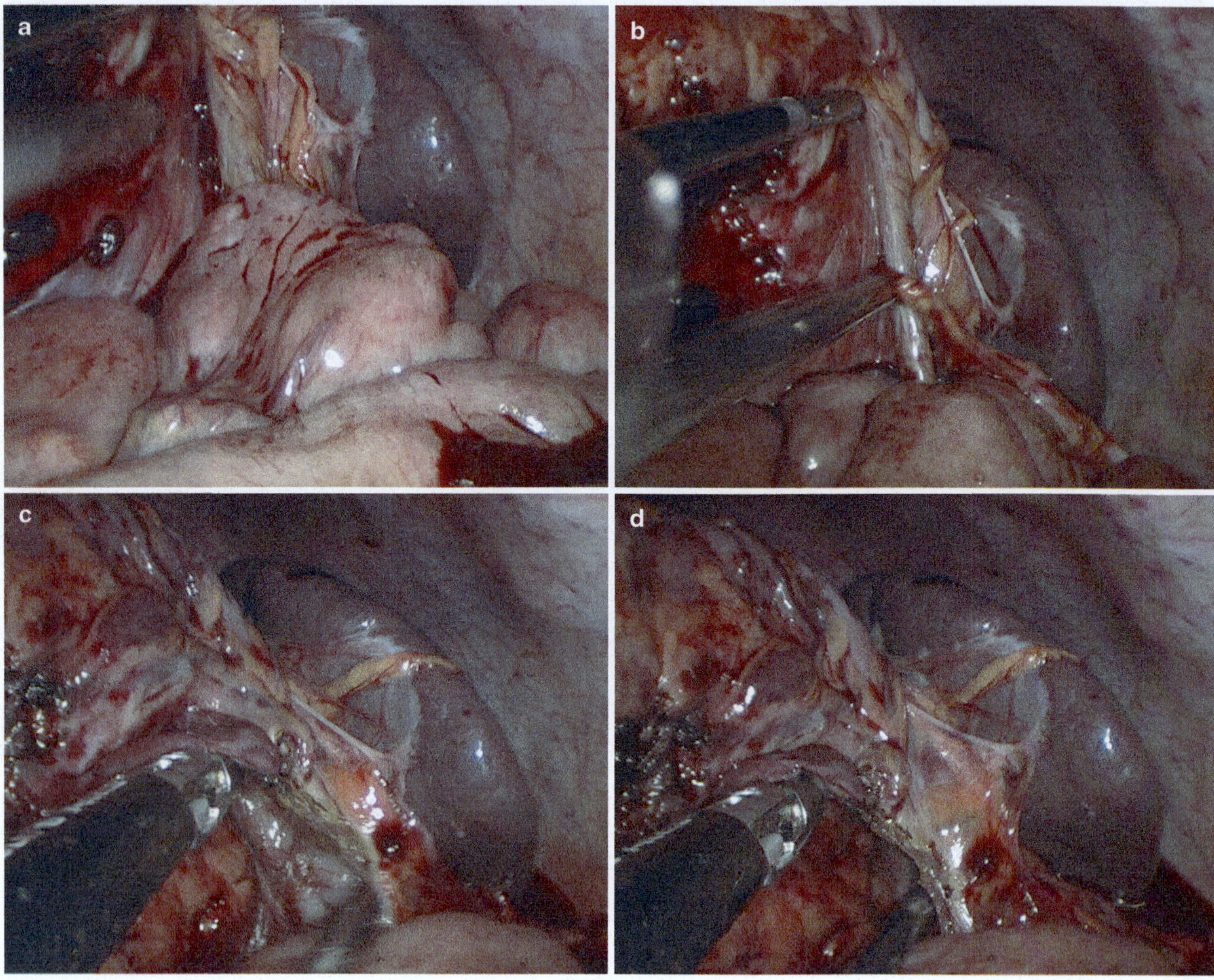

Fig. 11.6

The adhesion was divided and the transverse colon was exposed. Then the transverse colon was transected 3 cm away from the margin of lesion using Ligasure (Fig. 11.7a–h).

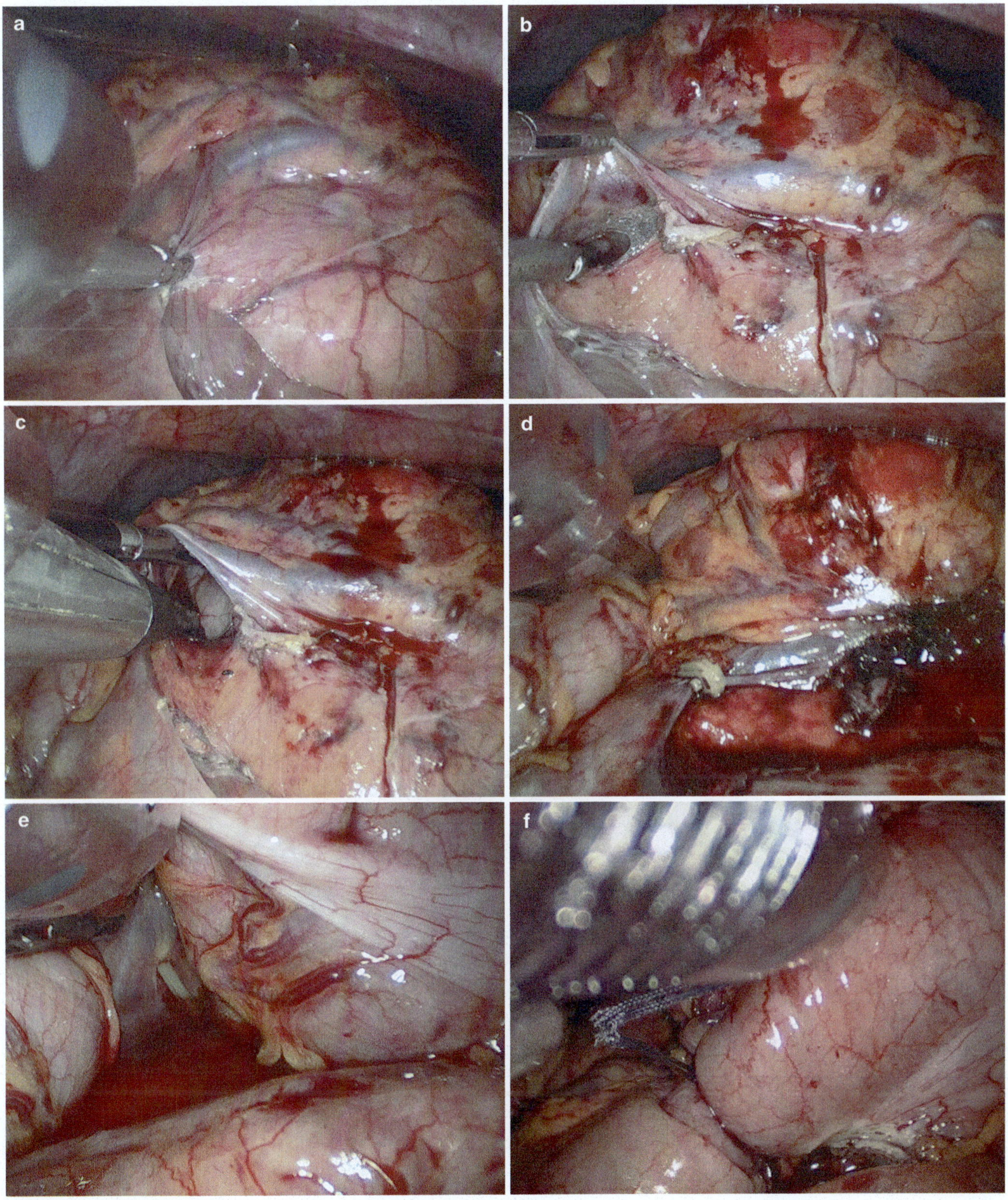

Fig. 11.7

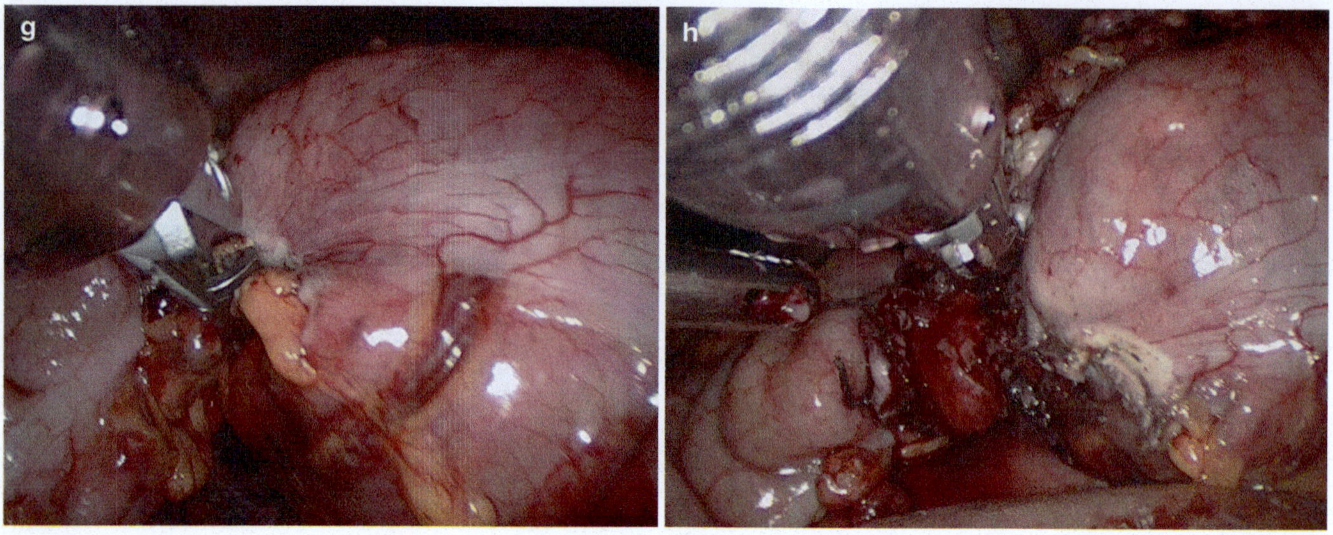

Fig. 11.7 (continued)

4. Resection of pancreatic body and tail
   The lesion infiltrated the pancreatic body and tail. Splenic artery and vein was dissected and cut at the proximal end of the tumor. Pancreas was dissected and transected using endoscopic linear cutter (Fig. 11.8a–h).

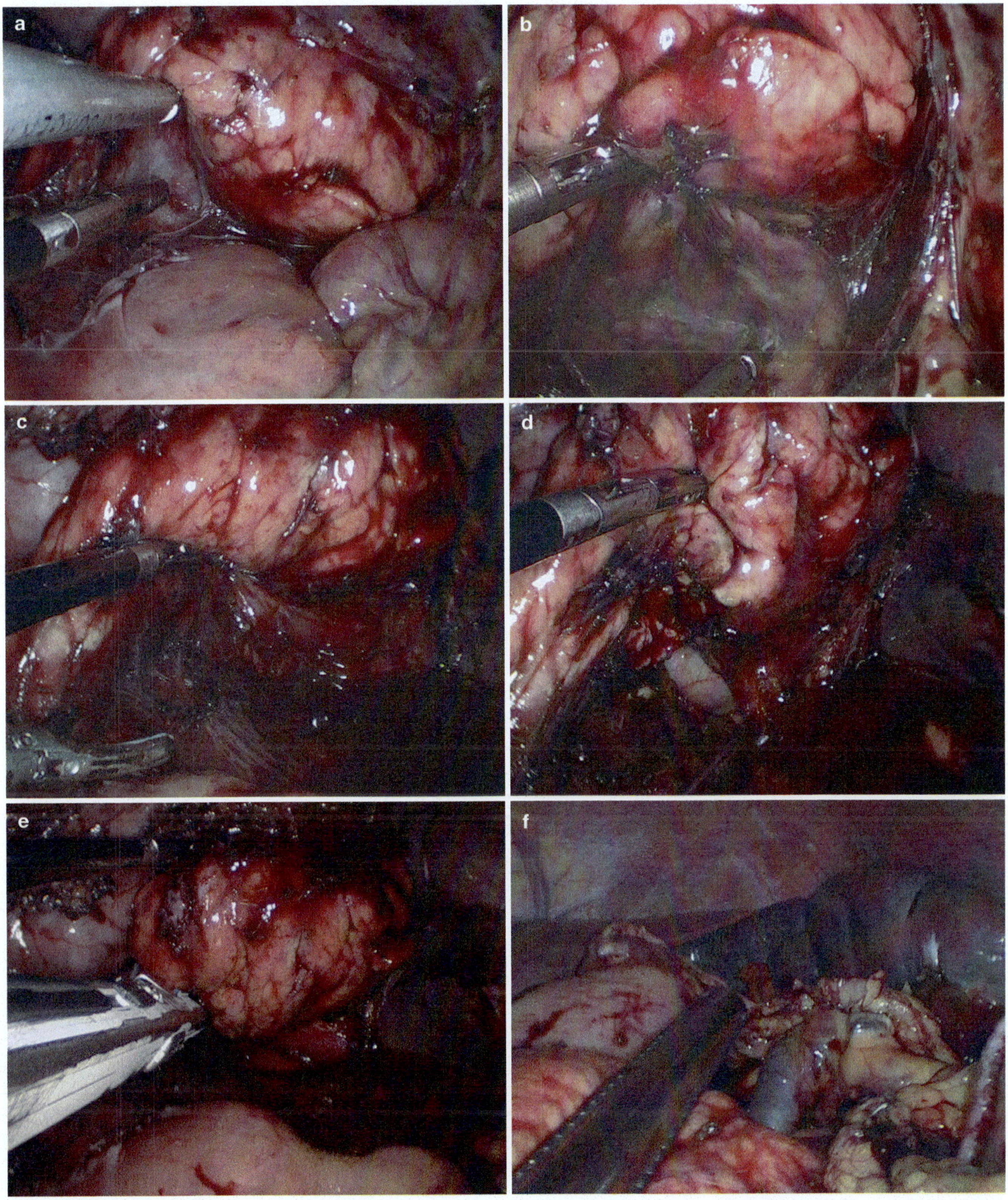

Fig. 11.8

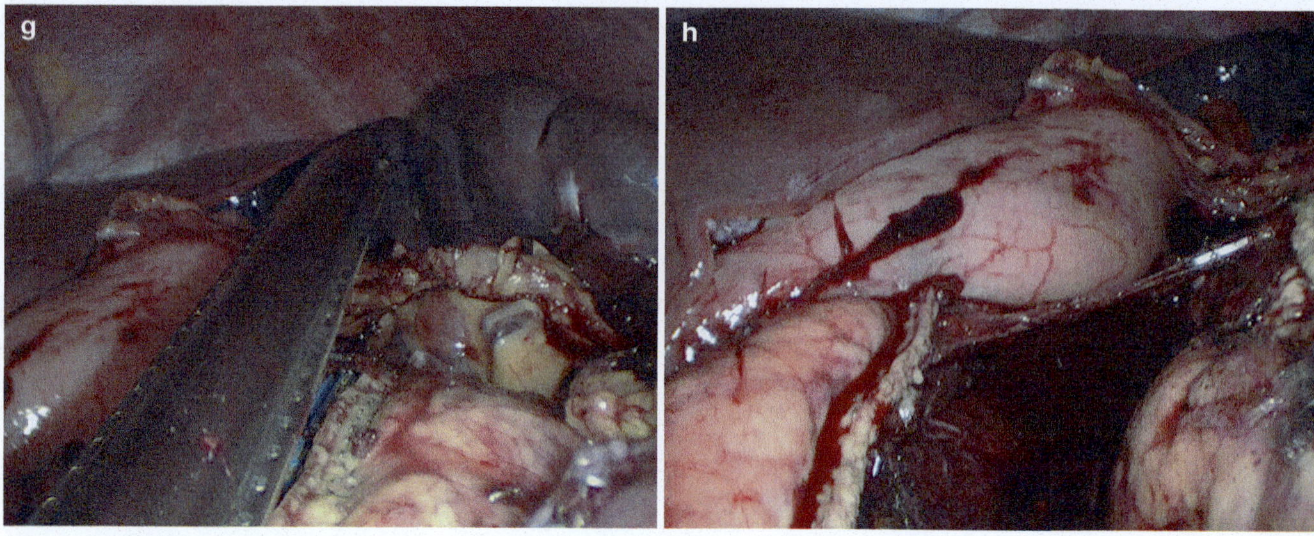

Fig. 11.8 (continued)

The tissue between pancreatic tail and splenic hilum was dissected carefully with the gastric short artery conserved. The tumor was removed with partial stomach, transverse colon, and pancreatic body and tail as an en bloc (Fig. 11.9a–f).

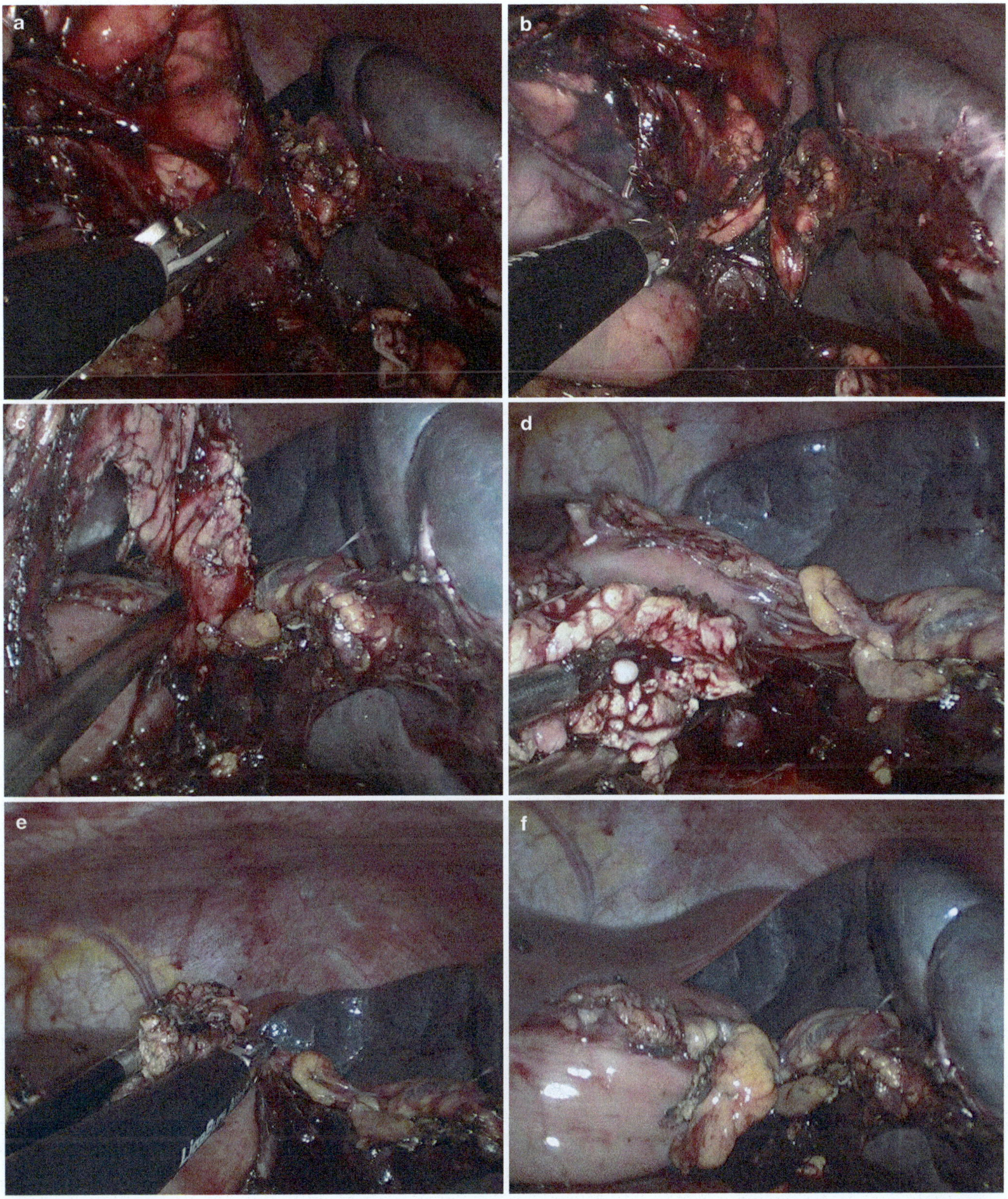

Fig. 11.9

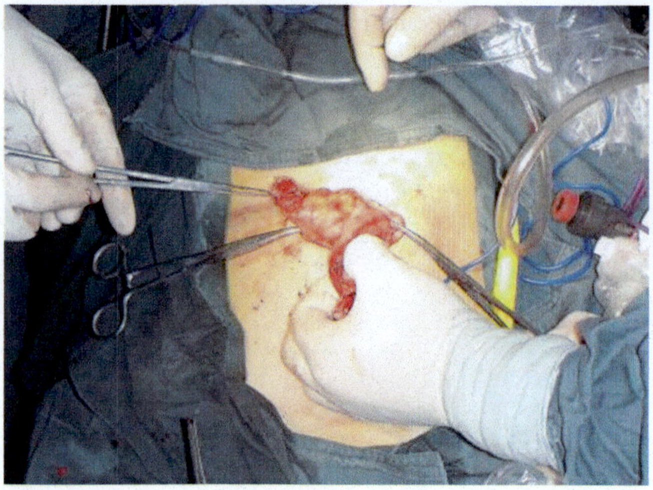

Fig. 11.10

5. Rebuilding of transverse colon
   The CO_2 was released and the trocars were removed. The umbilical incision was extended to 4–5 cm by cutting the tissue between 2 trocars. The incision was protected. The end-to-end anastomosis was performed extracorporeally. After the transverse colon was returned to the abdominal cavity, the incision was closed (Fig. 11.10).
6. Irrigation, drainage and closure of the incision
   The pneumoperitoneum was rebuilt then the abdominal cavity was checked carefully under laparoscopy. The anastomosis was solid with good blood supply (Fig. 11.11a–d).

   The abdominal cavity was irrigated, and then the wound surface was sprayed with glue. Two drainages were placed around Winslow hole and splenic hilum and out through the umbilical incision (Fig. 11.12).

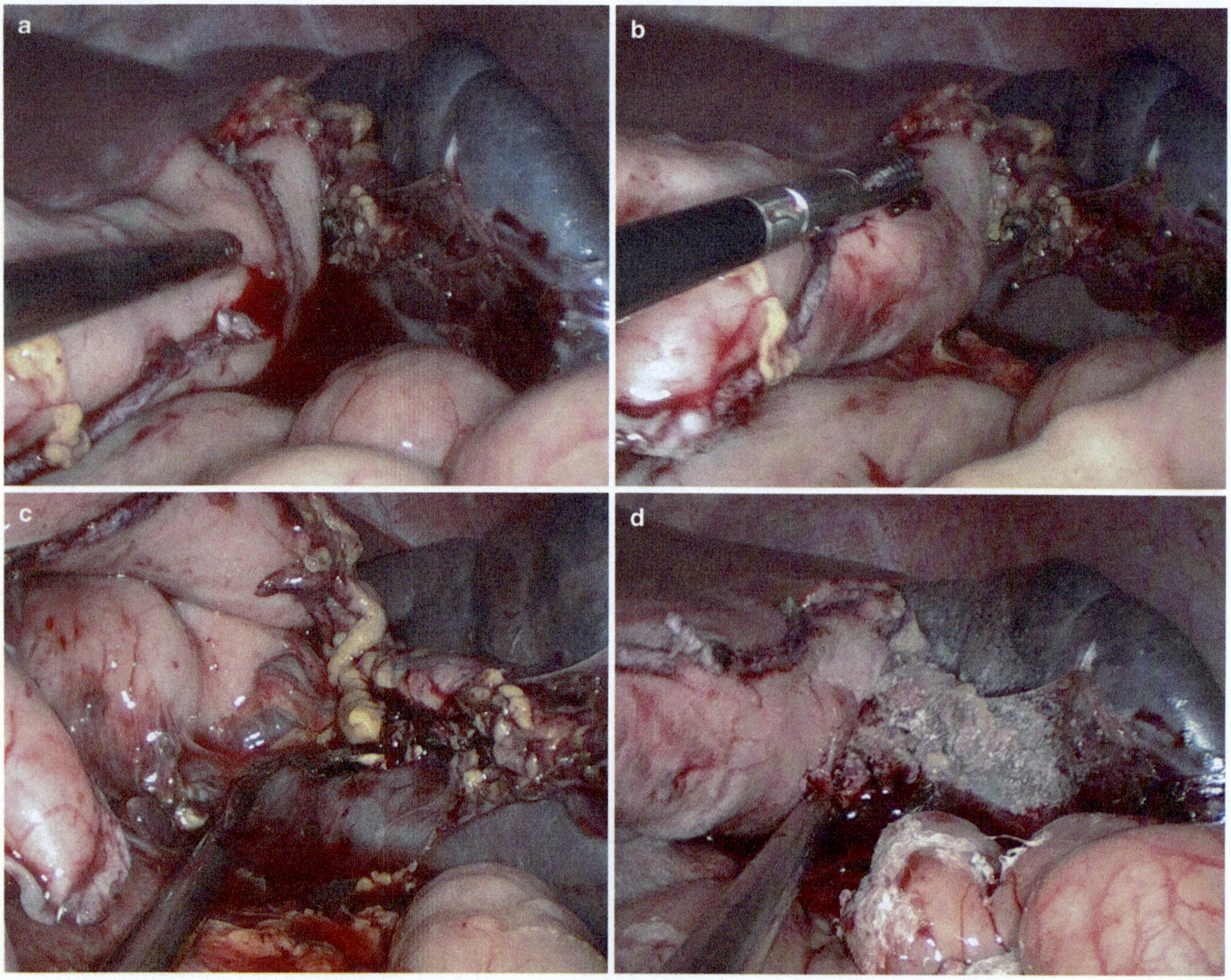

Fig. 11.11

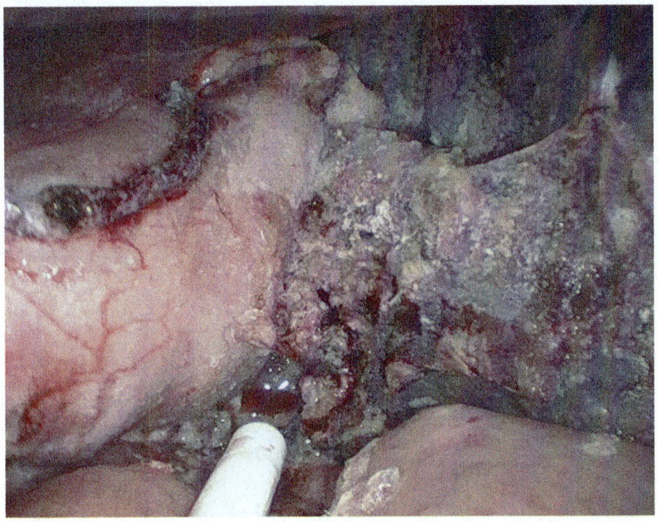

Fig. 11.12

11.7 Complications Analysis and Management

For the complications of SILS one-stage on multi-organ diseases, please consult the chapters of referred organs.

References

1. Kaiser AM, Corman ML. History of laparoscopy. Surg Oncol Clin N Am. 2001;10:483–92.
2. Ateş O, Hakgüder G, Olguner M, Akgür FM. Single-port laparoscopic appendectomy conducted intracorporeally with the aid of a transabdominal sling suture. J Pediatr Surg. 2007;42:1071–4.
3. Ponsky LE, Cherullo EE, Sawyer M, Hartke D. Single access site laparoscopic radical nephrectomy: initial clinical experience. J Endourol. 2008;22:663–5.
4. Castellucci SA, Curcillo PG, Ginsburg PC, Saba SC, Jaffe JS, Harmon JD. Single port access adrenalectomy. J Endourol. 2008;22: 1573–6.
5. Wu SD, Han JY, Tian Y. Single-incision laparoscopic cholecystectomy versus conventional laparoscopic cholecystectomy: a retrospective comparative study. J Laparoendosc Adv Surg Tech A. 2011;21:25–8.
6. Tian Y, Wu SD, Chen YS, Chen CC. Transumbilical single-incision laparoscopic cholecystojejunostomy using conventional instruments: the first two cases. J Gastrointest Surg. 2010;14:1429–33.
7. Kaouk JH, Palmer JS. Single port laparoscopic surgery: initial experience in children for varicocelectomy. BJU Int. 2008;102:97–9.
8. Mantke R, Wicht S. Single-port liver cyst fenestration combined with single-port laparoscopic cholecystectomy using completely reusable instruments. Surg Laparosc Endosc Percutan Tech. 2010; 20:28–30.
9. Cai W, Xu J, Zheng M, Qin M, Zhao H. Combined laparoendoscopic single-site surgery: initial experience of a single center. Hepatogastroenterology. 2012;59:986–9.

Integrated Multi-subject Surgery 12

12.1 Laparoscopic Sleeve Stomach Esophagoplasty

12.1.1 Major Instruments or Energy Sources

1. Laparoscopy System
2. Harmonic scalpel
3. Ligasure

12.1.2 Team Setup, Anesthesia and Position

Under general anesthesia, the patient was placed in supine position with the legs apart. The position of surgeon, assistants and nurses is shown in Fig. 12.1.

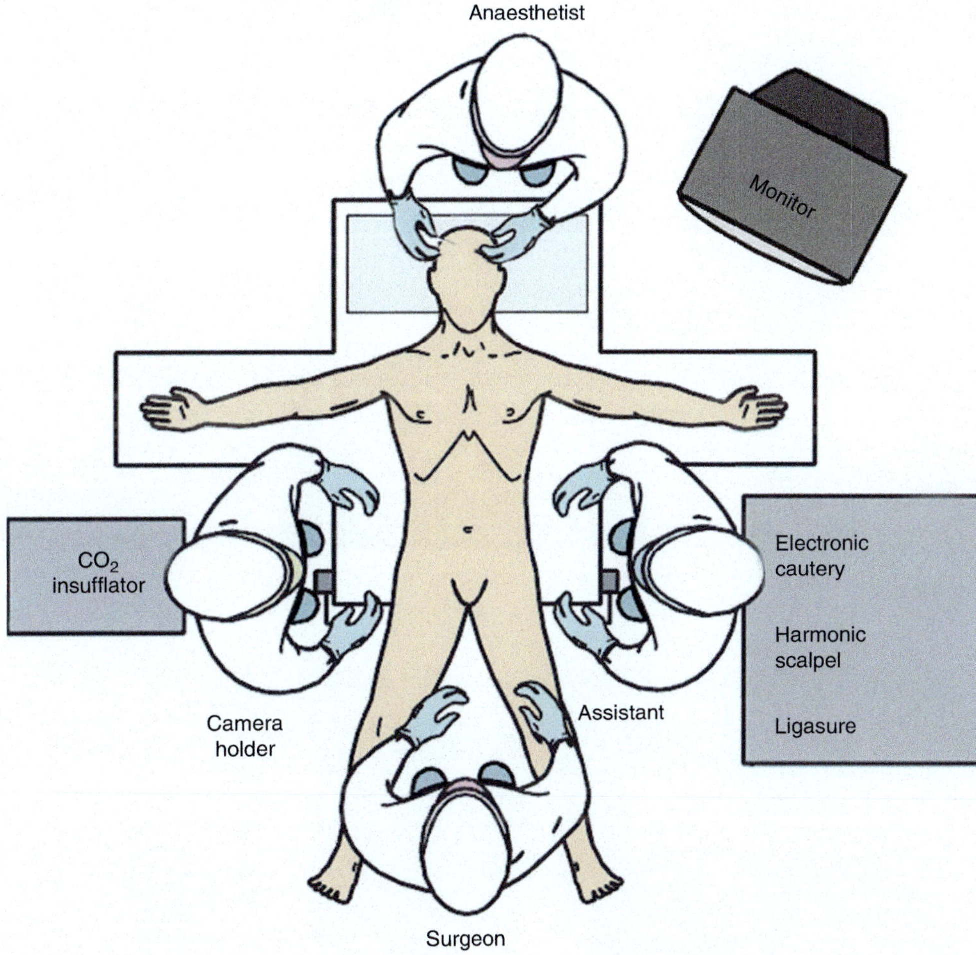

Fig. 12.1

S. Wu et al. (eds.), *Atlas of Single-Incision Laparoscopic Operations in General Surgery*,
DOI 10.1007/978-94-007-6955-7_12, © Springer Science+Business Media Dordrecht 2013

12.1.3 Key Steps

1. Dissection of the gastrocolic ligament
2. Dissection of the gastrosplenic ligament
3. Division of the left gastric artery
4. Dissection of the hepatogastric ligament
5. Mobilization of the lower esophagus

12.1.4 Surgical Techniques

1. Dissection of the gastrocolic ligament
   Greater curvature was retracted and gastrocolic ligament was divided along the greater curvature (Fig. 12.2a–d).

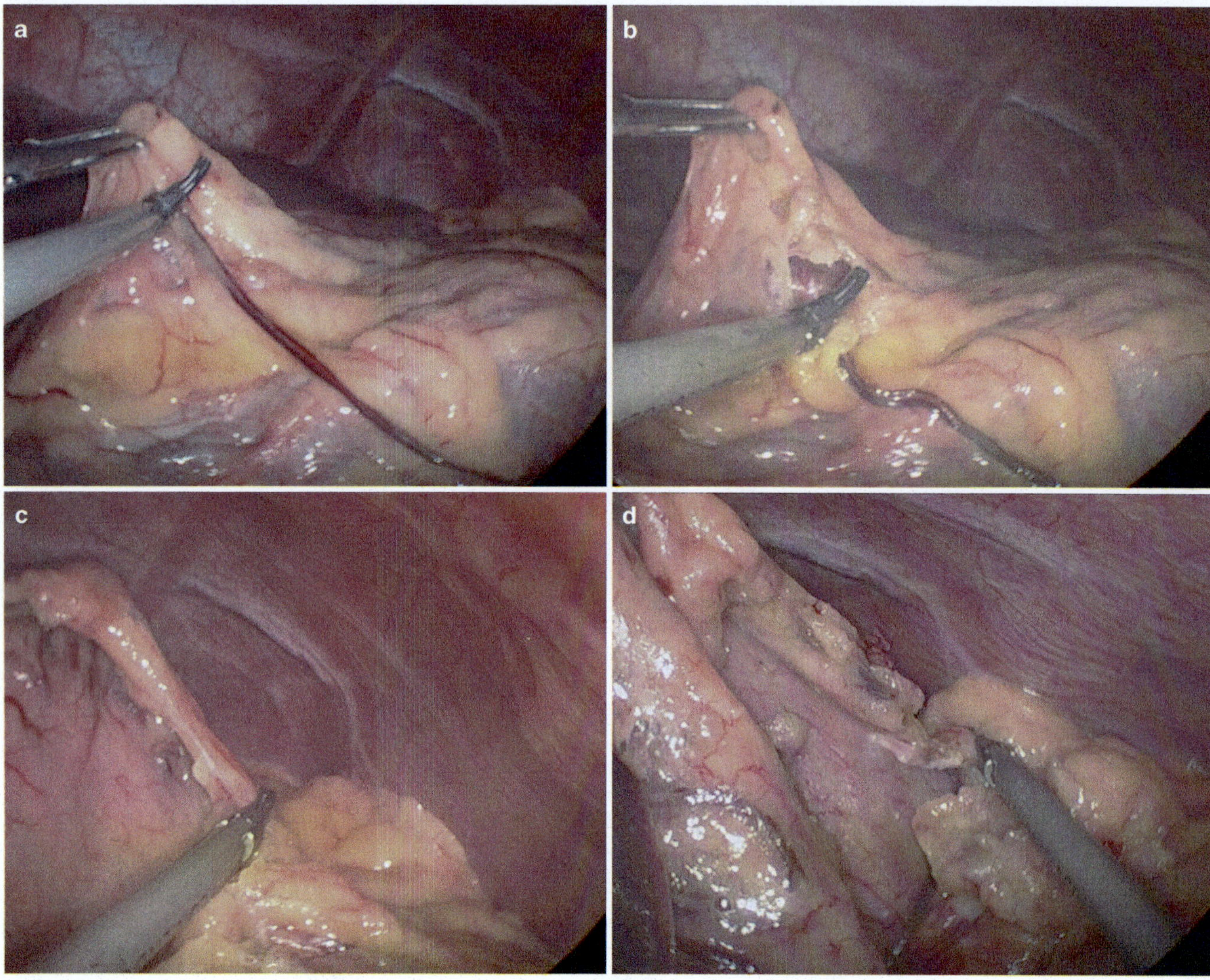

Fig. 12.2

2. Dissection of the gastrosplenic ligament
   Gastrosplenic ligament was divided along the greater curvature. The fundus of stomach was exposed. Then the gastrocolic ligament was divided caudally to the antrum of stomach (Fig. 12.3a–d).

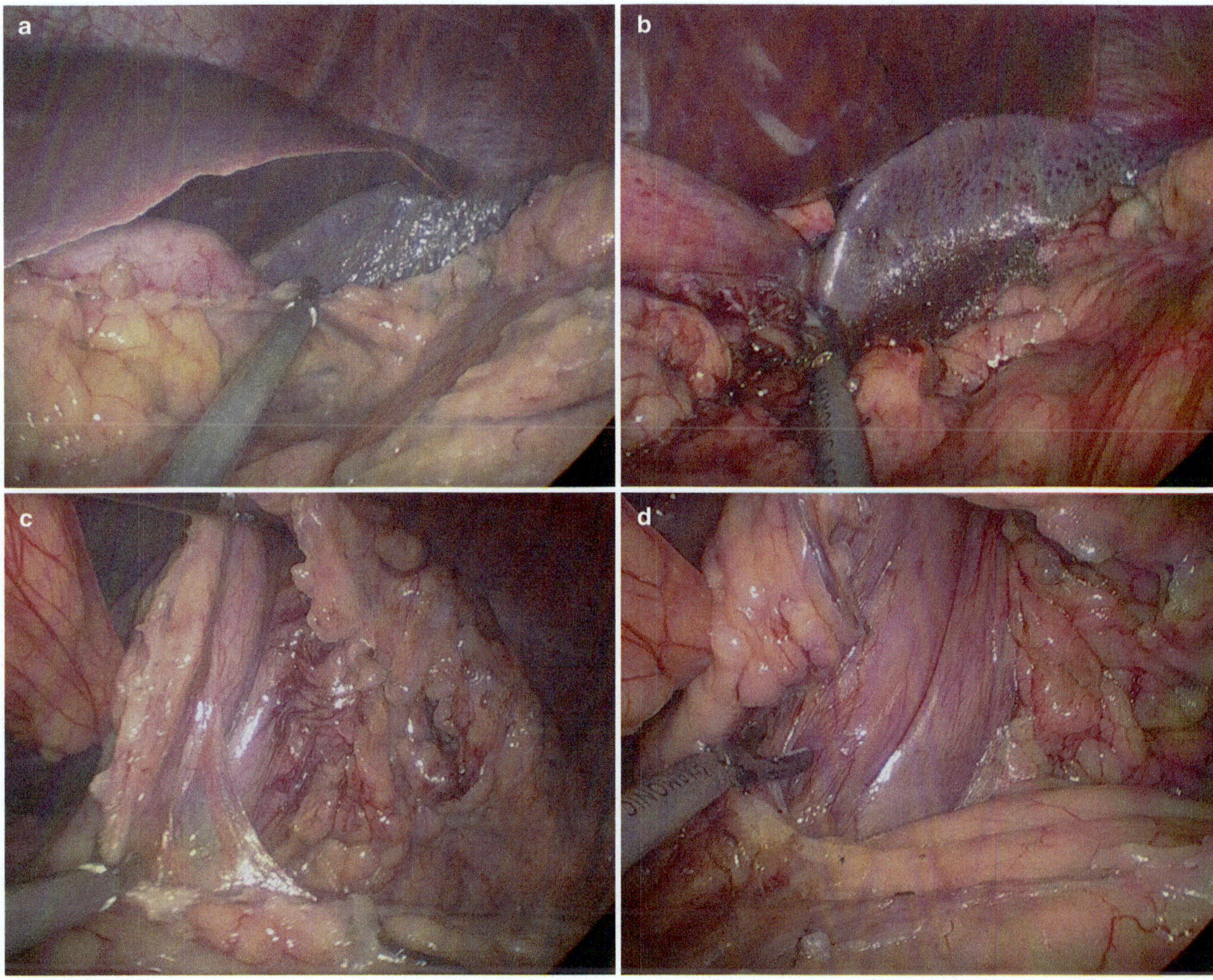

Fig. 12.3

3. Division of the left gastric artery
   The left gastric artery was identified and clamped (Fig. 12.4a–d).

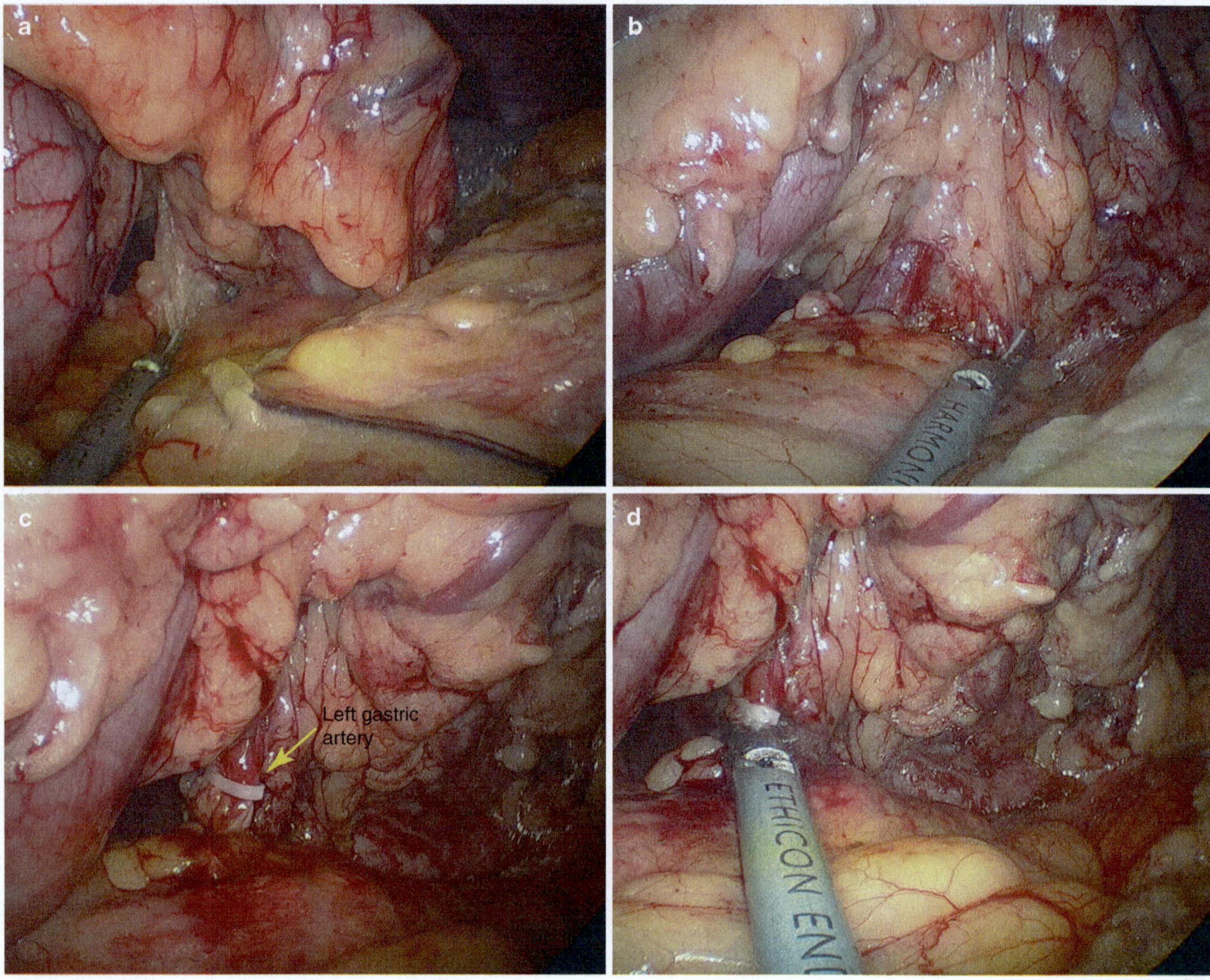

Fig. 12.4

4. Dissection of the hepatogastric ligament
   The left lateral lobe of liver was suspended to the diagram with glue. Then the hepatogastric ligament was divided using harmonic scalpel (Fig. 12.5a–f).

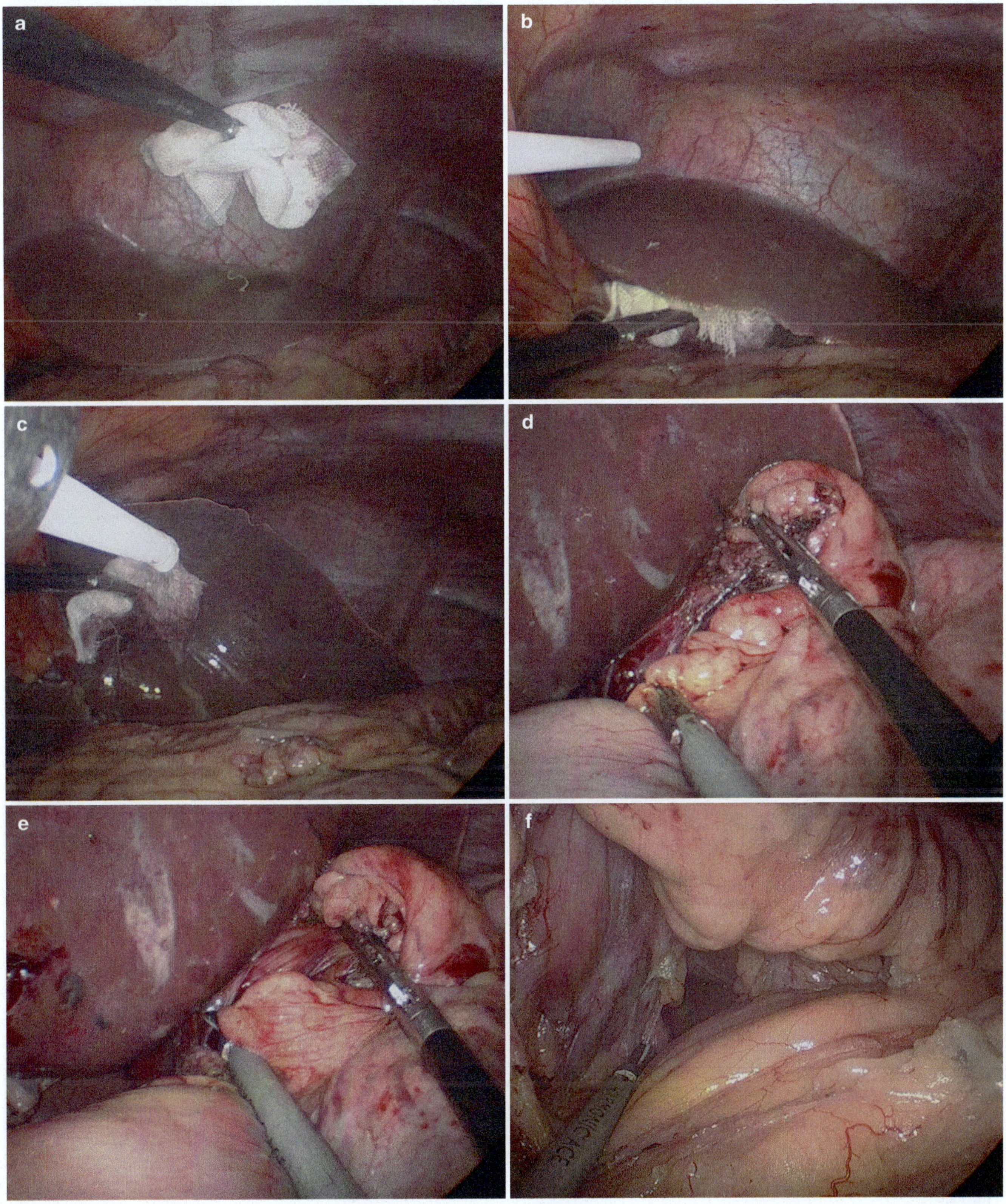

Fig. 12.5

5. Mobilization of the lower esophagus
   The peritoneum covering the esophagus was cut open, and then the lower part of the esophagus was mobilized along the left and right side. The diaphragmatic hiatus was extended so that the stomach could be lifted up to the thoracic cavity through it (Fig. 12.6a–i).

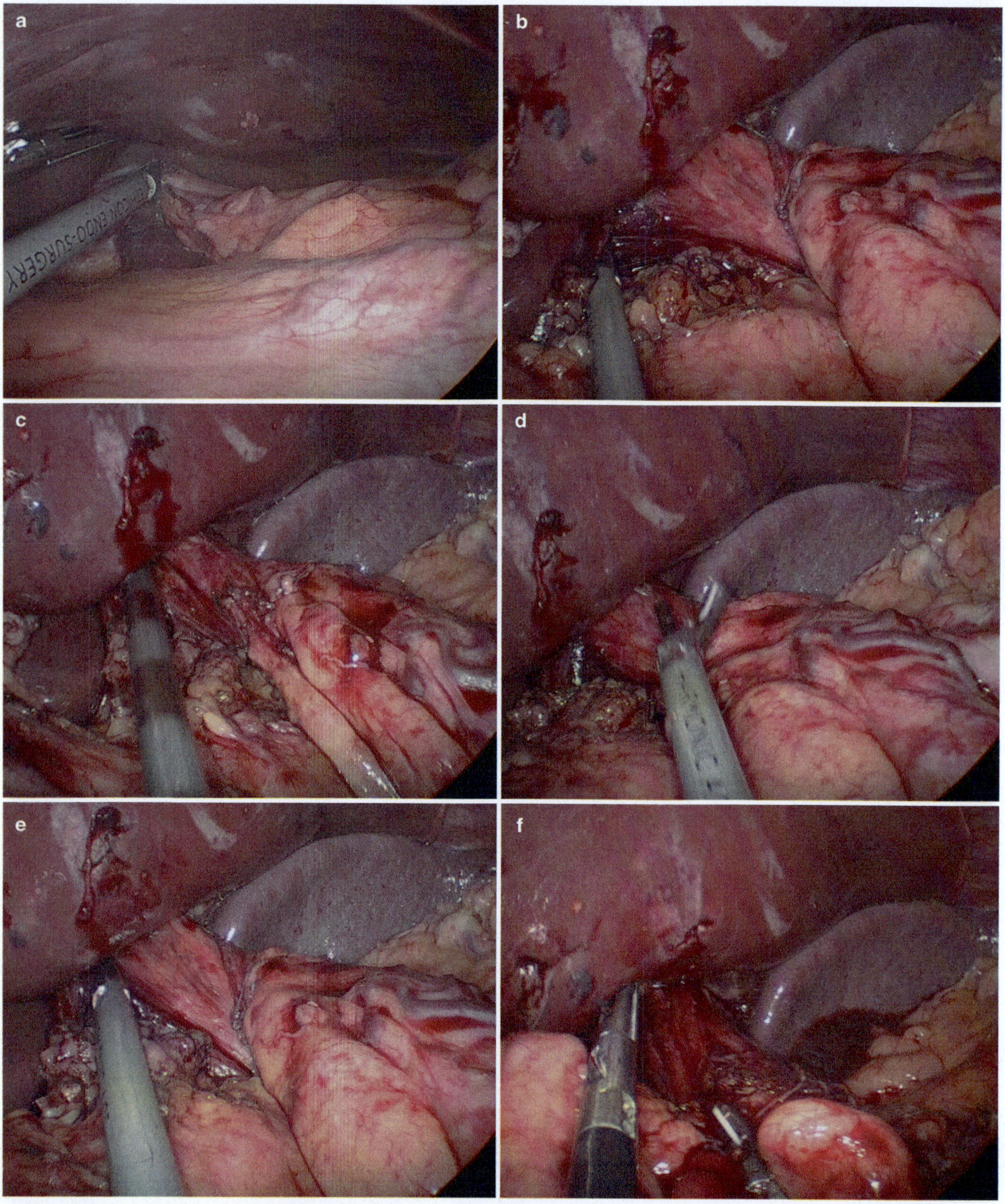

Fig. 12.6

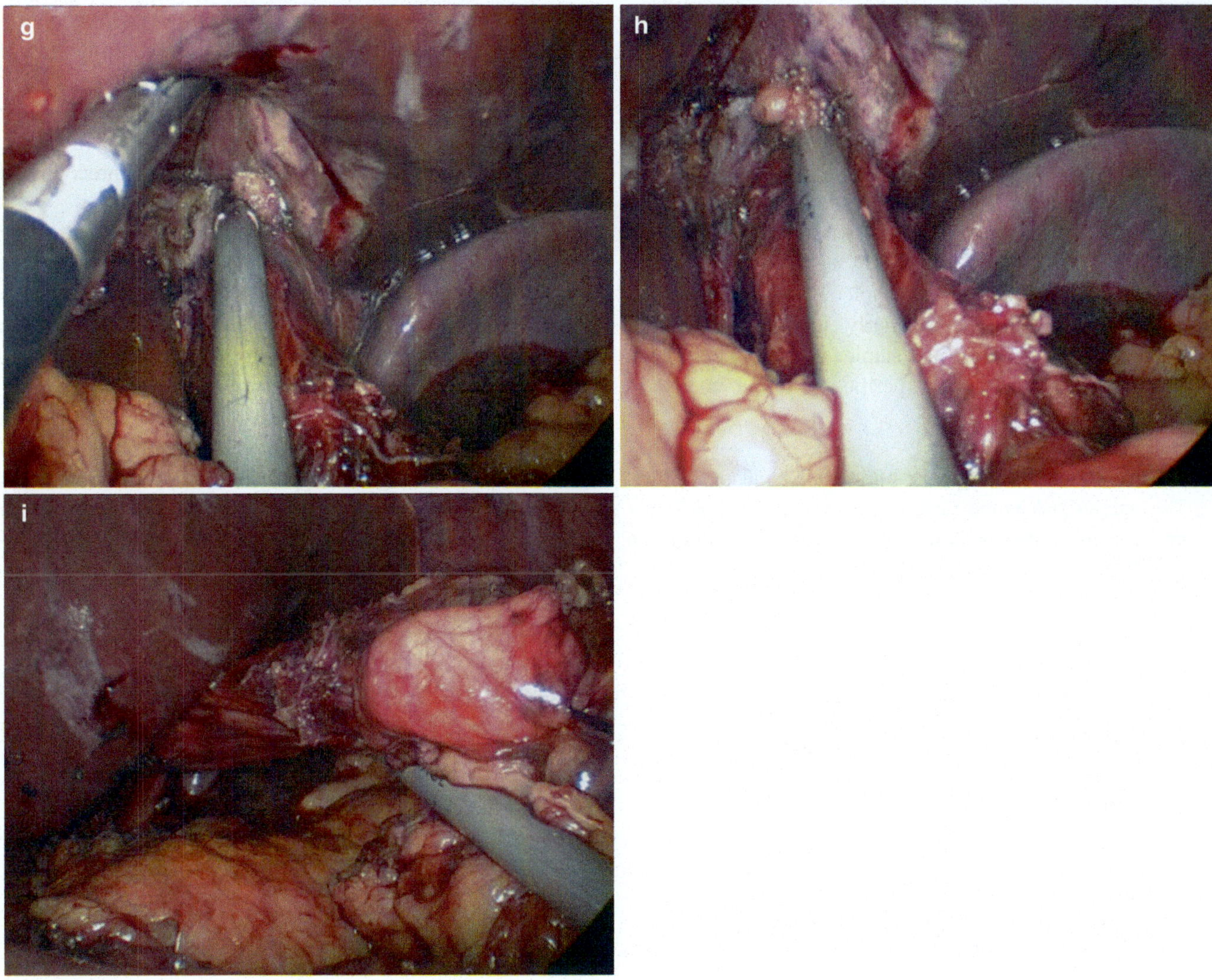

Fig. 12.6 (continued)

12.1.5 Complications Analysis and Management

1. Anastomotic leakage and anastomotic stenosis
   The tension of anastomotic stoma plays an important role in the formation of leakage. The residual stomach can be prolonged 5–8 cm by the sleeve stomach, which effectively decreases the tension of anastomotic stoma. A proper sleeve stomach can prevent the formation of anastomotic leakage. Reasonable choice and skilled application of staplers are particularly important to avoid anastomotic leak. When the stapler is fired, the surgeon should make sure that no peripheral tissue is tied to stapler.
2. Haemorrhage
   It is similar to SILS gastric and esophageal procedure. The greater risk is the violently tearing of venous structures, such as the azygous vein. Ultrasonic scalpel can directly cut off the vessels less than 1.5 mm in diameter. For the larger vessels, Ligasure or firing stapler is necessary for safe and effective hemostasis. Before the end of surgery, haemorrhage should be examined carefully, because there is also a risk of delayed bleeding from the short branches that feed the esophagus directly from the aorta, the short gastric vessels, or from an unrecognized splenic injury.
3. Reflux esophagitis and cardiopulmonary dysfunction
   Cutting-off the vagus nerve may decrease tension and evacuation of the intrathoracic stomach, which induces the reflux esophagitis. Compression of intrathoracic stomach is the reason of cardiopulmonary dysfunction, and the postoperative quality of life will be obviously affected. Thus, an appropriate volume is important in making sleeve stomach. A better sleeve stomach should be close to the original esophagus in appearance which is easily placed in esophageal bed to decrease the dilation and alleviate the gastroesophageal reflux and compression to the mediastinum or lung.

12.2 Laparoscopic Jejunum Pharyngoplasty

12.2.1 Major Instruments or Energy Sources

1. Laparoscopy System
2. Harmonic scalpel
3. Ligasure

12.2.2 Team Setup, Anesthesia and Position

Under general anesthesia, the patient was placed in supine position. The position of surgeon, assistants and nurses is shown in Fig. 12.7.

Fig. 12.7

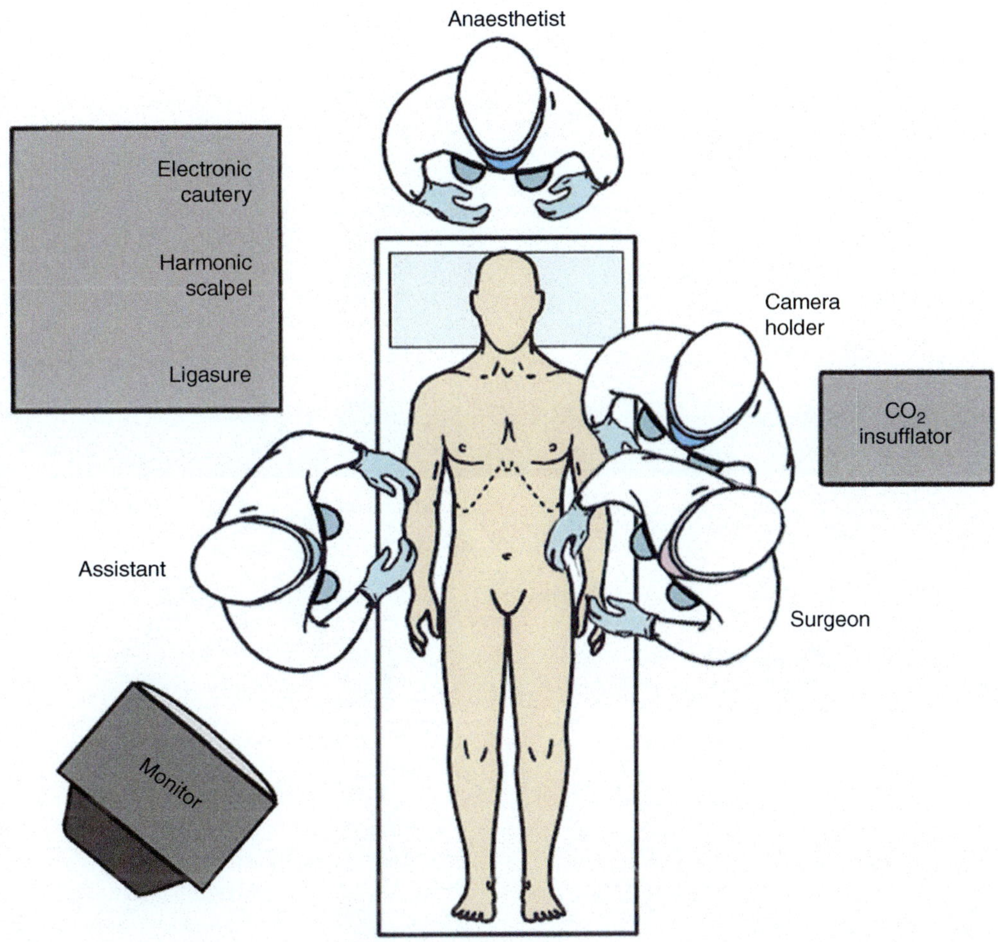

12.2.3 Key Steps

1. Identification of the Treitz ligament
2. Observation of the distribution of the jejunal artery
3. Isolation of the segment of jejunum
4. Anastomosis of the jejunum-jejunum
5. Pharyngoplasty by ENT doctor

12.2.4 Surgical Techniques

1. Identification of the Treitz ligament
   The transverse colon was retracted by non-invasive forceps. The Treitz ligament and proximal jejunum was identified (Fig. 12.8a–d).

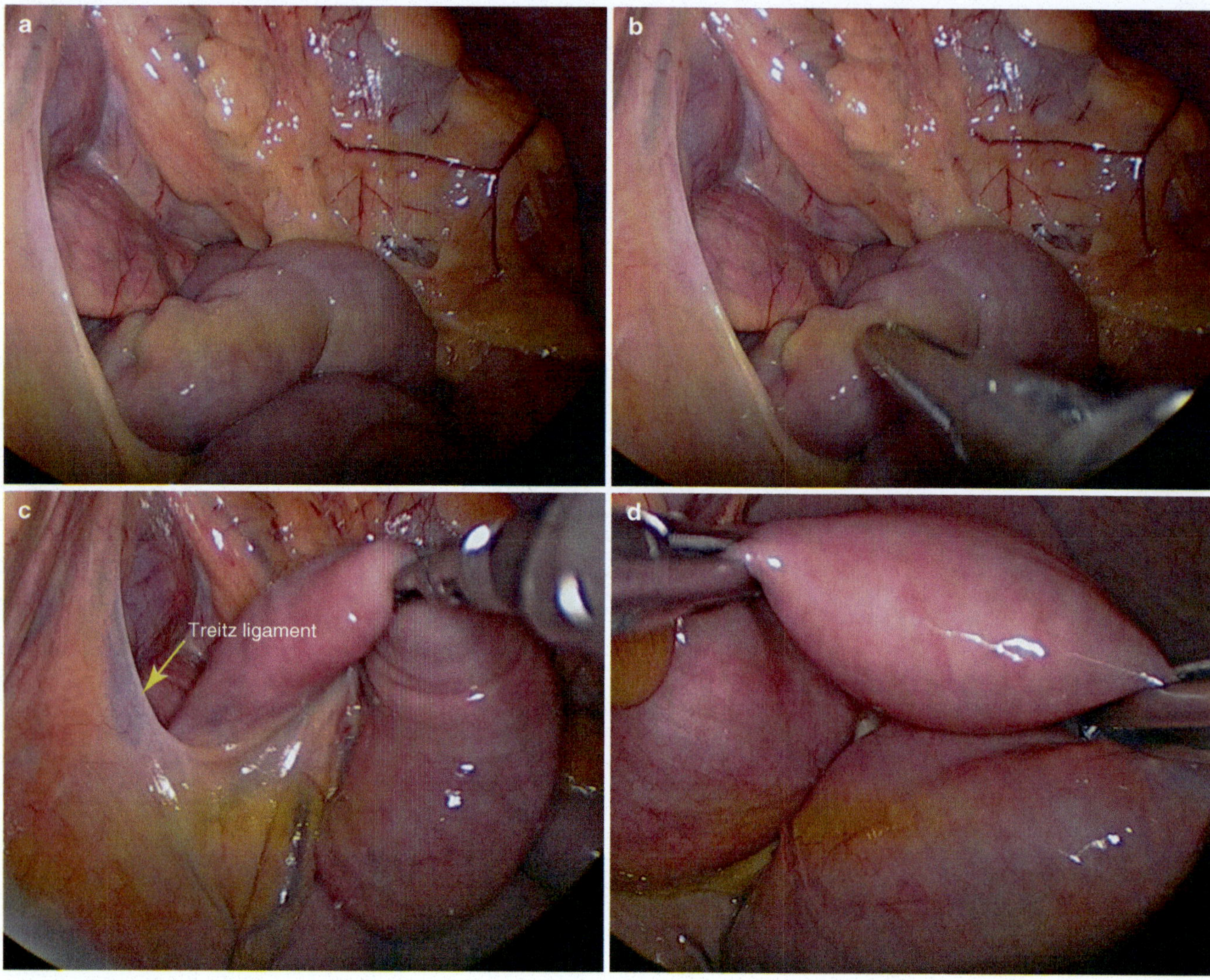

Fig. 12.8

2. Observation of the vessel distribution and choice of the appropriate segment of jejunum
   The jejunum was grasped and the mesentery was checked carefully to observe the distribution of the vessel so that the blood supply of the segment of jejunum was good (Fig. 12.9a, b).

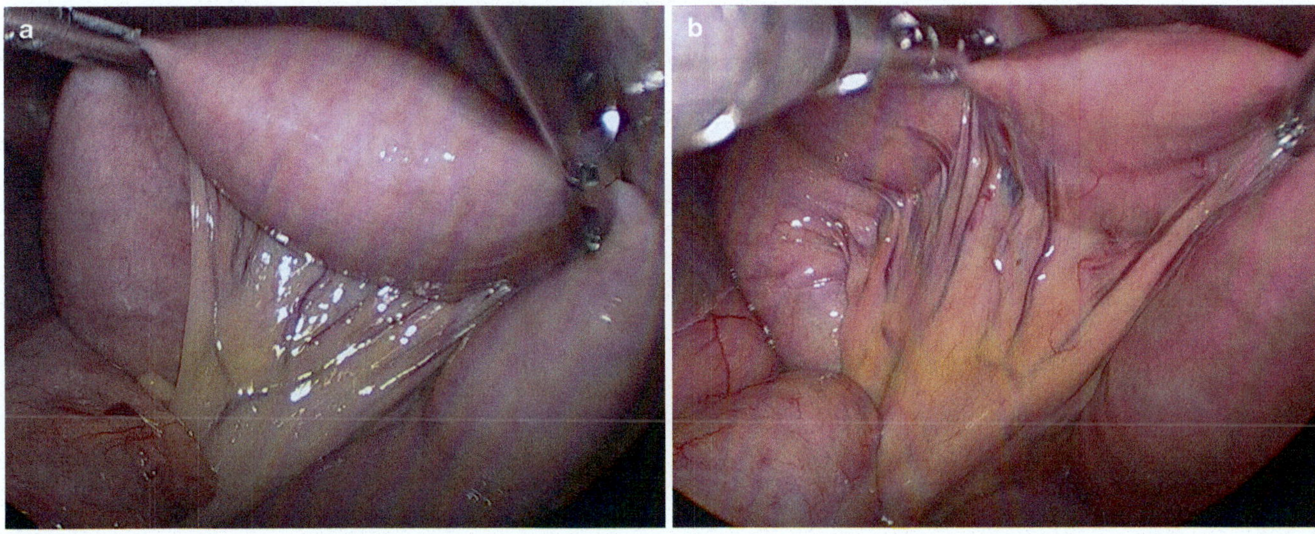

Fig. 12.9

3. Isolation of the segment of jejunum
   The peritoneum of mesentery was cut open and the vascular pedicle was made into the shape of fan. Good blood supply must be confirmed (Fig. 12.10a–d).

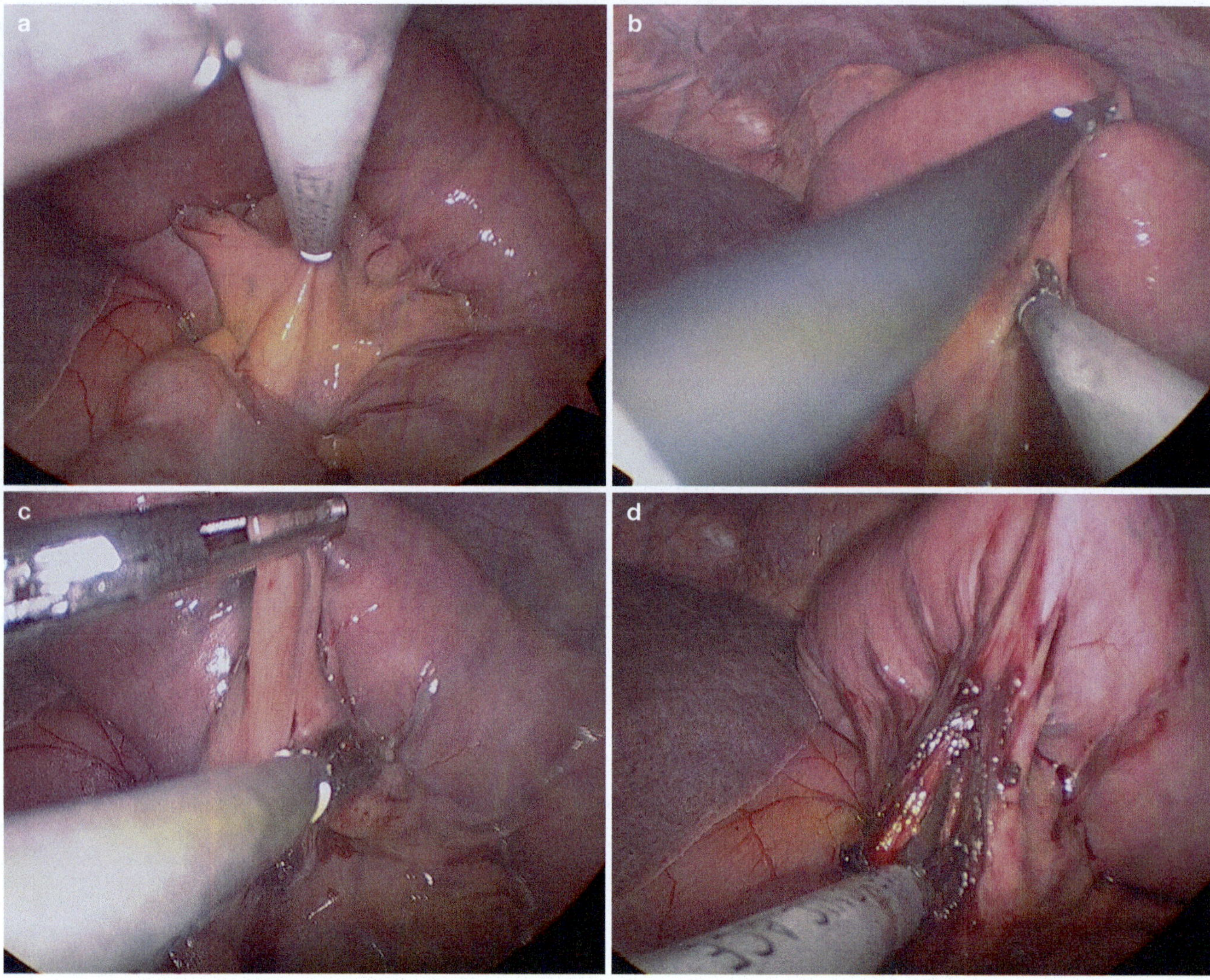

Fig. 12.10

The jejunum was transected using the linear cutter (Fig. 12.11a–c).

The proximal jejunum was labeled by suturing to avoid the wrong jejunal anastomosis (Fig. 12.12a, b).

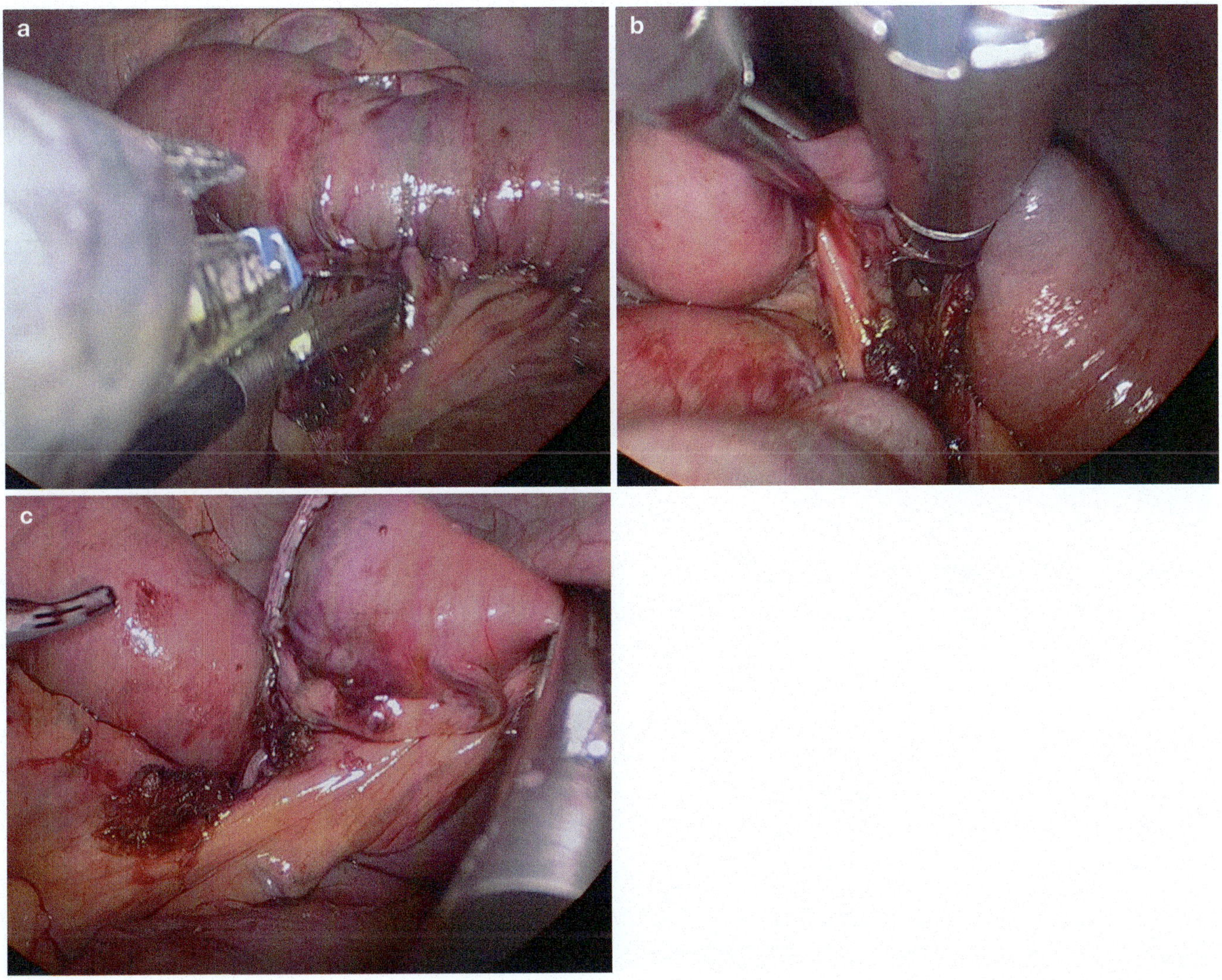

Fig. 12.11

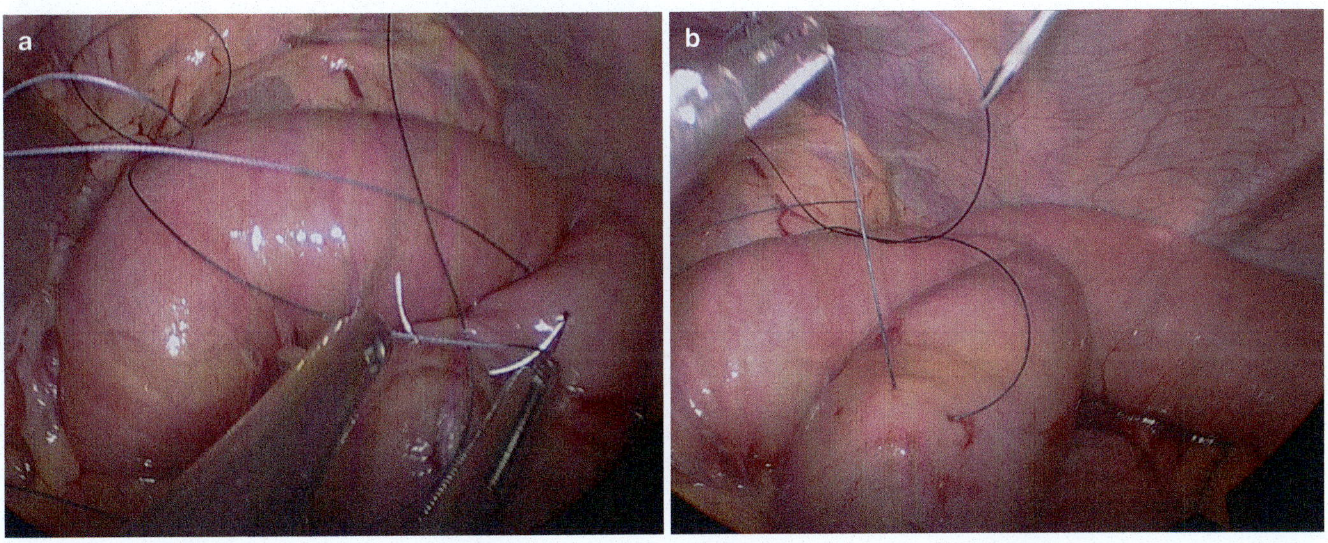

Fig. 12.12

The mesentery was further divided and the supply of blood vessel was kept completely (Fig. 12.13a–d).

The jejunum was transected using linear stapler to make a 20 cm segment of jejunum (Fig. 12.14a–f).

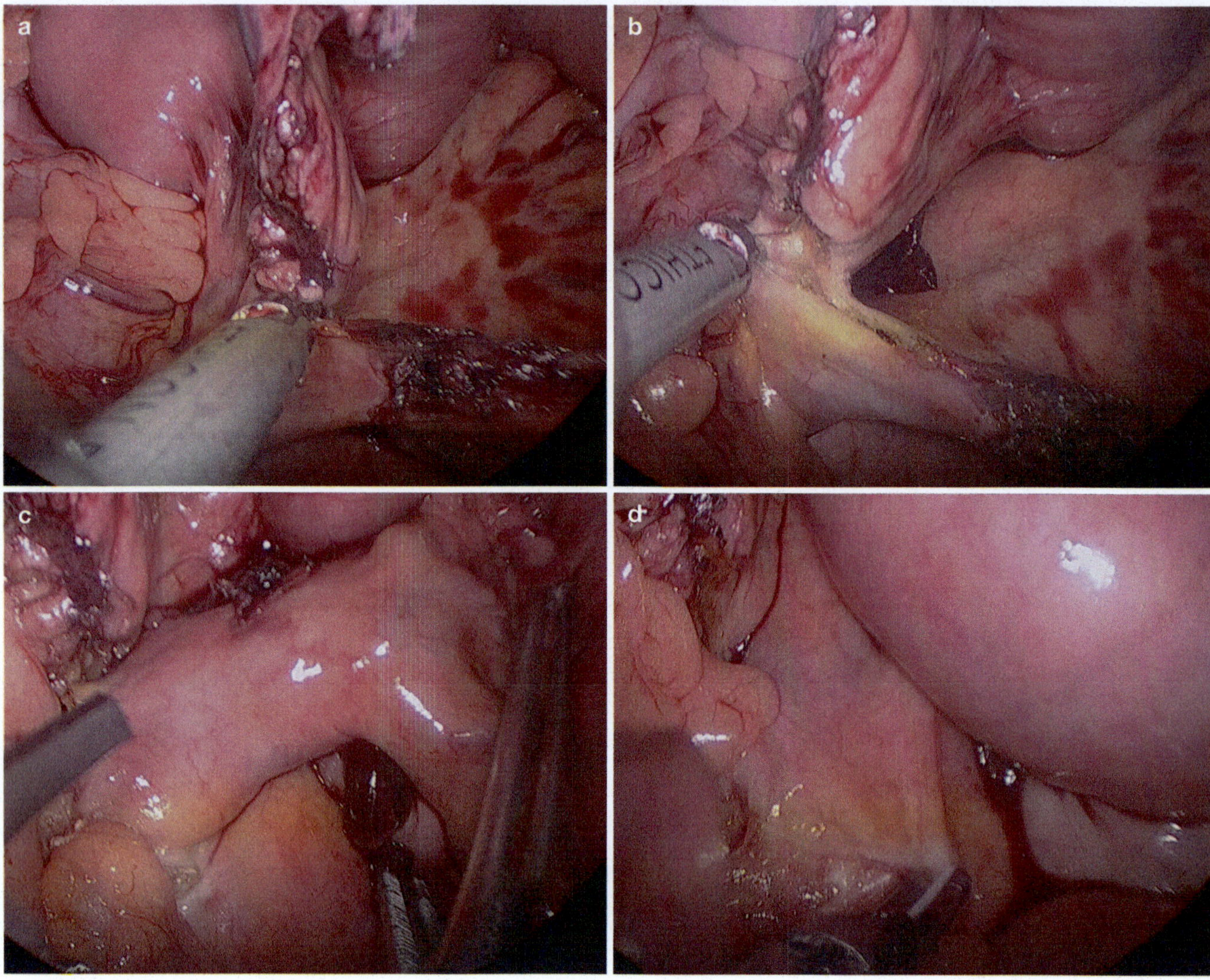

Fig. 12.13

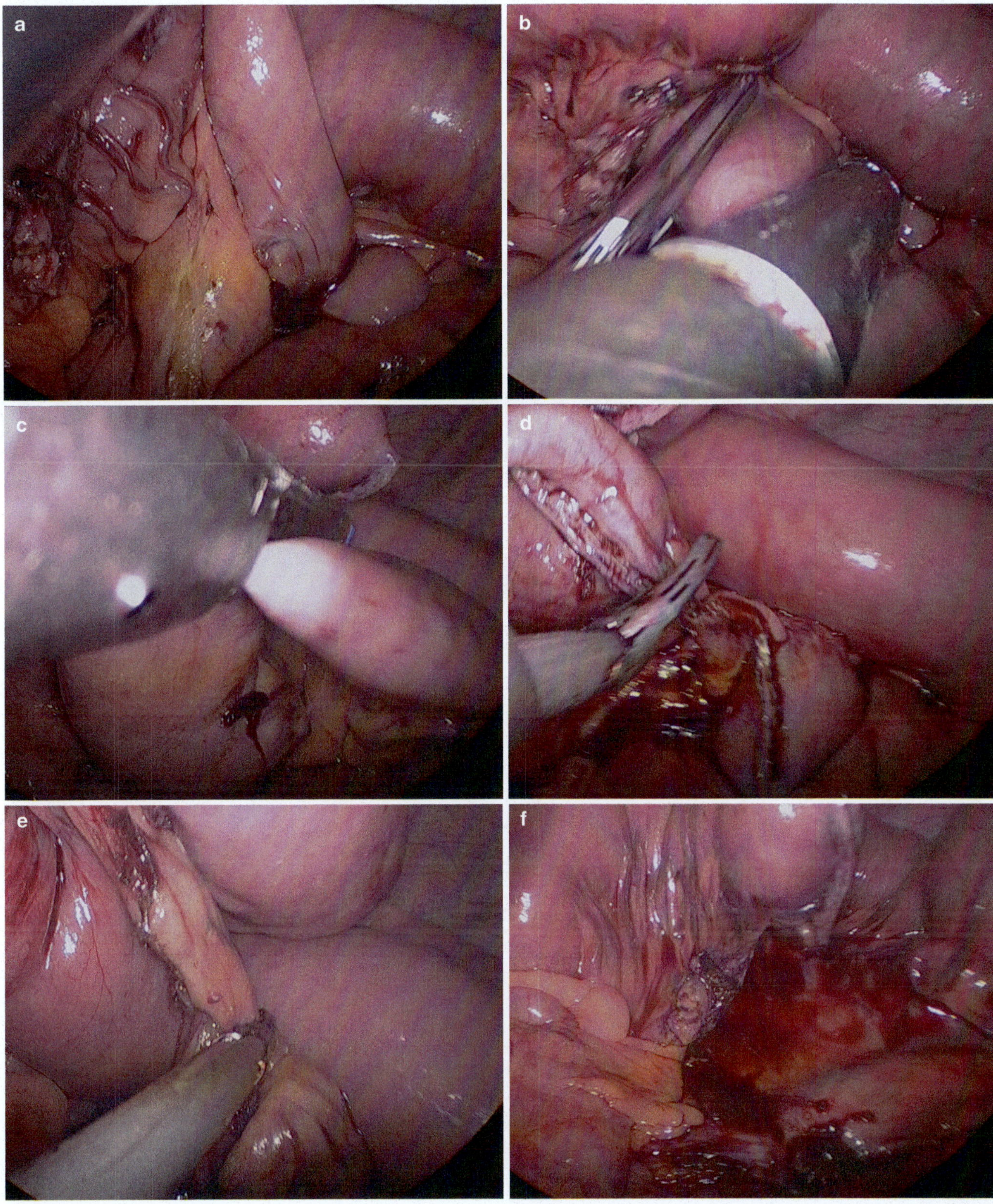

Fig. 12.14

The umbilical incision was extended and the segment of jejunum with the vascular pedicle was extracted out of the abdominal cavity for the pharyngoplasty (Fig. 12.15a–e).

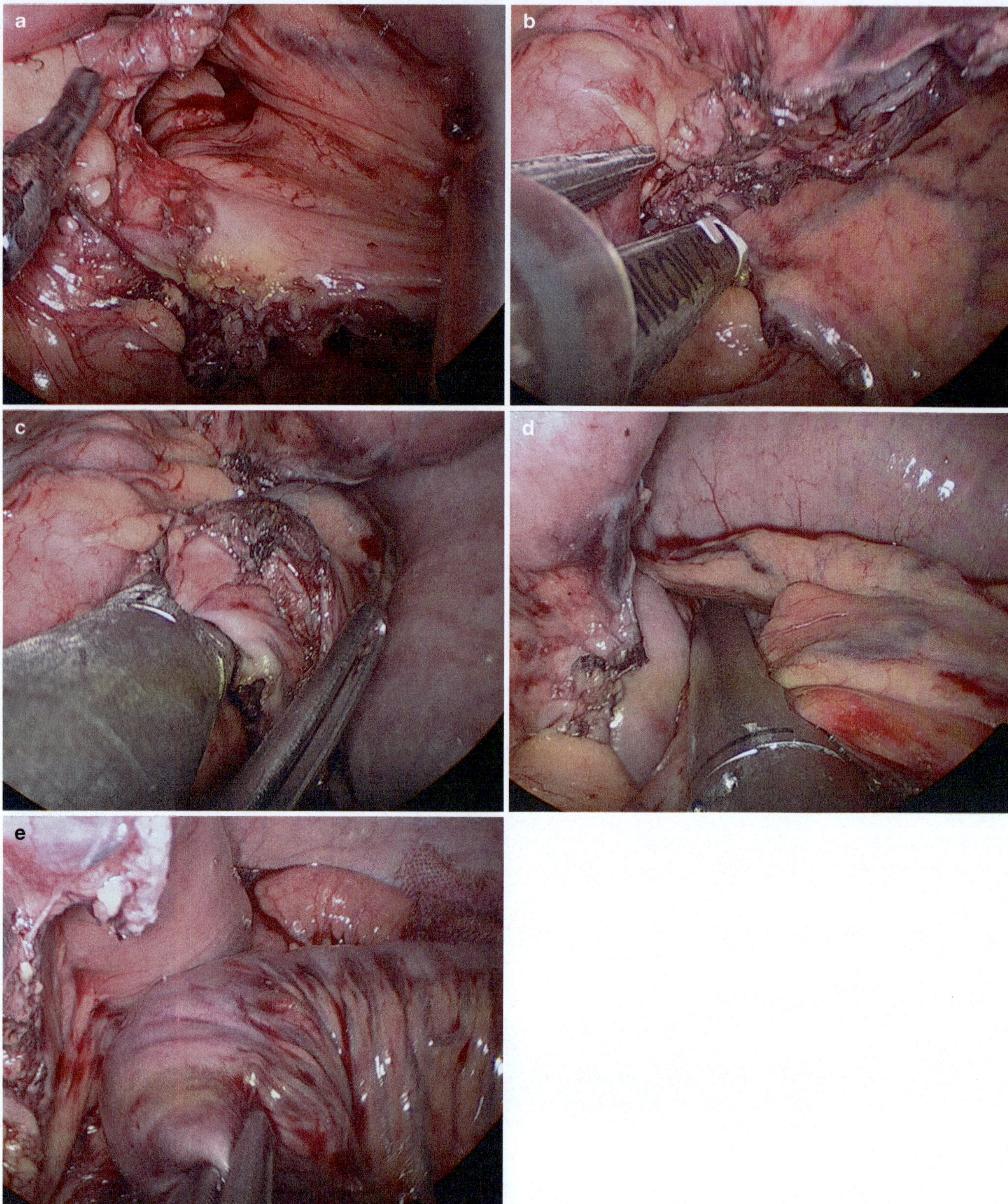

Fig. 12.15

4. Anastomosis of jejunum
   The proximal and distal jejunum were extracted out of the abdominal cavity and the anastomosis was performed extracorporeally. Then the jejunum was returned to the abdominal cavity (Fig. 12.16a–c).

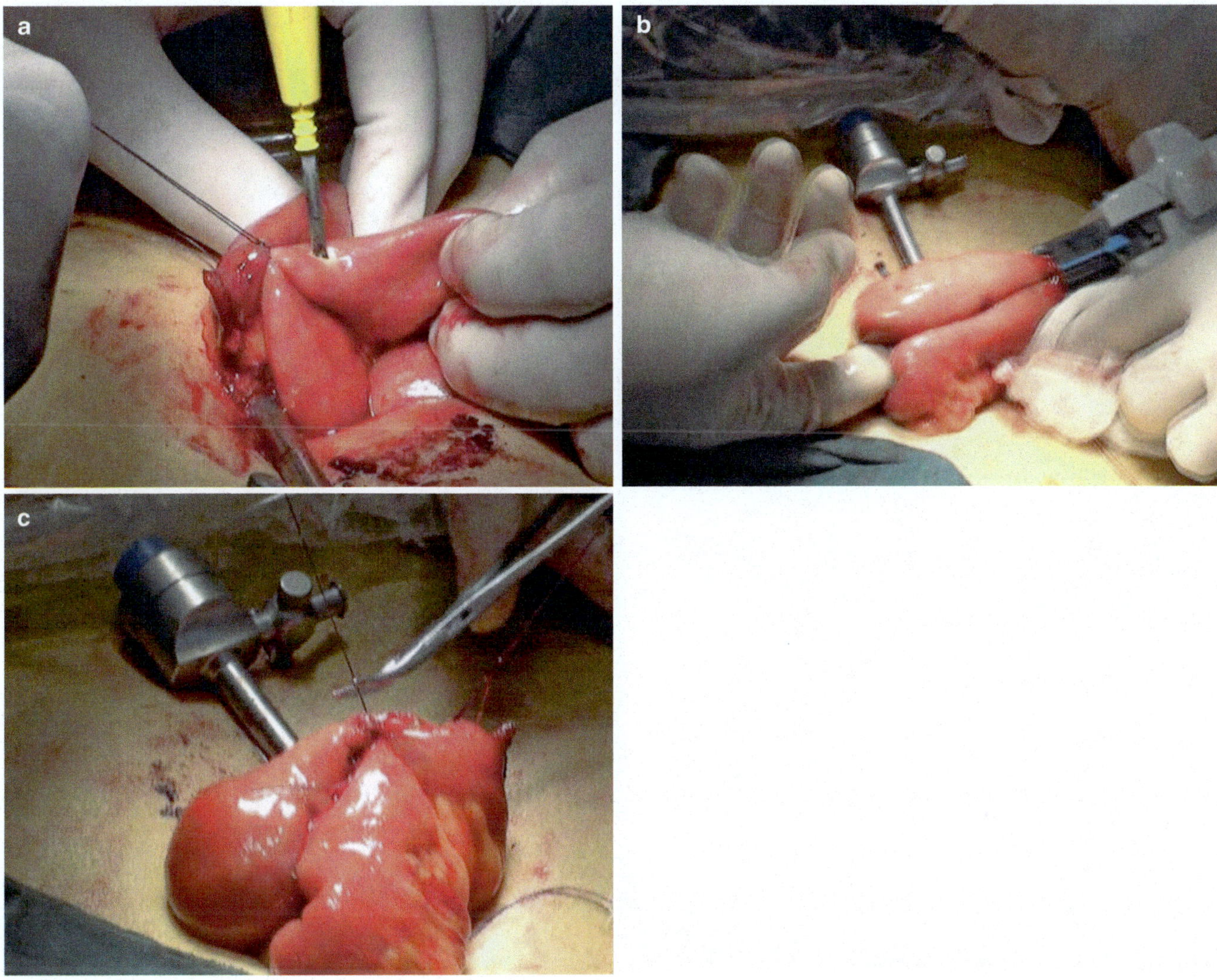

Fig. 12.16

The abdominal cavity was irrigated and the anastomosis was checked carefully. The drainage was placed (Fig. 12.17a–d).

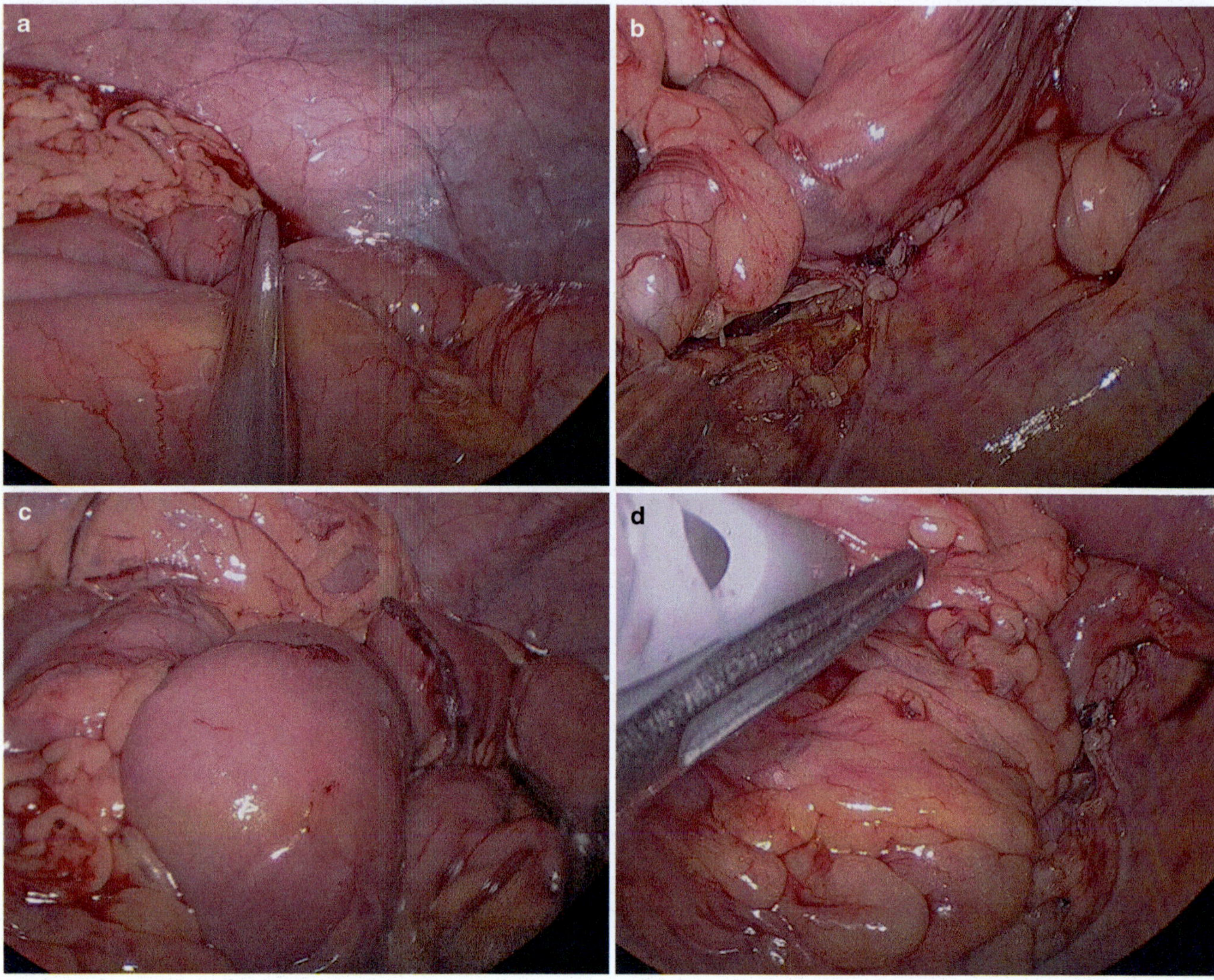

Fig. 12.17

5. Jejunum pharyngoplasty
   The segment of jejunum was repaired extracorporeally and the anastomosis was performed by the ENT doctor. The blood vessel was anastomosed by microsurgeon. The color and peristalsis of the jejunum was checked (Fig. 12.18a–f).

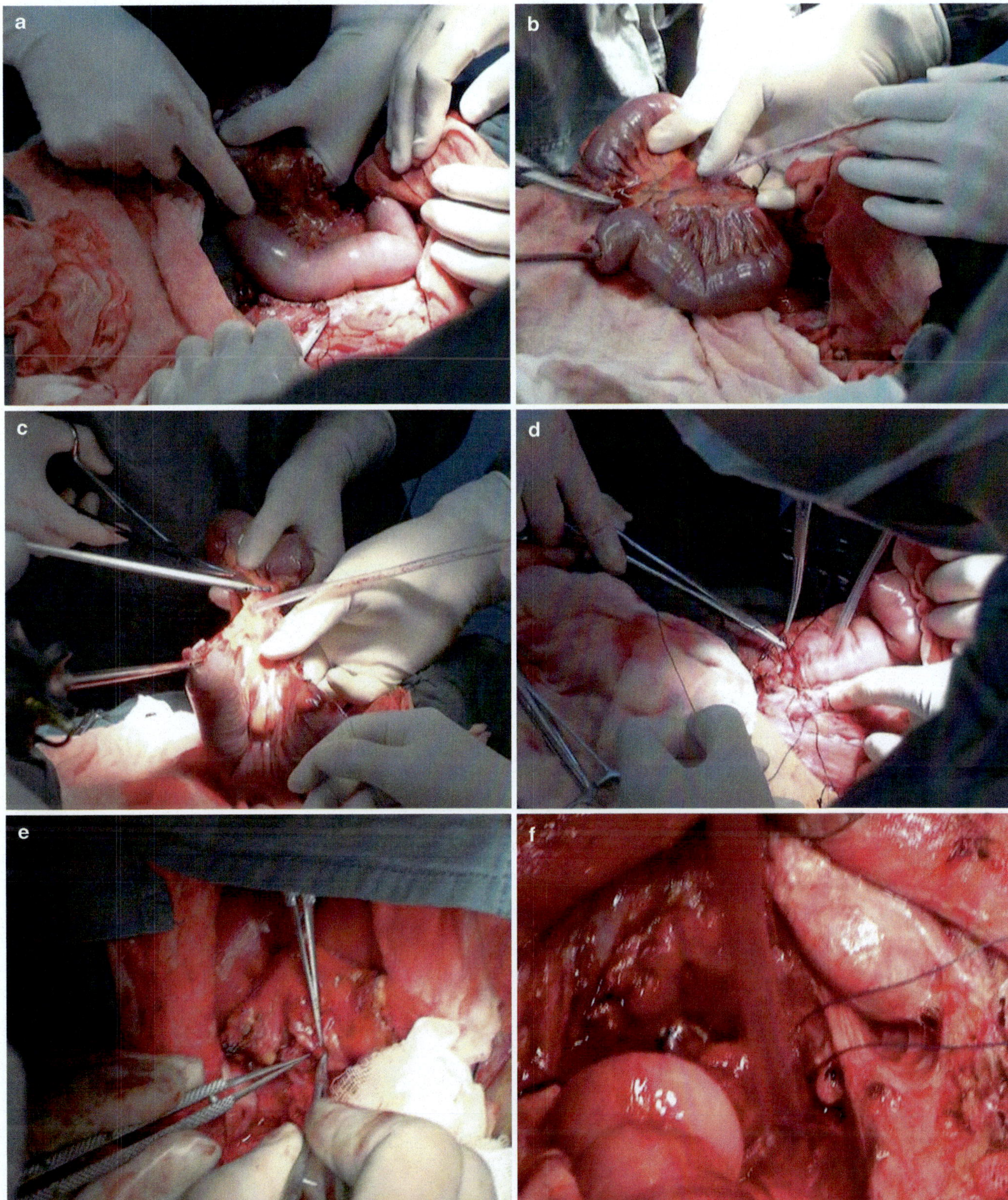

Fig. 12.18

12.2.5 Complications Analysis and Management

In the procedure of jejunum pharyngoplasty, SILS plays the role of resection of jejunum for repair. Haemorrhage, jejunal anastomotic leakage and internal hernia are possible complications. Hemostasis should be thorough. After side-to-side anastomosis, the residual hole for stapler must be carefully sutured. Closing the mesenteric gap of removal jejunum may prevent the formation of internal hernia.

12.3 Laparoscopic Sigmoid Colon Vaginoplasty

12.3.1 Major Instruments or Energy Sources

1. Laparoscopy System
2. Harmonic scalpel
3. Ligasure

12.3.2 Team Setup, Anesthesia and Position

The patient was positioned lithotomy under general anesthesia. The position of surgeon and assistant is shown in (Fig. 12.19).

12.3.3 Key Steps

1. Dissection of sigmoid colon
2. Isolation of the segment of sigmoid colon
3. Creation of the perineal incision
4. Creation of the pelvic incision
5. The anastomosis of the rectum and the sigmoid colon
6. Security of isolated segment of sigmoid colon and fixation of the neovagina
7. Irrigation and drainage

Fig. 12.19

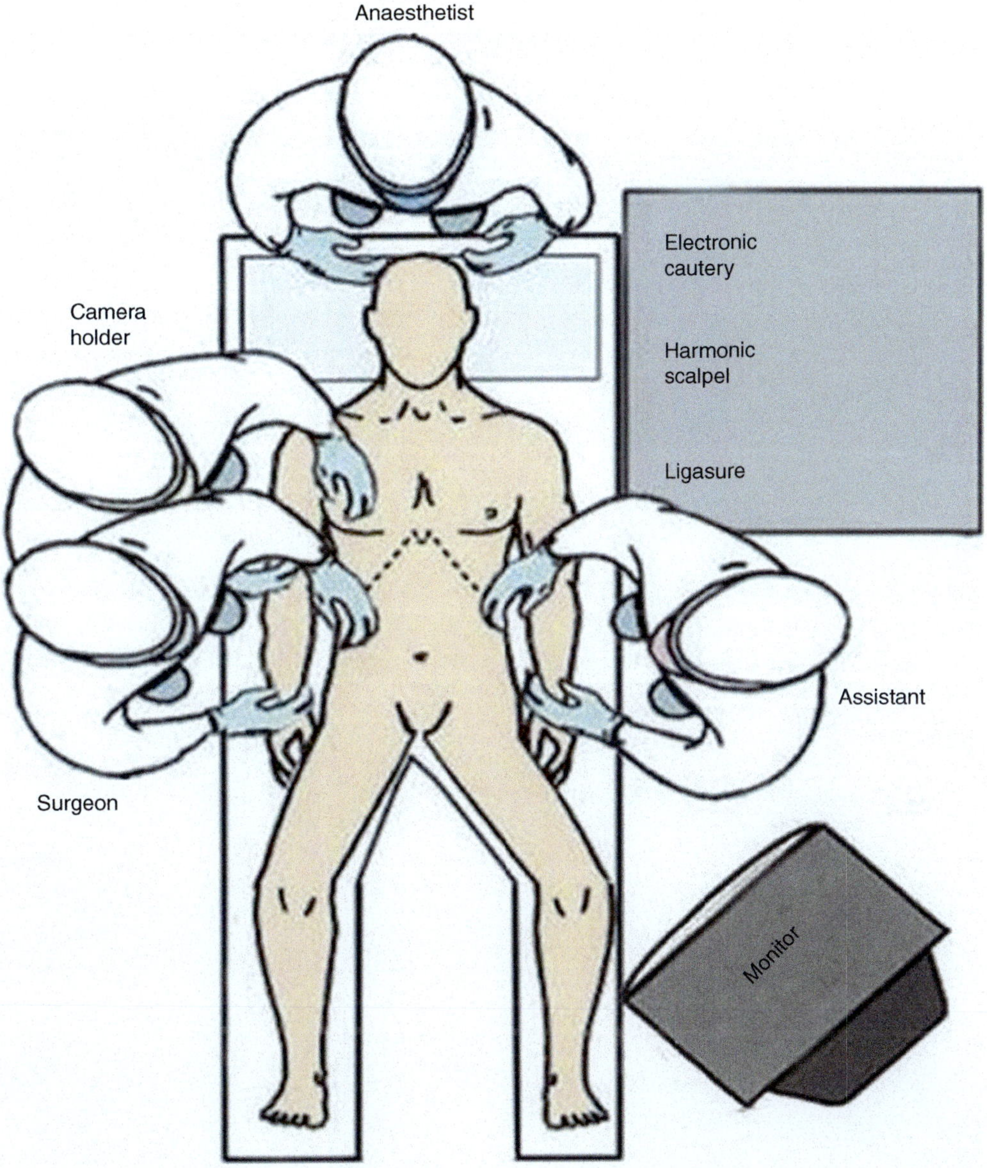

12.3.4 Surgical Techniques

1. Dissection of sigmoid colon
   The noninvasive forceps and Harmonic scalpel were inserted through the umbilical incision. The sigmoid colon was retracted to expose the mesocolon. Fifteen to 20 cm segment of sigmoid colon was mobilized with its vascular pedicle (Fig. 12.20a–f).

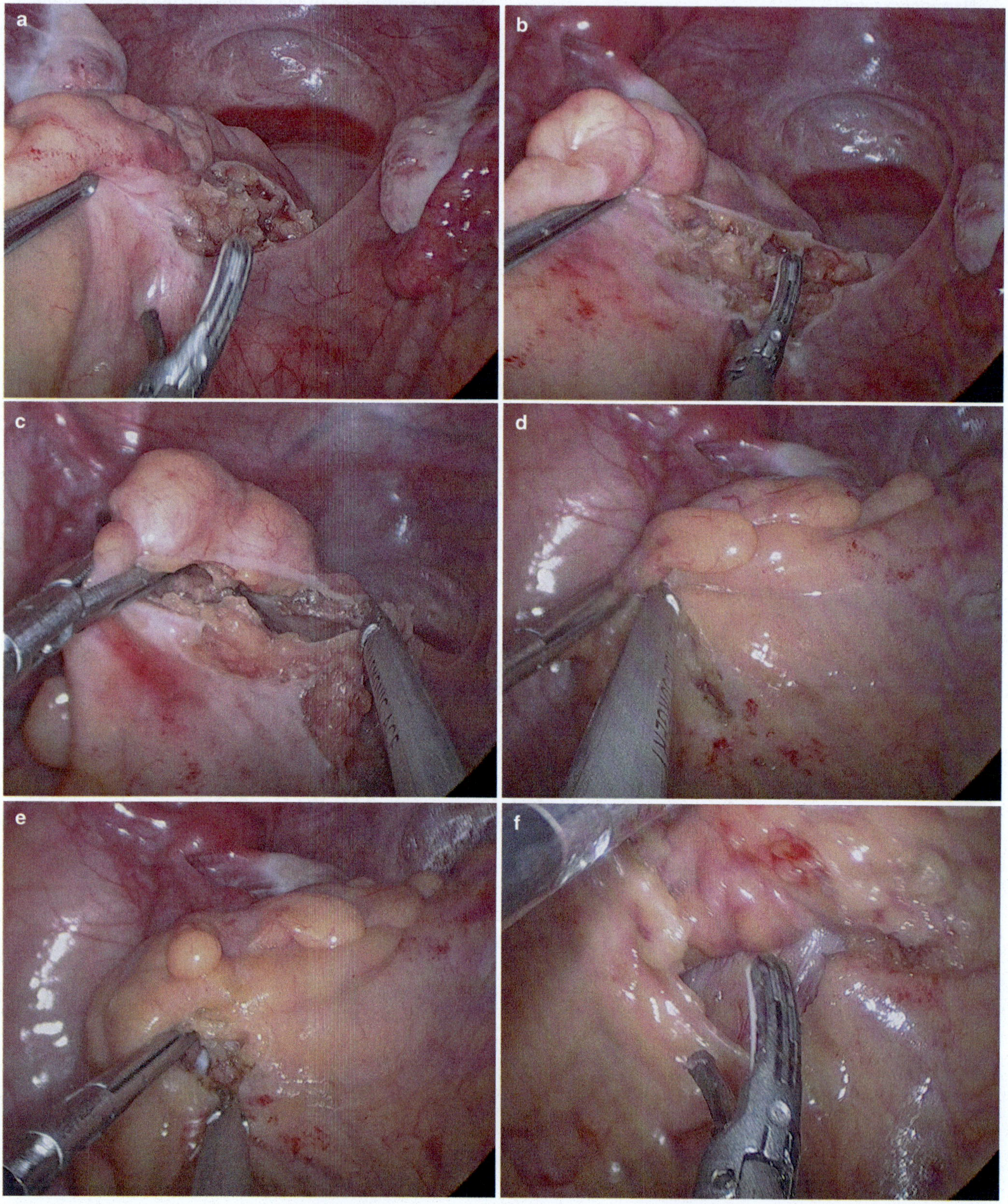

Fig. 12.20

2. Isolation of the segment of sigmoid colon
   The isolated segment of sigmoid colon was created by transecting the colon using the endoscopic linear cutter. The distal end of the sigmoid colon was located around 3 cm away from the peritoneal reflection. The blood supply was checked to guarantee the survival of the sigmoid colon (Fig. 12.21a–j).

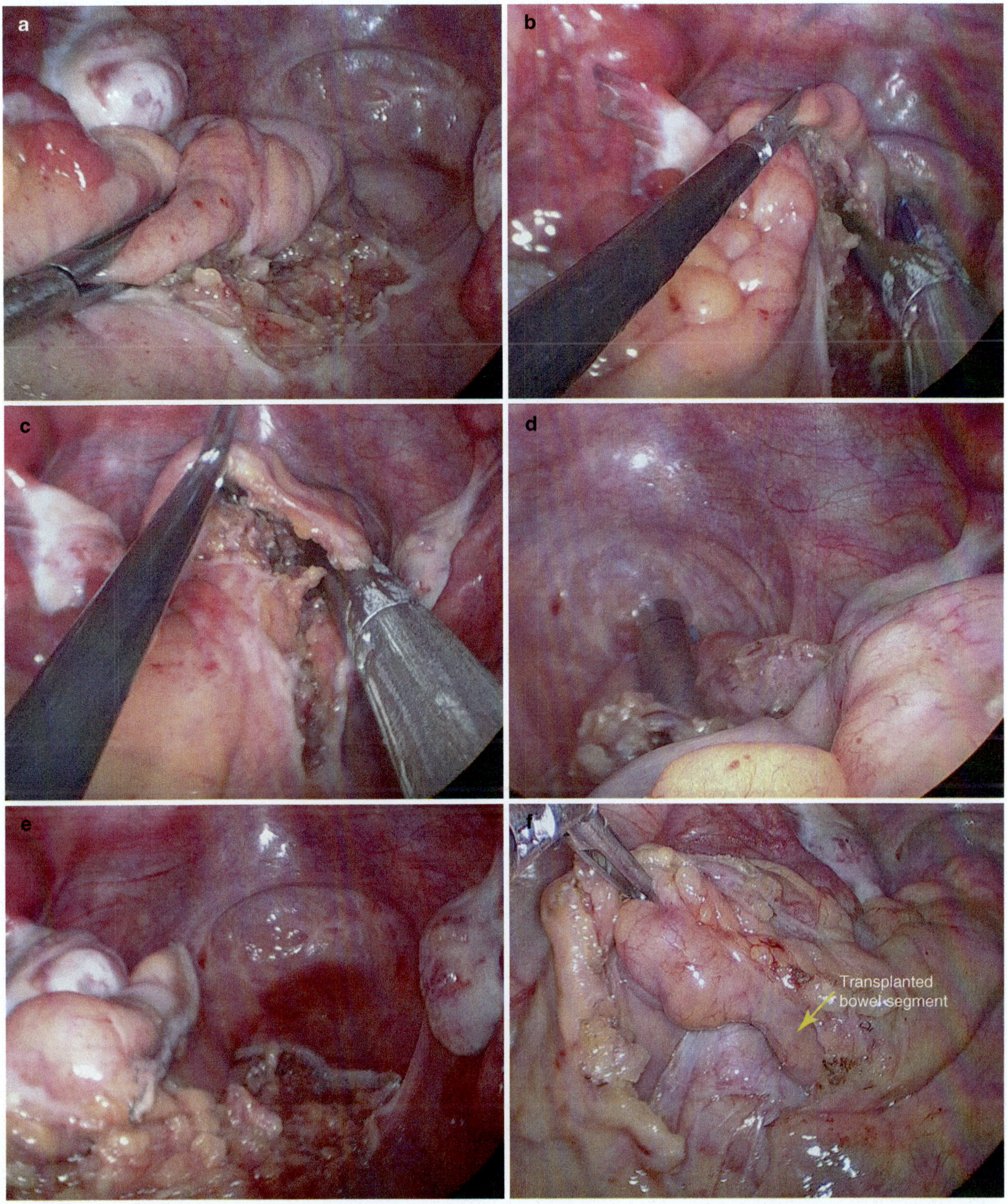

Fig. 12.21

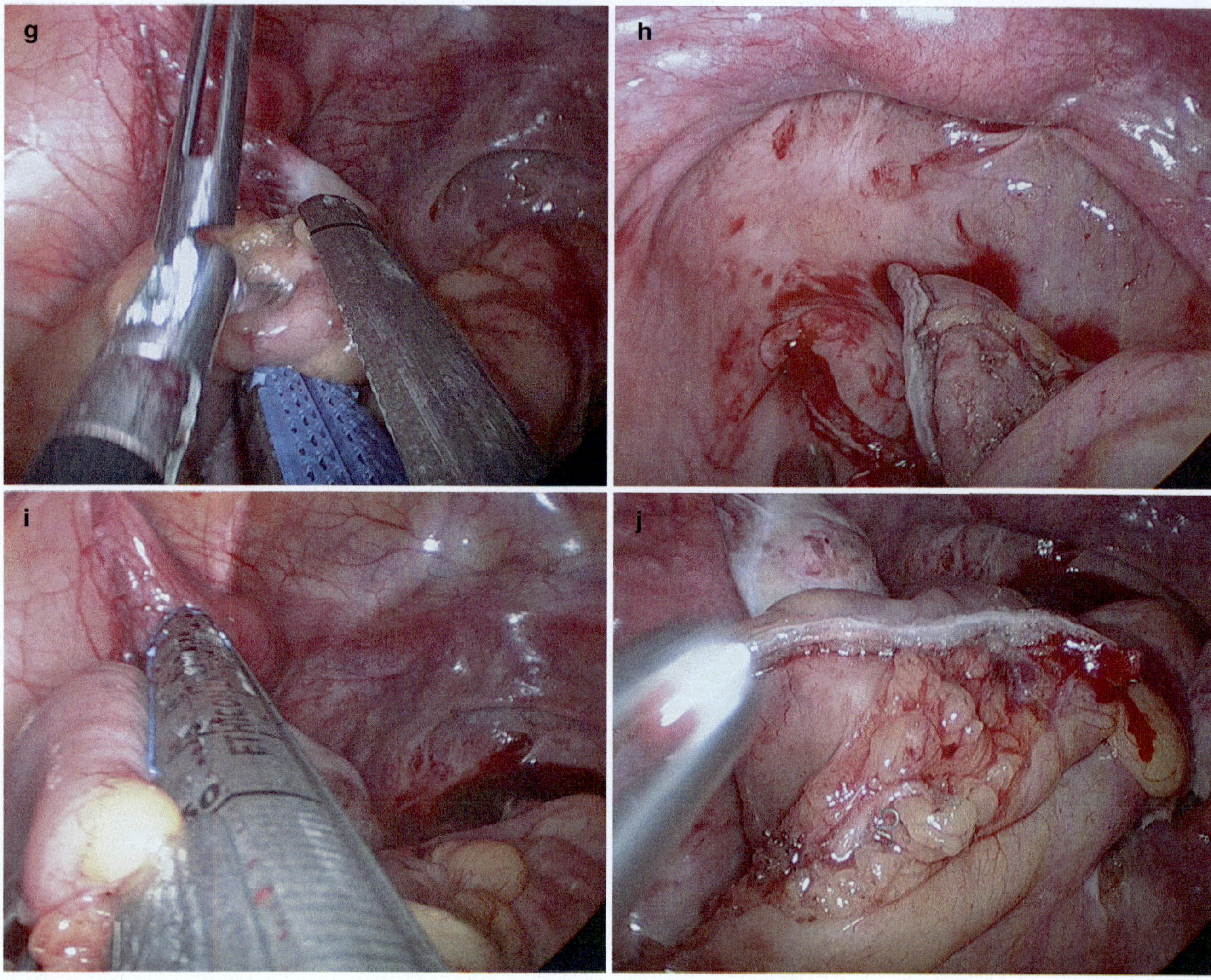

Fig. 12.21 (continued)

3. Creation of perineal incision
   The U shape incision was made under the external orifice of urethra. The tunnel was built and extended to three fingers wide so that the segment of sigmoid colon could be extracted through the incision (Fig. 12.22a, b).

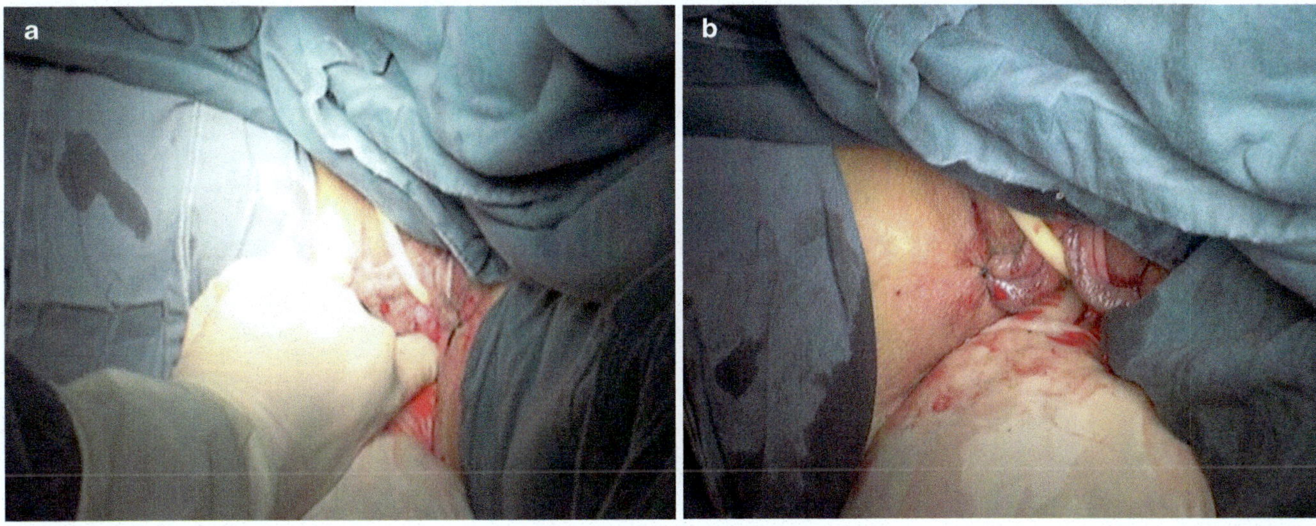

Fig. 12.22

4. Creation of pelvic incision

A 3 cm incision was made on the pelvic peritoneum between the anterior wall of rectum and posterior wall of bladder. Then the incision was extended to reach the perineal incision (Fig. 12.23a–h).

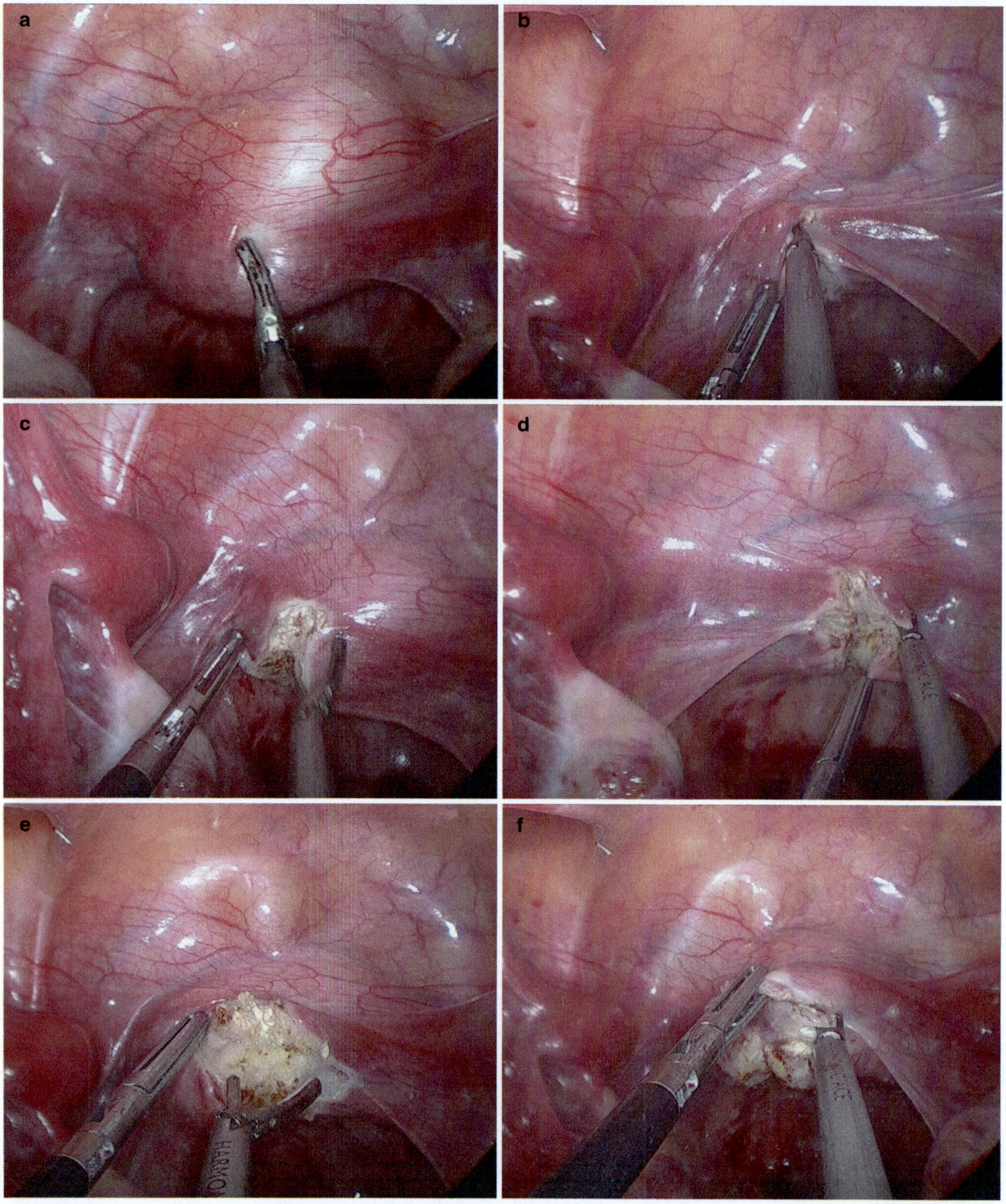

Fig. 12.23

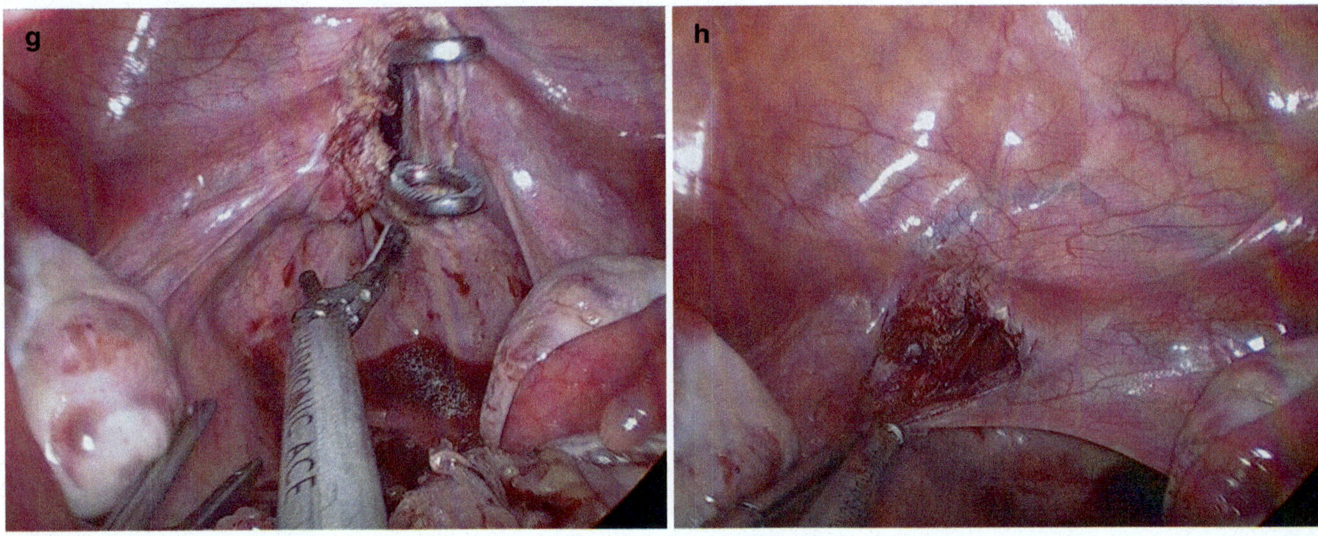

Fig. 12.23 (continued)

5. Anastomosis of proximal sigmoid colon and rectum
   The proximal colon was extracted from the tunnel. The head of the stapler was inserted and secured. Then the colon was returned to the abdominal cavity. The stapler was inserted through the anus. The anastomosis between the colon and the rectum was performed (Fig. 12.24a–z).

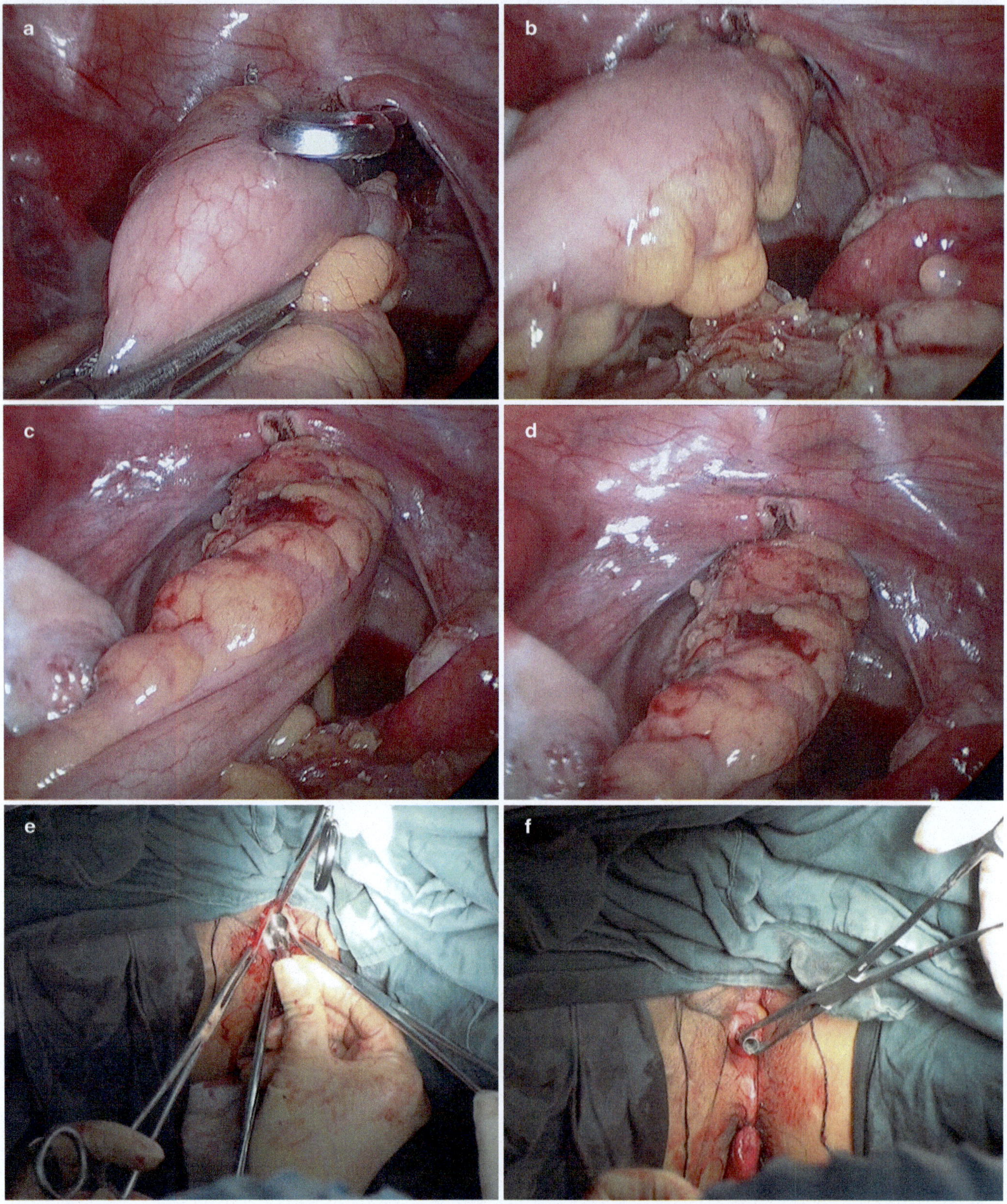

Fig. 12.24

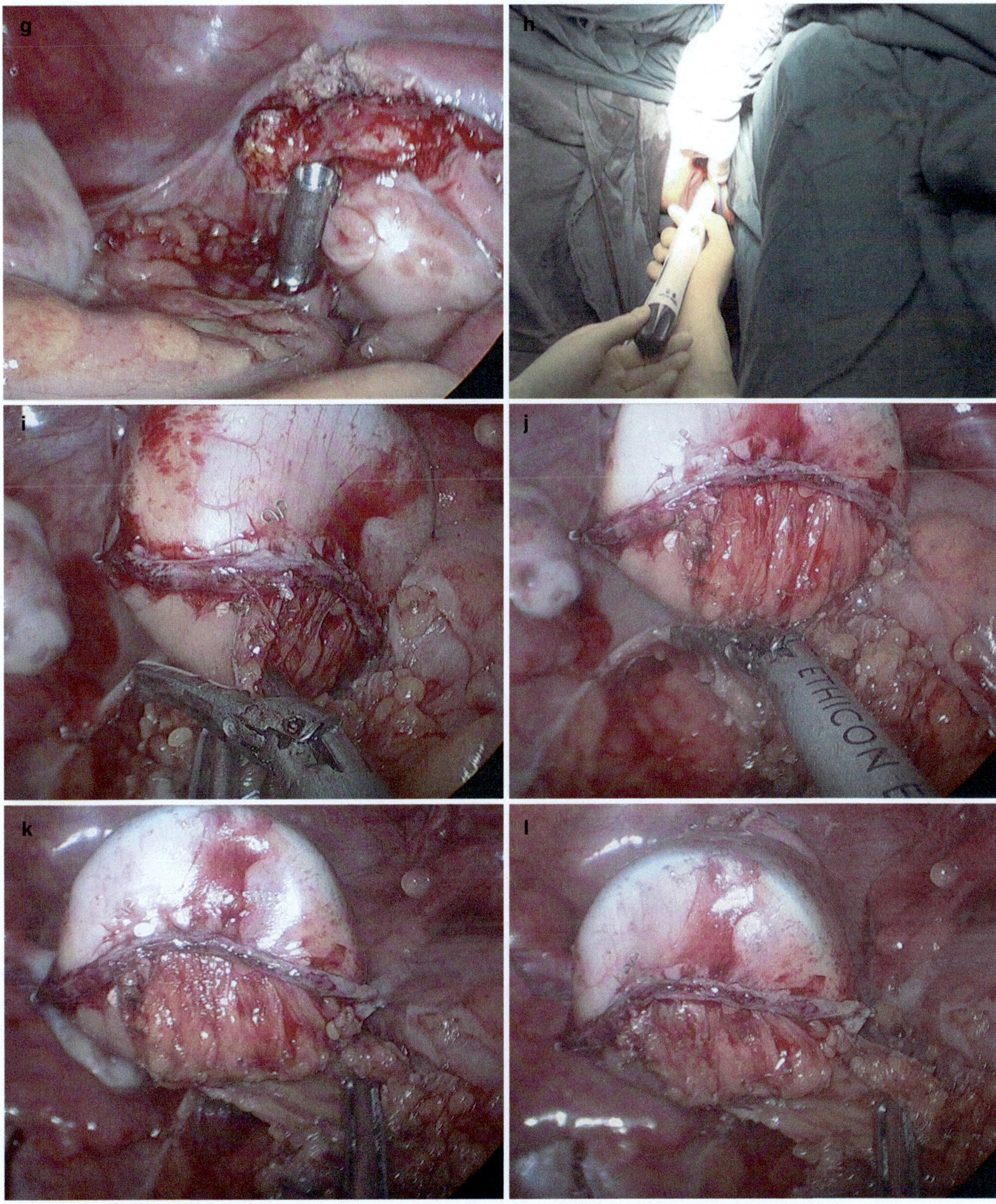

Fig. 12.24 (continued)

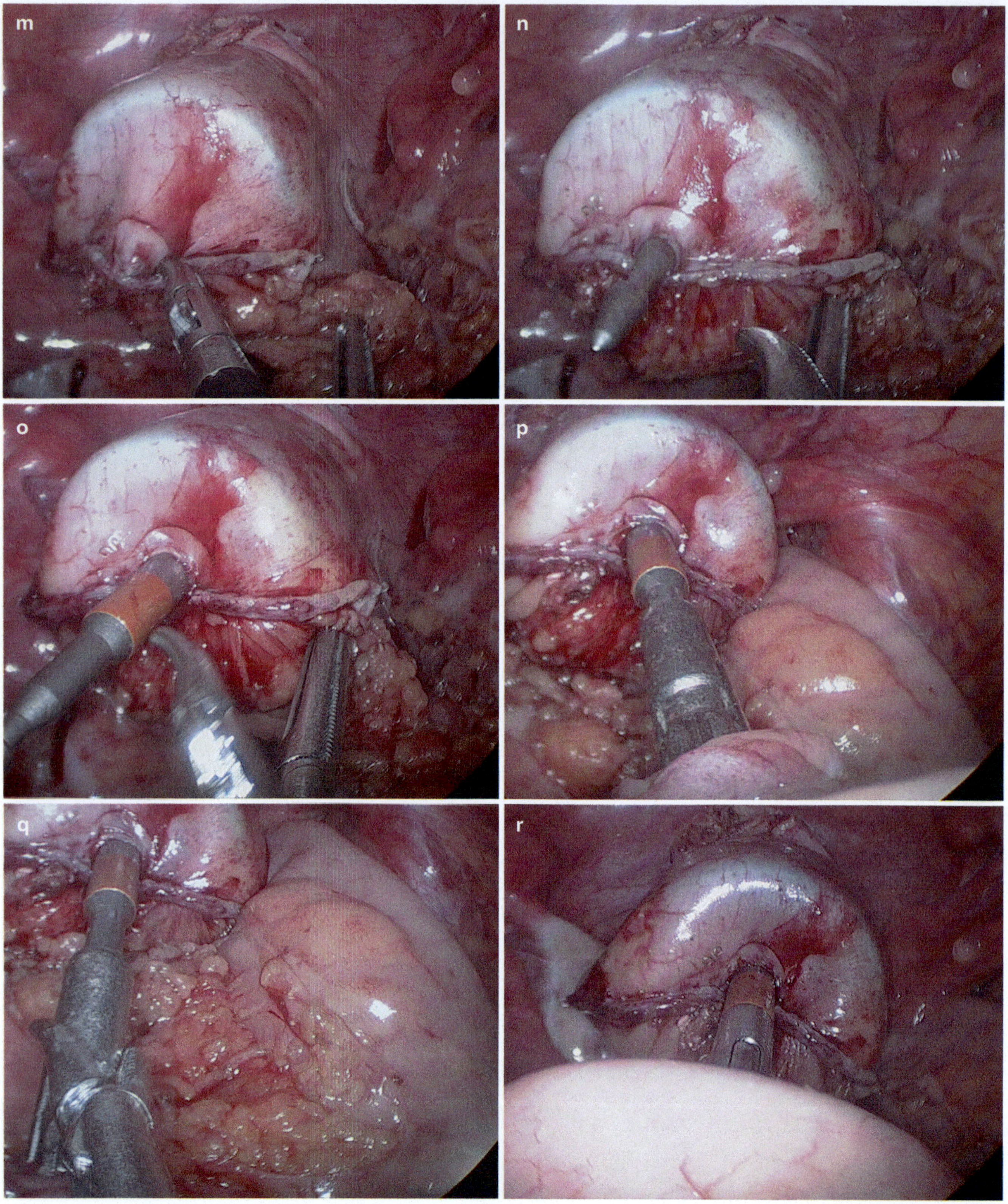

Fig. 12.24 (continued)

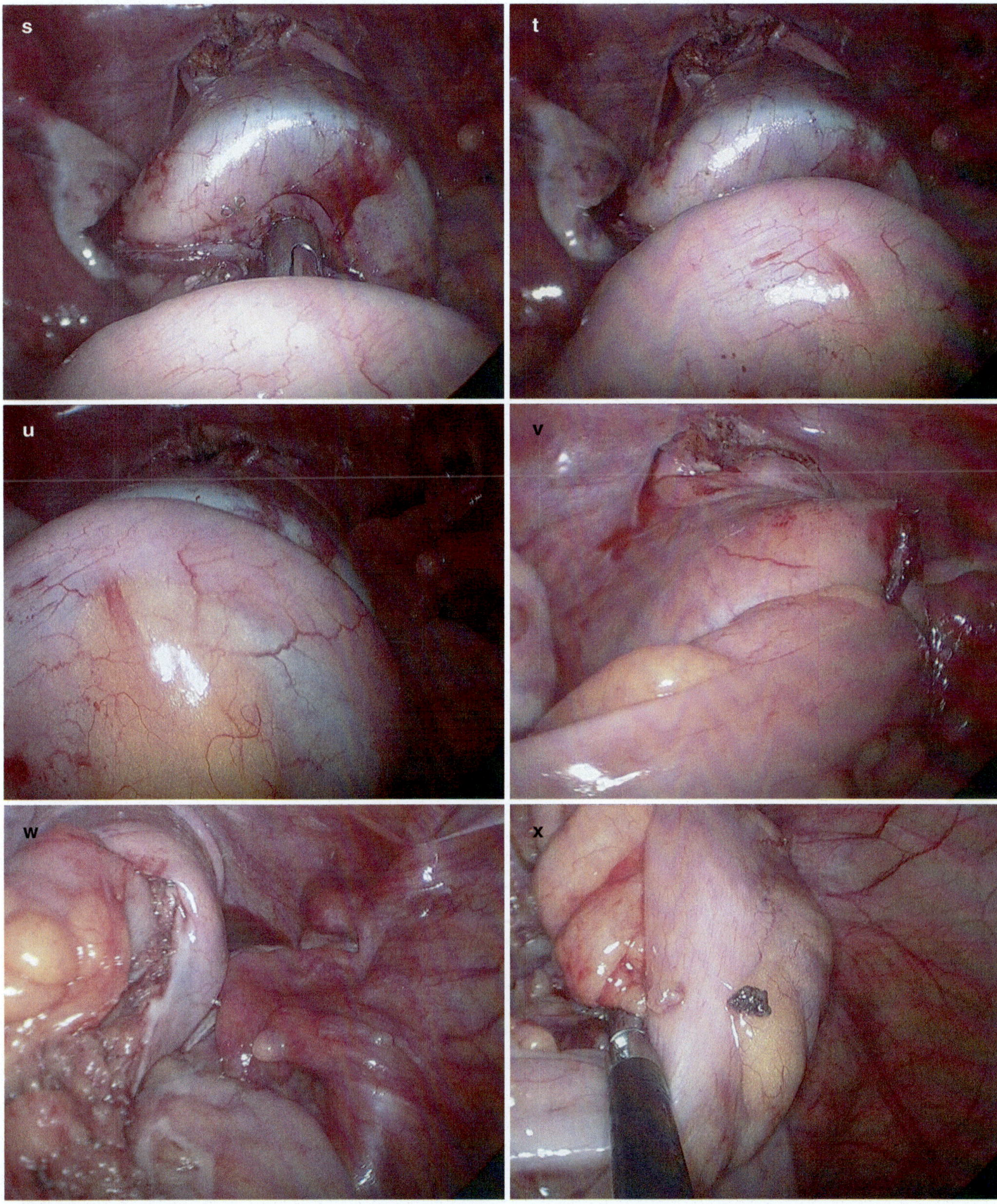

Fig. 12.24 (continued)

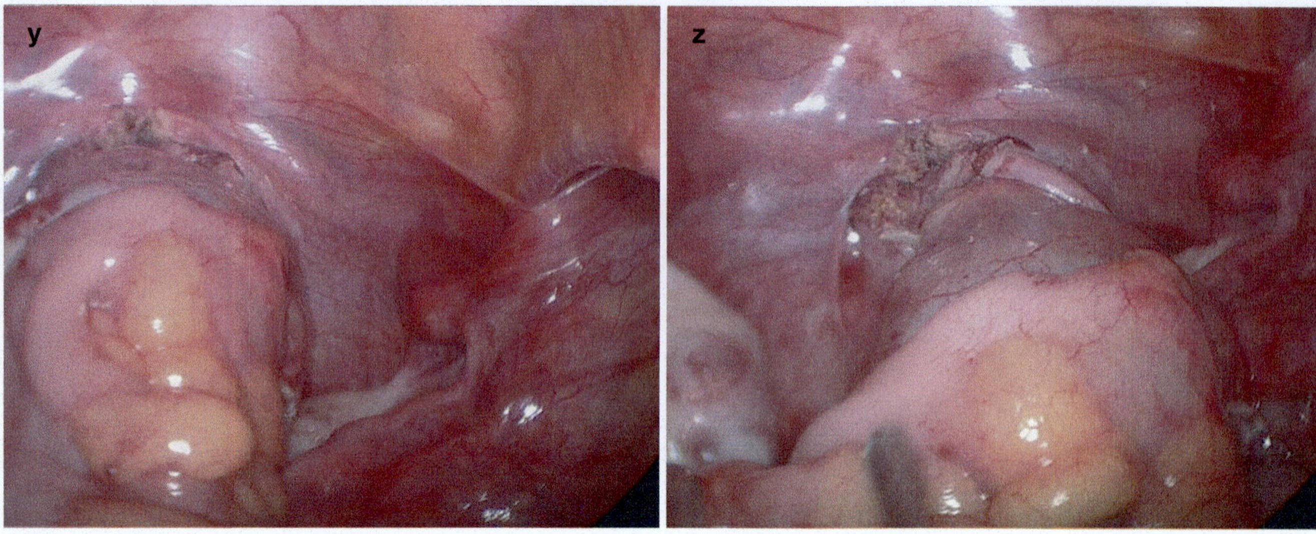

Fig. 12.24 (continued)

6. Security of isolated segment of sigmoid colon

   The isolated sigmoid colon was extracted out of the abdominal cavity through the man-made tunnel. The distal end of the isolated sigmoid colon was opened and the margin was sutured around the perineal incision. The segment of sigmoid colon was sutured and secured by suturing to the pelvic peritoneum to create the neovagina (Fig. 12.25a–p).

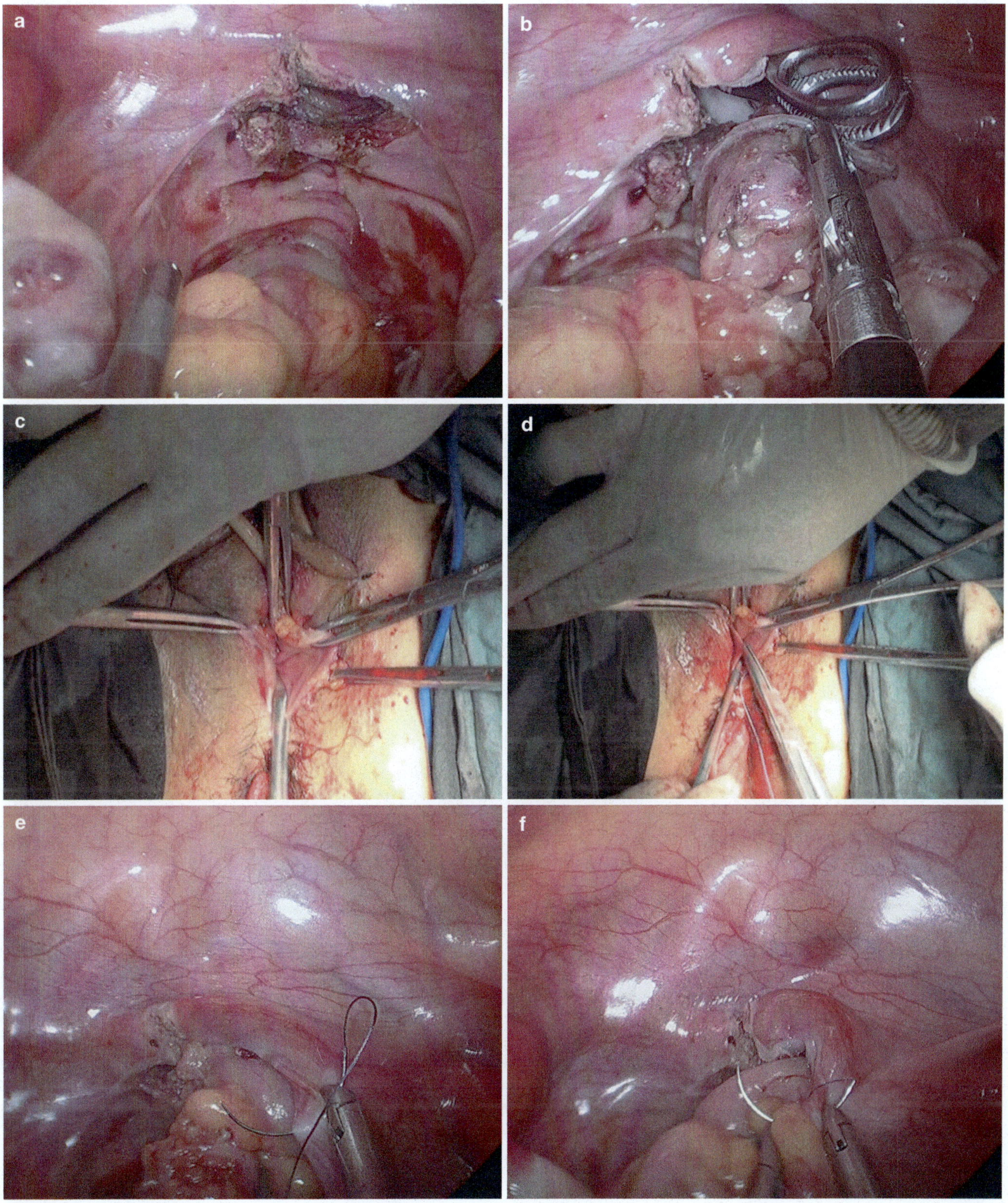

Fig. 12.25

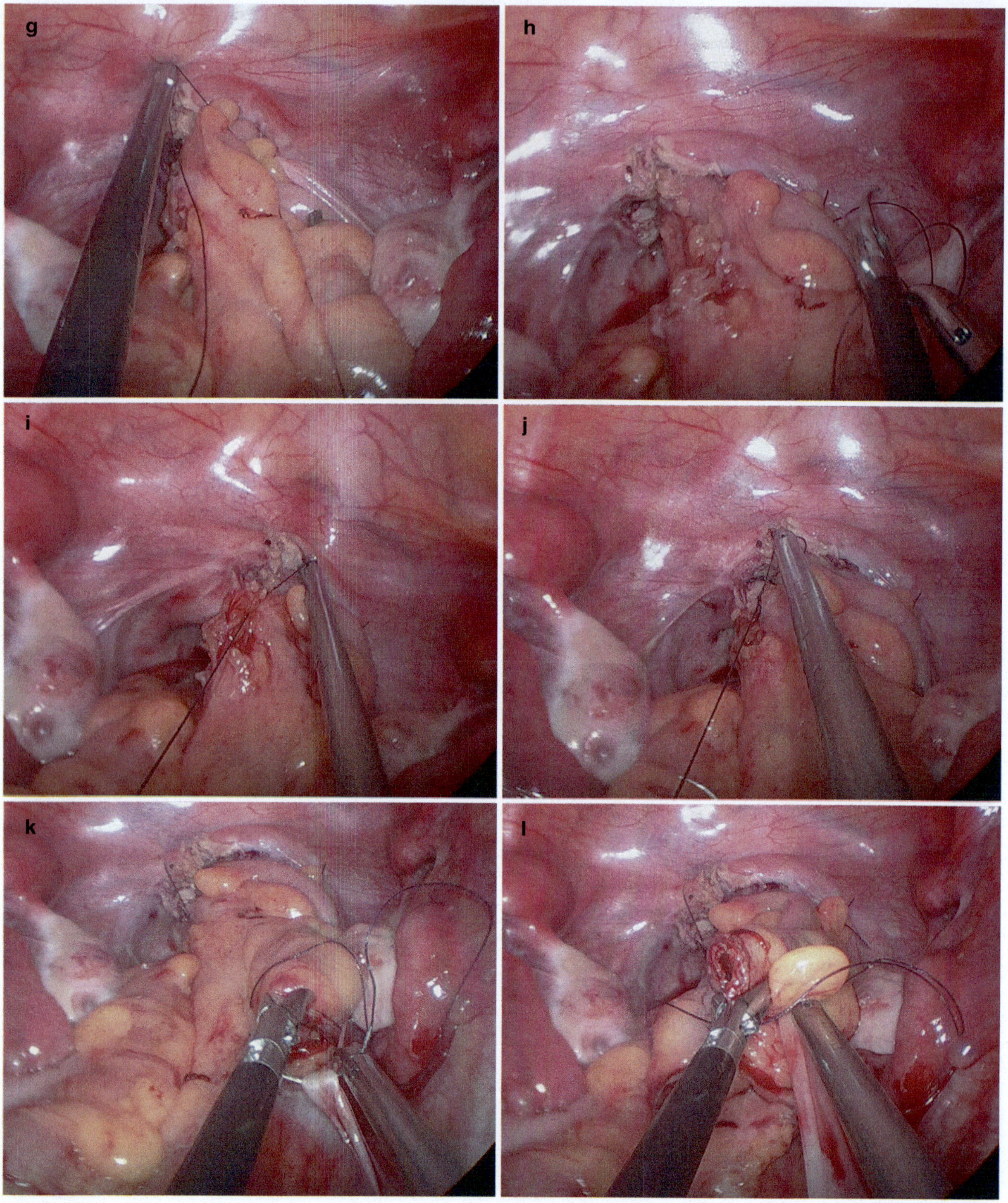

Fig. 12.25 (continued)

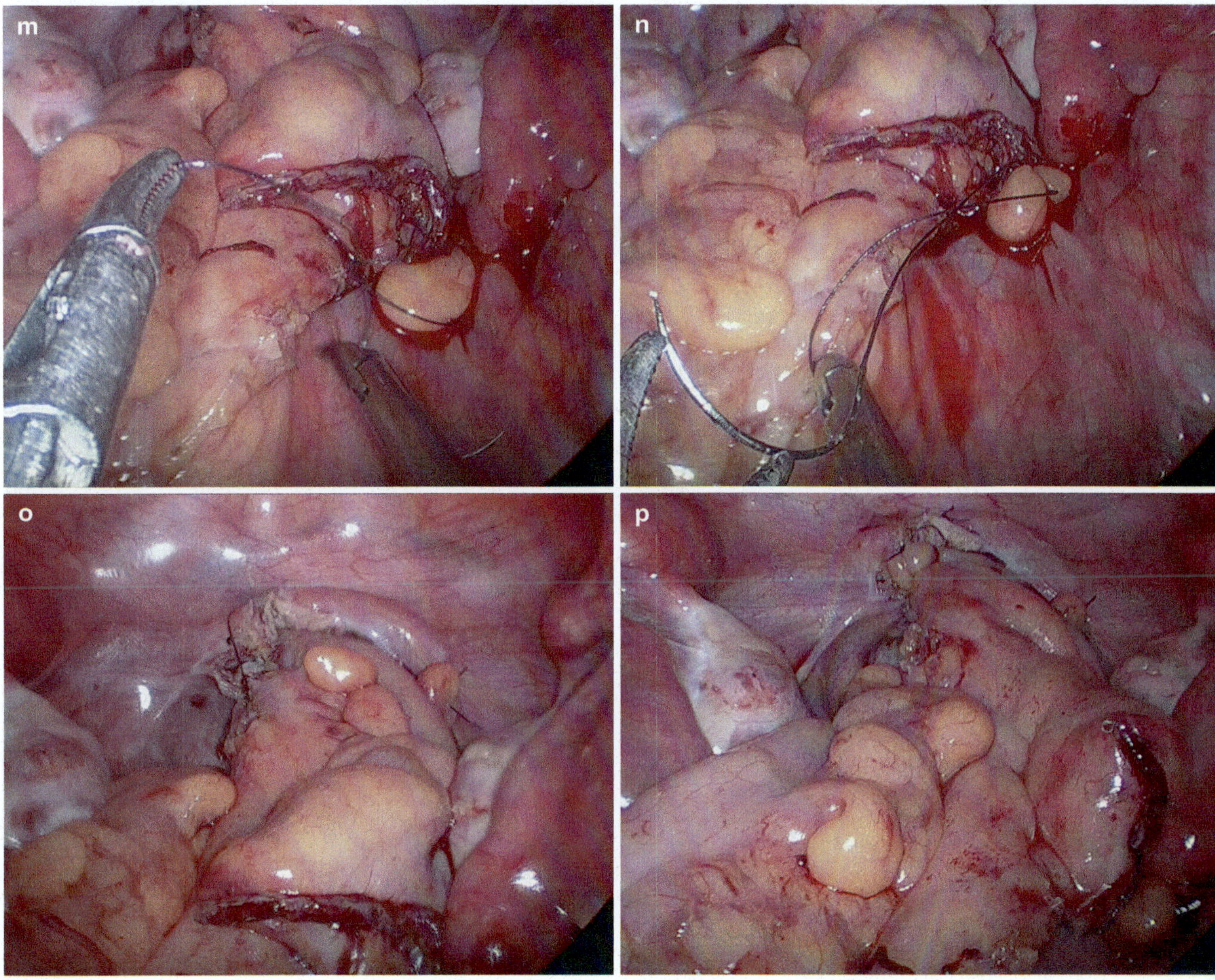

Fig. 12.25 (continued)

7. Irrigation and drainage
   The drainage was placed around the anastomosis and put out through the umbilical incision (Fig. 12.26a, b).

12.3.5 Complications Analysis and Management

In the procedure of laparoscopic sigmoid colon vaginoplasty, SILS plays the role of resection of sigmoid colon for repair. It is similar to SILS colorectal surgery; haemorrhage, anastomotic leakage and left ureteral injury are possible complications. Thorough hemostasis, avoiding violent operation, definite suture of residual hole for stapler and the anatomic level are effect methods to prevent these complications.

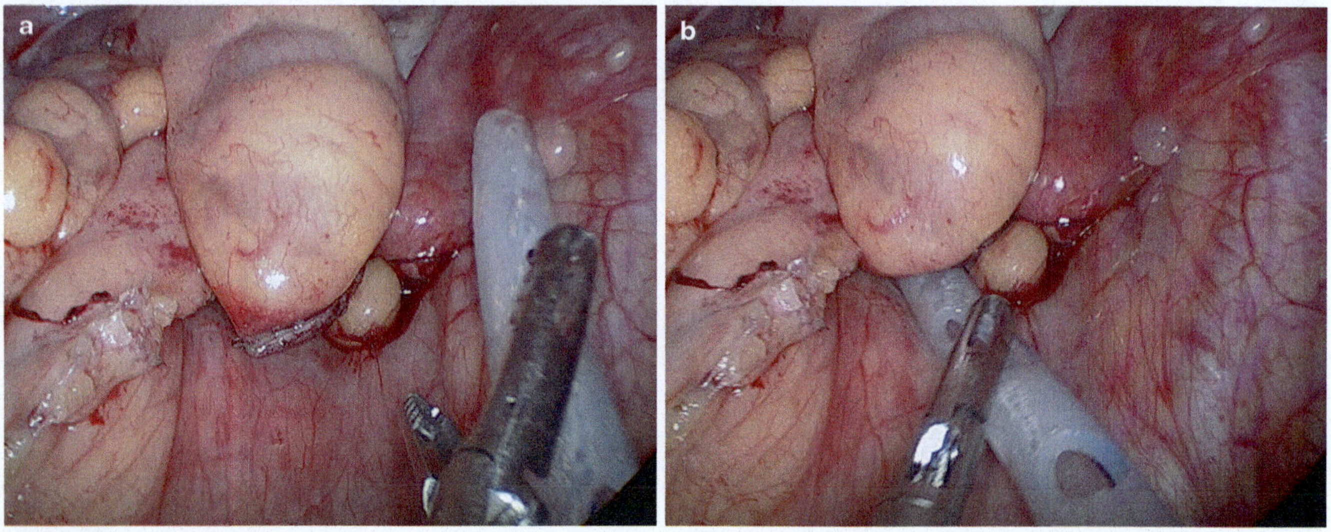

Fig. 12.26

NOTES: Transvaginal Endoscopic Appendectomy

13

Abstract

Natural orifice transluminal endoscopic surgery (NOTES) (Halim and Tavakkolizadeh, Int J Surg 6:273–276, 2008) is an surgical technique whereby "scarless" abdominal operations can be performed with an endoscope passed through a natural orifice (mouth, urethra, anus, etc.) then through an internal incision in the stomach, vagina, bladder (Lima et al., J Urol 176:802–805, 2006) or colon, thus avoiding any external incisions or scars (Baron, Br J Surg 94:1–2, 2007).

This technique has been used for diagnostic and therapeutic procedures in animal models, including transgastric (through the stomach) organ removal. Most recently, the transvesical and the transcolonic approaches have been advocated by some researchers as being more suited to access upper abdominal structures that are often more difficult to work with using a transgastric approach (Fong et al., Gastrointest Endosc 65:312–318, 2007; Pai et al., Gastrointest Endosc 64:428–434, 2006).In this sequence, a group from Portugal used transgastric and transvesical combined approach to increase the feasibility of moderately complex procedures such as cholecystectomy (Rolanda et al., Gastrointest Endosc 65:111–117, 2007). NOTES was originally described in animals by researchers at Johns Hopkins University (Dr. Anthony Kalloo et al.), and was recently used for transgastric appendectomy in humans in India (by Drs. G.V. Rao and N. Reddy). Auyang ED and colleagues reported human cholecystectomy using hybrid NOTES technique in 2009 (Auyang et al., J Gastrointest Surg 13:1149–1150, 2009). Totally transvaginal cholecystectomy has been described in experimental model without using laparoscopic assistance (Sánchez-Margallo et al., Minim Invasive Ther Allied Technol 17:361–364, 2008). In late 2008, surgeons from Johns Hopkins School of Medicine removed a healthy kidney from a woman donor using NOTES. The surgery was called transvaginal donor kidney extraction (Surgeons remove healthy kidney through vagina. InfoNIAC.com. http://www.infoniac.com/health-fitness/remove-healthy-kidney-through-vagina.html).

The transvaginal access to NOTES seems to be the most safe and feasible for clinical application. In early March 2007, the NOTES Research Group in Rio de Janeiro, Brazil, led by Dr. Ricardo Zorron, performed the first series of transvaginal NOTES cholecystectomy in four patients, based in previous experimental studies. With fewer potential complications, the procedure has a disadvantage of being possible only in women.

Proponents and researchers in this field recognize the potential of this technique to revolutionize the field of minimally invasive surgery by eliminating abdominal incisions. NOTES could be the next major paradigm shift in surgery, just as laparoscopy was the major paradigm shift during the 1980s and 1990s. Potential advantages include lower anesthesia requirements, faster recovery and shorter hospital stays, avoidance of the potential complications of transabdominal wound infections (e.g. hernias), less immunosuppression, better postoperative pulmonary and diaphragmatic function, and the potential for "scarless" abdominal surgery. Critics challenge the safety and advantages of this technique in the face of effective minimally invasive surgical options such as laparoscopic surgery.

Keywords
Natural orifice transluminal endoscopic surgery (NOTES) • Transvaginal • Appendectomy

13.1 Indications and Case Selection

1. Patients with acute, or chronic appendicitis.
2. Patients with purulent or gangrenous appendicitis.
3. Patients with acute episode of chronic appendicitis.

However, it's more indicated for patients who are obese, suffering from diabetes mellitus, old patients, acatalepsy, patients with much pus, or cosmetic requirements.

13.2 Contraindications

1. Absolute contraindications to performing transvaginal laparoscopic appendectomy include the inability to tolerate general anesthesia or pneumoperitoneum, suspicion of carcinoma, refractory coagulopathy, pregnancy or patients with hesitation for transvaginal surgery.
2. Relative contraindications to performing transvaginal laparoscopic appendectomy include advanced acute appendicitis, periappendical abscess formation, previous abdominal surgery, diffuse peritonitis, chronic obstructive pulmonary disease, morbid obesity.

13.3 Major Instruments or Energy Sources

1. Laparoscopy System
2. Harmonic scalpel
3. Ligasure

13.4 Team Setup, Anesthesia and Position

The patient was positioned lithotomy under general anesthesia. After the resection of vagina due to the gynaecologic disease, the general surgeon performed the transvaginal laparoscopic appendectomy. A 10 mm trocar and two 5 mm trocars was inserted through the orifice and the end of vagina. The three trocars were placed into a shape of inverted triangle. The pneumoperitoneum was up to 13 mmHg (Fig. 13.1a–c).

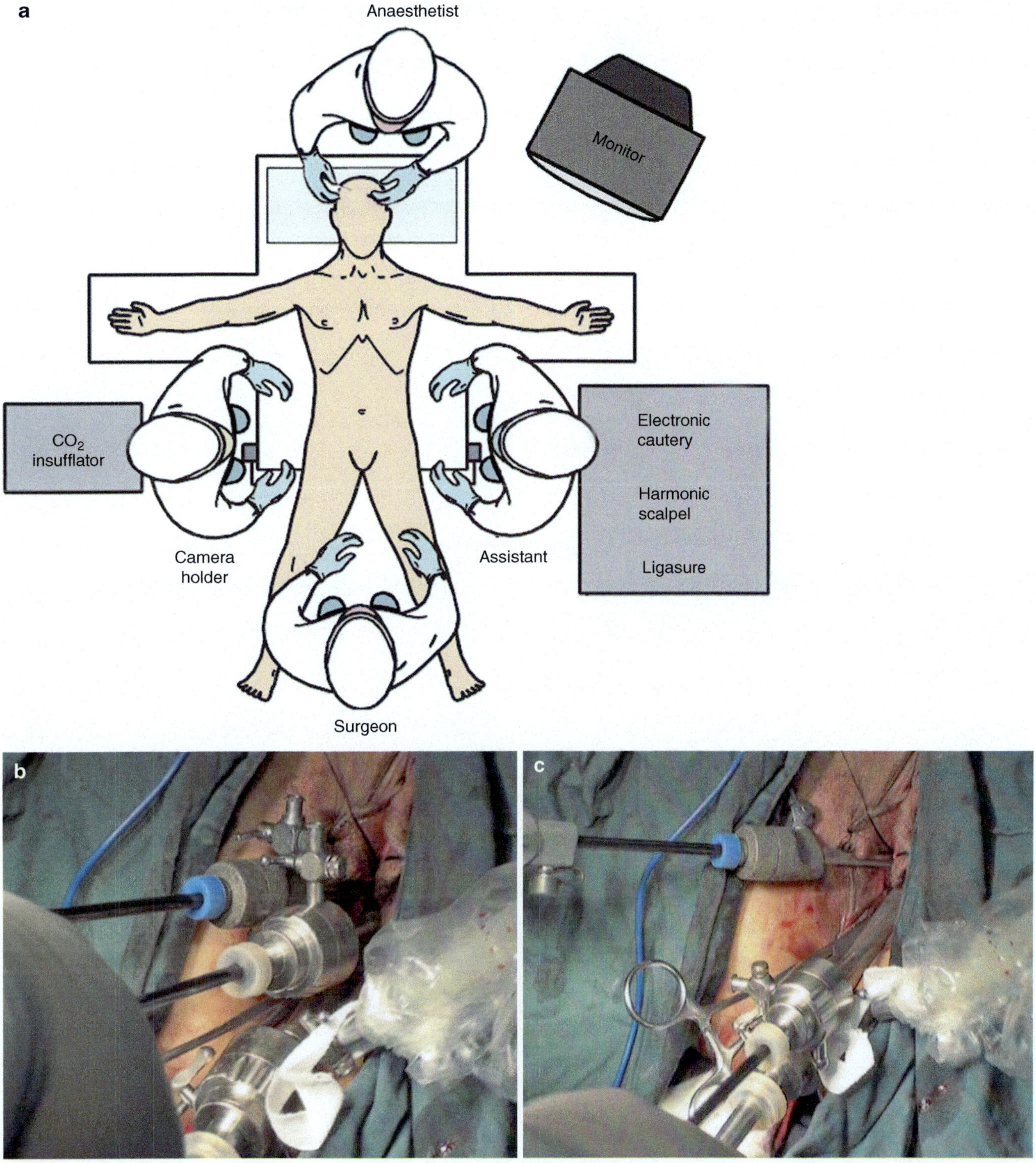
a
Anaesthetist
Monitor
CO_2 insufflator
Electronic cautery
Harmonic scalpel
Ligasure
Camera holder
Assistant
Surgeon
b
c

Fig. 13.1

13.5 Key Steps

1. Division of the mesoappendix
2. Closure of the root of appendix and resection of appendix
3. Retrieve of appendix from vagina
4. Closure of the end of vagina

13.6 Surgical Techniques

1. Abdominal exploration and division of the mesoappendix
   The abdominal cavity was explored and appendix was realized. The appendix was grasped with forceps (Fig. 13.2a–h).

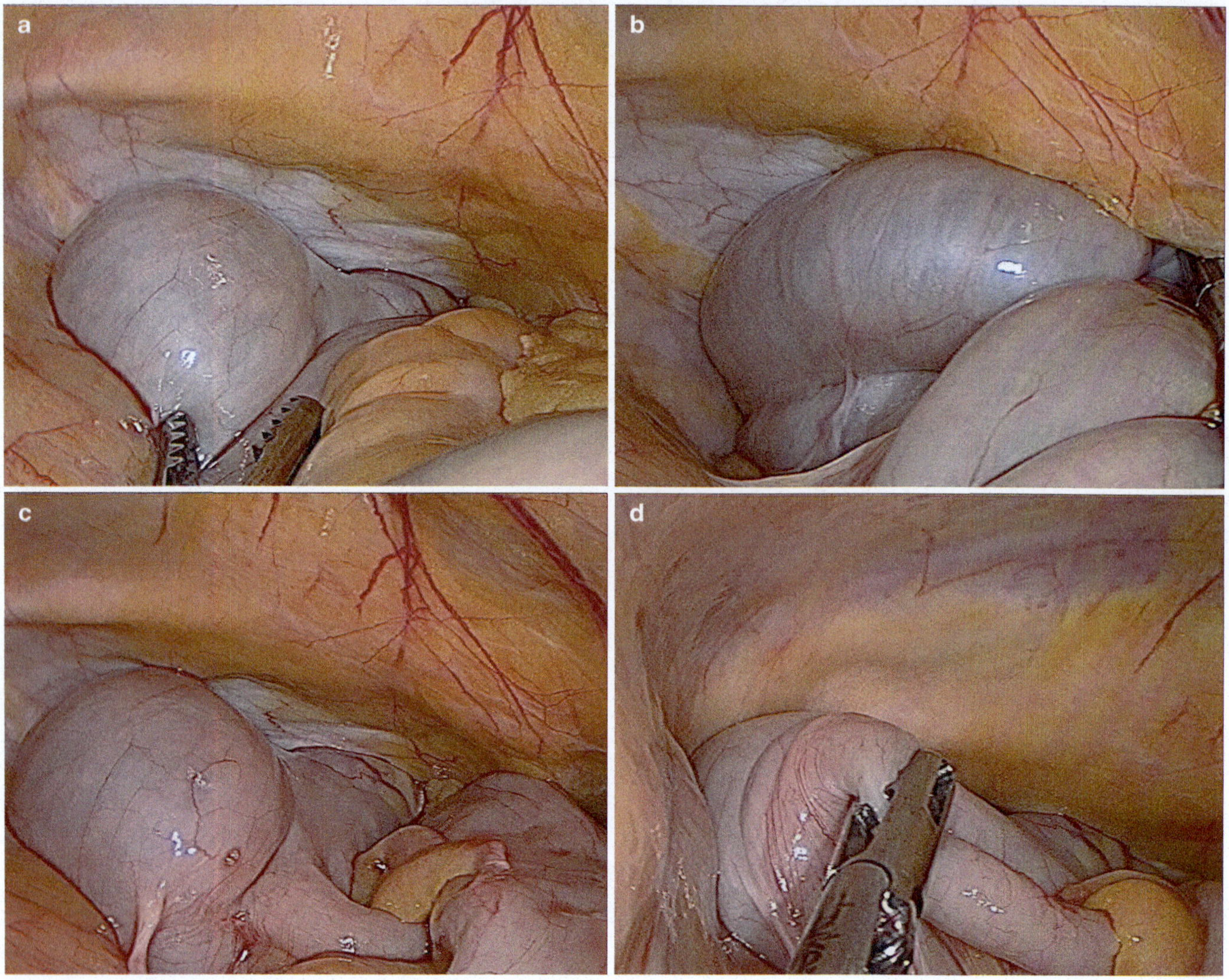

Fig. 13.2

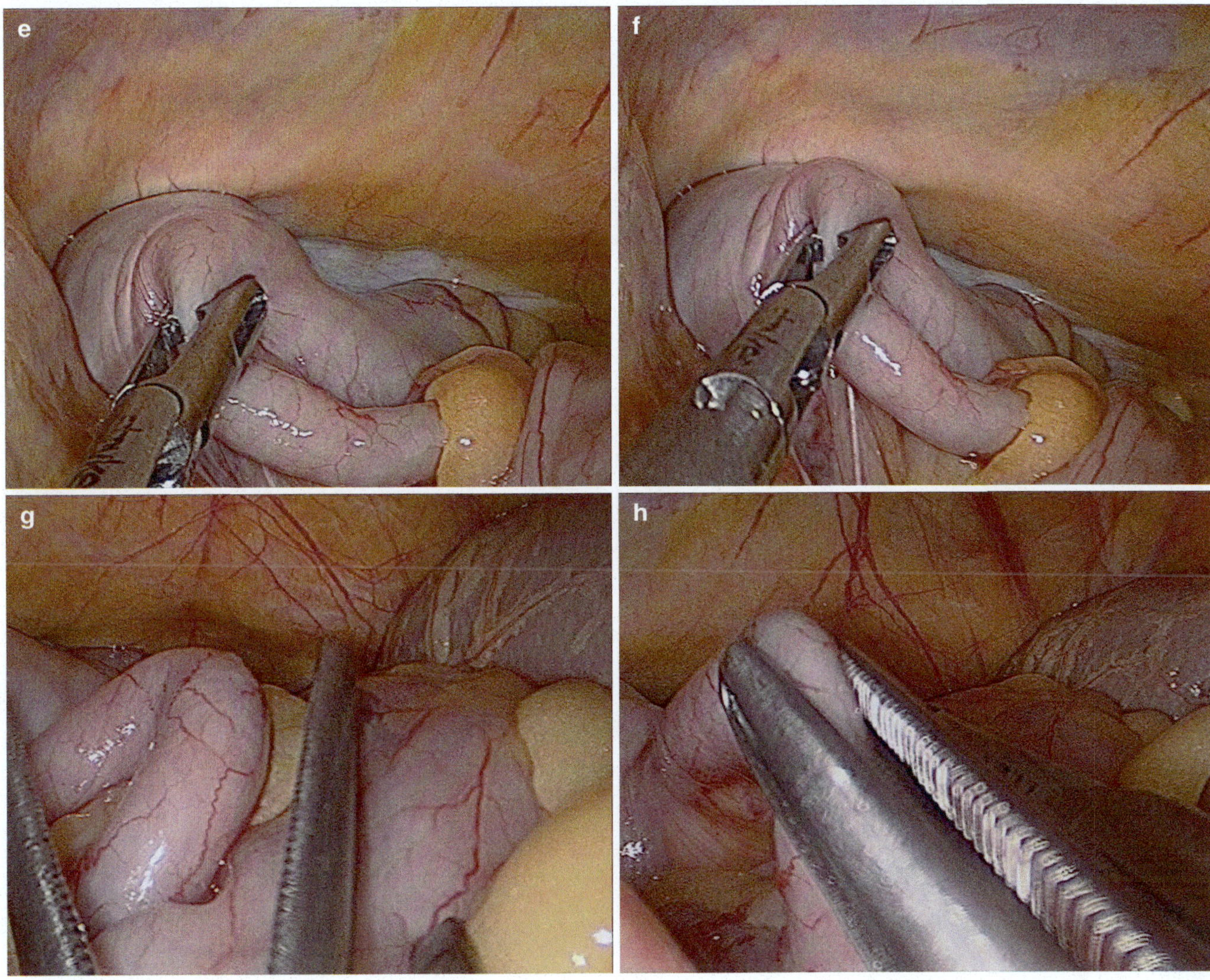

Fig. 13.2 (continued)

The mesoappendix and appendicular artery was divided with harmonic scalpel. The root of the appendix was dissected (Fig. 13.3a–f).

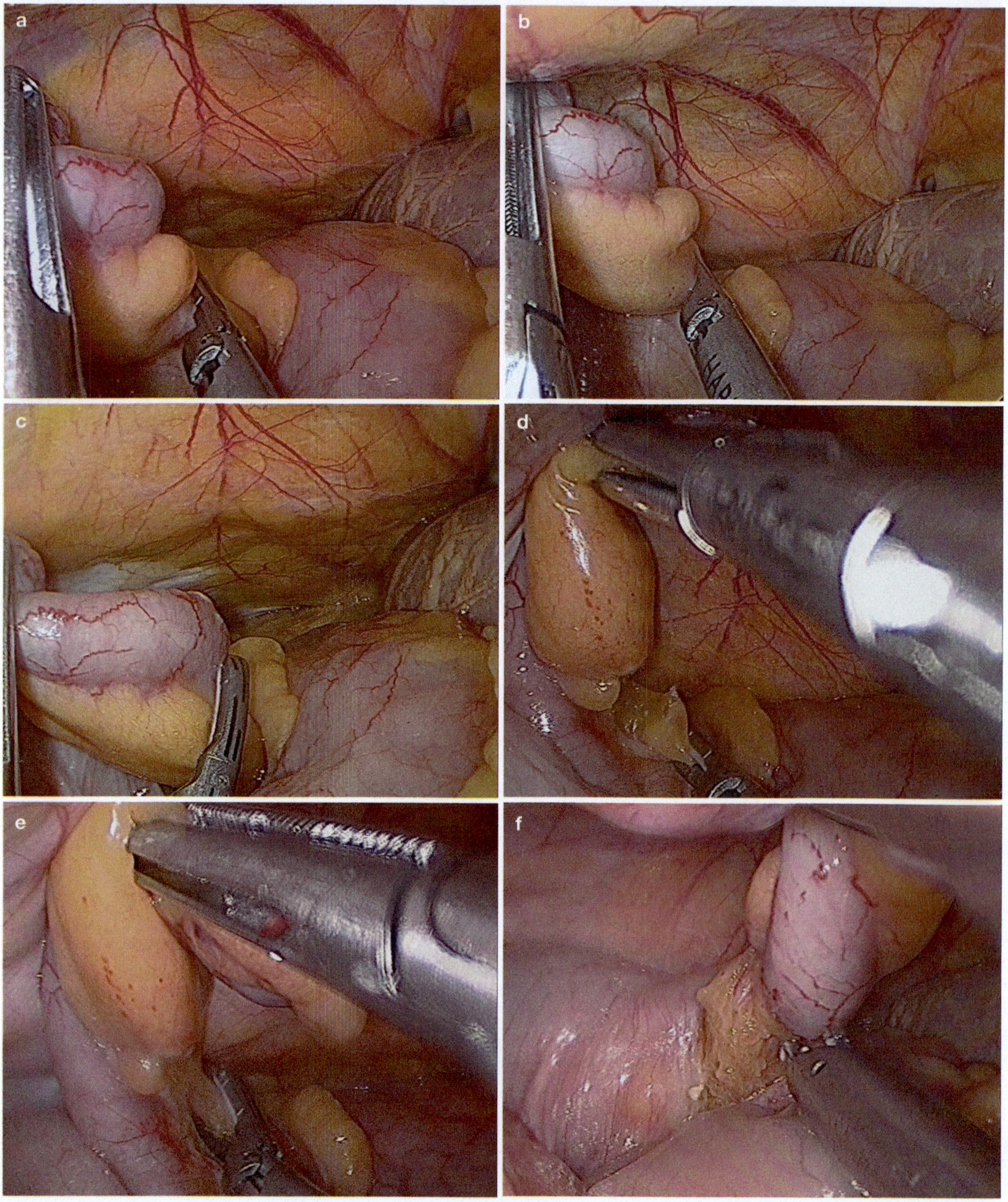

Fig. 13.3

2. Closure of the root of appendix
   The root of the appendix was clipped using hemolock clip and the appendix was divided with harmonic scalpel (Fig. 13.4a–d).
3. Retrieve of appendix from vagina
   The appendix was retrieved from vaginal incision and the incision was closed by suturing.
4. Closure of the end of vagina

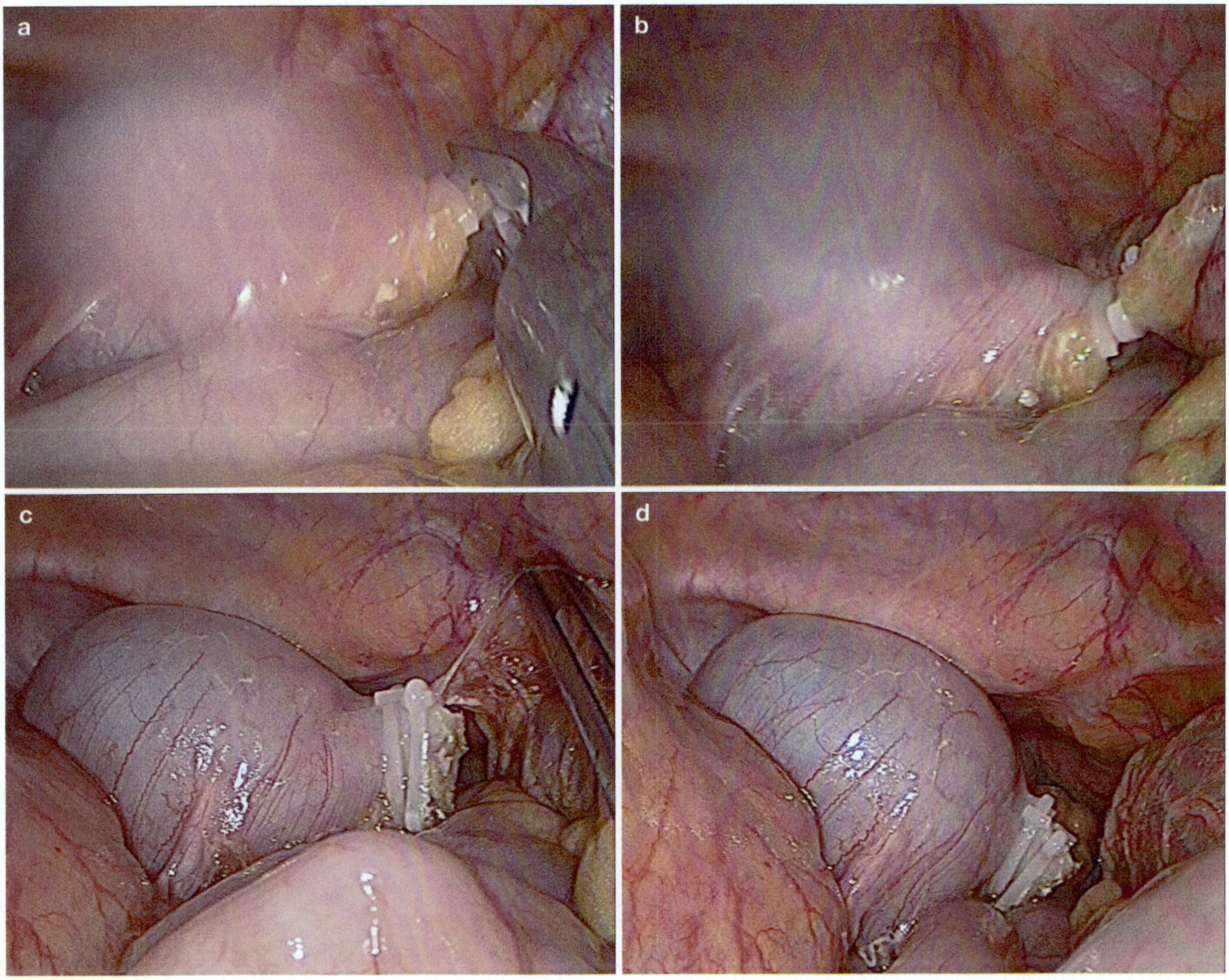

Fig. 13.4

13.7 Complications Analysis and Management

The complications of transvaginal endoscopic appendectomy are the same as SILS appendectomy. The specific complications of NOTES transvaginal access include rectal and colonic injuries, small bowel injuries, ureterovaginal fistula formation, vulvar lacerations, and bladder injuries. Assistance from a gynecologist experienced in transvaginal access should be considered, at least initially, in the performance of transvaginal NOTES. Sometimes, using simultaneous visualization of colpotomy creation with a transumbilical laparoscope may improve the safety of NOTES. The use of a uterine manipulator to anteriorly retract the uterus is another method to assist the procedure of NOTES.

References

1. Halim I, Tavakkolizadeh A. NOTES: The next surgical revolution? Int J Surg. 2008;6:273–6.
2. Lima E, Rolanda C, Pêgo JM, Henriques-Coelho T, Silva D, Carvalho JL, Correia-Pinto J. Transvesical endoscopic peritoneoscopy: a novel 5 mm port for intra-abdominal scarless surgery. J Urol. 2006;176:802–5.
3. Baron TH. Natural orifice transluminal endoscopic surgery. Br J Surg. 2007;94:1–2.
4. Fong DG, Pai RD, Thompson CC. Transcolonic endoscopic abdominal exploration: a NOTES survival study in a porcine model. Gastrointest Endosc. 2007;65:312–8.
5. Pai RD, Fong DG, Bundga ME, Odze RD, Rattner DW, Thompson CC. Transcolonic endoscopic cholecystectomy: a NOTES survival study in a porcine model (with video). Gastrointest Endosc. 2006;64:428–34.
6. Rolanda C, Lima E, Pêgo JM, Henriques-Coelho T, Silva D, Moreira I, Macedo G, Carvalho JL, Correia-Pinto J. Third-generation cholecystectomy by natural orifices: transgastric and transvesical combined approach (with video). Gastrointest Endosc. 2007;65:111–7.
7. Auyang ED, Hungness ES, Vaziri K, Martin JA, Soper NJ. Human NOTES cholecystectomy: transgastric hybrid technique. J Gastrointest Surg. 2009;13:1149–50.
8. Sánchez-Margallo FM, Asencio JM, Tejonero MC, Pérez FJ, Sánchez MA, Usón J, Pascual S. Technical feasibility of totally natural orifice cholecystectomy in a swine model. Minim Invasive Ther Allied Technol. 2008;17:361–4.
9. Surgeons remove healthy kidney through vagina. InfoNIAC.com. http://www.infoniac.com/health-fitness/remove-healthy-kidney-through-vagina.html. Retrieved 2009-02-03.

Postscript

It was my first witness of single-incision laparoscopic surgery technique when I attended the SAGES meeting in 2009 and I was deeply attracted. When laparoscopic cholecystectomy was first performed in China in 1990, I just carried out choledochoscope and duodenoscope. Though, very young and less experienced, I was deeply attracted by its minimal invasiveness and quick recovery. So, I traveled to Japan to study laparoscopic techniques. 3 years later, I returned to my country and gradually carried out laparoscopic operations. Reviewing the development course of laparoscopic surgery, I often think why the western colleagues can have such an innovation ability to transform an idea into productivity. I also often blames myself. So, when the single-incision laparoscopic surgery technique is in its infancy, I am unable to hold myself back to grasp this opportunity to extend this technique to general surgery and other subjects.

It is because of the impetus of this idea, the authors have carried out more than 1,000 cases and 40 categories single-incision laparoscopic operations in less than 3 years. We believe there is no essential difference between single-incision and conventional laparoscopic operations. Reduced injury and excellent cosmetic effect are its advantages. However, single-incision laparoscopic surgery requires high skills of the surgeon and should be performed by experienced laparoscopic surgeons. Its merits and shortcomings when compared to the conventional laparoscopic surgery are yet to be demonstrated in a prospective clinical study.

Upgrading of laparoscopic equipments is very rapid. This book benefited from the HD video recording system which can provide a more clear picture for the readers to facilitate learning and understanding.

Associate professor Ying Fan spent a lot of precious time on composing the book and I feel deeply grateful to him. Meanwhile, I also feel grateful to the domestic and foreign experts to give guidance and criticism to this book.

Shuodong Wu
Shenyang City, Liaoning Province, China

S. Wu et al. (eds.), *Atlas of Single-Incision Laparoscopic Operations in General Surgery*,
DOI 10.1007/978-94-007-6955-7,

Index

S. Wu et al. (eds.), *Atlas of Single-Incision Laparoscopic Operations in General Surgery*,
DOI 10.1007/978-94-007-6955-7, © Springer Science+Business Media Dordrecht 2013

The manufacturer's authorised representative in the EU is Springer Nature Customer Service Centre GmbH, Europaplatz 3, 69115 Heidelberg, Germany. If you have any concerns regarding our products, please contact ProductSafety@springernature.com

Printed and bound by CPI Group (UK) Ltd, Croydon, CR0 4YY
22/09/2026
02221073-0001